Manual of Pediatric Therapeutics

Fifth Edition

Department of Medicine
The Children's Hospital, Boston

Edited by John W. Graef, M.D.

Foreword by
David G. Nathan, M.D.
Robert Stranahan Professor of
Pediatrics,
Harvard Medical School;
Physician-in-Chief,
The Children's Hospital, Boston

Little, Brown and Company
Boston/New York/Toronto/London

Library of Congress Cataloging-in-Publication Data

Manual of pediatric therapeutics / Department of Medicine, the
    Children's Hospital, Boston ; edited by John W. Graef. —5th ed.
        p.   cm.
    Includes bibliographical references and index.
    ISBN 0-316-13875-4
    1. Children—Diseases—Treatment—Handbooks, manuals, etc.
I. Graef, John W., 1939–   . II. Children's Hospital Medical Center
(Boston, Mass.).   Dept. of Medicine.
    [DNLM: 1. Therapeutics—in infancy & childhood.   WS 366 M294
1993]
RJ52.M36   1993
615.5'42—dc20
DNLM/DLC
for Library of Congress   93-1126
                                                                 CIP

Printed in the United States of America

SEM

Sponsoring Editor: Elizabeth Thompson
Development Editor: Kristin Odmark
Production Editor: Karen Feeney
Copyeditor: Libby Dabrowski
Indexer: Betty Hallinger
Production Supervisor: Cate Rickard
Cover Designer: Tsuneo Taniuchi

To my wife, Gretchen, who is a
constant source of wisdom about
children in general, and our children
in particular, and who has patiently
endured the preparation of these
editions.

Contents

Foreword

This book represents a labor of love by John W. Graef, M.D. and his colleagues, all of whom are present or former members of the staff of The Children's Hospital in Boston. These fine pediatricians and an excellent gynecologist have banded together to develop this, the fifth edition of the *Manual of Pediatric Therapeutics,* an effort that was begun in 1970 by Thomas Cone, M.D.

For the past 23 years, the Department of Medicine of the Children's Hospital has been completely committed to the development and refinement of this volume. The Department believes that it must find ways to develop simplified but highly accurate and practical guides to diagnostic and therapeutic initiatives applicable in childhood. This new revision does that job well.

Dr. Graef has used his judgment and broad experience to choose first class authors of his chapters. In doing so he has thoroughly revised the fourth edition with particular emphasis on the many changes that have occurred in nephrology, gastroenterology, endocrinology, hematology, and acute care. We are all grateful to Dr. Graef for the excellence of this volume and his commitment to this task. It is a lasting tribute to his mentor, Tom Cone.

David G. Nathan, M.D.

Preface

In our profession, it is an honor to be asked by one's colleagues to assist in the task of caring for patients. The publication of this fifth edition of the *Manual of Pediatric Therapeutics* comes 23 years after I was honored by Dr. Thomas Cone when he asked me to assemble the first edition. While I expect to continue to play an active role in the preparation of future editions, it will be my pleasure to pass on the principal editing role to a colleague or colleagues at The Children's Hospital to breathe fresh ideas and new insights into future editions.

Throughout these editions, our goal has been to ask selected faculty and staff of The Children's Hospital who are active in patient care and knowledgable about new developments in their fields to focus their contributions on the specific area of patient management. Our authors have been encouraged to add those "pearls" that come with their experience and teaching.

This book has always been prepared with the assumption that its readers are familiar with concepts of pathophysiology and differential diagnosis. Those readers interested in the diagnostic aspects of patient care are referred to Dr. Kenneth Roberts' excellent book, *Manual of Clinical Problems in Pediatrics*. To the extent such material is present in our manual, it is for the purpose of ensuring that therapeutic recommendations are applied in the appropriate clinical setting.

While all chapters have been reviewed and updated, several chapters have been more extensively revised and in some cases, completely rewritten. These latter include the chapters on Acute Care, Renal Disorders, Cardiac Disorders, Disorders of the Endocrine System, Prepubertal and Adolescent Gynecology, Parasitic Infections, and Hematologic Disorders. Considerable new material is found in the chapters on Well Child Care, Poisoning, Management of the Sick Newborn, Gastroenterology, Allergic Disorders and Immunodeficiency, and Behavior. Parts of the introductory chapter have been rewritten. The chapters on Management of the Normal Newborn, Fluid and Electrolytes, Neurology, and the Formulary have been updated. We have retained the overall approach of providing general principles at the beginning of each chapter followed by discussion of management of specific conditions in an outline format emphasizing treatment.

Finally, the need to keep the manual a workable size means that some specific topics in general pediatrics are not included. Generally, the decision to exclude material has depended mainly on whether or not those conditions are treatable rather than merely to acknowledge their existence and/or describe them. On the other hand, a few untreatable conditions occur with such frequency or are of such compelling importance, such as HIV, that to omit them would undermine the comprehensiveness of the *Manual*.

We owe special thanks to a number of individuals for the preparation of this edition; especially Ms. Carol Donovan for her assistance in manuscript typing and Ms. Kristin Odmark of Little, Brown and Co. for her gentle prodding of this editor. As in the past, we welcome comments from our readers. We are grateful to those readers who have taken the time to notify us when an error has been found.

On behalf of the Department of Medicine of The Children's Hospital, we thank you for your continued support of this book. It is especially gratifying that the *Manual* is now translated into Spanish, Portuguese, Italian, Japanese, Greek, French, and even Farsi. Whatever language you prefer, we hope you will find this new edition helpful.

J.W.G.

Manual of
Pediatric
Therapeutics

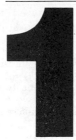

General Care of the Patient

John W. Graef,
Charles Berde, and
Frederick Mandell

I. **Caring for children.** Care must be taken to respect the modesty, integrity, and privacy of each child. A child's illness, regardless of severity, can be frightening for both child and parents. Children feel and react even at times when they might appear uninterested. They can be absorbed by apprehensions about their illness and the attendant hospital procedures. Because children are most likely to be afraid of situations that they do not understand, they should be told about their illness and its treatment in terms they can comprehend. Children quickly recognize insincerity, and deceiving a child only serves ultimately to alienate him or her. It should not be surprising to an understanding physician if a child reacts angrily to painful procedures or is frustrated at her or his own lack of progress. It is often the quiet and passive infant or child who may be a cause for concern. Older children, particularly, understand pain and even death and, like adults, can be made unnecessarily anxious by bedside staff conversations, which may be misinterpreted or misunderstood.

A wise pediatrician understands that parents know their children far better than those trying to help care for them. Both parents are seen by the child uniquely, especially when the child is sick. Listening to parents, carefully noting their observations, putting them at ease, and hearing out their worries even if they appear unrelated or disproportionate to the child's illness can help to provide them with the emotional resources needed to help their child and their child's caretaker. Impatience with or misunderstanding parents can impede their inclusion in the therapeutic process, particularly because parents will reassume care for the child after the illness—a point easily overlooked during the time of acute intervention. To make their participation easier, parents need objective advice from the physician. Although they should not be asked to make medical judgments, they have a legal and ethical right to be informed of the benefits and risks of therapy and to be included respectfully in the decision-making process.

Finally, a pediatrician's responsibility to a child does not end when the child has been cured of a physical illness. It is the privilege of those who care for children to help them fulfill their potential and take their rightful place as responsible adults. This may require the pediatrician to go beyond traditional medical intervention into the area of schools, environment, economic circumstances, and even government in the effort to assist the child.

II. **Principles of therapeutics.** Because of the intrinsic recuperative capacities of infants, children, and adolescents, it has been observed by experienced pediatric clinicians that, **in the large majority of patients, therapeutic intervention is either irrelevant or worse.** The remaining patients can be divided into those for whom an intervention would be helpful if only more were known about the disease and those for whom an appropriate intervention can affect the outcome beneficially. Thus, the most difficult decision is not which therapy to perform, but whether to intervene at all. In considering possible intervention, the clinician must assess the following: accuracy of diagnosis, relative effectiveness of possible therapies, risks to the patient of toxic effects, discomfort to the patient, and costs. These factors must be balanced against the risks and benefits of not intervening. Finally, follow-up and long-term observation should be anticipated.

   A. **Accuracy of diagnosis**

      1. After initial assessment is completed, a **working diagnosis** is established. As

new information becomes available, the working diagnosis should be **constantly reassessed.**

2. No therapy should be completed simply because it has been started. It is better to recognize an error in diagnosis than to continue a therapeutic regimen blindly based on flawed data or conclusions.

3. The most common error in diagnosis is attributing pathogenicity to an associated, but not causative, finding.

4. When a diagnosis depends on a laboratory test, the clinician should be aware of the relative accuracy of **that** test in **that** laboratory.

5. It is prudent to obtain the results of diagnostic tests **first hand.**

B. **Effectiveness of therapies**

1. Few therapeutic regimens are **completely** effective in **all** cases.

2. Data on effectiveness are usually comparative. The clinician should assess the **relevance** of available studies to the case at hand.

3. "Cures" are usually a combination of therapy and the patient's own defenses. Thus, the underlying condition of the patient may be the most important determinant of effectiveness.

4. Even an effective therapy such as hemodialysis may not be more effective than the patient's own physiology (e.g., renal clearance of a particular substance). Thus, the general application of an effective technique is not necessarily appropriate in all cases.

C. **Risks to the patient** are sometimes overlooked. This is particularly true when multiple pharmacologic agents are used.

1. Drug interactions should be known and anticipated.

2. Any worsening of the patient's condition should prompt a reevaluation of the therapy as well as the working diagnosis.

3. Do not **assume** that the patient has received the dose or the drug prescribed. Compliance studies indicate that patients may not participate as fully as expected in prescribed therapy. For hospitalized patients, daily routine should include careful checking of nurses' notes and medication orders.

4. The appearance, taste, and odor of a medication may have a profound effect on compliance. The clinician should be familiar with the available preparations, flavors, and unpleasant characteristics of particular medications. When in doubt, taste it yourself.

5. Therapeutic advice should be realistic. Patients may need reinforcement and support to comply or continue, despite adverse side effects or unpleasant taste, or both.

6. Potential side effects should be discussed fully with parents and, when appropriate, patients. Avoid medical jargon. Simply listing effects is not sufficient; be sure they are **understood.**

D. **Discomfort** for the patient is difficult to assess, but should be considered.

1. Physicians who have been patients testify to the discomfort of procedures considered routine. These include nasogastric tubes, some intravenous medications, and gastrointestinal (GI) discomfort associated with some drugs.

2. Discomfort is not, per se, a contraindication to a particular regimen.

3. When an uncomfortable regimen is chosen, parents and patients should be informed of the discomfort in optimistic terms regarding the duration of discomfort and steps to minimize it.

E. **Costs** must be considered.

1. A hospital or local pharmacist can usually provide costs of a pharmaceutical regimen.

2. Generic drugs are usually cheaper than trade preparations, particularly if the pharmacist has permission to interchange.

3. Prescribe enough medication to avoid repeated trips to the pharmacy, but not so much as to be wasteful. State laws may limit the prescription of controlled substances.

4. A particular regimen may have hidden costs. These include monitoring laboratory tests (e.g., serum levels), instability in storage, or use of preparations that provide less drug per unit cost.

5. Clinical decisions by physicians can add enormously to health care costs. Thus, a system that keeps the physician informed of therapeutic costs should be encouraged.

F. Follow-up and long-term care. After a therapeutic regimen has been completed, whether in or out of the hospital, a follow-up visit should be scheduled to begin the process of continuing observation. Physicians should be alert to recurrent symptoms as well as possible sequelae. Frequently, therapeutic regimens may produce their own sequelae, such as an alteration in renal or hepatic function, or both.

Most important, if acute care has been provided by a person or persons other than the patient's primary provider, an orderly return of responsibility to the primary provider should occur with the full knowledge of the patient and parents. Periodic follow-up study by acute care providers is appropriate and is enhanced by communication between the acute care and primary care providers.

III. The hospitalized patient

A. Medical orders. Written medical orders are the physician's instructions to the nursing staff concerning the care and treatment of the patient. They should be written clearly and accurately, with special attention to dosage calculation and decimal points. Each entry as well as each page (if there is more than one) should be correctly labeled with the time and date, and should be properly signed. An incorrect entry should be canceled by drawing a single line through it, and *error* should be written nearby, so that there will be no confusion at a later time. Although orders are the **legal responsibility** of the physician, nurses should be treated as colleagues, not as underlings. Nursing input in patient care decisions should be sought. Unusual orders should be discussed with the nurse at the time they are written and individualized for each patient. Properly written orders should provide for the patient's comfort and dignity during therapy. The following schemes can be utilized:

1. Diagnosis. List the diagnostic findings in order of significance. Indicate the condition of the patient, whether critical, guarded, fair, or satisfactory. When a patient's condition is listed as critical, the family should be informed **by the physician** to avoid misunderstanding.

2. Dispositions. This includes the frequency of monitoring vital signs and weighing the patient, permitted activities, special observations, isolation procedures, and environmental conditions.

a. Unnecessarily frequent determination of vital signs overburdens the nursing staff and may unnecessarily discomfit the patient.

b. Bed rest for an ill child is often more constraining than limited activity, and the social environment will also affect the degree of activity. Hospitalized children, even those in isolation, should not be denied social interaction.

3. Diet. Choose the diet with these considerations in mind: age, caloric needs, ability to chew, and special requirements necessitated by problems of absorption, intestinal irritation, residue, and transit time (see Chap. 10).

4. Diagnostic tests. Group in logic sequence (e.g., blood, radiographic). List all tests and the dates and times they are to be done. Standing orders for diagnostic tests should be reviewed frequently.

5. Drugs. Include generic name, dose, route, frequency, and length of time to be administered. Review orders for opioids *daily*. In general, separate drugs for specific therapy from drugs for symptomatic relief. Orders for respiratory or physical therapy must also be explicit as to duration, frequency, type, anatomic site of administration, and associated medication. Oxygen and aerosols require specific orders as well.

B. Analgesia and sedation (see also Chap. 3)

1. Analgesia

a. General principles. The following guidelines may be helpful:

(1) If pain is present in multiple sites, only the *single* most severe source will be recognized by the patient.

(2) Although it is sometimes assumed that pain is not felt as deeply by children, particularly small infants, or is easily forgotten, local anesthesia should be provided for diagnostic and therapeutic procedures whenever feasible.

(3) True analgesics such as morphine may mask pain, whereas sedatives such as phenobarbital will not. For this reason, sedatives may be helpful in elucidating pain and tenderness, particularly in examining the acute abdomen. In this case, sedation short of general anesthesia does not mask pain, but permits its elucidation by reducing surrounding anxiety and factitious tenderness.

(4) Postoperative pain, although generally of shorter duration in children than in adults, may still be severe enough to require medication for several days.

(5) Neonates also feel pain, but are less able to express it. Do not forget to order analgesia for neonates when pain is expected to be present. **Opioids in the newborn will necessitate increase of observation for respiratory depression.**

(6) For children with intravenous access, conscious sedation for painful procedures may be provided with short-acting anxiolytics such as midazolam (incremental intravenous doses of 0.03 mg/kg q 5 minutes x 2–3) alone or in combination with short-acting opioids such as fentanyl (incremental intravenous doses of 0.5–1 mcg/kg q 5 minutes x 2–3). When combinations of sedatives and opioids are used, there may be synergistic effects on sedation and respiratory depression, so that careful titration is warranted. A benzodiazepine reversal agent, flumazenil, is now available in the U.S., though it has received little pediatric use to date. Midazolam can also be given orally in apple juice or strawberry syrup (0.3–0.6 mg/kg to a maximum of 15 mg for adolescents) with good anxiolysis within 30 minutes in most cases. Patients receiving conscious sedation require constant observation for adequacy of respiration because clinical observation of cyanosis is imperfect, pulse oximetry is recommended as a monitor of adequacy of oxygenation. Resuscitative drugs, airway equipment, suction, and an oxygen source should be at hand.

b. Specific therapeutics

(1) Nonopioid analgesics (Table 1-1)

(a) Acetaminophen. Acetaminophen is now the drug of choice for mild pain and antipyresis in pediatrics. The routine oral dosage is 10–15 mg/kg/dose q4h. However, doses of 20/kg/dose q4h up to 2 weeks have been tolerated without toxicity and may be needed for adequate analgesia. To achieve adequate plasma levels, rectal doses of 20–25 mg/kg/dose may be needed. Peak blood levels are achieved in 2 hours (see Chap. 2, p. 34). Toxic effects include methemoglobinemia, anemia, and liver damage, but it does not cause hemolysis in glucose 6-phosphate dehydrogenase (G-6-PD) deficiency. Overdose can produce fulminant liver failure (see Chap. 4, p. 109).

(b) Acetylsalicylic acid (aspirin) has antipyretic properties as well (see Chap. 2, p. 34 for the dose and route of administration).

(i) Its analgesic properties are most suitable for the pain of headache, arthralgia, dysmenorrhea, or muscular ache. Doses in patients with acute rheumatic fever and juvenile rheumatoid arthritis are considerably higher (see Chap. 18, p. 509) than for simpler analgesia.

(ii) Enteric-coated preparations are available to reduce gastric irritation, but absorption of these preparations is variable.

(iii) Toxic effects include salicylism (see Chap. 4, p. 108), GI bleeding, iron deficiency anemia, abnormal clotting, altered thyroid function, decreased fasting blood sugar in diabetes, and increased cardiac load, which can aggravate incipient congestive heart failure and hemolysis in patients with G-6-PD deficiency.

Table 1-1. Narcotic and nonnarcotic analgesics and dosages for pediatric use

Analgesic	Dose
Nonnarcotic	
Acetylsalicylic acid	65 mg/kg/24 hr in 4–6 doses
Acetaminophen	Under 1 year 60 mg q4h
	1–3 years 60–120 mg q4h
	3–6 years 120–240 mg q4h
	Over 6 years 240–320 mg q4h
	or 10–15 mg/kg/dose q4h
Nonsteroidal antiinflammatory agents	See Chap. 18, p. 509ff
Narcotic	
Codeine phosphate	1 mg/kg PO or IM q3–4h
Meperidine	0.5–0.7 mg/kg IV slowly q2h
	0.6 mg/kg/hr continuous infusion IV or SC
	1–1.3 mg/kg IM q3–4h
Methadone	0.1 mg/kg IV or IM; 0.2 mg/kg PO; initial 2–4 doses at short intervals (3–4 hr); subsequent doses q6–12h *or,* occasionally, 24h as needed
Morphine sulfate	0.05–0.10 mg/kg IV slowly q2h
	0.06 mg/kg/hr continuous infusion IV or SC
	0.1–0.13 mg/kg IM q3–4h
Hydromorphone	0.01–0.015 mg/kg IV q2h
	0.015–0.025 mg/kg SC q3–4h
	0.05 mg/kg PO q4h
Oxycodone	0.5–1.5 mg/kg PO q3–4
Fentanyl	0.5–3 μg/kg IV slowly q1h or hourly by continuous infusion

     (iv) Because of the risk of Reye syndrome, the use of aspirin is contraindicated in the management of flu-like illness or varicella.

  (c) Nonsteroidal antiinflammatory agents are fully discussed in Chap. 18, p. 509. Their analgesic properties appear to be equivalent to those of aspirin and may be slightly greater than those of acetaminophen when inflammation is present. Liquid preparations of ibuprofen are available.

(2) Opioid analgesics (narcotics) (see Table 1-1) (morphine, meperidine, codeine, methadone, oxycodone, hydromorphone, fentanyl) provide effective analgesia with little or no myocardial depression at moderate doses. **However, they can cause reversible respiratory depression.** (For use of naloxone in the management of opioid overdose, see Chap. 4, p. 105).

  (a) For practical purposes, the available opioids have roughly proportional dose-response relationships for analgesia, sedation, and respiratory depression, that is, at equivalent doses, the incidence of respiratory depression (and most other adverse effects) is fairly similar.

  (b) Other **adverse effects** common to opioids include pruritus, urinary retention, ileus, constipation, nausea, and dysphoria.

  (c) Differences among opioids include:

    (i) Duration of action. Fentanyl is short acting, **meperidine** and

morphine are intermediate acting, and **methadone** is long acting.

(ii) Histamine release is greatest with morphine and least with fentanyl.

(d) In the use of opioids for ongoing pain, the most common error is administering them at intervals that are too prolonged. It is important to schedule administration at intervals short enough to avoid peaks and valleys in plasma levels. In this regard, continuous infusions or long-acting agents such as methadone are particularly useful. Conversely, when opioids are used for brief, painful procedures, IV boluses are helpful because of their short duration.

(e) Patient-controlled analgesia utilizes a computer-controlled pump activated by the patient to administer small doses of medication. It is safe and well tolerated, particularly among patients with postoperative pain, burning, or sickle cell crisis. It can be used safely by children as young as 6–7 years.

(f) Opioids can be effective for analgesia or sedation by an oral route if the GI tract is functioning and sufficient doses are given. Approximate oral/parenteral dosage ratios are: methadone, 2:1; meperidine, 4:1; hydromorphine, 4:1; and morphine, 6–10:1 in single doses and 3:1 in chronic doses.

(g) **Tolerance** to opioids may occur with repeated administration, though this is highly variable. If a patient who is chronically receiving opioids suddenly stops taking them, symptoms of withdrawal may occur (e.g., goose flesh, agitation, tachycardia, nasal stuffiness, diarrhea). These symptoms may be prevented by gradual tapering of opioid doses over a period of days.

(h) In contrast to dependence, tolerance, and withdrawal, **addiction** should be regarded as a largely psychological process characterized by drug-seeking, compulsive behavior. Addiction is **extremely** rare in children or adults who are given opioids for acute pain or cancer pain. There is no basis for giving opioids infrequently or in inadequate doses for acute pain because of a fear of addiction.

(i) **Codeine** is a morphine derivative. Its antitussive properties are well known, and it is frequently used for this purpose; however, there is risk of its abuse for this indication. It is frequently prescribed in combination with acetaminophen for moderate pain. Prolonged use of any opioid is constipating, which may be especially significant postoperatively.

(j) **Morphine** is perhaps the most important and widely used opioid analgesic and is effective in any age group. It has moderate sedative effect and produces concomitant euphoria.

(i) PO and PR preparations, although effective, are somewhat variable in absorption and metabolism. If PO preparations are indicated, individual dosage adjustment must be made. In children with cancer, timed-release oral morphine preparations provide prolonged analgesia. When used parenterally, *slow* IV drip may be preferable to SQ (20 min) or IM (20 min). Analgesia usually lasts 2–3 hours.

(ii) Morphine is excreted via the liver and **should be administered with caution to a newborn or a patient with liver disease.**

(iii) **Tolerance to morphine** includes tolerance to its central nervous system (CNS) depressive properties, so that increasing the dose does not increase the likelihood of respiratory toxicity.

(iv) **Toxic effects** include respiratory depression, increased in-

tracranial pressure, arterial hypotension, nausea and vomiting, pruritus, urinary retention, addiction, and constipation.
  (k) Meperidine (Demerol) is a commonly used analgesic. High dose or chronic use (more than several days) should be avoided because its metabolite, nonmeperidine, can produce convulsions and dysphonia (Table 1–2).
  (l) Methadone is included because of its widespread use in antiaddiction programs and in cancer patients with ongoing severe pain. Its analgesic potency IV is roughly equivalent to that of morphine in single doses, but its effect is more prolonged. It is effective PO. The elixir can be used as a substitute for timed-release oral morphine.
  (m) Fentanyl is a synthetic opioid agent. It differs from morphine by having a shorter duration of action and less vasodilation. In higher doses it may produce mild bradycardia and rigidity. Fentanyl is useful in small to moderate doses (1–3 μg/kg slowly IV) for **sedation** for brief, painful procedures such as painful dressing changes or bone marrow aspiration. In higher doses (5–50 μg/kg) fentanyl is used as an **anesthetic** with hemodynamic stability even in critically ill newborns.
(3) Local anesthetics (lidocaine, bupivacaine) are administered by infiltration before painful procedures are performed. These include, but are not limited to, placement of IV and arterial lines and chest tubes, arterial and lumbar punctures, suture of lacerations, bone marrow aspiration, newborn circumcision (via dorsal penile block), and intramuscular injection of large volumes.
Topical application of lidocaine is also useful for mucosal analgesia.
  (a) Dosage. Safe limits of total dosage for infiltration are:
    (l) Lidocaine without epinephrine, 4–5 mg/kg (in newborns, 3 mg/kg); with epinephrine, 5–7 mg/kg (in newborns, 4 mg/kg)
    (ii) Bupivacaine without epinephrine, 2 mg/kg (in newborns, 1.5 mg/kg); with epinephrine, 2.5 mg/kg (in newborns, 2 mg/kg)
  (b) Toxic reactions can occur if local anesthetics are injected intravascularly or if total dosage exceeds safe limits. These include

Table 1-2. Sedatives and dosages for pediatric use

Drug	Dose
Alcohol	10 ml brandy in 30 ml/H_2O in infants
Chloral hydrate	10–50 mg/kg/dose q6–8h
Paraldehyde	0.15 ml/kg/dose
Antihistamines	
Diphenhydramine	5 mg/kg/24 hr in 4 divided doses
Promethazine	0.5 mg/kg/dose q6h
Hydroxyzine	2 mg/kg/24 hr in 4 divided doses
Chlorpromazine	2 mg/kg/24 hr in 4–6 divided doses
Barbiturates	
Amobarbital (Amytal)	6 mg/kg/24 hr in 3 divided doses
Secobarbital (Seconal)	6 mg/kg/24 hr in 3 divided doses
Pentobarbital (Nembutal)	6 mg/kg/24 hr in 3 divided doses
Phenobarbital	6 mg/kg/24 hr in 3 divided doses
Demerol compound 25 mg meperidine 6.25 mg chlorpromazine 6.25 mg promethazine in 1 ml	1 ml/15 kg IM, not to exceed 2 ml per dose

tinnitus, metallic taste, lethargy, irritability, headache, and, in severe cases, seizures, hypotension, and potentially fatal dysrhythmias.

(c) **Topical** administration of lidocaine or diclonine is useful for mucosal analgesia.

(d) **Transdermal** application of abdocaine/prilocaine (EMLA) mixture is effective for analgesia for venipuncture, IV placement, and subsequent infiltration of other local anesthetics.

(e) A combination of tetracaine, epinephrine, and cocaine (TAC) applied by drip to open wounds is used to facilitate suture of lacerations. This mixture can cause ischemia due to vasoconstriction if used in proximity to endarterial blood supply. Administration near mucosal surfaces can result in excessive absorption and toxic effects including seizure.

2. **Sedation**

a. **General principles.** Among the most important characteristics of childhood are curiosity and the drive to explore and learn. Sedation can interfere with the child's capacity to interact with and learn from the environment.

(1) **Indications for sedation in children are few.** They include **preanesthesia;** painful **diagnostic procedures** such as bone marrow aspiration; **agitation** that contributes to morbidity, as in respiratory diseases such as asthma or croup (in which sedation should be used only with **extreme caution**); **intubation** or **tracheostomy** for respiratory assistance; **intractable pain;** and occasionally in the **evaluation** of severe visceral pain (e.g., acute appendicitis).

Sedation may be indicated for procedures that require immobility. For example, computed tomographic (CT) scans are not painful for toddlers, but mild sedation may be required to accomplish an adequate study. *In sicker children, sedation deep enough to provide immobility may produce airway obstruction or hyperventilation. In many such circumstances, general anesthesia with a controlled airway is safer than deep sedation.*

Any child who is paralyzed, either iatrogenically or by disease, may still be aware of his or her surroundings, with all of the fear and pain as well as the loss of control entailed. Sedation in such a case is an important part of acute care.

In children, sedation is *not* the treatment of choice in insomnia or hyperactivity and should be used only as a last resort.

(2) **The reaction of children to sedatives,** particularly barbiturates and sometimes antihistamines, is unpredictable. At the toddler stage, sedatives may cause agitation. Agitation is particularly likely to occur when sedatives are given in the presence of ongoing, acute pain. In these circumstances, if sedation is indicated, an opioid analgesic should be employed, either alone or in conjunction with a sedative. In children receiving parenteral sedation, constant observation and availability of facilities (oxygen, suction, bag and mask) and skill to provide airway maintenance and assisted ventilation in the event of overdosage are essential. Pulse oximetry is prudent.

The choice of drugs for sedation depends on the age, clinical condition, and procedure contemplated; routine formulas should not be applied without consideration of the particular situation. The route of drug administration chosen depends on the clinical condition, availability of IV access, and duration of the procedure contemplated. If oral medications are used, they should be given at least 90 minutes before the planned procedure. For most purposes, the *weakest* effective sedative, such as hydroxyzine, is safe and least liable to cause unwanted side effects.

b. **Specific therapeutics** (see Table 1-2)

(1) **Chloral hydrate** is probably the safest sedative and is inexpensive. It has a wide margin of safety, with the acceptable dose from 20–40 mg/kg/24 hr PO or PR. Although the aftertaste is bitter, it seems to be well tolerated by children, particularly if offered in a small glass of juice. Peak activity usually occurs within 30–60 minutes of administration. **Caution should be exercised in patients with liver disease. Aspiration can produce fatal laryngospasm.**

(2) **Antihistamines** have a variety of clinical uses that have varying degrees of success.

  (a) Antihistamines with the most effective sedative properties include promethazine (Phenergan), diphenhydramine (Benadryl), and hydroxyzine (Atarax). Hydroxyzine and diphenhydramine may reduce pruritus, possibly as a result of their sedative properties.

  (b) **Serious side effects** are few, and the drugs are well tolerated PO.

(3) **Benzodiazepines** (diazepam, midazolam) are effective in providing amnesia and diminished anxiety. They do not provide analgesia. Respiratory depression is mild but variable. **Both respiratory depression and sedation are markedly increased in the presence of opioids.** Occasional dysphoria may be seen, especially in patients with pain. Because of prolonged clearance of diazepam and its active metabolites, prolonged somnolence may also be a problem. Midazolam is now more widely used for short-term sedation.

(4) **Neuroleptic drugs** include butyrophenones (haloperidol, droperidol), phenothiazines (chlorpromazine, prochlorperazine), and similar agents used primarily as antiemetics (promethazine, metoclopramide). These compounds provide sedation, usually mild but dose related, and secondarily an antiemetic effect.

  (a) **Side effects** include mild respiratory depression and vasodilation.

  (b) **Adverse reactions** include reversible **extrapyramidal reactions** (oculogyric crisis, stiffness) seen commonly with large or long-term dosage, **tardive dyskinesias,** and **dysphoria.**

    (i) Extrapyramidal reactions can largely be reversed (and often prevented) by administration of antihistaminic/anticholinergic agents. These include diphenhydramine, 0.5–1.0 mg/kg IV, PO, or IM, and benztropine, 0.02–0.04 mg/kg IV, PO, or IM.

    (ii) Tardive dyskinesias are uncommon with single doses of phenothiazines, but may have very prolonged effects when the drugs are discontinued after long-term use.

    (iii) The dysphoria associated with neuroleptic agents used for sedation can be quite unpleasant. These drugs have been referred to as "chemical strait jackets." These unpleasant recollections are less common when these drugs are used in small doses and especially when they are administered in combination with opioids and benzodiazepines.

(5) **Barbiturates** are true hypnotic agents. In adequate doses, they can produce unconsciousness, if this is desirable. Respiratory depression is usually mild but variable. In addition to sedation, barbiturates can produce excitement or delirium, particularly in lower doses and in patients with pain; the concomitant use of opioids makes this less likely.

  (a) Phenobarbital is used most widely in the control of seizure disorders. For a detailed discussion of this use, see Chap. 19, p. 534. It is a very weak sedative in therapeutic doses.

  (b) Secobarbital and pentobarbital are probably more useful sedative hypnotics because of their rapid action and are widely used as preoperative medication. They are not analgesics, so that pentobarbital in particular can be helpful in evaluating abdominal pain in the anxious small child.

  (c) All three agents are available for use PO, PR, or parenterally.

    (d) For PR administration of barbiturates, a suppository should be used; even then, effective absorption is variable. IM or IV injection is more reliable, but the individual reactions to a given dose preclude prediction of its effect.

    (e) Because of respiratory depression, extreme caution should be used in administering barbiturates IV, although pentobarbital produces relatively little respiratory depression for the hypnotic dose used.

  (6) Ketamine is used to induce sedation for procedures. It produces relative immobility and a "dissociative" state with some analgesia and amnesia. Ventilatory support and airway protection must be at hand. Standard dose is 0.5–1.5 mg/kg IV or 1.5–3.0 mg/kg IM.

The major adverse effect of ketamine is the occurrence of unpleasant dreams. These occur more commonly in adults and adolescents, but may be seen at any age. The incidence and severity of bad dreams can be diminished by prior concomitant administration of benzodiazepines and by warning the patient that dreams may occur.

IV. The pediatric consultation. Pediatricians may be asked to consult with colleagues from other medical specialties (e.g., surgery, internal medicine), other pediatric providers (e.g., family practitioners, child psychologists), or other pediatricians. The following guidelines may be helpful:

  A. Respond as soon as possible. A colleague seeking consultation is usually in need of prompt assistance unless otherwise specified. If necessary, a suitable substitute should be offered. Do not provide a substitute without the knowledge of the requesting colleague, since this may create confusion.

  B. Determine what questions require your assistance and respond specifically to them.

  C. Your colleague has asked for assistance, not replacement. Explain the limits of your role to patients and parents at the onset and maintain those limits, particularly if the consultation requires follow-up.

  D. Successful consultation is best accomplished by meticulous attention to detail. Do not assume that you have more knowledge than a requesting colleague. You may, however, have more time. Frequently, the answer to a clinical dilemma lies in elucidating the temporal relationships of illness events or in finding an overlooked detail on physical examination.

  E. Do not comment on a colleague's management in the presence of the patient or parents. Such comments are frequently misunderstood, blown out of proportion, or both.

  F. The best consultation provides the requesting colleague with information on which to base clinical decisions. Inform—do not attempt to dictate patient care.

  G. Discuss your findings with the requesting colleague and request her or his permission **before** discussing them with patient and family.

Medical practice is, at best, inexact. Part of good medical judgment is knowing when to ask for help. Consultation provided in a prompt and helpful manner assures a patient of an extra measure of knowledge and concern, with the added benefit of enhancing the knowledge of all participants.

V. Death of a child (see also *Pediatrics* 62:96, 1978). In the first week of life, more deaths occur than in any subsequent period of childhood. Between the first week of life and 1 year of age, the sudden infant death syndrome is the most common cause of death. (For a complete discussion of this syndrome, see Chap. 3, p. 75.) After 1 year of age, accidents exceed all other acquired causes.

The strongest of all grief reactions occurs when parents have lost a child. Much of parental grief is based on the concept of parent-infant bonding. The reciprocal interaction between a parent and a young infant results in mutual investment of growing intensity. The death of a child brings a sudden and drastic end to that relationship. When a child has a fatal disease, the parents and immediate family face the loss of all their expectations for the child and an extended period of sadness. Parents react to the death of their child in a manner that reflects their family life, emotional structure, individual attachment, and degree of specific circumstances associated with the loss. What health professionals do during this period is usually based on their own feelings as well as on assumptions that arise from customs, traditions, state and hospital health rules, and even research interests. Thoughtful and caring medical personnel can share and help to lighten the family's burden. After learning of the diagnosis of terminal illness, parents usually cannot absorb the detailed information they are given about the disease and its clinical course. They require sufficient time and privacy to formulate their questions, and they need guidance to establish realistic expectations, especially if referral to a large medical center is to be made. Often, their questions are repetitious; sometimes they completely avoid certain topics.

One or both parents may seem to limit their requests for help, or, even more often, such requests after the loss of their child are not recognized by health professionals. Given a chance to express their feelings, parents can utilize support constructively. If possible, the same physician should talk with both parents together or separately, or both, about the child's progress and remain aware of their individual needs.

Following a child's death the physician's first responsibility is to inform the parents in a direct, sensitive manner; warmth and understanding provide a closeness with the family. Unless there are exceptional circumstances, a parent should *never* be informed of a child's death by telephone. An important prerequisite in talking to parents about their child's death is knowledge of the circumstances in which it occurred. Not being given this information may reinforce parents' doubts and guilt. It may be helpful to provide sedation or a quiet place for the parents, who may prefer to be alone. The hospital staff can also help with funeral arrangements, inform other family members, or arrange transportation. Similarly, viewing and touching the body may be important, to help the parents grasp the actuality of their child's death. They may need time alone to hold and talk to the deceased child as their last gestures of caring. In the case of a newborn, seeing the body is especially important to the parents. Though these parents have had little physical contact with their child, they have experienced pregnancy and have formulated plans and expectations that are suddenly ended. During the pregnancy they may also have had the normal fears about deformed infants, and mothers may often recall incidents during pregnancy that they feel could have influenced the eventual outcome. To quiet those fears, they may need to see that their baby was not grossly abnormal.

Not only the parents but surviving children may need help with their grief. Children under the age of 5 years view the death as a temporary and reversible situation. Children between 5 and 10 years of age may look at death in terms of responsibility—something or someone was responsible. By the time children are about 10 years old, they are able to understand that death is inevitable and irreversible. Surviving older children appear to be able to resolve the problem of loss, and do substantially better when they are included in the grief process. For this reason parents can be advised to be as open as possible with their explanations and their own reactions. Clinicians may need to clarify that a sibling died of a special illness or one that affects only infants and not older children or parents. Children may also need to be reassured that their health is good and that the same event will not happen to them. In the course of normal sibling rivalry, children might wish an infant brother or sister to die. Small children indulge in magical thinking; they believe they can cause events to occur by wishing them. In this way they may implicate themselves and need assurance that they did nothing to cause the death. Some children mourn losses for a long time. Their grief may be exhibited in school difficulties, sleep problems, or special fears. These should be addressed individually, with the knowledge that sibling loss almost certainly plays a significant role in these behavioral changes.

Follow-up visits with parents are important. If an autopsy has been performed, a visit to discuss the findings should follow its completion. Irrespective of an autopsy, visits should be made at 6 weeks and 6 months to gauge the progress of grieving, anticipate unusual problems in adjusting to the child's death, and answer the many questions about the circumstances of the death and how to help siblings adjust to their feelings. Friends and relatives usually tire of discussing the death long before parents have worked through their own feelings.

When parents have lost a child, the decision to have another is complex. If they are able to complete the grief process, the psychological environment for the subsequent newborn will be healthier. Parents are too often advised to have a "replacement" child quickly. There is no replacement for a lost child, and it may be better advice to parents to allow more time following a loss before a subsequent pregnancy. The physician who was so intimately involved can not only be open to such discussions, but also can help to correct the inevitable distortions of events caused by grief. Finally, physicians must be aware of and deal with their own feelings about the death of a patient. A feeling of failure is often present, particularly when complicated management did not suffice. There may be a desire to "make it up" to the family because of possible uncertainty surrounding the physician's participation. There is nothing wrong with feeling a sense of loss at the death of a patient or with the need to grieve, but it is the physician's hard task to put his or her own grief aside until the needs of the parents and family have been met.

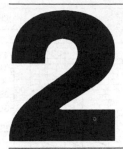

Well Child Care

Lewis R. First and
Ann McGravey

I. General principles. The chief functions of the well child visit are **health assessment, prevention,** and **screening.**
  A. **Goals of well child visits**
    1. Establish relationship of trust and open communication.
    2. Gain an understanding of the child's cultural, ethnic, religious, and socioeconomic background.
    3. Inquire about the child's environment.
    4. Detect stresses that affect the family.
    5. Determine risks of genetically transmitted diseases.
    6. Detect early disease by a history, physical examination, and screening tests.
    7. Detect early developmental and behavioral problems and monitor their remediation.
    8. Provide health maintenance (i.e., immunizations, information on nutrition).
    9. Provide appropriate counseling and anticipatory guidance.
  B. **Frequency of visits**
    The American Academy of Pediatrics (AAP) recommends a minimum of five health supervision visits from birth to 2 years of age, three supervision visits from 2 to 6 years of age, and four supervision visits from 6 to 18 years of age. The current consensus is visits at: 1–2 weeks, 2 months, 4 months, 6 months, 9 months, 12 months, 15 months, 18 months, 2 years, 3 years, 4 years, and 5 years, with visits every 2 years thereafter.
    Increased visit frequency is recommended for: parents with a particular need for guidance or education, those who come from a disadvantaged social or economic environment, and patients with perinatal disease, congenital defects, or acquired illness of a chronic nature.
II. Specific considerations
  A. **Purpose of the visit**
    1. **Assess growth**
      Height and weight charts. Height and weight should be plotted at each well child visit on a National Center for Health Statistics (NCHS) growth chart (Figs. 2-1 through 2-4). Head circumference should be recorded for at least the first 12 months of life. The NCHS charts include a graph of the weight-to-height ratio, which can be helpful in judging whether a child is underweight or overweight for height. Sequential measurements are much more useful than single determinations of weight and height in giving an overall picture of the child's growth pattern. When in doubt, incremental growth charts should be used.
    2. **Assess development**
      Simple screening tests, such as the Denver Developmental Screening Test (DDST) (Fig. 2-5), can be used to detect infants who require further evaluation for possible motor delays in the gross motor, fine motor, language, and social skills. The abbreviated revised DDST is a more efficient screen that requires only 5–7 minutes to administer. Table 2-1 summarizes usual ages of attainment of developmental milestones.
    3. **Screening**
      Screening for early disease or problems that may be diagnosed in an

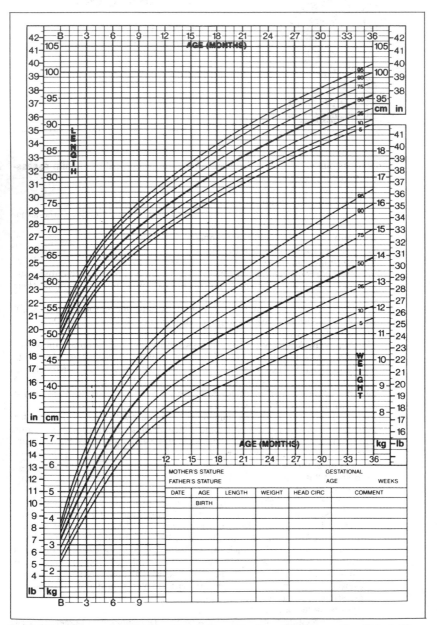

Fig. 2-1. Physical growth of girls from birth to 36 months of age. NCHS percentiles. (Adapted from P.V.V. Hamill et al., Physical growth: National Center for Health Statistics percentiles. *Am. J. Clin. Nutr.* 32:607, 1979. Data from the Fels Research Institute, Wright State University School of Medicine, Yellow Springs, Ohio. © 1982 by Ross Laboratories, Columbus, OH)

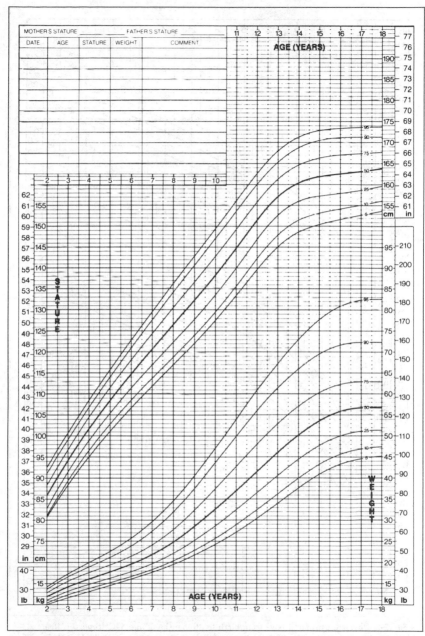

Fig. 2-2. Physical growth of girls from 2 to 18 years of age. NCHS percentiles. (Adapted from P.V.V. Hamill et al., Physical growth: National Center for Health Statistics percentiles. *Am. J. Clin. Nutr.* 32:607, 1979. Data from the National Center for Health Statistics, Hyattsville, Maryland. © 1982 by Ross Laboratories, Columbus, OH)

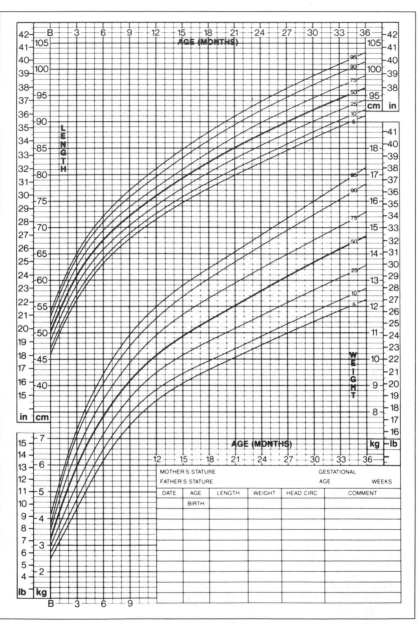

Fig. 2-3. Physical growth of boys from birth to 36 months of age. NCHS percentiles. (Adapted from P.V.V. Hamill et al., Physical growth: National Center for Health Statistics percentiles. *Am. J. Clin. Nutr.* 32:607, 1979. Data from the Fels Research Institute, Wright State University School of Medicine, Yellow Springs, Ohio. © 1982 by Ross Laboratories, Columbus, OH.)

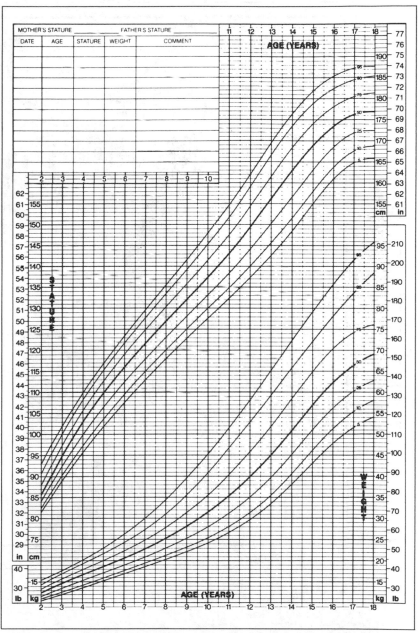

Fig. 2-4. Physical growth of boys from 2 to 18 years of age. NCHS percentiles. (Adapted from P.V.V. Hamill et al., Physical growth: National Center for Health Statistics percentiles. *Am. J. Clin. Nutr.* 32:607, 1979. Data from the National Center for Health Statistics, Hyattsville, Maryland. © 1982 by Ross Laboratories, Columbus, OH.)

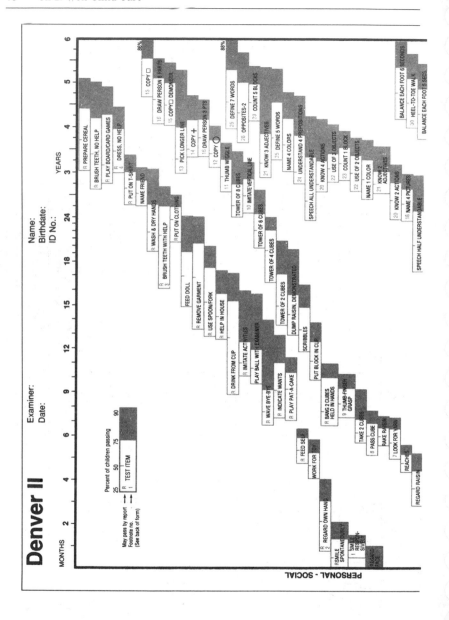

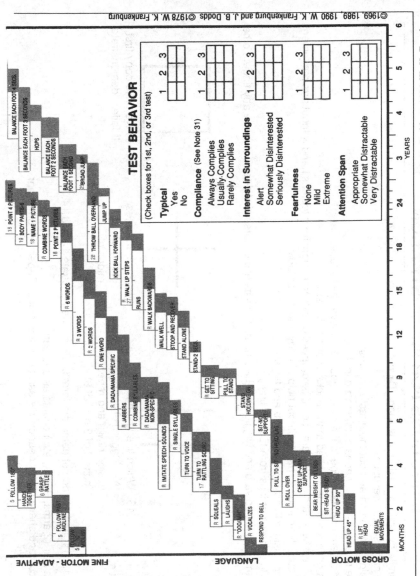

Fig. 2–5. Denver Developmental Screening Test. © 1969, 1989, 1990 W. K. Frankenburg and J. B. Dodds © 1978 W. K. Frankenburg

DIRECTIONS FOR ADMINISTRATION

1. Try to get child to smile by smiling, talking or waving. Do not touch him/her.
2. Child must stare at hand several seconds.
3. Parent may help guide toothbrush and put toothpaste on brush.
4. Child does not have to be able to tie shoes or button/zip in the back.
5. Move yarn slowly in an arc from one side to the other, about 8" above child's face.
6. Pass if child grasps rattle when it is touched to the backs or tips of fingers.
7. Pass if child tries to see where yarn went. Yarn should be dropped quickly from sight from tester's hand without arm movement.
8. Child must transfer cube from hand to hand without help of body, mouth, or table.
9. Pass if child picks up raisin with any part of thumb and finger.
10. Line can vary only 30 degrees or less from tester's line.
11. Make a fist with thumb pointing upward and wiggle only the thumb. Pass if child imitates and does not move any fingers other than the thumb.

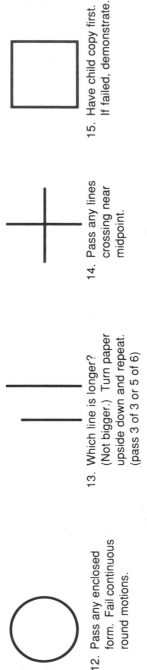

12. Pass any enclosed form. Fail continuous round motions.

13. Which line is longer? (Not bigger.) Turn paper upside down and repeat. (pass 3 of 3 or 5 of 6)

14. Pass any lines crossing near midpoint.

15. Have child copy first. If failed, demonstrate.

16. When giving items 12, 14, and 15, do not name the forms. Do not demonstrate 12 and 14.
17. When scoring, each pair (2 arms, 2 legs, etc.) counts as one part.
18. Place one cube in cup and shake gently near child's ear, but out of sight. Repeat for other ear.

18. Point to picture and have child name it. (No credit is given for sounds only.)
    If less than 4 pictures are named correctly, have child point to picture as each is named by tester.

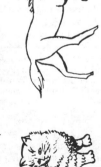 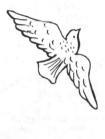 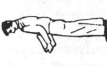 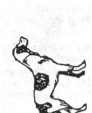

19. Using doll, tell child: Show me the nose, eyes, ears, mouth, hands, feet, tummy, hair. Pass 6 of 8.
20. Using pictures, ask child: Which one flies?... says meow?... talks?... barks?... gallops? Pass 2 of 5, 4 of 5.
21. Ask child: What do you do when you are cold?... tired?... hungry? Pass 2 of 3, 3 of 3.
22. Ask child: What do you do with a cup? What is a chair used for? What is a pencil used for?
    Action words must be included in answers.
23. Pass if child correctly places and says how many blocks are on paper. (1, 5).
24. Tell child: Put block on table; under table; in front of me, behind me. Pass 4 of 4.
    (Do not help child by pointing, moving head or eyes.)
25. Ask child: What is a ball?... lake?... desk?... house?... banana?... curtain?... fence?... ceiling? Pass if defined in terms
    of use, shape, what it is made of, or general category (such as banana is fruit, not just yellow). Pass 5 of 8, 7 of 8.
26. Ask child: If a horse is big, a mouse is ___? If fire is hot, ice is ___? If the sun shines during the day, the moon shines
    during the ___? Pass 2 of 3.
27. Child may use wall or rail only, not person. May not crawl.
28. Child must throw ball overhand 3 feet to within arm's reach of tester.
29. Child must perform standing broad jump over width of test sheet (8 1/2 inches).
30. Tell child to walk forward, 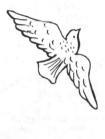 heel within 1 inch of toe. Tester may demonstrate.
    Child must walk 4 consecutive steps.
31. In the second year, half of normal children are non-compliant.

OBSERVATIONS:

Fig. 2–5. (continued)

Table 2-1. Usual ages of attainment of developmental milestones

Age	Type	Milestone	Age	Type	Milestone
1 mo	GM	Head up in prone	9 mo	GM	
	FM			FM	Object constancy
	LAN	Social smile (6 wks)			Bang cubes together
2 mo	GM	Chest up in prone			Rings bell for fun
	FM	Follows across midline		LAN	Gesture games
	LAN	Coos	10 mo	LAN	Dada (discriminately)
3 mo	GM	On elbows in prone	11 mo	FM	Plucks pellet
	FM	Follows in a circle		LAN	First word (other than
		Blinks to visual threat			ma/da)
	LAN		12 mo	GM	Walks independently
4 mo	GM	Up on wrists in prone		FM	Places pellet in bottle
		Rolls prone to supine			Voluntary release
	LAN	Orients to voice (E)			Marks with a crayon
		Laughs out loud (4½)		LAN	Immature jargon
5 mo	GM	Rolls supine to prone			Imitates squeezing a
		Transfers		P.S.	doll (E)
	FM	Pulls down ring			Drinks from a cup
	LAN	Orients to sound (E)			Assists with dressing
6 mo	GM	Sits (unsupported)	15 mo	GM	Runs
	FM	Unilateral reach		FM	Dumps pellet from
	LAN	Babbles			bottle
7 mo	GM	Comes to sit (7.5)		LAN	Directed pointing
	FM	Attempts pellet			4–6 words
	LAN		18 mo	FM	Scribbles spontaneously
8 mo	GM	Crawls; pulls to stand			Uses tools
	FM	Attains pellet			3-cube tower
		Inspects bell		LAN	3 body parts
	LAN	Understands "no"			Parallel play
		Dada (indiscriminate)			Domestic imagery
					7–20 word vocabulary
					Mature jargon (16 mo)
				P.S.	Uses spoon
			21 mo	LAN	2-word phrases
					50-word vocabulary
					Points to pictures (E)
				FM	3-cube train
			24 mo	LAN	2-word sentences

FM = fine motor/problem solving; GM = gross motor; LAN = language; P.S. = personal/social. Gross motor and personal social milestones are historical. Fine motor/problem solving are elicited. Language milestones are historical save where noted by examiner (E). Source: Reprinted with permission from R. Dershewitz (Ed.), *Ambulatory Pediatric Care*. Philadelphia: Lippincott, 1988.

"asymptomatic" state is important. Because parents often notice abnormalities before they become evident to the pediatrician, the best screening test is a good history.
Examples include:
a. Physical examination
  (1) Strabismus
  (2) Heart murmurs
  (3) Abdominal masses
  (4) Orthopedic anomalies (i.e., internal tibial torsion, congenital hip disorder)

    (5) Hypertension
    (6) Dental problems
  b. **Simple testing**
    (1) Decreased visual or hearing acuity
    (2) Tuberculosis
  c. **Simple laboratory tests**
    (1) Anemia
    (2) Lead poisoning
    (3) Pyuria
  Guidelines for appropriate times for these screens are suggested by the AAP.
4. **Immunizations**
  The AAP has recommended a schedule for routine active immunization of normal infants and children. This schedule was modified in 1992 to include immunization of infants with *Haemophilus influenzae* vaccine and hepatitis B vaccine (Table 2-2). This schedule is appropriate for premature and low-birth-weight infants with the exception that oral polio vaccine (OPV) should always be given after discharge from the hospital. Table 2-3 includes

Table 2-2. Recommended schedule for active immunization of normal infants and children, including prematures[1]

Recommended age	Vaccine[2]	Comments
Newborn	Hep B	
2 months	DPT, OPV, HbCV, Hep B	DPT and OPV can be initiated as early as 4 weeks in areas of high endemicity; Hep B may be given at 1 or 2 months depending on the hepatitis B status of mother
4 months	DPT, OPV, HbCV	2-month interval desired for OPV to avoid interference
6 months	DPT (OPV), HbCV, Hep B	OPV optional for areas where polio might be imported; Hep B may be given at any time from 6–18 months depending on hepatitis B status of mother.
15 months	Measles, mumps, rubella (MMR), HbCV	DPT, OPV may be given at 15 months or 18 months if desired
15–18 months	DPT, OPV	May be given simultaneously with MMR and HbCV; acellular pertussis vaccine can be given at 15–18 months and 4 years in place of whole cell vaccine.
4–6 years[3]	DPT, OPV	Preferably at or before school entry
11–12 years	MMR	At entry to middle school unless second dose given previously
14–16 years	Td	Repeat every 10 years for lifetime

[1] Adapted from the American Academy of Pediatrics. *Report of the Committee on Infectious Diseases,* 22nd edition, 1991.
[2] Note: For all products used, consult manufacturer's brochure for instructions for storage, handling, and administration. Abbreviations: Hep B = hepatitis B vaccine; DPT = diphtheria and tetanus toxoids with pertussis vaccine absorbed; OPV = oral, attenuated poliovirus vaccine which contains poliovirus. Types 1, 2, and 3; MMR = live measles, mumps, and rubella viruses in a combined vaccination; Td = adult tetanus toxoid (full dose) and diphtheria (reduced dose) in combination; HbCV = Haemophilus b conjugate vaccine.
[3] Up to seventh birthday.

Table 2-3. Recommended immunization schedules for children not immunized in first year of life[1]

Recommended time	Immunization(s)	Comments
Less Than 7 Years Old		
First visit	DPT,[3] OPV, MMR HbCV	MMR if child ≥ 15 months old; tuberculin testing may be done (see Tuberculosis)
Interval after first visit		
2 months	DPT, OP, HbCV	Second dose of HbCV only in children less than 15 months old
4 months	DPT (OPV)	OPV is optional (may be given in areas with increased risk of poliovirus exposure)
10–16 months	DPT, OPV	PV is not given if third dose was given earlier
Age 4–6 years (at or before school entry)	DPT, OPV	DPT is not necessary if the fourth dose was given after the fourth birthday; OPV is not necessary if recommended OPV dose at 10–16 months following first visit was given after the fourth birthday
Age 11–12 years	MMR	At entry to middle school
10 years later	Td	Repeat every 10 years throughout life
7 Years Old and Older		
First visit	Td, OPV, MMR	
Interval after first visit		
2 months	Td, OPV	
8–14 months	Td, OPV	
11–12 years	MMR	At entry to middle school
10 years later	Td	Repeat every 10 years throughout life

[1] Reproduced with permission from the *Report of the Committee on Infectious Diseases.* American Academy of Pediatrics, 22nd edition, 1991.

[2] *Haemophilus b* vaccine can be given, if necessary, simultaneously with DPT (at separate sites). The initial three doses of DPT can be given at 1- to 2-month intervals; so, for the child in whom immunization is initiated at 24 months old or older, one visit could be eliminated by giving DPT, OPV, MMR at the first visit; DPT and HbCV at the second visit (1 month later); and DPT and OPV at the third visit (2 months after the first visit). Subsequent DPT and OPV 10–16 months after the first visit are still indicated.

[3] The acellular pertussis vaccine can be used in children older than 15 months and younger than 7 years (in place of whole cell vaccine).

a schedule for primary immunization of children not immunized in infancy. In children more than 6 years of age, the adult-type diphtheria tetanus (Td) vaccine is preferred over the diphtheria-pertussis-tetanus (DPT) vaccine. Because recommendations are often revised, one should consult the *Morbidity and Morality Weekly Reports* or the AAP's *Report of the Committee on Infectious Diseases* (The Redbook) for the most current information.

a. Informed consent

The AAP has emphasized the importance of providing patients and parents with benefit and risk statements about vaccine in lay terminology. The Centers for Disease Control has developed "Important Information" statements about vaccines, which are available from the immunization divisions of state health departments. Current recommendations from the AAP state that *parents' signatures on a form are not as important as making sure the information is understood and consent given.* Consent should be documented in the medical record.

   b. **Scheduling—other considerations**
      (1) **Acute febrile illness:** Postpone immunization; do not postpone for minor nonfebrile illnesses such as upper respiratory infections.
      (2) **Unknown immunization status:** Consider child susceptible and immunize.
      (3) **Lapse in routine immunization schedule:** This does not interfere with immune response. It is unnecessary to repeat doses. Do not give any reduced dosages, as this may induce inadequate immune response.
      (4) **Prior anaphylactoid reaction** to same or related vaccine: Defer immunization until skin testing is performed.
   c. **Contraindications to live virus vaccines** (TOPV, MMR)
      (1) **Immunodeficiency.** Patients infected with human immunodeficiency virus (HIV) should receive measles, mumps, rubella (MMR) vaccine, as the risk of measles is thought to outweigh the risks of the vaccine. Immunodeficient patients or children living in a household with an immunodeficient person can be given killed polio vaccine (IPV). Hospitalized children should not be given oral polio vaccine because of the possibility of transmission of the vaccine virus to an immunosuppressed infant.
      (2) **Immunosuppressed individuals,** including those receiving radiation therapy, steroids, or antimetabolites. Children receiving alternate-day steroids at low to moderate doses or those on short-term steroid usage (i.e., asthmatics) can be immunized.
      (3) **Pregnancy.** Pregnant women should not receive live viral vaccines. However, it is permissible to give live vaccine to a household contact of a pregnant woman.
   d. **Contraindications to pertussis vaccine**
      (1) **Absolute**
         (a) Encephalopathy within 7 days of receiving DPT
         (b) Seizure with or without fever within 3 days of receiving DT
         (c) Persistent inconsolable screaming or crying for 3 or more hours or an unusual high-pitched cry within 48 hours
         (d) Shock-like state (hypotonic-hyporesponsive episode) within 48 hours
         (e) Temperature of 40.5°C (104.9°F) or greater, unexplained by another cause within 48 hours
         (f) An allergic (anaphylactic) reaction to vaccine
      (2) **Relative** (i.e., reason to defer temporarily)
         (a) Evolving neurologic disorders
         (b) Personal history of seizure—begun recently or not well controlled; this does *not* include a family history of seizures.
   e. **Common side effects** of vaccine
      Parents should be advised that side effects may occur, but that the incidence and severity of these side effects are far exceeded by the risks and damages of the diseases against which vaccines afford protection.
      (1) **Pertussis** (symptoms occur within 48–72 hours of injection).
      (2) **MMR.** Temperature of 39.4°C (103°F) or more may develop between the 6th and 10th day after vaccination and last 1–2 days. Transient rashes and arthralgias may occur.
      (3) ***Haemophilus influenzae* type B (HIB).** Mild local reactions (erythema or swelling) may occur and usually resolve within 24 hours. Systemic reactions are rare.

(4) TOPV. Minute risks of producing poliomyelitis

(5) IPV. Mild local reactions only

f. **Natural immunity**

Children who have incurred the natural disease of pertussis, measles, mumps, or rubella develop lifelong immunity and do not need to receive the vaccine. However, receipt of the vaccine, even when prior immunity to these diseases exists, will cause no problem. Infection with *Hemophilus influenzae* B in children <24 months of age **does not confer immunity and these children should be immunized.**

g. There are no known problems with the **simultaneous administration** of DPT, TOPV, or IPV, MMR, and HIB (*MMWR* 37:13–16, 1988). They must be given at different sites.

h. The use of the HIB vaccine conjugated with diphtheria toxoid does not reduce immunity to diphtheria. Routine immunizations with DPT must be done. Children not immunized as infants should receive the vaccine when first seen up until the age of 5 years. Revaccination is not presently recommended if a dose of the vaccine has been received on or after 15 months of age.

i. **Pneumococcal vaccine.** A 23-valent vaccine containing polysaccharide antigens from the serotypes causing nearly 100 percent of pneumococcal bacteremia and meningitis in children is available. Infants or toddlers may have a poor or unpredictable antibody response; hence, the vaccine is not recommended for children under 2 years of age. High-risk children with sickle cell disease, functional or anatomic asplenia, or nephrotic syndrome, and those about to undergo cytoreduction therapy for Hodgkin's disease, should be vaccinated.

j. **Hepatitis B vaccine.** Two recombinant vaccines (Recombivax HB and Energix-B) are licensed and produced in the United States. They induce more than 90 percent protection against hepatitis B virus (HBV) infection, and adverse effects are minimal, consisting primarily of soreness at the injection site. Previously, both the AAP and the U.S. Public Health Service Immunization Practices Advisory Committee recommended selective vaccination of high-risk populations and serologic screening of all pregnant women for hepatitis B surface antigen (HBsAg). Since identifying high-risk individuals and getting them to utilize preventive health care are difficult, this strategy made little impact on the control of hepatitis B (HBV). Current recommendations state that the highest priority should be immunization of high-risk children and all infants, followed by immunization of adolescents living in high-risk areas, and then all adolescents. A summary of recommendations is as follows:

(1) Routine serologic screening of all pregnant women for HBsAg should continue.

(2) All newborn infants should be immunized with HBV vaccine. The appropriate doses are listed in Table 2-4.

(a) For infants born to **HBsAg-negative mothers:** Administer first dose to newborn (0–2 days) before discharge from the hospital; administer second dose at 1–2 months of age, followed by the third dose at 6–18 months of age.

Infants who did not receive a dose of vaccine at birth should receive three doses by 18 months of age. The minimal interval between the first two doses is 1 month and between the second and third doses is 3 months, but 4 months or more may be preferable. An alternative schedule of immunizations at 2, 4, and 6–18 months of age, although not preferred, is acceptable, provided the infant's mother is HBsAg negative.

(b) Infants born to **HBsAg-positive women** must be immunized at or shortly after birth and should receive one dose of Hepatitis B surface antigen positive (HBIG) as soon as possible after birth. The second dose should be administered at 1 month and the third

Table 2-4. Recommended doses of licensed hepatitis B vaccines

	Vaccine	
Patients	Recombivax HB Me	Energix-B
Infants of HBsAg-negative mothers and children < 11 years	0.25	0.5
Infants of HBsAG-positive mothers (HBIG should also be given)	0.5	0.5
Children, adolescents 11–19 years	0.5	1.0
Adults ≥ 20 years	1.0	1.0
Dialysis and/or immunosuppressed patients	1.0	2.0

Source: Adapted from the 1991 *Report of the Committee on Infectious Diseases*, 22nd ed.

dose at 6 months. These infants should have their serologic status checked at 9 months of age. If their anti-HBs titer is less than 10 mIU/ml, they can receive up to two more doses of vaccine.

(c) If the mother's **HBsAg status is unknown** at the time of delivery, the infant should be immunized at birth with the dose of vaccine recommended for infants born to HBsAg-positive mothers. The mother should be screened as soon as possible to determine the need for HBIG if she is HBsAg positive.

(3) Older children, adolescents, and adults at increased risk of HBV infection (Table 2-5) should be immunized with HBV vaccine.

(4) Routine immunization of all adolescents against HBV should be implemented when feasible.

The vaccine can be given simultaneously with DPT, *Hemophilus influenzae* type B, polio, and/or MMR vaccines without interference. They should not be mixed in the same syringe, but can be given one or more inches apart in the same thigh or deltoid. The volume should be administered intramuscularly.

k. **Varicella vaccine.** A live alternated varicella vaccine has been studied.

Table 2-5. High-risk groups who should receive hepatitis B immunization regardless of age

Hemophiliac patients and other recipients of certain blood products
Intravenous drug abusers
Heterosexual persons who have had more than one sex partner in the previous 6 months and/or those with a recent episode of a sexually transmitted disease
Sexually active homosexual and bisexual males
Household and sexual contacts of HBV carriers
Members of households with adoptees from HBV-endemic, high-risk countries who are HBsAg positive
Children and other household contacts in populations of high HBV endemnicity
Staff and residents of institutions for the developmentally disabled
Staff of nonresidential day care and school programs for the developmentally disabled if attended by a known HBV carrier; other attendees in certain circumstances
Hemodialysis patients
Health care workers and others with occupational risk
International travelers who will live for more than 6 months in areas of high HBV endemnicity and who otherwise will be at risk
Long-term inmates of correctional facilities

Source: Adapted from the 1991 *Report of the Committee on Infectious Diseases* (see pp 246–249 for further details and explanation). Committee on Infectious Diseases, 1991–1992.

Both seroconversion rates and protective efficacy were greater than 90 percent when the vaccine was administered to healthy children and adults. Seroconversion rates were 80 percent when the vaccine was administered to children with leukemia in remission, and the vaccine either prevented or modified varicella in these high-risk children (*Pediatrics* 78:742–747, 1986). Use of the vaccine may be approved soon.

  I. **Acellular pertussis vaccines.** The Food and Drug Administration has approved an acellular pertussis vaccine (Acelimune). In clinical trials, children who received Acelimune experienced fewer and milder local systemic side effects than those receiving the whole cell vaccine. It is currently not recommended for children younger than 15 months of age, so the whole cell vaccine must still be used at 2-, 4-, and 6-month dosing of the five-dose DPT regimen. Pediatricians can decide for the 18-month and 5-year immunization whether the decreased incidence of side effects outweighs the added cost (at least double) of the acellular vaccine over the whole cell one.

5. **Anticipatory guidance**
A well child visit is incomplete without adequate time for anticipatory guidance. The AAP has issued two companion manuals, *Guidelines for Health Supervision* and *Health Supervision Visit,* which address anticipatory guidance for each visit. More abbreviated comments are given here.
   a. **Prenatal visit:** Parents and physician get acquainted. Discussion of practice arrangements, philosophy of care, feeding—breast vs. bottle, circumcision—pros and cons, support for parents, safety issues, car seat and crib selection, smoke detectors, etc.
   b. **Newborn visit** (1–2 weeks): reassurance that adequate weight gain is occurring and that the baby is healthy. Encouragement is also provided.
   c. **2-month visit:** reassurances that breast milk or formula without additional foods supplies adequate nutrition (see sec. **B.1.a.**)
   d. **4-month visit:** introduction of solids (see sec. **B.1.c**). Accident prevention—baby becoming mobile (Table 2-6). Teething (see sec. **B.3**).
   e. **6-month visit:** review of developmental milestones reached or soon to be reached; sitting without support, holding objects, babbling. Accident prevention (see Table 2-6). Supply Poison Center telephone number and possibly ipecac sample.
   f. **9 to 12 month visit:** introduction of finger foods, increasing autonomy, accident prevention (see Table 2-6)
   g. **18-month–2-year visit:** discussion of temper tantrums, toilet training, and limit-setting techniques

B. **Common management issues**
1. **Feeding:** The early discussion of variability in feeding patterns, both in quantity and quality, helps to allay future concerns.
   a. **Breast feeding.** Breast-feeding mothers often benefit from additional counseling by the physician or nurse to help with mechanics. Particular points that need discussion include the following:
      (1) **Feeding frequency** should be determined by the baby's demand, usually every 2–3 hours during the first 2–3 weeks. The duration of each feeding is usually 5–10 minutes per breast. The mother should alternate the breast on which the nursing is begun at each feeding to keep milk production and consumption fairly even. "Bubbling" or "burping" should be done at least between breasts or possibly more frequently as needed. Milk supply is low for the initial 2–5 days, and the new mother needs reassurance that her milk will "come in," that she should continue to put the baby to breast, and that the baby will be fine until that time.
      (2) **Nipple soreness** is a common early problem that may be helped by keeping initial feeding periods brief in the first 24–48 hours, using only water to cleanse nipples, and changing position to assure proper "latching on," which will minimize soreness and prevent cracking of nipples at pressure points.

Table 2-6. Accident prevention in childhood

Age and cause of morbidity	Prevention
0–6 months	
Auto accidents	Use authorized car seat until child is 3 years old; then use seat belts
Crib injuries	Be sure that crib meets consumer protection specifications; refrain from using pillow in crib
Burns/fire	Install smoke detector; lower water tank temperature to 120° F
6–12 months	
Falls	Use childproof barriers for stairs and doors; have screens and locks on windows
Foreign body ingestions	Check toys for small removable parts and discard; keep floors clear of coins, buttons, nails, tacks, etc.
Shocks	Insert plastic covers into electric outlets
Pica	Remember that paint on walls and ceilings—and yard dirt —may contain lead
Crib injuries (from falling)	Ascertain that height from the mattress to the top of crib rail is 21 inches or more
12–24 months	
Burns	Keep hot beverages away from table edge; use rear burners of stove whenever possible; keep matches out of reach
Ingestions	Keep all medicines, cleaners, and chemicals out of reach in a locked cabinet; have ipecac and the telephone number of the poison control center on hand at home
Car accidents (as pedestrian)	Buy suitable toys—two wheelers, skateboards, rollerskates, and even some tricycles cannot be controlled by a typical toddler; supervise play near streets or have the child play in a fenced-in area
24–48 months (same as for 12–24 months)	
Burns/fire	Begin fire hazard education, especially fire escape route and "drop and roll"
School age	
Sports injuries	Maintain adult supervision in contact sports; buy appropriate protective equipment for contact sports

(3) **Breast engorgement** may begin 2–3 days postpartum and can be alleviated by a supportive bra, compresses (cool at first, warm if no relief), and oral analgesics.

(4) **Alveolar engorgement** may occur on days 3–4 postpartum as the result of milk secretion unresolved by proper letdown and emptying. Treatment involves facilitating the letdown reflex by ensuring maternal comfort and the manual expression of enough milk to relieve some fullness.

(5) The breast-fed baby may require 2 and occasionally even 3 weeks to regain birthweight. **Inadequate weight gain** at 2 weeks is best assessed by observing the mother and infant during feeding. Usually, decreasing the frequency of feeds and assuring that support systems are available to the mother so that she can get adequate physical and emotional rest will suffice. The weight should be rechecked within a few days.

(6) Jaundice is more likely to occur in the breast-fed baby than in the formula-fed infant. Jaundice from breast feeding generally occurs with the onset of the milk coming in and peaks at about 10–14 days of age. All other causes of jaundice should be excluded. If the bilirubin gets dangerously high (≥20), the mother should stop breast feeding for 12–48 hours. If the etiology of the jaundice is the milk, the bilirubin level will fall, even as much as 2 mg/dl in 12 hours. Breast feeding can then be reinstituted. Generally, the bilirubin does not rise to its previous high point. The mother should pump her breasts if an observation period is necessary, so that breast feeding will not be compromised when reinstituted. Since there are no reported cases of kernicterus associated with breast milk jaundice, breast feeding should never have to be discontinued on this basis.

(7) Supplementation with formula can be used after nursing is established (3–6 weeks), but the mother should understand that, as suckling at the breast decreases, so will milk production. If the breast milk supply seems inadequate, formula can be offered after nursing to supplement; this still assures the suckling stimulus to continued milk production.

(8) Breast milk pumping allows the woman who works outside the home to continue to provide breast milk for her infant. Breast milk can be refrigerated for 24 hours or frozen for 2 weeks. Pumping can be done 1 to 2 hours after feeding or from the alternate breast. Weaning should be done gradually to prevent painful breast engorgement. One breast milk feeding should be replaced at a time with a few days in between.

(9) Breast-fed infants should usually be **supplemented** with **fluoride drops.** (For dosage, see Table 2-7.) There is some disagreement over the necessity of **vitamin D.** If given, the common preparations of multivitamins containing 400 IU/day in combination with 1,500 IU vitamin A and 50 mg vitamin C are generally used. Breast milk is adequate in all other nutritional requirements as the sole intake for the first 4–6 months of life. Contraindications to breast feeding are well discussed in J. Cloherty and A. Stark (Eds.), *Manual of Neonatal Care*, Boston; Little, Brown, 1991, and a summary of drugs contraindicated in breast feeding is given in *Pediatrics* 84:924–936, 1989 (Tables 2-8 and 2-9).

b. Formula feeding

(1) A **cow's milk–based** formula containing iron (12 mg elemental iron/liter) is recommended for the first 9–12 months of life. Powdered or concentrated formula mixed with tap water is recommended for babies in communities with fluoridated water. There is no need to boil

Table 2-7. Supplemental fluoride dosage schedule (mg/day[a])

Age[b]	Concentration of fluoride in drinking water (ppm)		
	<0.3	0.3–0.7	>0.7
2 weeks–2 years	0.25	0	0
2–3 years	0.50	0.25	0
3–16 years	1.00	0.50	0

[a] Fluoride content of 2.2 mg sodium fluoride is 1 mg fluoride.
[b] Schedule of the Council on Dental Therapeutics of the American Dental Association initiates fluoride supplements at birth and continues them until 13 years.
Source: Adapted from *Pediatric Nutrition Handbook.* Evanston, IL: American Academy of Pediatrics, 1985.

Table 2-8. Drugs that are contraindicated during breast feeding

Drug	Effect
Amphetamine	Irritability, poor sleep
Bromocryptine	Suppresses lactation
Cocaine	Cocaine intoxication
Cyclophosphamide, cyclosporine, doxorubicin, methotrexate	Possible immune suppression, unknown effect on growth, or association with carcinogenesis, cyclophosphamide and methotrexate may cause neutropenia
Ergotamine	Vomiting, diarrhea, convulsions
Heroin	Addiction
Lithium	$1/3$ to $1/2$ therapeutic blood concentration in infants
Nicotine (smoking)	Shock, vomiting, diarrhea, rapid heart rate, restlessness; decreased milk production
Phencyclidine (PCP)	Potent hallucinogen

Source: Adapted from American Academy of Pediatrics Committee on Drugs, Transfer of drugs and other chemicals into human milk. *Pediatrics* 84:924, 1989

the water in most municipal water supplies. If ready-to-feed formula is used or bottled water is mixed with powder or concentrate, the infant should be supplemented with fluoride drops (see Table 2-7).

(2) **Soy-based formulas** can be used initially for babies with a strong family history of atopic disease. All soy formulas currently contain iron, so there is no need to supplement infants who are fed these formulas.

(3) Most newborns require approximately 5 oz formula/kg/day, based on caloric needs of 100 calories/kg/day and formula caloric density of 20 calories/oz. Infants of any age rarely require more than 32 oz of formula per day, because caloric requirements decline with age and alternate food sources become available to the older infant.

(4) **Whole cow's milk** can be introduced between 9 and 12 months of age, provided that the infant is consuming one third of calories as supplemental foods that provide adequate sources of iron and vitamin C. Defatted cow's milk is **not recommended** in children less than 2

Table 2-9. Drugs that have caused significant effects on some nursing infants and should be used with caution

Drugs	Effect
Aspirin (salicylates)	Metabolic acidosis (dose related); may affect platelet function; rash
Clemastine	Drowsiness, irritability, refusal to feed, high-pitched cry, neck stiffness
Phenobarbital	Sedation; infantile spasms after weaning from milk containing phenobarbital; methemoglobinemia
Primidone	Sedation; feeding problems
Psychotropic drugs	Antianxiety, antidepressant, antipsychotic; have an unknown effect, but are probably of special concern when given to nursing mothers for long periods

Source: Adapted from American Academy of Pediatrics Committee on Drugs, Transfer of drugs and other chemicals into human milk. *Pediatrics* 84:924–936, 1989.

years of age, since 30–40 percent of dietary calories should be in the form of fat.

c. **Introduction of solids**

(1) The timing of introducing solids varies widely. Somewhere around 3–6 months is probably the most uniformly accepted age. This timing should be based on the attainment of developmental milestones, i.e., adequate head control, loss of the tongue thrust, and some ability to express hunger and satiety. Some intake and growth factors can be considered, i.e., intake of formula greater than 32 oz per day, doubling of the birth weight, and/or an unacceptable increase in frequency of feedings.

(2) Iron-fortified cereals are recommended as the first solid foods. Fruits and vegetables in a blenderized or strained form are begun next. A 2 to 4-day period should separate the introduction of each new food to mark the occurrence of specific food intolerance or allergy.

(3) Although specific food intolerance or allergy is unusual during the first year of life, parents of infants with family histories of allergy might delay introduction of the more troublesome foods, i.e., egg whites, citrus fruits, strawberries, chocolate, and fish. Delayed exposure has been shown to reduce sensitivity reactions.

(4) During the second half of the first year of life, infants begin to like "finger foods," which allow some independence in feeding (before the development of dexterity, it is still necessary to feed the baby with a spoon).

(5) After one year of age, parents should offer a varied diet including each of the four major food groups. Periods of apparent decreased food intake may occur at 7–9 months, when the desire of babies to feed themselves begins; at 2–3 years, when there is a further need for independence; and at 5–6 years. In general, parents can be reassured during these periods by demonstrating the child's continued adequate weight gain on growth charts. *Forced feedings are never useful at any age.*

2. **Crying.** Parents need to understand that babies normally cry for as many as 4 hours per day. It takes time to understand their babies' cries and what they mean. Parents also need reassurance that sometimes there is no discernible cause and allowing the infant to cry is acceptable.

a. **Colic** refers to paroxysmal abdominal pain of intestinal origin, but the term is used loosely and includes moderate to severe and otherwise unexplained bouts of crying. It occurs in 10–15 percent of infants, usually between the ages of 3 weeks and 3 months.

(1) **Etiology.** There is no single cause. **Persistent** crying signals distress and should stimulate efforts for an explanation. Hunger, swallowed air, milk intolerance, or an acute illness must be excluded. The **typical pattern** is that of a usually calm and placid infant who suddenly screams, draws knees up to abdomen, and may pass flatus or feces. An episode can last 10 minutes to 2 hours.

(2) **Management**

(a) Underfeeding and overfeeding should be discontinued. Air swallowing may be prevented by altering feeding and burping techniques. If the infant is formula fed, enlarging the nipple holes may help improve flow of the formula.

(b) **Listening and lending support are the cornerstones of management.** The baby who is often fussy and crying provokes anxiety and tension, and the parents need an outlet for their own concerns and feelings, often of inadequate parenting.

(c) Holding a fussy infant with colic is recommended. Gentle rocking, holding the baby close to the body in a front pack, and using soothing words are helpful. Sometimes an automobile ride, if available, works wonders.

(d) Parents need reassurance that allowing the infant to cry is an acceptable option if all soothing techniques have failed. This simple "giving of permission" may lessen parental anxiety and tension, resulting in a calmer infant.

(e) When parents are especially tired or anxious, it is important to ask whether they are afraid of hurting the baby, and definite strategies for respite time may need to be established.

(f) Sedative and anticholinergic drugs are ineffective, and the hazards of overdosage and toxicity are such that use of these drugs is not recommended. The use of simethicone drops as an antiflatulent has not been proved effective, but they are safe and acceptable on a trial basis.

(g) Devices that attach to the crib and cause vibration are available and may be of benefit in selected infants.

3. Teething
a. General considerations
(1) Teething is defined as the natural eruption of teeth. The symptoms that accompany the process begin from the 1st to the 15th month and may continue off and on into the third year of life.

(2) Teething is probably never responsible for *significant* fever, rhinorrhea, rashes, or diarrhea.

(3) The normal appearance at age 4 months of oral exploration and consequent salivation and drooling is frequently attributed to, but rarely due to, teething. A gingival inflammation that occurs with actual eruption of a tooth may produce an increase in this activity, as well as periods of irritability.

(4) The lower central incisors are generally the first teeth to erupt and usually do so at 5 months of age. For an appropriate chronology of deciduous tooth eruption, see Table 2-10.

b. Management
(1) Rubbing swollen gums or giving the infant a cold, hard object to bite may provide relief of discomfort.

(2) Application of commercially available topical analgesics and gels at best provides limited and very transient relief.

(3) When discomfort and irritability are clearly related to teething, acetaminophen may be useful.

4. Organic problems
a. Fever

Table 2-10. Chronology of eruption of deciduous teeth

Deciduous tooth	Mean age at eruption in months ± (SD)
Maxillary	
Central incisor	10 (8–12)
Lateral incisor	11 (9–13)
Canine	19 (16–22)
First molar	16 (13–19, boys; 14–18, girls)
Second molar	29 (25–33)
Mandibular	
Central incisor	8 (6–10)
Lateral incisor	13 (10–16)
Canine	20 (17–23)
First molar	16 (14–18)
Second molar	27 (23–31, boys; 24–30, girls)

Source: Adapted from J. M. Davis et al., *An Atlas of Pedodontics* (2nd ed.). Philadelphia: Saunders, 1981.

(1) General considerations

(a) Most fevers in infants and children are caused by acute viral infection. Fever, unless exceptionally high—over 41.1°C (106°F)—does no specific harm to the patient. Indeed, there is evidence to suggest that fever may play a role in the natural body defenses against infection.

(b) The physician's concern should be aroused when patients fail to act and look better when less febrile. Actual response to antipyretics in terms of a decrease in the degree of fever is not predictive of the significant source of the infection.

(c) The presence of fever in an infant under 3 months of age should prompt the physician to see that child without delay.

(d) In the neonatal period, a temperature below normal is probably of as much concern as an elevated temperature.

(e) The height of the fever does not necessarily correlate with the severity of its cause.

(2) Management

(a) The treatment of temperature elevation should be aimed at making the patient comfortable. **The mere presence of fever does not always mandate treatment.** However, the child with a **history of febrile seizures** should have fever promptly treated.

(b) Adequate hydration of the patient with oral fluids and increased ambient fluid content of the air may help prevent dehydration.

(c) Exposure of the skin to the air by removal of clothing and sponging the body with tepid water promote heat loss. Alcohol or ice water should **never** be used for this purpose, since they cause a rapid lowering of the skin temperature, with resulting vasoconstriction and prevention of heat loss.

(d) Antipyretics

(i) Acetaminophen has both antipyretic and analgesic properties. Children's preparations are available in drops, syrup, chewable tablets, and suppositories. The dosage is 10–15 mg/kg every 4 hours. At therapeutic dosages, acetaminophen should have no adverse effects. Acetaminophen intoxication may cause serious hepatic injury. For management of overdose, see Chap. 4, p. 109.

(ii) Nonsteroidal antiinflammatory agents. Children's liquid preparations of ibuprofen have recently been approved. They have antipyretic, analgesic, and antiinflammatory properties. Although, there are not thought to be any significant side effects, they are currently considered second-line treatment for fever, with acetaminophen still being recommended as first choice. The dose is 10–15 mg/kq/dose every 6–8 hours.

(iii) Aspirin, or acetylsalicylic acid, probably no longer has a role in the management of pediatric fever. Its side effects as well as possible association with Reye syndrome when used in children with viral illness make it an unnecessarily risky choice.

b. Constipation

(1) Diagnosis

(a) Constipation may be diagnosed by history with the findings of fecal contents on abdominal or rectal examination. Abdominal pain may suggest it.

(b) Although constipation may accompany many syndromes (see Chap. 20, p. 553), it more often represents too little free water in the diet, inadequate intake of high-residue food, disruption of the child's daily habits, or a painful anal fissure that causes withholding of the stool.

(c) Passing a daily stool does not exclude constipation as a problem.

Large, hard, or painful stools, sometimes large enough to clog the toilet, are significant signs even if they occur daily by history. Conversely, infrequent stools, even once every 3–7 days, can be normal in breast-fed infants, and are even common in formula-fed infants.

(2) Treatment. A stepwise approach follows.

(a) To assist the child under age 2 to pass a hard stool:
(i) Glycerine suppository
(ii) Dilation with a lubricated rectal thermometer or finger

(b) To assist the child over age 2 to pass a hard stool:
(i) **Glycerine or bisacodyl (Dulcolax) suppository (one only)**
(ii) *Pediatric* **Fleet's enema (can be repeated once)**
(iii) Mineral oil, 15 ml PO. Magnesium sulfate or sodium sulfate may help in passing a hard stool and softening a forming stool.
(iv) Manual disimpaction, which is unpleasant for both child and physician, may be necessary. There is no known simple or pleasant way to perform this time-honored physician's chore.
(v) Soapsuds or milk and molasses slurry enemas are helpful to resistant cases. Gastrografin or Mucomyst enemas can be useful in the impaction of cystic fibrosis, but have serious potential side effects, including electrolyte disturbances, intravascular depletion, and toxic absorption, and are expensive.

(c) To increase bulk and soften the stool:
(i) Increased intake of free water
(ii) Natural dietary lubricants (e.g., prune juice, olive oil, tomatoes, and tomato juice)
(iii) High-residue foods (e.g., fruits and green vegetables). The addition of bran and whole grain products is optimal for lifelong dietary changes.
(iv) Pharmacologic stool softeners, such as dioctyl sodium sulfosuccinate (Colace), malt soup extract (Maltsupex), or senna concentrate (Senokot), may be useful. The dosage of stool softeners is as follows: age 1 month–1 year, ½ tsp bid; age 1–5 years, 1 tsp bid; 5–15 years, 2 tsp bid.
Large initial doses are essential; when the stools become soft, the dosage can be reduced. Regular daily dosage is continued for about 2–3 months and slowly reduced as bowel tone and regular bowel habits are reacquired. Relapses are common, and prolonged follow-up study is advisable. Initially, Senokot, in particular, may produce cramping.

(d) To assist the child with anal fissures:
(i) A glycerine or bisacodyl suppository may be necessary (one only).
(ii) Soften the stool as described.
(iii) Sitz baths tid for small children

(e) If anatomic lesions have been ruled out:
(i) Establish a pattern of bowel movement after meals (gastrocolic reflex) or at other times—but at the same time each day—by sitting the child on the toilet whether or not a bowel movement results.
(ii) Be sure that emotional stress and anxiety have been carefully excluded as causes.

(f) If constipation persists and encopresis occurs, a psychiatric evaluation is indicated, and long-term management by the pediatrician is required (see Chap. 20, sec. **IV.B**).

c. Cough

(1) General considerations

(a) A cough is a reflex directed at clearing the upper and lower

airway of irritating secretions or foreign material. Many parents have the misconception that cough itself is harmful and **must** be treated. An explanation can be offered of the usefulness and protective benefits of coughing in lieu of a prescription.
  (b) Only in a few specific conditions (croup, perhaps foreign bodies, pertussis) do the characteristics of the cough itself help to make the diagnosis.

(2) **Management**
  (a) Treatment should be directed at the underlying cause, e.g., infection, allergy, foreign body, irritants such as cigarette smoke.
  (b) Humidification of an otherwise dry environment may be beneficial in enhancing expectoration.
  (c) One may consider use of a codeine-containing (or dextromethorphan) cough suppressant for the irritative cough that interferes with sleep. Dextromethorphan is a nonnarcotic analogue that, with adequate dosing, can be considered equipotent to codeine but without the narcotic side effects.
  (d) Expectorants, though thought to increase the flow of respiratory tract secretions, have never been clinically proved to be more effective in decreasing sputum viscosity or easing expectoration over a placebo or simply good hydration. Thus, they should not be routinely recommended for pediatric usage.
  (e) See Table 2-11 for symptomatic medications (see Formulary)

Table 2-11. Symptomatic medications

Medication	Dosage
Antitussives	
Dextromethorphan	
Available as: liquid (5–30 mg/5 ml depending on preparation)	1 mg/kg/24 hr Divide into 3 doses
Codeine phosphate	
Available as: syrup (10 mg/5 ml); tablets (15, 30, and 60 mg)	1–1.5 mg/kg/24 hr Divide into 6 doses
Decongestant	
Pseudoephedrine	
Available as: liquid (15–30 mg/5 ml depending on preparation); tablets (7.7, 30, or 60 mg)	5 mg/kg/24 hr Divide into 4 doses
Antihistamines	
Brompheniramine maleate	
Available as: tablets (4 mg) prolonged-action tablets (8 and 12 mg); elixir (2 mg/5 ml)	0.5 mg/kg/24 hr Divide into 3–4 doses
Diphenhydramine	
Available as: liquid (12.5 mg/5 ml)	5 mg/kg/24hr Divide into 3–4 doses
Chlorpheniramine maleate	
Available as tablets (4 mg); prolonged-action tablets (8 and 12 mg); syrup (2 mg/5 ml)	0.35 mg/kg/24 hr Divide into 4 doses 0.2 mg/kg single dose (prolonged action)
Nasal spray	
Oximetazoline	
Available as: solution 0.0590 (20 ml drops bottle) spray 0.05% (15 ml squeeze bottle)	> 6 yr 2–3 qts or 1–2 sprays each nostril bid

d. **Coryza (upper respiratory infection)**
   (1) **General considerations**
      (a) The symptom of persistent mucous drainage from the nose is most often called a "cold" and is by far the most frequent illness encountered in pediatric practice.
      (b) The illness is most often caused by a virus, produces a clear nasal discharge, and, when uncomplicated, lasts 3–5 days and disappears.
      (c) Such viral infections may lower local resistance in the nose and throat, which may in turn lead to secondary bacterial invasion (e.g., otitis, sinusitis, pneumonia).
      (d) Coryza can be due to excessively dry air or irritants such as allergens.
   (2) **Management in the infant**
      (a) Remove mucus with a suction bulb. A 3-oz bulb is most efficient.
      (b) Increase the humidity in the environment by using a cold mist humidifier or by placing a pan of water on the radiator.
      (c) Thin nasal mucus with a few drops of saline solution made by dissolving 1 tsp salt in an 8-oz cup of water. Place two to three drops of the solution into one nostril at a time, wait 2 minutes, and then suction that nostril. This should be done before meals and before sleep as needed.
      (d) If the discharge becomes purulent and is associated with fever, consider secondary bacterial infection.
      (e) Decongestants contain cardiotonic agents and should not be used in infants under 6 months of age. In any case their value remains unproven. (See Table 2-11 for symptomatic medications.)
   (3) **Management in the older child**
      (a) Treat as for the infant, except that gentle nose blowing can also be attempted.
      (b) A vasoconstricting nose drop can be prescribed, but should not be used chronically because of "rebound phenomenon," in which vasodilation and further edema of the turbinates can occur with repeated usage.
      (c) Oral decongestants (sympathomimetics) have not been established as effective drugs; however, in some children they may relieve profuse coryza. The benefits must be weighed against the possible side effects of irritability and drowsiness. Occasionally, paradoxical hyperactivity may occur. Antihistamines have no place in treatment of viral coryza, but can be useful in an allergic rhinitis.
      (d) See Table 2-11 for symptomatic medications.
e. **Vomiting**
   (1) **General considerations**
      (a) Vomiting is a common symptom. Table 2-12 includes the differential diagnosis for the causes of vomiting in infants, older children, and adolescents.
      (b) Common causes of vomiting are viral gastroenteritis and improper feeding technique.
      (c) In monitoring the adequacy of hydration (see Chapter 7) (a major complication of vomiting along with electrolyte abnormalities), the physician should question the parents as to the frequency of urination, the degree of moistness of the mucous membranes, the presence or absence of tears with crying, and the child's activity level. The parental perception of how sick the child is between episodes of vomiting will help in determining how soon the child needs to be seen.
      (d) Always be alert for intestinal obstruction, either partial or complete, or for increased intracranial pressure as causes of

vomiting. This vomiting can often be sudden or projectile, or both, and not associated with feelings of nausea.
  (e) Medicines such as theophylline and erythromycin can cause vomiting.
  (f) Anorexia nervosa and bulimia must be considered in adolescents with persistent vomiting.
  (2) **Management of nonobstructive vomiting**
    (a) Initiate frequent (every 30–60 min) small (1–2 oz) amounts of easily digested clear fluids. The volume can be increased as the symptom decreases.
    (b) Formula intolerance may be due to the sugar or to the protein in the formula. A change to a soy product that does not contain lactose or to a casein-based formula may be helpful.
    (c) The assessment of improper feeding technique requires first-hand observation in the office and continuing follow-up by telephone.
    (d) If vomiting is due to simple gastroenteritis in a child over 2 years of age, a **single** dose of an antiemetic such as prochlorperazine IM or PR may provide relief.
  f. **Diarrhea** (see also Chap. 10, p. 274)
  (1) **General considerations**
    (a) Causes include local intestinal factors; viral, bacterial, and parasitic infections; antibiotics; inflammatory bowel disease; or extraintestinal infections, such as otitis media, pneumonia, and urinary tract infection.
    (b) Important facts in the history include the general condition of the patient; presence of fever; number, consistency, and size of the stools; presence or absence of blood in the stool; and diarrhea in family members. When seeing a child with gastroenteritis, always **record a weight,** noting the clothing worn.
    (c) Evaluate the state of hydration (skin turgor, mucous membranes, fullness of the fontanels, presence of tears), activity level of the child, and presence or absence of infection other than in the gastrointestinal tract.
  (2) **Treatment**
    (a) Because most cases of gastroenteritis are caused by self-limiting

Table 2-12. Causes of vomiting in infancy, childhood, and adolescence

Infants	Children	Adolescents
Overfeeding	Food poisoning	Food poisoning
Infection (bacterial or viral)	Drug ingestion	Drug ingestion
Neuromuscular incoordination	Infection (bacterial or viral)	Infection (bacterial or viral)
Formula intolerance	Cyclic vomiting	Pregnancy
Esophageal dysfunction	Esophageal dysfunction	Esophageal dysfunction
Intestinal obstruction	Intestinal obstruction	Intestinal obstruction
Increased intracranial pressure	Increased intracranial pressure	Increased intracranial pressure
Peptic ulcer disease	Peptic ulcer disease	Peptic ulcer disease
Reye syndrome	Reye syndrome	Reye syndrome
Inborn error of metabolism	Heavy-metal poisoning	Neurosis (i.e., self-induced)
Uremia		Inflammatory bowel disease
Rumination		

Source: Developed by Jeffrey Hyams, M.D., Department of Pediatrics, Hartford General Hospital, Hartford, CT.

viral infections, an initial period of dietary treatment is helpful, with daily telephone contact to follow the patient's progress. Initially (for the first 12–24 hr), clear liquids, such as oral electrolyte solutions, are given in small amounts if the child is vomiting.

   (b) After 12–24 hours, when the vomiting has stopped and diarrhea alone is present, early refeeding with breast milk, a gradually strengthened soy-based formula, or lactase-treated cow's milk, in addition to the oral electrolyte solution, will prevent starvation, stooling, and a deficit of protein and calories, and will stimulate repair of intestinal mucosa.

   (c) After 24–48 hours, a bland diet (banana, rice cereal, applesauce, and unbuttered toast) can be introduced.

   (d) Kaopectate and antispasmodics should not be used. Such medications make many parents lose sight of the importance of a restrictive, clear-fluid diet. Even with a decrease in the number of stools, continual fluid loss into the gut may persist.

g. Thrush

   (1) General considerations

   (a) Thrush is an infection of the mouth caused by *Candida albicans*. It commonly occurs in infants who have been intimately exposed to the fungus during passage through the birth canal. It may often be associated with a diaper rash caused by the same organism and in such cases may well imply stool colonization with the fungus. A nursing mother may have concomitant surface infection of the nipples and areolae, which may require topical antifungal treatment.

   (b) Persistence of extensive oral candidiasis after the age of 3–4 months is distinctly unusual and should prompt an evaluation of cell-mediated immunity.

   (2) Management

   (a) Thrush is most easily treated with nystatin (Mycostatin) solution (100,000 units/ml), given as 1–2 ml in each cheek qid after meals. The dose can be divided, with half swabbed directly onto the affected area and the other half swallowed. Parents should be cautioned to continue therapy despite apparent resolution of the infection to prevent recurrence. Treatment is continued for 10–14 days.

   (b) Nystatin ointment (occlusive) or cream (nonocclusive) can be used on the diaper rash tid for 1–2 weeks. In many cases it may take several weeks to eradicate this condition. Oral nystatin solution can be used as well should the rash recur after discontinuation of the ointment (even if oral thrush is not visible).

5. Functional problems

   a. Sleeping habits (see also Chap. 20)

   (1) General considerations. After the first few months of life, sleeping patterns are, in large part, learned responses. By 3–4 months of age, most babies have learned to sleep in an apparently uninterrupted stretch of 6–8 hours, generally at night if their feeding, bathing, and play time are scheduled in the daytime. By 7–12 months, babies should be accustomed to taking their long sleep period at the family's convenience, namely, at night.

   (2) Management

   (a) It is best to remove the baby's crib from the parents' room by 3–6 months, so that the periodic awakening of most young infants at night does not escalate into a prolonged wakeful time.

   (b) After 6–9 months of age, the baby's waking at night, despite having been fed, tucked in, and diapered, needs to be handled with a resolute firmness and consistency, so that by experience the baby learns that there is a quiet time for **all** members of the family.

(c) If the child cries on being placed in the crib at night after the bedtime routine (and is otherwise healthy), or awakes crying in the middle of the night as a means of getting attention or food, then the parent should be encouraged to reassure the child with a minimal amount of physical contact (e.g., standing at the door to the room) and/or refreshment. The parent should then leave the room and return after longer and longer intervals. This technique often allows the child to establish his or her own ability to fall back to sleep without any significant parental intervention.

(d) Nightmares and night terrors (3–4 years of age) are common and need to be handled with reassurance and gentle comforting in the dimly lit bedroom. Frequent episodes should be investigated with regard to possible daytime environmental factors that might be precipitating these frightening nighttime dreams (see also Chap. 20, p. 557). A child is not apt to remember being afraid in the setting of a night terror, whereas a nightmare is often remembered with vivid detail. Parents may be frustrated by their inability to comfort the child with a night terror, but should be reassured that their being there is sufficient support for the child (who will be less concerned the following morning than the parent). On the other hand, discussion of the nightmare with the child by the parent can be reassuring for both parties (see Chap. 20, p. 558).

(e) The young child should grow up with the firm conviction that he or she is to stay in his or her bed until morning. This is a safe habit and also allows the parents the privacy and comfort of their own bed and bedroom. Be firm about **not** allowing the child to come into the parents' bed. If the child must be comforted for a special reason, it should be done in his or her own room and bed.

(f) Many children are able to give up their crib by 2 years of age, and some even by 18 months. Do not advise parents to make the change too early, because they might be losing a "safe place" for the child at night. If a bed move is planned due to the arrival of a new sibling, that move should occur several weeks before or after the arrival of the new baby so as not to convey to the child the sense of being "evicted" or "displaced" by the new family member.

b. **Eating habits or "the picky eater"**

(1) **General considerations.** Concerns about feeding, especially pertaining to the amount and variety of food, commonly arise during the second year. Children are now feeding themselves, have become discriminating, and are beginning to respond to behavioral feedback from parents who feel they should exercise control over the amount and type of food eaten. In general, **children eat only when they are hungry.** The child who refuses to eat a given meal will **not** become ill or hypoglycemic or be undernourished by the next meal—merely hungry. Therefore, the child need not be permitted to manipulate and thus dictate his or her diet.

(2) **Management**

(a) When introducing solids to an infant, one might want to introduce vegetables before fruits so as to broaden the palate of the infant, and allow for a greater variation in preferred tastes, rather than just the sweeter ones.

(b) Milk is not essential beyond 1 year of age, provided protein, calcium, and vitamin D are available from other sources. Vegetables are not essential in a diet that contains fruit, grains, and meats. Vitamin supplements are generally not necessary for children who are growing well, except in instances of the most restrictive diets.

(c) Growth charts and "nutrition diaries" may occasionally be useful in reassuring parents that the child who "doesn't eat enough to keep a bird alive" actually eats enough to keep a child alive, permitting normal growth and development at the same time.

(d) Regular morning and afternoon snacks should be considered the norm, especially for toddlers. As long as these snacks are nutritious (e.g., cheese, yogurt, fruit) and occur at the same time every day, they will not interfere with mealtime and will help the "picky eater" to improve total caloric intake.

(e) Anticipating and discussing normal eating patterns before parental anxiety and mealtime tension develop is time well spent. Attempting to force a child to eat when he or she does not wish to can set the stage for more damaging parent-child conflict. The best advice to parents on this point is: "Don't fight wars you can't win."

(f) Parents should also be encouraged to eat similar foods as they want their children to eat so as to set a good example for them.

(g) If parents believe their toddlers do not eat enough, or are just "picky," encouraging parents to put small portions on large plates (and refill these plates as needed) rather than large portions on small toddler plates may be a more successful feeding maneuver than verbal encouragement to "eat more."

c. **Toilet training**
   (1) **General considerations.** All normal children will toilet train themselves. Most parents, however, have difficulty in waiting for this to happen. The parents can **help** the child achieve this goal and should think of it in this manner, not that they are actually training the child. Remind parents that there is no earthly way for them to keep their child from becoming toilet trained, but unfortunately they can do all sorts of things to delay the process.
   (2) **Management**
      (a) The best time to start is between **2 and 3 years** of age, which is the time when many children begin to train themselves. Before this age, they have to learn by association, coincidence, luck, and fleet parental feet. Children who voice their displeasure with a full diaper and are interested in watching others in the bathroom are usually ready to begin training.
      (b) **Bowel control** is much simpler for a child to master than control of urination because the former involves much less complicated muscle coordination and occurs far fewer times during the day. It might help to put the child on the potty or toilet just after a meal when the gastrocolic reflex occurs.
      (c) **Urine training** should begin when the frequency of urination decreases and the child begins to awaken dry after a nap, usually around 2.5–3 years of age.
      (d) Any child who has been trained and then develops urinary or fecal incontinence should be evaluated.

d. **Fears**
   (1) **General considerations.** Expression of fear, either in action or in words, is part of normal development. Fears become abnormal only when they interfere with or severely inhibit the child's day-to-day functioning.
   (2) **Management**
      (a) Fear of **strangers** may appear at 5–8 months. Gently remind strangers to keep at a distance until the child becomes used to their presence.
      (b) Fear of the **bathtub** or of bathing may arise between 1 and 2 years

of age and may occasionally derive from a negative experience, e.g., soap in the eyes or slipping in the water. Advise parents not to insist on a bathtub bath, but to try an alternative—a dishpan bath or sponge bath.

(c) Fear of **separation** is one of the most common and, for parents, most distressing developmental reactions of childhood. It appears around 2 years of age when a sensitive, dependent child is suddenly separated from his or her major caretaker. The manifestations usually worsen at bedtime. Encourage the parents to allow the child to develop independence, in carefully controlled circumstances, at an early age. Accustom the child to a babysitter gradually; a half-hour "warm-up period" before the parents leave may be helpful. Above all, when it is time to leave, parents should act with confidence. If the child is inconsolable, giving the child an object that belongs to a parent (e.g., a mother's scented handkerchief) to keep until the parent returns may reinforce to a child that the parent has not left permanently and will return soon.

(d) Imaginary worries arise at 3–5 years of age. Dogs, the dark, fires, and death all figure prominently. Such patterns may be seen in children who are tense from battles over toilet training or feeding, but need not be ascribed to these causes. Frightening stories, warnings, or television shows may also stimulate these fears. Management involves parental reassurance and an understanding acceptance of the child's aversions. Above all, never force the child to face fears abruptly. Instead, encourage him or her to play games about the fears. Letting the child take an active role in dealing with the fears (e.g., by spraying his/her room with water that he/she believes is "monster spray" to prevent monsters, or by drawing a picture of a "scarier monster" to ward off the ones in the room) often lead to successful eradication of these fears.

(e) The fear of **injury** occurs at or beyond 3 years of age and is often triggered by seeing crippled or deformed people. The child is quick to perceive that something is wrong and quickly puts himself or herself in the injured person's place. A child may interpret the physical differences between the sexes as an injury. The best treatment is simply to offer an explanation appropriate to the child's age and comprehension.

e. **Thumb and finger sucking**
   (1) **General considerations**
      (a) Sucking is an instinctual behavioral pattern. Most young infants suck on their fingers for varying periods of time. This behavior should be considered normal.
      (b) Thumb sucking is strongly related to the emotional satisfaction of the infant or young child. Finger sucking will not have any detrimental effect on the position of the permanent teeth, as long as the habit is discontinued **before** the second teeth have erupted.
   (2) **Management.** The majority of children give up the habit of finger sucking, except in moments of severe stress, by the time they reach school age. In most cases, thumb sucking represents a **greater problem to the parents than to the child.** The history usually reveals that the child does not do an unusual amount of thumb sucking; it is the parent who is made anxious by the behavior. Ordinarily, information, reassurance, and support will relieve the parents and thus prevent secondary emotional problems in the child. The child may benefit from the use of positive reinforcements for not sucking the thumb rather than negative statements regarding the behavior.

f. **Self-stimulation**
   (1) **General considerations.** What parents report as "self-stimulation"

usually consists of the normal self-soothing habits of children that arise in early infancy. Such behaviors appear in two forms:

(a) **Rhythmic habits,** including rocking, head rolling, and head banging. Appearing in the second half of the first year, these behaviors usually occur at times of fatigue, sleepiness, or frustration, and serve to comfort the child.

(b) **Genital exploration or manipulation.** The extent of this behavior is directly correlated with age. In an infant or young child, genital manipulation is a manifestation of wholesome curiosity, while in the 3- to 6-year-old, it is an expression of a normal interest in sex. At this stage, genital stimulation should arouse no concern if the child is outgoing, sociable, and not preoccupied with the activity. Excessive stimulation usually indicates underlying high-level anxiety or family conflict, or may be a sign of emotional disturbance. In the latent stage, from 6 years to puberty, such behavior, in general, is suppressed naturally.

(2) **Management**

(a) Management of concerns regarding rhythmic behavior is directed toward averting injury and reducing noise. No attempt should be made to discipline or restrain the young child once the behavior has started.

(b) Management of concerns regarding masturbation is directed toward reassuring parents that masturbation is part of normal development. Parents should be advised that gentle inhibition or distracting the child is more appropriate than calling attention to the activity. **Attempts to suppress the activity, especially if punitive, may produce potentially damaging psychological sequelae.**

6. **Common complaints in the older child**

a. **Headache** (see also Chap. 19, p. 536)

(1) **General considerations.** Headache is a common complaint of children, and repeated evaluations may be needed. Associated symptoms and signs that mandate evaluation are vomiting; hypertension; abnormal neurologic findings, including motor or visual abnormalities; nocturnal or early-morning awakening; or frequent school absences.

(a) Depending on the location and pattern of symptoms, dental disorders, occult sinusitis, and systemic infection should be considered.

(b) Poor vision is a rare cause of headache.

(c) Psychogenic or muscle contraction headaches are commonly felt as "pressure" or aching occipital pain. They may be accompanied by signs of anxiety or depression.

(d) Migraine headaches are experienced as paroxysmal, throbbing, or pounding bifrontal-temporal pain. They are commonly associated with nausea, pallor, irritability, and photophobia. The child usually has a family history of migraine headaches.

(2) **Management**

(a) A thorough neurologic examination, blood pressure check, and fundoscopic examination are essential for evaluation of headache.

(b) Psychogenic headaches can be treated with the judicious use of analgesics. Attempts should be made to uncover any personal, social, or family conflicts.

(c) Migraines (see Chap. 19, p. 536)

b. **Abdominal pain**

(1) **General considerations.** Abdominal pain is most frequent in the school-age child. An organic cause is identified in no more than 5 percent of cases of recurrent abdominal pain; the diagnosis is usually suggested by the clinical presentation, and appropriate investigation and treatment are indicated when the cause is organic.

(2) Management of nonorganic abdominal pain

(a) The diagnosis of pain of emotional origin should be supported by evidence of emotional disturbance, not merely by lack of an organic cause. In this respect, the history tends to be more revealing than the physical examination or laboratory tests.

(b) Commonly, evidence of other emotional disturbances, such as school or sleep problems or difficulties with family or peers, is found. Frequently, the family history will reveal other members with emotional or psychosomatic problems, often taking similar form.

(c) Laboratory investigations should be kept to a minimum and should be reasonable (e.g., urine and stool studies).

(d) For the child or adolescent with pain of short duration, the reassurance afforded by normal findings may be curative.

(e) In cases of more severe, chronic, and incapacitating pain, management should be directed at the underlying emotional disturbance.

7. Common complaints of parents of older children and adolescents
   a. Television
      (1) General considerations
         (a) The physician should include questions about the television habits of his or her patients and their families in the general checkup.
         (b) There is some evidence that watching violent scenes produces aggressive behavior in young people.
         (c) Television advertisements encourage conflict and confrontation between parent and child.
      (2) Management
         (a) Parents should be encouraged to set limits on television viewing by their children and should monitor their own viewing habits.
         (b) Excessive television viewing is potentially a mental and physical health hazard and can significantly compromise the child's functioning in school and in the social sphere. As for any health hazard, the key is prevention.
         (c) Guidelines for television viewing can be obtained from the San Francisco Committee on Children's Television, Inc.; the American Academy of Pediatrics; or Action for Children's Television, Newton, MA.
   b. Cigarettes
      (1) General considerations
         (a) The pediatrician can influence behavior patterns and growth through repeated encounters with the child, and early and repeated discussions of drug issues, including cigarette smoking, may influence future usage patterns.
         (b) Areas to be emphasized are the effects of prenatal usage on the unborn baby, including low birth weight for gestational age and its concomitant problems; the effects on the incidence and severity of respiratory infection and pulmonary function in children exposed to smoking parents; and the known increase in cigarette usage among the children of smoking parents.
      (2) Management
         (a) Physicians and nurses can obviously act as examples by not smoking and by not permitting smoking in their offices.
         (b) The key is **prevention.**
   c. Alcohol and drugs (see also Chap. 4)
      (1) General considerations
         (a) Attitudes toward alcohol and drugs are learned first at home. Children later apply these attitudes in peer groups.

(b) When parents are in agreement, they constitute a powerful and important factor affecting the child's point of view.

(c) Adolescents consider the use of alcohol and drugs as the mark of being an adult. Thus, getting deliberately intoxicated for the first time is seen as an act of autonomy and independence.

(d) Factors in the history that are indicators of alcoholism or drug abuse, or both, include:

(i) Drunkenness at an early age; drinking to become drunk

(ii) Truancy, school expulsion, dropping out of school, job problems

(iii) An alcoholic parent

(iv) Automobile accidents or arrests

(2) Management

(a) The subject should always be approached as an issue of health, not of morals. A nonthreatening discussion of chemical use and abuse should begin at least by age 12.

(b) As the patient grows older, any problems with alcohol or drugs should be discussed openly and directly as the pediatrician becomes aware of high intake or frequent use.

(c) Discussion should include the effects of alcohol and drugs on others' lives and how drug or alcohol abuse affects one's ability to relate to family and friends.

(d) Make appropriate referrals for drug counseling when necessary.

(e) Confidentiality is important. If the patient's parents are to be involved, the patient should be so informed.

(f) The patient's needs are the physician's first consideration. However, a distinction should be made between caring for a "user" and a "dealer." Dealing in drugs is a federal offense that carries severe penalties; the use of drugs, antisocial though it may be, can be managed as an illness. The pediatrician should be informed of legal constraints in his or her locality.

d. Sex education and activity

(1) General considerations

(a) The parents are the natural people to educate their child about sex, but many are reluctant or unable to do so. Under these circumstances the roles of the pediatrician and school become important.

(b) Sex education should begin when first questions arise, usually at age 3–4 years. The child should be thoroughly educated before puberty in the anatomic and physiologic functions of the sexes.

(c) While understanding the goals of parents to maintain family morals and social standards, the physician should help parents realize that the main tasks of adolescence are separation from the family and adjustment to sexuality.

(d) Adolescent behavior is influenced by peers and in many ways reflects prevalent subcultural values and practice. Every adolescent must come to terms with the pressure of sexuality; his or her response may range from attempts at total suppression to indiscriminate promiscuity.

(e) The importance of sexuality can be either underestimated or highly exaggerated by the adolescent, the parent, or the physician.

(2) Management. To relieve sources of anxiety, many concerns can be discussed as an accepted part of a routine physical examination.

(a) Early adolescence. Young adolescents are preoccupied with their body changes and worry over any perceived deviations from normal. They require open communication and reassurance.

(i) Somatic changes; breast development, menstruation, nocturnal emission, and erections

(ii) Anticipatory concerns about sexual intercourse and contraception
(iii) Masturbation as normal behavior
(iv) Homosexuality. Fear or suspicion of homosexuality must be differentiated from its actual presence. Attraction to same-sex adults is a common occurrence for young adolescents as they begin separation from their parents. Early homosexual episodes do not predict eventual sexual preference.
(v) AIDS education
(b) **Mid to late adolescence**
(i) Relationships
(ii) Contraception. Patient confidentiality is important. When the physician is faced with the dilemma of dispensing contraceptives without parental knowledge, this situation is best handled by working within the value constraints of the family. However, the physician has the responsibility to challenge the attitudes and values of either or both parties when the welfare of the patient is at stake.
(iii) Venereal disease (see Chaps. 12 and 14)
(iv) Homosexuality. Homosexual adolescents face many personal, social, and family stresses. Discussions should include medical considerations, especially the high incidence of sexually transmitted diseases. Referral for psychological counseling may be warranted, particularly when parental and social disapproval create a fundamental conflict within the family.
(v) AIDS education

III. Speech and language delay
  A. The **etiology** includes hearing deficit, overall developmental delay, oral motor planning problems (dyspraxia), autism, environmental deprivation, plumbism, and primary language disorder.
  B. **Diagnosis and evaluation** (Table 2-13.)
    1. All children with language delay should have their hearing formally evaluated. This can be done at any age in specialized facilities.
    2. Developmental evaluation should be done using age-appropriate tools (i.e., DDST, Early Language Milestone Scale, Bayley Scales of Infant Development). Language delay must be regarded as a part of overall delay in development.
    3. History and observations should include the child's means of communicating

Table 2-13. Indicators of significant language delays*

Age (months)	Indicators
12	Limited babbling; quiet child
18	Does not understand specific words, his name, or names of common objects; cannot follow simple commands such as "Come here," "Sit down"
24	Uses few single words; is not imitating words
30	Does not know names of common objects or simple body parts; cannot point on command to familiar objects or get an object on request not directly in visual field; no true two word combinations such as "No cookie," "More milk"; child is often misunderstood
36	No simple sentences (subject, verb, object); does not seem to understand simple explanations or discussions of events in past or future

* Children with these findings would be significantly behind normal developmental expectations.

his or her needs without language. Those with a hearing deficit, oral motor planning problems, and primary language disorders may act out their needs, whereas children with developmental delay and autism will not.

4. Feeding problems and inability to imitate tongue movements should be examined in evaluating for oral motor planning problems.

5. Comparison between levels of receptive and expressive language may be helpful.

6. The history should involve a description of the home environment and child's interactional style (to look for environments with low levels of language stimulation).

7. **Caution**—Many children will not show their best language skills with strangers. Diagnosis often must be suggested by the history.

C. Treatment

1. Referral to a speech pathologist for isolated language delay or to an audiologist for hearing problems is often appropriate after the initial workup.

2. Mild delays can be treated in many cases by educating and encouraging parents to use language more pervasively in a play context, with frequent modeling of words.

3. Early intervention (under 3 years old) or language-centered classrooms in public schools (over 3 years) may be helpful for these children.

Acute Care

Richard Saladino and
Michael McManus

I. Cardiopulmonary resuscitation (CPR)

A. The **diagnosis** of cardiorespiratory arrest must be made rapidly (absent pulse and respirations). Prompt and orderly resuscitative efforts are essential, and assignment of responsibilities is mandatory.

1. The **first person** at a cardiorespiratory arrest must establish the diagnosis. If the patient is unresponsive, a patent airway is established via a chin lift or jaw thrust; **two slow** breaths are given, and then the carotid-brachial-apical pulse is palpated. If the patient remains unresponsive, help is called and the "ABCs" of resuscitation are started (see sec. **I.C**).

2. **The resuscitation team** includes the following:

a. The **leader** (the most experienced person) is in charge, makes **all** therapeutic decisions, assigns others their roles, and continually reassesses the quality of the resuscitation. The leader should immediately appoint persons for **airway management** and **cardiac compression**.

b. **Vascular access** should be accomplished by the next available person.

c. **Medications** and **recording**. Appropriate doses of medications are prepared. The dosages and times of giving medications, as well as any procedures or diagnostic tests, are documented.

d. The **float/circulator** obtains and monitors the blood pressure, adequacy of cardiac compressions, and chest movement during ventilation and assists wherever help is needed.

e. **Historian.** One person must obtain a history from the parents or caretakers and keep them informed of events.

f. The **electrocardiogram** must be monitored. Persons responsible for CPR must be familiar with ECG equipment.

B. The following equipment *must* be available:

1. **Airway.** Oxygen, suction and Yankauer suction catheters, adult- and pediatric-size masks, oral and nasal airways, flow-dependent anesthesia and self-inflating bags, endotracheal tubes, laryngoscopes with pediatric and adult blades, McGill forceps, stylets, benzoin, and tape

2. **Drugs** (Table 3-1)

3. **Vascular access.** Intravascular, catheters, syringes, intraosseous needles, cutdown tray, tourniquet, and tape

4. **Other.** Blood pressure cuff, thermometer, glucose-specific coated strips (Dextrostrip), ECG machine and leads, defibrillator, chest tubes and Pleurivacs, Foley catheter, nasogastric tubes, and cardiac pacemaker

C. **The ABCs of resuscitation** (adapted from the American Heart Association recommendations)

1. **Airway (A)**

a. Immobilize the cervical spine if spinal cord injury is a possibility.

b. Clear the oropharynx with a Yankauer suction or bulb suction. **Avoid blind finger sweeps.**

c. The jaw-thrust or chin-lift maneuver removes obstruction caused by the tongue and soft tissues of the neck.

d. The head must be in the midline. Because the larynx in a child is more anterior and superior than in an adult, the child should be put in the "sniffing" position by placing a folded towel under the occiput; avoid hyperextension of the neck as this may obstruct the airway. Oral airway placement may improve airway status.

2. **Breathing (B).** Begin mouth-to-mouth or bag-to-mouth ventilation with 100% oxygen. **Assess the adequacy of the ventilation by observing chest wall excursion.** If chest wall excursion is insufficient, endotracheal tube placement is indicated.

3. **Circulation (C)**
   a. The patient is placed on a hard, solid surface, and external cardiac compressions are started *immediately.*
   b. **Ventilation/compression.** The ventilation/compression ratio is 1 : 5 with a 1- to 1.5-second pause for ventilations to allow for adequate inspiratory time. The rate of compressions is at least 100 per minute for the infant and for the younger and older child. The rate of compressions in the newborn is at least 120 per minute, with a 1 to 3 ventilation/compression ratio.
   c. **Technique.** Compressions for the **infant** are performed using one of two methods. The **two-finger** technique utilizes two fingers of one hand for sternal compressions. The preferred **hand-encircling** technique is performed using two hands; the infant is grasped with the fingers supporting the back and the thumbs over the middle third of the sternum. Compressions in the infant are done one fingerbreadth below the nipple line. For the **toddler,** the heel of one hand is used and in the **older child,** two hands interlaced are used; in both cases, compressions are done two fingerbreadths above the xiphoid.
   d. The **adequacy** of cardiac compressions is assessed by palpating femoral or brachial pulses, or both. Counting aloud should be done by the rescuer doing chest compressions.
   e. An ECG monitor can be attached when help arrives.

4. **Drugs**
   a. As indicated in Table 3-1, several drugs can be delivered via the endotracheal tube. Vascular access should be attempted after help arrives. At this time, a brief history and physical examination are performed. Temperature, blood glucose (e.g., Chemstrip, Dextrostix), and hematocrit are measured.
   b. Peripheral venous access should be attempted percutaneously at the **antecubital fossae, saphenous vein, dorsum of the hands, and femoral areas.** Proceed quickly to **intraosseous needle placement** at the proximal tibia if peripheral access requires more than 1–2 minutes. **Central access (femoral)** is best achieved using the Seldinger catheter-over-a-guidewire technique.
   c. **Asystole** is treated with epinephrine and atropine; bicarbonate is used in prolonged arrests and for documented **acidemia.** Calcium is used to treat documented **hypocalcemia. Bradycardia** is treated with atropine. Intravenous glucose is given to correct **hypoglycemia.** (see Table 3-1).

5. **Electrical energy**
   a. **Cardioversion**
   (1) **Indication: tachydysrhythmias**
   (2) **Supraventricular tachycardia (unstable):** synchronized cardioversion; dose, 0.25–0.50 watt-sec/kg; double the dose if unsuccessful.
   (3) **Ventricular tachycardia:** synchronized cardioversion; dose, 2 watt-sec/kg; double the dose if unsuccessful. Treat with lidocaine, 1–2 mg/kg IV.
   (4) **Ventricular fibrillation (rare in children):** nonsynchronized defibrillation; dose, 2 watt-sec/kg. Repeat at twice the dose if unsuccessful; give epinephrine, 10 μg/kg IV, intraosseously (IO), or via endotracheal tube; and continue CPR. Precede subsequent defibrillation attempts with intravenous lidocaine or bretylium. Maximum dose is 360 watt-sec.

Table 3-1. Drugs used in a resuscitation*

Drug	Dose (adult dose)	Preparation	Route	Indication
Atropine	0.02 mg/kg (0.4 mg); 1.0 mg max	0.4 mg/ml	IV, IM, ETT	To treat bradycardia and to block vagally mediated bradycardia
Bicarbonate	1–2 mEq/kg (same)	1 mEq/ml; 0.5 mEq/ml available for infants	IV	Metabolic acidosis
Elemental calcium	10–20 mg/kg (300 mg)	CaCl = 27 mg/ml; calcium gluconate = 9 mg/ml	IV	Electromechanical dissociation: for positive inotropy and to increase vasomotor tone
Dextrose	0.5 gm/kg (same)	25% D/W and 50% D/W	IV	Presumed hypoglycemia
Epinephrine	0.1 ml/kg (10 ml)	Epinephrine 1:10,000 (10 ml = 1 mg)	IV, ETT	Asystole, bradycardia, hypotension, to coarsen ventricular fibrillation before countershock
Lidocaine	1–2 mg/kg (50–100 mg)	100 mg/10 ml	IV, ETT	Ventricular ectopy
Naloxone hydrochloride (Narcan)	0.01 mg/kg (0.4 mg)	0.4 mg/ml	IV	Opiate intoxication

ETT = via endotracheal tube; D/W = dextrose in water.
* See sec. II for a discussion of cardiotonic infusions.

b. Paddle placement

(1) Interface: Electrode cream, electrode paste, and saline-soaked gauze can all be used; **do not use alcohol pads.**

(2) Paddle placement: one paddle at the right parasternum at the second intercostal space, one paddle in the midaxillary line at the level of the xiphoid.

(3) Safety: Be certain that no one is in contact with the patient or the table; announce **"clear the table"** before discharge.

c. Cardiopulmonary resuscitation is immediately reestablished until effective cardiac output is achieved.

D. If the resuscitation does not establish cardiac output, the cause of the "arrest" should be evaluated for correctable mechanical or metabolic insults, or both, such as the following:

1. **Hypothermia.** The patient may appear dead and/or unresponsive to pharmacologic management if the temperature is less than 30°C. Rewarming must accompany meticulous CPR (see sec. **VIII.C**).

2. **Tension pneumothorax or hemothorax**

3. **Cardiac tamponade**

4. Profound **hypovolemia** (see Chap. 7)

5. Profound **metabolic imbalance** (see Chap. 13)

6. **Toxin ingestion** (see Chap. 4)

7. **Closed head injury** with resultant increased intracranial pressure (see sec. **V.B**).

E. Common iatrogenic complications include:

1. **Trauma** from closed chest massage: rib fracture causing pneumothorax or hemothorax; splenic and hepatic rupture

2. **Pneumothorax** from subclavian and internal jugular cannulation or from positive pressure ventilation.

3. **Bleeding** and **pericardial tamponade** from intracardiac injections

F. After successful resuscitation the patient must be **closely monitored.** The following should be continually assessed:

1. **Cardiovascular system**

   a. Continuous ECG monitoring and a 12-lead ECG

   b. Blood pressure via radial artery catheter

   c. Central venous pressure (CVP) catheter to assess the intravascular volume status

2. **Pulmonary system**

   a. Arterial blood gases (ABGs) to document the adequacy of ventilation and oxygenation.

   b. Chest x-ray for evidence of aspiration, pneumothorax, and rib fracture

3. **Central nervous system.** Observe for seizures and signs of increased intracranial pressure.

4. **Renal system.** The renal lesion most commonly seen is acute tubular necrosis (see Chap. 8, p. 216).

5. **Miscellaneous injuries**

   a. Hypoxic injuries to the GI tract. Monitor stool guaiac and liver function tests.

   b. Disseminated intravascular coagulation (see Chap. 16, p. 477)

   c. If trauma is suspected, evaluate with appropriate radiographs and serial hematocrits.

   d. Sepsis or serious local infection may be a precipitating cause of the original arrest and can be anticipated from emergency "dirty" procedures.

II. Shock

A. Definition. Shock is defined as failure of the cardiac output to meet the metabolic demands of the body's tissues. Shock in children is not distinctly present or absent. Early shock may be subtle, and the diagnosis requires a careful history and physical examination for signs of compromised cardiac output. Compensatory mechanisms in the child are extraordinarily effective and blood pressure is often maintained until late shock becomes refractory. Early recognition and treatment are paramount.

B. Etiology (Table 3-2)

C. Evaluation

1. The **history** should include specific details of the acute illness, hydration status (intake and losses, i.e., vomit, stool, urine), and information about chronic disease and medication.

2. **Physical examination.** An accurate weight and temperature must be obtained. Particular attention should be paid to the cardiopulmonary systems: pulse and heart sounds, respiratory rate and auscultatory sounds, blood pressure with orthostatic changes, and peripheral perfusion. Neurologic status should be assessed, including level of consciousness and pupillary response. Serial observations are important to assess status and effectiveness of treatment.

3. **Laboratory studies** include:
   a. ABGs
   b. Complete blood count (CBC)
   c. Electrolytes, blood sugar, calcium, blood urea nitrogen (BUN), creatinine, cardiac enzymes, liver function tests, toxic screen, prothrombin time, partial thromboplastin time, and fibrin split products
   d. A chest x-ray to evaluate cardiac size and pulmonary vasculature

D. Monitoring

1. **Vital signs.** The following must be continuously monitored and recorded on flow sheets:
   a. Temperature
   b. Respiratory rate
   c. Continuous ECG
   d. **Blood pressure.** In infants and children, arterial cannulation is the best way to monitor blood pressure continually. If this method is not possible, blood pressure can be obtained with a blood pressure cuff; often, a Doppler is required for auscultation.
   e. **Intake and output records.** Measurement of hourly urine output, as well as nasogastric losses, and iatrogenic blood losses

2. Swan-Ganz catheterization and CVP measurement may be required.

E. Treatment of shock

1. An adequate airway must be maintained; **oxygen** should be administered to every patient with signs of shock. Intubation and ventilatory support may be necessary.

2. **Volume resuscitation.** In shock without congestive heart failure, rapidly give a 10- to 20-ml/kg intravenous or intraosseous bolus of isotonic fluid (normal saline or lactated Ringer's solution).
   a. If this volume replacement produces no clinical improvement, a CVP catheter is placed before further therapy is begun.
      (1) If the CVP is less than 5 mm Hg, further volume resuscitation is continued until the CVP is greater than 5 mm Hg.
      (2) If the CVP is greater than 5 mm Hg with no clinical improvement, the following procedures should be considered:
         (a) Pharmacologic support with inotropes (Table 3-3)
         (b) An ECG to evaluate the possibilities of myocarditis, pericardial tamponade, metabolic imbalance, or arrhythmias
         (c) An echocardiogram to evaluate ventricular function
         (d) A Swan-Ganz catheter

3. **Drugs** (see Table 3-3)

4. Evaluate and treat the precipitating event.

III. Respiratory emergencies

A. Upper airway obstruction may result from (1) **swelling** of normal tissues (as in traumatic, infectious, and allergic processes), (2) **aspiration** of foreign objects, (3) anatomic abnormalities, or (4) loss of neurologic function and soft tissue tone.

Table 3-2. Causes of shock in infants and children

Type of shock	Newborn	Older child
Hypovolemic		
Loss of intravascular volume		
Blood	Intracerebral hemorrhage; placental hemorrhage; twin-twin, fetal-maternal transfusion	Trauma: Hemophilia, splenic-hepatic rupture, pelvic or long bone fracture
		Epistaxis, ectopic pregnancy, GI hemorrhage, sickle cell sequestration crisis
Fluid	Gastroenteritis, gastroschisis, omphalocele, meningomyelocele	Gastroenteritis, severe burn, diabetes mellitus and insipidus, cystic fibrosis with profound sweat loss, nephrotic syndrome
Loss of vascular resistance	Sepsis, adrenogenital syndrome, CNS injury	Sepsis, anaphylaxis, adrenal crisis, CNS injury, drug ingestion
Hypervolemic, normovolemic		
Myocardial failure	Endocardial fibroelastosis, viral infections, congenital heart disease, sepsis, hypoglycemia	Viral infections, cardiotropic drugs, coronary insufficiency, sepsis, hypoglycemia, hypocalcemia
Outflow obstructive lesions	Coarctation, critical aortic stenosis, malignant hypertension	Coarctation, aortic stenosis or idiopathic hypertrophic subaortic stenosis, pulmonary embolism, cor pulmonale as seen with asthma, cystic fibrosis, malignant hypertension
Arrhythmias	Paroxysmal atrial tachycardia and other arrhythmias, drug intoxication, sepsis	Paroxysmal atrial tachycardia and other arrhythmias, drug intoxication
Increased metabolic demands	Severe anemia, hyperthyroidism	Severe anemia, hyperthyroidism, ingestion

Table 3-3. Drugs used in the treatment of shock

Drug	Dose	Maximum adult dose	Mechanisms of action	Indications	Limitations
Epinephrine	0.1–1.0 µg/kg/min	1–4 µg/min	α- and β-adrenergic, increases heart rate, increases systemic vascular resistance, positive inotropy	Anaphylaxis, hypotension, diminished cardiac contractility, bradycardia	Ventricular arrhythmias, decreases coronary blood flow, decreases renal blood flow
Norepinephrine	0.1–1.0 µg/kg/min	1–4 µg/min	α- adrenergic, increases heart rate, increases systemic vascular resistance	Hypotension without preexisting vasoconstriction	Ventricular arrhythmias, decreases coronary blood flow, decreases renal blood flow
Isoproterenol	0.1–1.0 µg/kg/min	1–4 µg/min	β-adrenergic, increases heart rate, positive inotropy, decreases vasomotor tone	Bradycardia, diminished cardiac contractility	Ventricular arrhythmias, hypotension if the patient was hypovolemic
Dopamine	1–5 µg/kg/min	Same	Delta, increases renal, coronary, splanchnic flow	Poor tissue perfusion, to attempt to increase renal perfusion	
	5–15 µg/kg/min	Same	β-adrenergic, increases heart rate, positive inotropy	Bradycardia, decreased myocardial contractility	Ventricular arrhythmias
	15–20 µg/kg/min	Same	α- and β-adrenergic, increases heart rate, increases systemic vascular resistance, positive inotropy	Hypotension, bradycardia, decreased myocardial contractility	Ventricular arrhythmias, decreases coronary blood flow, decreases renal blood flow
Dobutamine	1–20 µg/kg/min	Same	Similar to dopamine, but no delta effect; less α-effect, possibly less chronotropic	Diminished myocardial contractility	Ventricular arrhythmias

1. **Evaluation**
   a. **History**
      (1) **Onset.** Acute or gradual
      (2) The nature and course of **symptoms,** including fever, dyspnea, stridor, wheezing, dysphagia, dysphonia or aphonia, and cough
      (3) **Precipitating event or condition,** including choking on a foreign body, trauma to the upper airway, and an acquired or congenital abnormality of the airway
      (4) Current **medications**
      (5) **Allergies**
   b. The **physical examination** should quickly assess the adequacy of ventilation and oxygenation and identify the cause and site of airway obstruction.
      (1) **General appearance,** including alertness, distress, anxiety. Restlessness, altered mental status, pallor, or cyanosis suggests **hypoxia.**
      (2) **Vital signs**
      (3) **Cardiorespiratory findings.** The nature and adequacy of air movement and adventitious sounds, including stridor, dysphonia, and wheezing. Tachycardia out of proportion to the level of anxiety is often present in the child with a compromised airway. **Hypotension and bradycardia occur in association with severe impairment of air movement.**
2. **Specific conditions**
   a. **Epiglottitis** is a rapidly progressive bacterial cellutitis of the supraglottic tissues that can result in total airway obstruction. **It is a true medical emergency.**
      (1) **Etiology.** *Haemophilus influenzae* type B (Hib) has traditionally been the cause of 95 percent of cases. The incidence of epiglottitis due to Hib has declined sharply with the advent of effective immunization against Hib. Group A streptococci, pneumococci, *Corynebacterium diphtheriae,* or *Mycobacterium tuberculosis* are rarely isolated as causal agents.
      (2) **Evaluation and diagnosis**
         (a) **To prevent death, the diagnosis must be made and definitive airway maintenance established quickly.**
         (b) The onset of respiratory difficulty is usually acute, with rapid progression over several hours. Drooling, dysphagia, fever, toxicity, inspiratory stridor, protruding jaw, and extended neck are seen.
         (c) Epiglottitis is most often seen in children 3–6 years old; children under 2 years of age may occasionally become infected and the diagnosis confused with croup.
         (d) In some centers, definitive diagnosis is obtained via direct or fiberoptic visualization of the epiglottis conducted in the emergency room by experienced personnel. Under most conditions, however, **no attempt should be made to visualize the epiglottis or to carry out any other procedure until the airway has been secured.** Any manipulation, including aggressive physical examination or venipuncture, **may precipitate complete obstruction.**
         (e) The *presumptive* diagnosis can be made on clinical grounds alone when needed, and if the child is in little distress, lateral neck x-rays may assist in the *definitive* diagnosis. These should be done under controlled conditions, with the required staff and equipment for immediate intubation or tracheostomy in attendance. In younger children, special care must be taken that the film is truly lateral, as even slight rotation may produce "smudging" of the epiglottic shadow.
      (3) **Therapy**
         (a) **Initial stabilization** requires placement of a secure artificial air-

way under controlled conditions (i.e., in the operating room after induction of general anesthesia). Intubation may be required for 1–3 days.

(b) Nasotracheal intubation is preferred over oral intubation as being more secure and comfortable for the patient. An oral endotracheal tube is initially placed and then changed if this can be done easily.

(c) Very rarely, when intubation cannot be carried out, tracheostomy is indicated.

(d) After intubation, the epiglottis can be examined and swabs for culture can be taken. At the same time, blood cultures can be drawn and IV fluids begun.

(e) Antibiotic therapy. Ampicillin/sulbactam (Unasyn) 200 mg/kg-/day should be started immediately. Alternatively, ceftriaxone, 50 mg/kg/day or cefotaxime, 150–200 mg/kg/day, can be used.

(f) Other foci of infection should be ruled out and the patient maintained in respiratory isolation for 24 hours after initiation of antibiotic therapy.

b. Croup, or **viral laryngotracheobronchitis,** is marked by glottic and subglottic edema, resulting in loss of voice and airway cross-sectional area. Inflammation and obstruction to air flow result in characteristic barking cough and stridor.

(1) Etiology. Parainfluenza, influenza, respiratory syncytial virus, and, less commonly, adenovirus are typical causes. Bacterial infection has been increasingly recognized but remains unusual.

(2) Evaluation and diagnosis

(a) History. A coryzal prodrome is common, with increasing barking cough and hoarseness. Often, it is worse at night and usually occurs in children under 3 years of age.

(b) Physical examination is directed at assessing the extent of airway narrowing. **Inspiratory stridor, tachypnea, retractions, and diminished breath sounds indicate critical narrowing.** Restlessness, tachycardia, altered mental status, or cyanosis suggests **hypoxia.**

(c) Laboratory data. A lateral neck x-ray will rule out epiglottitis. An anteroposterior neck film will show subglottal narrowing (the classic *steeple* sign). In serious cases, arterial oxygen saturation can be monitored continuously by pulse oximetry and adequacy of ventilation by ABG.

(3) Therapy

(a) Home care. Most cases of croup are mild and can be managed at home. Therapeutic measures include a cool mist vaporizer, increased fluids, and careful observation. Parents should be instructed to call their physician if the child's respiratory distress worsens.

(b) Hospital care. Humidified oxygen should be administered in a quiet room where parents can stay with the child. Elimination of all but the most necessary procedures will help reduce the child's anxiety and associated increased respiratory work. Continuous pulse oximetry is desirable.

(c) Aerosolized **racemic epinephrine** is usually sufficient: 0.25–0.75 ml racemic epinephrine diluted with 2 ml normal saline (2.25%) and administered by standard passive aerosol equipment. However, rebound worsening often occurs approximately 30–60 minutes after use. Therefore, its use **requires** hospitalization.

(d) While some controversies remain, steroid administration is now generally accepted as helpful in reducing the severity of croup and diminishing the need for intubation. While dosage recommendations vary widely, dexamethasone (0.5–0.6 mg/kg 1 m) may be used in moderate to severe cases.

(e) When respiratory compromise is severe and respiratory failure is present or imminent, intubation under controlled conditions is indicated. **The need for frequent administration of racemic epinephrine may indicate impending respiratory failure.**

c. **Foreign body aspiration** is the leading cause of accidental deaths in toddlers. The neurologic sequelae of aspiration depend on the relative compromise of air movement. The respiratory sequelae depend on the material aspirated and the extent and character of associated inflammation.

(1) **Etiology.** Poorly designed or age-inappropriate toys or food products, including peanuts, hard candy, and gum, are usually involved. **Balloons** are a particular hazard in younger children, who may bite the inflated toy and aspirate fragments as they startle on its rupture.

(2) **Evaluation and diagnosis** are directed at assessing the adequacy of air movement and locating the site of obstruction.

(a) The **history** should identify the acuteness of onset and the circumstances surrounding aspiration. Choking, gagging, high-pitched wheezing, dysphonia, or aphonia may be noted. A history of fever and the clinical course will help differentiate acute aspiration from an infectious obstructive process (epiglottitis, croup, bacterial tracheitis).

(b) The **physical examination** should first establish the adequacy of the airway.

(c) **Laboratory data.** Anteroposterior and lateral neck and chest roentgenograms will reveal radiopaque foreign bodies and occasionally provide clues as to the location of radiolucent objects. Obstruction of the upper airway from foreign bodies usually occurs at the laryngeal level. Inspiratory and expiratory films and fluoroscopy are sometimes very useful in patients with negative radiographic findings.

(3) **Therapy** should be responsive to the acuteness and severity of the obstruction.

(a) If the child is in stable condition, pink, coughing, and vocalizing well, attempts to remove the foreign body (laryngoscopy or bronchoscopy) should await controlled conditions.

(b) **A conscious, actively choking, aphonic child with minimal air movement requires immediate noninvasive procedures.**

(i) If the victim is a child (> 1 yr), the **Heimlich maneuver** (4–6 subdiaphragmatic abdominal thrusts) is recommended.

(ii) If the victim is an infant (< 1 yr), **the Heimlich maneuver should be avoided because of potential intraabdominal injury.** In this age group, a combination of up to 5 back blows and 5 chest thrusts is recommended.

(iii) **Blind finger sweeps are contraindicated in the infant and child because they can advance a foreign body further down the airway.**

(iv) An unconscious child with inadequate respirations should receive 100% O_2 by face mask. When staff members experienced in laryngoscopy are present, immediate direct laryngoscopy may allow visualization and removal of the foreign body. When this is not possible, or if laryngoscopy is difficult or prolonged, then **emergency cricothyrotomy** with a large-bore (e.g., 14-gauge) catheter (for insufflation of 100% oxygen), or tracheostomy, is indicated. Occasionally, **endotracheal intubation** will bypass a soft foreign body or move the object into a main-stem bronchus and permit ventilation of the contralateral lung.

d. **Peritonsillar abscess**

(1) **Etiology.** Gram-positive bacteria, especially streptococci

(2) Evaluation and diagnosis
  (a) Usually occurs in children over age 8. If spontaneous rupture occurs, **aspiration pneumonia or death may follow.**
  (b) A soft-palate bulge is usually seen, with deviation of the uvula to the opposite side.
  (c) The tonsil is inflamed and pushed medially.
  (d) There is marked trismus with drooling because of the obstructive enlargement of the tonsils.
  (e) A **"hot-potato"** voice is characteristic.
(3) Therapy
  (a) Hospitalization is required in children and most adolescents.
  (b) Incision and drainage are accomplished through the soft palate **above** the tonsil (rather than lateral to the tonsil, in proximity to the internal carotid artery) and are preferable to needle aspiration. Obtain bacterial cultures at this time.
  (c) IV antibiotics. Give penicillin G, 100,000 units/kg/day q4–6h. When cultures are available, select an appropriate antibiotic on the basis of culture results (see Table 14-2).
  (d) Give IV fluids; NPO.
  (e) Administer a cool mist via face mask or croup tent.
  (f) Elevate the head of the bed 30 degrees.
  (g) Because of the frequency of recurrence, tonsillectomy is indicated after the acute episode.
e. Diphtheria pharyngitis
  (1) Etiology. *Cornyebacterium diphtheriae*
  (2) Evaluation and diagnosis
    (a) Intense inflammation of the tonsils and pharynx is seen. The structures may be covered by a thick, dirty-gray *pseudomembrane* that is densely and tenaciously adherent to underlying structures. Its removal yields brisk bleeding.
    (b) The membrane can occlude the airway.
    (c) Involvement of the larynx must be ruled out.
    (d) Bacteriologic examination is necessary for diagnosis.
  (3) Treatment
    (a) Ensure an **airway.** If the larynx is involved, **tracheotomy** may be necessary to minimize laryngeal stenosis.
    (b) IV antibiotics. Give penicillin G (see Table 14-2).
    (c) Antitoxin must be given **early** to prevent tissue fixation by the toxin.
f. Retropharyngeal abscess is suppurative adenitis of the nodes of Henle in the buccopharyngeal and prevertebral fascia. Because these nodes atrophy after the age of 5, the abscesses occur before this age.
  (1) Etiology. Gram-positive cocci and anaerobes are the causative organisms. There may be antecedent otitis media.
  (2) Evaluation and diagnosis
    (a) The abscess is almost always unilateral.
    (b) A bulge of the posterolateral pharyngeal wall may be seen.
    (c) The head and neck may be extended or the neck flexed with prevertebral muscle spasm; the head is extended for a better airway.
    (d) Drooling and dysphagia are present.
    (e) The retropharynx should not be palpated because of the risk of rupture, aspiration or mediastinitis, and death.
    (f) Anteroposterior and lateral soft tissue neck **x-rays** will support the diagnosis, especially if gas is seen in the retropharyngeal area. **Fluoroscopy** may be helpful.
  (3) Therapy
    (a) Surgical drainage is performed under general anesthesia.
    (b) IV antibiotics (see Table 14-2)

g. **Bacterial tracheitis** is an acute, infectious airway disease with clinical features common to both croup and epiglottitis.
   (1) **Etiology.** *Staphylococcus aureus* is the most common pathogen. Streptococcus and *H. influenzae* have also been reported.
   (2) **Evaluation**
      (a) **History.** There are usually upper respiratory symptoms, which progress within hours or days to severe respiratory distress.
      (b) **Physical examination** reveals fever, barking cough, and inspiratory stridor.
      (c) **Laboratory examination.** A lateral neck **radiograph** obtained to rule out epiglottitis shows irregular tracheal margins with a blurring of the tracheal air column. **Culture** of tracheal secretions should be positive. Blood cultures are usually negative.
   (3) **Treatment**
      (a) Humidified oxygen in a croup tent
      (b) Antibiotics with adequate staphylococcal coverage (see Table 14-2)
      (c) **Endotracheal intubation** may be required for pulmonary toilet and relief of obstruction. Endoscopy with direct tracheal suctioning has been beneficial in some cases.
B. **Lower airway disease** includes impaired gas exchange in the lung, or a portion of the lung, caused by viral and bacterial infections, foreign bodies, or intrinsic bronchospastic disease.
   1. **Asthma** is a condition in which bronchospasm, mucosal edema, and mucous secretion and plugging contribute to significant narrowing of the large airways and subsequent impaired gas exchange.
      a. **Evaluation and diagnosis**
         (1) The **history** should include age, duration, and course of the present attack, the course and severity of previous attacks, and a list of all medications (with doses) previously administered. Foreign body aspiration and anaphylaxis should be ruled out.
         (2) The **physical examination** should assess the adequacy of air exchange.
            (a) Altered mental status is a sign of marked impairment of gas exchange.
            (b) **Vital signs** should be measured often. *Tachypnea* and *tachycardia* are common. An abrupt *decline* in respiratory rate may indicate impending respiratory failure.
            (c) Measure and follow *pulsus paradoxicus.*
            (d) Assess the quality of breath sounds, degree of dyspnea, and retractions. Pallor and cyanosis may be observed in severe cases.
            (e) Assess hydration.
            (f) Palpate for the presence of subcutaneous emphysema in the neck and upper chest.
         (3) **Laboratory tests and ancillary studies** should be done concomitant with starting therapy.
            (a) Measurement of ABGs is particularly helpful in evaluating response to therapy in patients with severe symptoms. Pulse oximetry confirms suspected desaturation.
            (b) Spirometry, particularly peak expiratory flow rate (PEFR) and 1-second forced expiratory volume (FEV_1), provides good indications of the state of respiratory function in children.
            (c) Chest roentgenograms are useful only when the cause is in question (e.g., foreign body aspiration), when an associated pneumonia is considered likely, or when complications such as pneumothorax or pneumomediastinum are suspected.
            (d) Serum theophylline concentration in children taking theophylline should be followed.
      b. **Therapy**
         (1) **Oxygen. Asthmatic patients are hypoxic.** Give humidified oxygen by nasal cannula or face mask to deliver at least 30–40% oxygen.

(2) Subcutaneous medication
   (a) Epinephrine. Give 0.01 ml/kg (1 : 1,000 dilution) SQ, with a maximum of 0.3 ml/dose. If a beneficial effect is obtained, the injection can be repeated twice at 20-minute intervals. When complete clearing of the attack is achieved, give 0.005 ml/kg Sus-Phrine (epinephrine in 1 : 200 thioglycolate suspension) 20 minutes after the last dose for action of longer duration. If the patient is still suffering from significant bronchospasm after three doses of epinephrine or deteriorates after its administration, **do not give further doses. Excessive or inappropriate use of epinephrine can induce serious cardiac arrhythmias and cause increased restlessness and anxiety.**
   (b) Terbutaline. When adverse effects of epinephrine are prohibitive for further use in older children, terbutaline, 0.01 ml/kg of 0.1% (1 mg/ml) solution SQ, with a maximum dose of 0.30 mg, can be used.
(3) Inhalation therapy
   (a) Nebulized bronchodilators have surpassed subcutaneous agents as initial treatment of choice for reactive airway disease. Continuous or aggressive intermittent administration of beta-2 agonists often provides efficacy equal to or greater than parenteral therapy with fewer side effects.
   (b) Selective beta-2–specific bronchodilators such as *albuterol* and *terbutaline* are preferred over less selective agents such as *isoetharine* (Bronkosol), yet individual patients may occasionally respond more favorably to the latter. *Isoproterenol,* though potent, has a narrow therapeutic index as compared to more selective agents.
   (c) After initial assessment and administration of oxygen, begin nebulized albuterol, 0.1–0.25 mg/kg (up to 5 mg/dose) every 20 minutes × 3 or until measured peak flow normalizes.
   (d) Alternatively, nebulized terbutaline (intravenous preparation in nebulizer), 0.3 mg/kg up to 5 mg/dose, can be administered similarly.
   (e) Continuous or frequent administration of less beta-2–specific agents is not recommended until safety and efficacy have been established. In more limited use, isoetharine (Bronkosol) and isoproterenol (Isuprel, 1 : 200 preparation), 0.25–0.5 ml, can be diluted in 2 ml normal saline (NS) and delivered by an oxygen-driven nebulizer.
(4) Steroids
   (a) Administration of steroids is indicated when there is no response to initial nebulized treatment or when response to repeated treatments is incomplete.
   (b) Oral or parenteral equivalents of methylprednisolone, 1–2 mg/kg/dose, are begun and repeated every 6 hours.
(5) Hydration. The acutely ill asthmatic child will have increased fluid requirements.
   (a) Oral fluids are usually adequate in mild attacks.
   (b) In severe attacks, oral fluid may precipitate vomiting, and a stable IV line should be placed. Generally, an infusion of 5% dextrose in water (D/W) in NS with 20–40 mEq/liter KCl at 1.5 times maintenance for the first 12 hours is adequate. Adjustments should be made depending on clinical status.
(6) Intravenous infusions of bronchodilation are indicated when the initial clinical presentation is one of severe distress, when oral medications are not tolerated, or when SQ or aerosol treatment has failed.
   (a) Aminophylline. Methylxanthines do not enhance the effects of

continuous or frequently repeated beta-2 agonists, yet may produce additive bronchodilation otherwise.

   (i) Before starting aminophylline it is important to document any recent oral theophylline administration. In some situations a theophylline level is helpful.

   (ii) Intravenous aminophylline can be given as a **bolus** or a **constant infusion**. In **bolus** therapy, 5–8 mg/kg is infused over 20 minutes and is repeated every 6 hours. Further dosage can be adjusted after measuring postinfusion peak serum levels 30–60 minutes after the bolus. A **constant infusion** can be started following a routine loading dose. The usual dosage range for an infusion is 0.9–1.2 mg/kg/hr.

   (iii) Serum levels can be measured any time during an infusion. All aminophylline doses should be tailored to achieve a serum theophylline level of 10–20 μg/ml. Generally, 1 mg/kg IV bolus will raise serum concentration 2 μg/ml.

   (iv) Theophylline **toxicity** includes severe headache, tachycardia, tremors, gastritis with frequent vomiting, and seizures (for management see Chap. 4). **Note: Rapid IV infusion of aminophylline can lead to cardiac arrhythmias, hypotension, and death. When aminophylline is administered in combination with beta agonists, constant cardiac monitoring is essential.**

   (b) In severe cases, **intravenous beta-2 agonists** are indicated. Such therapy is conducted in an intensive care unit setting with continuous cardiorespiratory and hemodynamic monitoring via arterial line.

   (i) Terbutaline is administered IV using bolus-infusion technique: 10 μg/kg over 10 minutes followed by 0.4 μg/kg/min. Dosage is increased incrementally 0.2 μg/kg/min as necessary (expect to use 3–6 μg/kg/min).

   (ii) **Because of potential dysrhythmias, intravenous aminophylline and terbutaline should not be given concurrently. Complications** of terbutaline therapy include tremulousness, tachycardia, and hypokalemia.

(7) **Aerosols**

   (i) **Isoetharine (Bronkosol)**, 0.25–0.5 ml diluted in 2 ml NS should be delivered by an oxygen-driven nebulizer. Treatments can be repeated in the same manner as SQ epinephrine.

   (ii) **Isoproterenol**, 0.25–0.5 ml of a 1 : 200 preparation with 2 ml NS via oxygen-driven nebulizer

   (iii) Metaproterenol, salbutamol, terbutaline, and other more selective beta-2–specific agents may play a role in the management of severe attacks. In some countries, they are considered first-line drugs in *severe, acute* asthma. **Note: Intermittent positive pressure breathing administration of aerosol medication has not been found to be more effective than passive systems and is more likely to cause paradoxical bronchospasm and pneumothorax.**

2. **Bronchiolitis** is a syndrome of acute, small airway obstruction in young infants.

   a. **Etiology.** It is usually viral in origin (commonly respiratory syncytial virus).

   b. **Evaluation** should include assessment of hydration and respiratory distress.

   c. The **diagnosis** is suggested by the onset of coryza, cough, and dyspnea and by prominent wheezing, hyperinflation of the lungs, and retractions. Fever may not be present.

d. Therapy

(1) Humidified **oxygen** (40% or more). In severe cases, oxygenation should be followed with transcutaneous PO_2 monitors, pulse oximeters, or ABGs.

(2) Adequate **hydration** is important. Whether fluids are administered PO or IV depends on the severity of the respiratory distress. Infants in severe respiratory distress often cannot adequately and safely hydrate themselves orally.

(3) In severe cases, assisted **ventilation** may be required.

(4) Antibiotics are not routinely given, but are indicated if associated otitis media or pneumonia is present.

(5) **Bronchodilators** given parenterally or by inhalation are sometimes effective.

(6) Antiviral therapy with aerosolized ribavirin (see Chap. 14, p. 430) is indicated for those with respiratory failure, immunosuppression, or severe coexisting disease.

3. Foreign body aspiration (see also sec. **III.A.2.c**) must always be considered in children who have an initial episode of wheezing or recurrent or unresponsive pneumonia. Note: A foreign body in the esophagus can cause significant respiratory symptoms.

a. Evaluation. Roentgenographic studies will identify radiopaque foreign bodies or suggest **bronchial foreign bodies by paradoxical movement of the diaphragms or ipsilateral obstructive emphysema with a mediastinal shift to the contralateral side.**

b. Therapy. Aspirated foreign bodies are true emergencies **only** when air exchange is significantly compromised or when the foreign body may imminently migrate into a more dangerous position. Emergent mechanical efforts to dislodge a foreign body should be attempted **only** when air exchange is inadequate to sustain life.

(1) **Bronchoscopy** is the definitive therapy.

(2) Antibiotics are useful when infection is present (see Chap. 14).

(3) Persistent atelectasis, pneumonitis, pneumonia, or emphysema should raise the question of a remaining fragment or second foreign body.

4. Pneumonia may present with significant respiratory distress secondary to impaired gas exchange.

a. General supportive measures include 30–40% oxygen by face mask, and intubation if respirations are inadequate.

b. Monitoring of ABGs and pulse oximetry is advised.

c. For specific therapy, see Chap. 14, p. 406.

5. Pneumothorax

a. Etiology. Spontaneous pneumothorax may be an idiopathic occurrence in a previously healthy person, or it may be a complication of underlying pulmonary disease.

b. Evaluation and diagnosis

(1) **History.** The onset of severe respiratory distress is usually acute.

(2) **Physical examination.** Decreased fremitus, decreased breath sounds, and hyperresonance are present on the affected side. Asymmetric chest movement and displaced point of maximal impulse may be noted. Percussion over the clavicles on opposite sides reveals minor differences in percussion tones. In patients with very abnormal lung compliance, such as severe cystic fibrosis, the physical findings may be minimal.

(3) **Chest roentgenogram.** Sometimes, an expired posteroanterior view will aid diagnosis when the pneumothorax is small.

(4) **Classification.** Generally, a small pneumothorax is well tolerated after an initial period of distress because of an adjustment of perfusion to ventilation. However, **under positive pressure ventilation or during air transport with reduced in-flight cabin pressure, a pneumothorax may rapidly enlarge and become life threatening.**

(a) **Minor to moderate.** Less than 30 percent collapse
(b) **Major.** 30–70 percent collapse
(c) If **complete collapse** occurs, the possibility of tension pneumothorax should be suspected.
c. **Treatment.** (For infants, see Chap. 6, p. 151ff.)
(1) **If the clinical condition is critical, immediate lifesaving maneuvers
become more important than diagnostic procedures.**
(2) If the leak is in the **visceral** pleura, **positive pressure breathing can
aggravate the situation.** If there is a leak in the **parietal** pleura (flail
chest), on the other hand, positive pressure may be lifesaving.
(3) **Simple observation** will suffice if the clinical condition is stable and
the radiologic diagnosis is "minor."
(4) **Cough suppression.** If necessary, dextromethorphan, codeine, or
morphine should be used to suppress coughing. **The use of respiratory
depressants is dangerous and necessitates frequent ABGs.**
(5) **Thoracentesis.** Needle aspiration of air inserted at the second anterior intercostal space is lifesaving whenever tension pneumothorax is
present. Under positive pressure ventilation, a sealed system is
unnecessary. Later, a closed thoracostomy drainage system will be in
order.
(6) **Thoracostomy.** Tube thoracostomy is indicated when the pneumothorax is likely to reaccumulate. The term *closed thoracostomy* is used
to designate a thoracostomy tube connected to a water-seal bottle.
With a water seal (which can be improvised by placing the end of the
tube under the surface of sterile NS contained in any container with
an air vent), air (and also fluid) drains from the chest. Air cannot
reenter the submerged tube tip **if the end of the tube and water seal
are below the level of the patient's chest.** It is customary to place the
"bottle" on the floor. If the system is functioning well, the fluid will be
lifted a few centimeters up the tube as the patient breathes and
produces negative (subatmospheric) inspiratory pressure. Later, when
the visceral and parietal pleura are adherent, this will not be seen.
6. **Exacerbations of chronic pulmonary disease**
a. **Bronchopulmonary dysplasia** (BPD) is a chronic pulmonary disorder
characterized by squamous metaplasia and hypertrophy of small airways
with subsequent alveolar collapse and air trapping.
(1) The **etiology** is related to the prolonged mechanical ventilation of
premature infants with high inflation pressures and oxygen tensions.
(2) **Evaluation and management** will depend on the severity.
(a) Multiple systems are secondarily affected, including the respiratory, cardiovascular, and immunologic systems, as well as growth
and development.
(b) **Radiographic chest abnormalities** are common. Areas of hyper-
aeration and atelectasis may be chronic, making the diagnosis of
new infiltrate difficult. Comparison with previous films is helpful.
(c) Respiratory reserve is minimal in this condition. Hospitalization
is often required.
(3) **Complications include** chronic **respiratory insufficiency,** requiring
home use of continuous oxygen therapy, **right-sided congestive heart
failure** secondary to pulmonary hypertension, and **pneumothorax.
Nonspecific findings,** including lethargy and poor feeding, may
indicate worsening respiratory status. **Reactive airways disease** is
similar to that in bronchiolitis. ABGs may show moderate hypoxia or
compensated hypercarbia. Acute deterioration of the respiratory
status is not uncommon. **Sudden infant death syndrome** is more
common in infants with BPD (see sec. **VI.C**).
(4) **Lower respiratory infections** caused by usually benign viral agents
may cause severe respiratory distress. The child should be isolated
from others with viral illnesses.

      (5) **Sepsis** requires management similar to that in a febrile neonate (see Chap. 6).

   b. Cystic fibrosis (see also Chap. 10)

      (1) **Reactive airways disease** similar to bronchiolitis may cause severe respiratory distress in infants. Respiratory support and bronchodilator therapy may be required.

      (2) **Subacute respiratory deterioration** with decreasing exercise tolerance and increasing respiratory distress is a common problem. Chest x-rays usually reveal increased infiltrative changes. Hospitalization for chest physiotherapy, O_2, and antibiotic therapy is usually required. *Pseudomonas aeruginosa* and *Staph. aureus* are frequently isolated from sputum cultures.

      (3) **Pneumothorax** is common and should always be considered when acute chest pain or respiratory deterioration occurs.

IV. Cardiac failure (see also Chap. 9, p. 245)

  A. Congestive heart failure

    1. High output failure is seen with severe anemia, hyperthyroid storm, and sepsis. Low output failure is caused by either **myocardial disease** (ischemia, infection, congenital heart disease, metabolic imbalances, arrhythmias) or **obstructive disease** (coarctation of the aorta, critical aortic stenosis, malignant hypertension).

    2. **Evaluation**

      a. Common symptoms

        (1) Poor weight gain

        (2) Difficulty in feeding, anorexia

        (3) Chronic unproductive cough unrelated to other upper respiratory symptoms

        (4) Increased perspiration

        (5) Fatigue and poor exercise tolerance

      b. Physical examination. Attention is given to the following:

        (1) Chronic malnutrition

        (2) Cardiovascular findings, including tachycardia, an S_4 gallop, "thready" pulses (indicating narrowed pulse pressure), poor perfusion, rales, and tender hepatomegaly. The quality of femoral pulses and presence of murmurs must be evaluated to diagnose anatomic heart disease.

        (3) Respiratory distress

        (4) Evidence of infection, hyperthyroidism, or severe anemia

      c. Laboratory studies

        (1) Chest x-ray

        (2) ECG and echocardiogram

        (3) ABGs, CBC, electrolytes, blood sugar, calcium, toxic screen, and thyroid function tests if indicated. Measurement of cardiac enzymes (CPK, SGOT, LDH) may be helpful.

    3. **Treatment**

      a. The patient is positioned upright in bed to facilitate breathing; infants are placed in a chalasia chair.

      b. Supplemental oxygen is given. Intubation and mechanical ventilation with positive end-expiratory pressure when indicated

      c. Patients with severe **anemia** should be carefully transfused.

      d. Arrhythmias should be treated (see Chap. 9, pp. 249).

      e. The patient should be made comfortable and light **sedation** (morphine, 0.05–0.10 mg/kg/dose) provided if necessary to decrease systemic demands. In extreme cases, paralysis may be required.

      f. Maintain **normothermia** to avoid the added demands of excessive tachycardia or shivering.

      g. Diuretics (see also Chap. 8, p. 221) such as furosemide (Lasix), 1 mg/kg/dose, should be given if the electrolytes are within normal limits.

Chronic therapy may include chlorothiazide, 10–20 mg/kg/bid and spironolactone, 1–4 mg/kg/day.
h. Positive **inotropic** agents (dopamine, dobutamine, amrinone, epinephrine, and digoxin) can be used to support the myocardium. **Doses** are as follows:
   (1) **Dopamine,** 5–20 μg/kg/min IV titrated to effect
   (2) **Dobutamine,** 5–20 μg/kg/min, alone or in addition to dopamine
   (3) **Amrinone** (see also Chap. 8) is a phosphodiesterase inhibitor providing afterload reduction and mild inotropic support that can be used as an additional agent in severe, refractory congestive failure. Load normovolemic patients cautiously with 0.5 mg/kg followed by 5–10 μg/kg/min.
   (4) **Epinephrine,** 0.1–1.0 μg/kg/min, may be useful in patients whose condition is refractory to other agents, but will produce unwanted tachycardia and increased afterload.
   (5) **Digoxin.** A total digitalizing dose is given over the first 24 hours as follows: 40 μg/kg (use two thirds of this dose if given parenterally). Give one half of this dose immediately; one fourth at 8 hours, and one fourth at 16 hours. The maintenance dose is one fourth of the total digitalizing dose, divided bid. The total digitalizing dose for adults is 1 mg IV, and the adult maintenance dose is 0.125–0.250 mg/kg in divided doses bid.

B. **Pericardial tamponade**
   1. **Definition:** an accumulation of fluid in the pericardial space, producing cardiac compression and inadequate disastolic filling and leading to a small, fixed stroke volume and low output heart failure
   2. **Etiology**
      a. **Primary pericardial disease,** including viral, bacterial, and rheumatic pericarditis
      b. **Systemic disease** that can cause secondary pericardial tamponade, including congestive heart failure (CHF), uremia, tumor, or collagen vascular disease
   3. **Evaluation**
      a. **Vital signs** demonstrate tachycardia, tachypnea, and hypotension.
      b. **Physical examination**
         (1) Evidence of low output cardiac failure includes thready pulses, cool extremities, mottled gray skin, and oliguria.
         (2) **Cardiac examination** reveals muffled heart sounds, pericardial friction rub, jugular venous distention, and passive hepatic congestion.
      c. **Diagnostic studies**
         (1) The **chest x-ray** shows a bulbous cardiac silhouette.
         (2) The **ECG** shows S-T segment elevation, low voltage, and T-wave inversion.
         (3) An **echocardiogram** shows the effusion.
   4. **Therapy. Emergency decompression** by pericardiocentesis or surgery (pericardial window or pericardial stripping), or both, is lifesaving. **Cardiovascular status is fragile, and sedation or positive pressure ventilation may precipitate collapse. Pericardiocentesis should be performed by the most experienced person available.**
      a. The patient's ECG should be continuously monitored.
      b. **Equipment.** A 10-ml syringe and a 1-in. 20-gauge needle are adequate for an infant or toddler, whereas a 30-ml syringe and 3-in. spinal needle (20-gauge) should be used in an adult.
      c. Prepare the subxiphoid area with a povidone-iodine (Betadine) and alcohol wash.
      d. Using sterile technique, insert the needle in the subxiphoid area at a 30-degree angle, aiming for the left-mid scapula. Slight negative pressure should be maintained on the syringe. When the pericardium is entered, fluid will appear in the hub of the syringe; this fluid can be distinguished from intracardiac blood by its lower hematocrit and absent clotting.

    e. ECG monitoring shows ST changes with myocardial injury.
    f. Complications include pneumothorax, arrhythmias, coronary laceration, and myocardial puncture.
C. Tetralogy of Fallot spells
  1. Etiology. Caused by an acute increase in right ventricular outflow resistance, leading to an increase in the intracardiac right-to-left shunt. Such spells can last minutes to hours, resolving spontaneously or leading to progressive hypoxia, acidosis, and death.
  2. Evaluation
    a. Acute cyanosis, restlessness, and agitation may be present.
    b. Physical examination
      (1) A regular rhythm with good pulses is usually present.
      (2) The murmur of a **ventricular septal defect** will be heard frequently; the murmur of **pulmonary stenosis** may decrease an acute spell.
      (3) Rales and wheezes are absent.
  3. Treatment is aimed toward rapidly raising oxygen saturation and decreasing shunt fraction before hypoxia and acidosis occur.
    a. Oxygen is administered.
    b. The child is comforted and quieted.
    c. The child is positioned or held in the knee-to-chest position to increase the systemic resistance.
    d. Morphine sulfate (0.1mg/kg IM or IV) is given for sedation and subpulmonic relaxation.
    e. Volume is administered as a 10 ml/kg bolus of NS.
    f. Systemic resistance may be increased further by administration of phenylephrine (Neosynephrine), 5 μg/kg, or epinephrine, 5–10 μg/kg IV.
    g. Metabolic acidosis should be corrected.
  4. The best treatment of tetralogy of Fallot spells is *prevention*.
    a. Treat all hypovolemic states *early* with volume expansion.
    b. During procedures on a child with tetralogy of Fallot, employ adequate sedation and analgesia, and have a parent available to comfort the child.
V. Central nervous system (CNS) emergencies
A. Seizures. Minimizing the morbidity and mortality of seizures depends primarily on attention to the "ABCs" of resuscitation, with anticonvulsant therapy as a secondary concern.
  1. Etiology (see Chap. 19, p. 529)
  2. Evaluation and diagnosis
    a. The history should identify any underlying disease process. Careful attention should be paid to:
      (1) The quality and length of the seizure
      (2) The presence of fever or other symptoms (headache, stiff neck, poor feeding, irritability)
      (3) History of recent trauma
      (4) Past and family history of seizure or other chronic conditions
      (5) Prescribed medications and compliance
      (6) Possibility of ingestion
    b. Physical examination should assess the extent of impairment of cardiorespiratory status and illuminate a direct cause for the seizure activity. Include the following:
      (1) Vital signs
      (2) Air movement and chest wall excursion
      (3) Skin color (perfusion, cyanosis, hypopigmented areas)
      (4) Evidence of trauma (bruises, laceration, swelling)
      (5) Evidence of sepsis (purpura, petechiae)
      (6) Pupil size and reaction
      (7) Disk margins and retinal field (papilledema, hemorrhage)
      (8) Quality of the fontanel and transillumination of the skull in children under 18 months of age
      (9) Muscle tone, reflexes

(10) Observation of seizure activity

c. Laboratory tests

(1) Blood for immediate bedside glucose determination (Dextrostix), CBC, electrolytes, BUN, glucose, calcium, magnesium, toxic screen (including lead), pH and TCO_2, anticonvulsant levels when appropriate, and ABGs when indicated

(2) Urine for urinalysis, and an immediate pregnancy test when appropriate

(3) Lumbar puncture for cerebrospinal fluid (CSF) examination when signs of CNS infection are present and increased intracranial pressure (ICP) and mass effect have been ruled out. (See sec. **B.2**; see also Chap. 19, p. 530ff).

(4) Roentgenographic studies

(a) Skull films are indicated only with evidence of trauma or when metabolic disease associated with bony abnormalities is suspected.

(b) A **computed tomographic (CT) scan** is indicated when head trauma, increased ICP, or a mass lesion is suspected.

3. Therapy is based on ensuring adequate **ventilation and oxygenation** and terminating seizure activity.

a. Airway management is of paramount importance. Respiratory failure may occur secondary to loss of a patent airway or as a side effect of anticonvulsant therapy.

(1) Establish a patent airway via a chin lift or jaw thrust; protect the C-spine if trauma is suspected or known.

(2) Administer 100% oxygen.

(3) Place an oral airway if obstruction due to the tongue and soft tissues is present.

(4) Suction as necessary.

(5) If air movement is inadequate despite the preceding steps, artificial ventilation by bag and mask with 100% O_2 is indicated until spontaneous respirations improve. Intubation may be required when bag-and-mask ventilation is insufficient or when long-term ventilation seems probable.

b. Intravenous access should be established.

(1) Hypoglycemia is treated with intravenous dextrose, 0.25–0.50 gm/kg, using 25% dextrose in water.

(2) The intravenous line can be kept open with normal saline or any standard IV solution.

(3) When increased ICP is suspected, fluid administration should be minimized, assuming adequate blood pressure.

c. Anticonvulsant therapy

(1) Benzodiazepines

(a) Lorazepam (Ativan): rapid-acting anticonvulsant with longer half-life and less respiratory depressant effect than diazepam

(i) The initial **dose** is 0.05–0.10 mg/kg with a maximum dose of 4 mg; given over 1–4 minutes. A second dose of 0.10 mg/kg can be given if there is no response to the initial dose.

(ii) Respiratory depression is a possible side effect of benzodiazepines and sometimes, in part, due to rapid administration; airway equipment and skilled personnel should be present before administration.

(b) Diazepam (Valium): rapid-acting anticonvulsant with a short half-life and greater respiratory depressant effect than lorezapam

(i) The initial **dose** is 0.1–0.2 mg/kg, with a maximum dose of 10 mg; given over 1–4 minutes. A second dose of 0.25–0.4 mg/kg with a maximum dose of 15 mg can be given if there is no response to the initial dose.

(2) Phenytoin is effective, and its relatively long duration of action makes it a useful adjunct to a benzodiazepine administration. However, the onset of action is usually in 10–30 minutes. Therefore, it should not be used as a primary drug if immediate cessation of the seizure is paramount.

(a) Phenytoin should be infused as soon as a benzodiazepine has been given. The dosage is 15–20 mg/kg IV in NS over 20 minutes (not faster than 1 mg/kg/min).

(b) Cardiac arrhythmias and hypotension are the most important complications. Take care that infusion is not too rapid. Cardiac monitoring is essential.

(c) Phenytoin must be given directly into the IV tubing without dilution, as this may cause precipitation of the drug.

(3) Paraldehyde can be used as an adjunct to diazepam and phenytoin if further therapy is required. In addition, because paraldehyde is administered rectally, it can be used when an IV line cannot be started. The dosage is 0.3–0.4 ml/kg (maximum 8 ml) mixed in peanut or corn oil at a 10 : 1 (oil-paraldehyde) ratio and administered PR via rectal tube.

(4) Phenobarbital can be used when the preceding therapy has not terminated seizure activity.

(a) The dose is 10 mg/kg IV given slowly over 10–15 minutes. If no effect is evident after 20–30 minutes, this dose can be repeated twice.

(b) The combined respiratory depressant effect of phenobarbital and a benzodiazepine is greater than either drug alone, and care must be taken when giving these medicines in conjunction with one another.

d. With prolonged or refractory seizures, **underlying conditions must be ruled out.** The possibility of trauma, intracranial infection, increased ICP, bleeding vascular anomalies, or ingestion of toxic substances or medication should always be reconsidered.

4. Specific disorders

a. Febrile seizures are the most common form of childhood convulsive disorder. *Simple febrile seizures* are brief (less than 15 minutes duration), generalized, almost always occur in the first 24 hours of the febrile illness, and are seen in children between the ages of 6 months and 5 years without CNS infection or metabolic disorders. *Complex febrile seizures* are greater than 15 minutes in duration, and may be focal or occur in children with known epilepsy.

(1) Evaluation and diagnosis

(a) The **history** should elicit details as above and should include history of trauma, current illnesses, and family history of seizures.

(b) The **physical examination** should be directed to uncovering the cause of the fever, ruling out a CNS infection or residual neurologic signs, or both.

(c) Laboratory investigations should be determined by the child's age, history, and physical findings. In children under 24 months of age, meningeal signs are unreliable in detecting meningeal irritation. Febrile seizures that last **more than 15 minutes are focal** in nature or are associated with transient or permanent **neurologic abnormalities,** have a higher probability of being associated with an underlying infection or metabolic or traumatic disorder. These "complex" febrile seizures therefore require more aggressive diagnostic testing.

(2) Therapy

(a) For an ongoing seizure, anticonvulsant therapy is that for seizures as discussed previously (see sec **A.3**). "Make haste slowly" in stopping a febrile seizure. Note the time that anticonvulsant therapy is given to evaluate the length of seizures.

(b) Administer antipyretics and tepid sponge.
(c) Prophylaxis (see Chap. 19, p. 531)
b. Hypoglycemia (see also Chap. 11). **Hypoglycemic seizures are a medical emergency.**
   (1) Provide general supportive measures as outlined in **3.**
   (2) Look for Medic-Alert bracelet or other evidence of insulin use.
   (3) After withdrawing an aliquot of blood for glucose and other determinations, give intravenous dextrose, 0.25–0.50 gm/kg as 25% dextrose in water.
   (4) Begin an IV infusion of 4–6 mg/kg/min glucose.
   (5) Investigate the cause of the hypoglycemia.
c. Hypertension
   (1) Provide the general supportive measures outlined previously.
   (2) Rapid therapy for hypertension is required (see Chap. 8, p. 220ff).
   (3) Ongoing seizures can be treated acutely as outlined in **3** for general seizure disorders. Investigate the cause of the hypertension.
d. Meningitis or encephalitis
   (1) Provide the general supportive measures outlined previously.
   (2) Anticonvulsant therapy is that outlined for a general seizure disorder (see **3.c.**).
   (3) Rapid institution of antibiotic therapy is critical.
   (4) Treat evidence of shock with intravenous isotonic fluids (normal saline or lactated Ringer's solution), 10–20 ml/kg. To minimize any possible associated cerebral edema, fluid administration should then be carefully monitored and kept at the minimum rate required to maintain cardiovascular stability (usually at 75% of maintenance) (see Chap. 7, p. 201).

B. Increased ICP
  1. The **etiology** includes:
   a. Cerebral edema due to hypoxia and ischemia, Reye syndrome, or toxins (e.g., lead)
   b. Increased CSF volume due to hydrocephalus or an obstructed ventricular shunt
   c. Increased intracranial blood volume due to infection (meningitis and encephalitis), trauma (intraparenchymal bleeding, subdural hematoma), or arteriovenous malformations
   d. Space-occupying lesions due to tumor or abscess
  2. Evaluation
   a. A complete **history** should include any evidence of infection, trauma, hypoxic events, previous seizures, CNS insults, and medications. Neurologic symptoms should be carefully documented, with detailed accounts of the duration and progression.
   b. Physical examination
    (1) Vital signs should be taken and recorded frequently. The Cushing reflex (bradycardia, hypertension, slow and irregular respirations) is uncommon in children.
    (2) The **physical examination** should attempt to be directed toward finding the causes of the increased ICP, e.g., evidence of trauma, infection, hepatic disease, cyanotic heart disease, or systemic hemangiomas.
    (3) Neurologic examination. See Table 3-4 (Glascow Coma Scale). Complete and serial neurologic examinations are essential. Include pupillary and fundoscopic examinations. Look for focal neurologic deficits and listen for intracranial bruits. In the infant and toddler, measure the head circumference, feel for split sutures, and transilluminate the head.
   c. Laboratory studies include:
    (1) A CT scan, once the patient's condition has stabilized
    (2) Skull x-rays are helpful for eliciting splitting of the sutures, calcification, or bone erosion secondary to prolonged increased pressure.

Table 3-4. Glasgow Coma Scale[a]

Response	Score
Eyes	
Open	
Spontaneously	4
To verbal command	3
To pain	2
No response	1
Best motor response	
To verbal command	
Obeys	6
To painful stimulus[b]	
Localizes pain	5
Flexion withdrawal	4
Flexion abnormal (decorticate rigidity)	3
Extension (decerebrate rigidity)	2
No response	1
Best verbal response[c]	
Oriented and converses	5
Disoriented and converses	4
Inappropriate words	3
Incomprehensible sounds	2
No response	1
Total	3–15

[a] The Glasgow Coma Scale, based on eye opening and verbal and motor responses, is a practical means of monitoring changes in the level of consciousness. If the response on the scale is given a number, the responsiveness of the patient can be expressed by summation of the figures. The **lowest** score is 3; the **highest** is 15.
[b] Apply knuckles to sternum; observe arms.
[c] Arouse patient with painful stimulus if necessary.

   (3) A **lumbar puncture** is done **after** the CT scan (to rule out a mass lesion) for pressure measurement, and to aid in the diagnosis of infection or hemorrhage. **A lumbar puncture carries a risk of central herniation in the patient with increased ICP.** At times, however, examination of the CSF is essential, and the benefits outweigh the risks of the procedure. In these situations, great care should be taken to have:
   (a) Another person available to monitor the patient
   (b) The smallest spinal needle
   (c) An IV line in place
   (d) Mannitol at the bedside
 3. Therapy. The goal of therapy is to decrease the ICP by decreasing one or more of the component volumes.
   a. All correctable lesions are treated.
   b. The initial therapy includes:
   (1) Position. To avoid venous obstruction the patient's head should be kept midline, with the head of the bed at a 30-degree upward slant.
   (2) Oxygen and airway. The PaO_2 should be maintained above 100 mm Hg by whatever means required.
   (3) Hypocapnia. Endotracheal intubation and hyperventilation to a $PaCO_2$ 25 to 30 mm Hg will cause vasoconstriction and hence a decrease in the intracranial blood volume. Some patients will hyperventilate spontaneously and do not require mechanical ventilation.

(4) Osmotherapy. Attempt to achieve an osmolarity of 300–320 mOsm/ liter, as follows:

    (a) Calculate osmolarity if direct laboratory measurement is not available (mOsm = $[2 \times Na^+] + BUN/2.8 +$ blood glucose/18). The calculated value will be falsely low if other osmotic agents are present in the blood (i.e., mannitol, glycerol) (see also Chap. 7, p. 195).

    (b) Limit the amount of fluid intake (PO and IV).

    (c) Give **mannitol**, 0.25–0.50 gm/kg, as a bolus q2–4h.

    (d) Give **furosemide** (Lasix), 1 mg/kg q6–8h.

    (e) During osmotherapy, an accurate record should be kept of intake and output; urine output should not fall below 0.25–0.5 ml/kg/hr.

(5) Seizure control is important to avoid a sudden, massive increase in cerebral metabolism.

(6) Normothermia must be maintained to avoid increased blood flow and volume.

(7) Corticosteroids are effective in reducing the edema that surrounds brain tumors, but their benefit in intracranial hypertension from other causes has not been demonstrated. Dexamethasone (Decadron), 1 mg/kg/day in three divided doses, has been used. **Corticosteroids are contraindicated in the treatment of Reye syndrome because of their catabolic effects.**

  c. Maximum increased therapy. If the preceding maneuvers fail to control the increased ICP, more invasive monitoring in the form of a central venous pressure (CVP) line and an ICP monitoring device is required. The following therapeutic maneuvers can then be tried.

    (1) Muscle relaxation. Muscle relaxants (pancuronium [Pavulon], 0.1 mg/kg q1–2h) will prevent intracranial hypertension associated with movement and muscle strain.

    (2) Sedation. Sedation is helpful in controlling ICP spikes due to agitation or noxious stimuli. Sedation can be achieved with narcotic and benzodiazepine combinations; tolerance can occur, especially with short-acting agents (see also Chap. 1, p. 3).

      (a) Short-acting agents: fentanyl (2–5 µg/kg/hr) infusion and midazolam (0.05–0.3 mg/kg/hr) infusion, or intermittent doses of these agents

      (b) Longer-acting agents: morphine (0.1 mg/kg/hr) infusion with lorazepam (0.05–0.10 mg/kg q2–6h)

    (3) The duration of maximum increased ICP therapy can extend to weeks. The process of weaning the patient from therapy is started when the ICP is consistently in a normal range. The patient is first weaned from sedation and then from pancuronium and mechanical hyperventilation; osmotherapy is the last to be discontinued. The pace of weaning is dictated by the ICP response.

C. Spinal cord lesions. The patient usually presents with neurologic dysfunction below the level of the lesion. The most common lesions are discussed here.

  1. Trauma, usually as the result of hyperextension, hyperflexion, or vertical crush injuries. The fractures or dislocations most commonly occur at the level of T12–L1, C5–C6, and C1–C2.

    a. Evaluation. Patients may experience a *total loss* of function distal to the lesion (as in cord transections), or **temporary and completely reversible** loss (as seen in localized edema).

      (1) The **history** of the injury should be documented, with meticulous details of the progression and degree of neurologic loss.

      (2) The **physical examination** should include:

        (a) The adequacy of ventilation and cardiovascular status

        (b) Examination for associated injuries

        (c) The **neurologic examination** will usually demonstrate:

(i) Loss of **motor and sensory function** below the level of the lesion

(ii) **Areflexia** for 2–6 weeks, often with a return to some reflex activity at a later date

(iii) Total **flaccidity** is initially present; **spasticity** follows weeks after the insult.

(iv) Urinary retention can also be a feature.

(3) **Laboratory studies** include:
  (a) Radiographs of the spine
  (b) CT scan of the affected region
  (c) A myelogram may be indicated.

  b. **Treatment**
    (1) Locate the lesion and attempt to minimize any further damage.
    (2) The neck should be immobilized in a neutral position.
    (3) **Respiratory function** must be supported as required. Patients with a lesion at C1–C2 will require mechanical assistance.
    (4) The **cardiovascular system** must be supported as required; hypovolemia can result from associated autonomic dysfunction.
    (5) A Foley catheter is placed to avoid bladder distention.
    (6) Traction or surgical decompression, or both, is usually attempted in an effort to minimize any further damage.

2. **Epidural abscess.**
  a. **Etiology.** Usually *Staph. aureus*. The anatomy of the dura localizes the infection to the dorsal compartment.
  b. **Evaluation** may reveal exquisite back pain and a preference for the back to be held rigid. There may be distal muscle weakness and radicular pain. The **laboratory examination** includes:
    (1) Plain radiographs
    (2) A CT scan
    (3) Sedimentation rate, CBC, and blood cultures
    (4) If a lumber puncture is performed, it will reveal a pleocytosis and increased CSF protein.
  c. **Therapy** includes:
    (1) Surgical drainage
    (2) Antibiotics (see Chap. 14)

3. **Transverse myelitis.** Transverse myelitis is a destructive process at any level of the spinal cord and presents either acutely or insidiously. Both sensory and motor function losses can occur.
  a. **Etiology:** likely autoimmune process following a viral illness, such as measles, mumps, upper respiratory illness, gastroenteritis
  b. The **evaluation** of this lesion is the same as outline in **1.b.** All other spinal cord lesions must be ruled out.
  c. The **therapy** is controversial, with very equivocal results.
    (1) Supportive therapy is the mainstay, determined by the level of the lesion.
    (2) A *trial* of a corticosteroid (dexamethasone, 1–2 mg/kg, maximum 100 mg, followed by 0.5 mg/kg q6 h), should be given until cord compression secondary to tumor is ruled out.
    (3) Plasmapheresis is currently under consideration as a possible therapeutic maneuver.

D. **Hydrocephalus** is an increase in the CSF component of the intracranial volume, caused by a blockage in normal CSF flow and resorption (rarely, overproduction of CSF can also cause hydrocephalus).
  1. The **etiology** includes:
    a. **Hemorrhage.** Intraventricular, traumatic, and secondary to arteriovenous malformation
    b. **Tumor.** Particularly a posterior fossa tumor that directly blocks the third and fourth ventricle
    c. **Infection,** including:

(1) Congenital TORCH infections (toxoplasmosis, rubella, cytomegalic inclusion virus, herpes)

(2) Ventriculitis

(3) Tuberculous meningitis

    d. **Anatomic abnormality**

2. **Evaluation.** Signs and symptoms of ICP vary with the age of the patient.

    a. **History**

        (1) **Children under 2 years of age** usually demonstrate the following lethargy with poor sucking and poor feeding, apnea, spasticity, high-pitched cry, and/or vomiting.

        (2) **Children over age 2** usually present with headache that is worse in the early-morning hours, vomiting, and/or lethargy.

    b. **Physical findings**

        (1) **Children under a few years of age**

            (a) Increased head circumference, with split sutures, dilated scalp veins, and bulging fontanel

            (b) Lower-extremity spasticity with opisthotonos

            (c) Optic atrophy

            (d) Pseudobulbar palsy

        (2) **Children over a few years of age**

            (a) Lower-extremity spasticity

            (b) Papilledema

            (c) Gait disturbance

    c. **Laboratory examination**

        (a) **Plain skull radiographs** may demonstrate split sutures, intracranial calcifications, and bony erosions.

        (b) A **CT scan** is the best diagnostic tool. With it, ventricular size can be directly evaluated.

        (c) **Ultrasound** of the head can be used in children under the age of 1 year.

3. **The therapy** must be tailored to each clinical situation, but usually will include:

    a. **Decompression** of the spinal fluid compartment either by an external or an internalized shunt

    b. **Systemic corticosteroids** are used to decrease tumor-related edema (dexamethasone, 1 mg/kg/day in three divided doses).

E. **Complications of intraventricular shunts.** Ventriculoperitoneal (VP) or ventriculoatrial (VA) shunts are placed for decompression of the ventricles. The most common medical emergencies associated with these shunts are:

1. **Mechanical obstruction,** which presents with the symptoms and signs of ICP (see **B**). When obstruction occurs, neurosurgical consultation should be sought to determine the need for immediate percutaneous tapping of the shunt versus operative revision.

2. **Infection.** The shunt is a foreign body and serves as a nidus for infection. **Treatment** includes antibiotics and very often surgical removal of the shunt. If the shunt must be removed, emergency and perhaps temporary ventricular decompression can be effected by an indwelling ventricular catheter externalized through a burr hole.

VI. **Special problems in the emergency department**

A. **Evaluation of the febrile infant in the first 90 days of life** (see also Chap. 6). Elevated temperature ($\geq 38.0°C$) in the infant most commonly indicates infection, whether viral or bacterial in origin. This may signify sepsis (nonlocalized, widespread infection) in a host with an immature immune system. Overwhelming viral infection can be as devastating as bacterial infection in this age group.

1. **Etiology.** Viral causes are present in up to 95 percent of cases. Group B streptococci, *Escherichia coli,* and *Listeria monocytogenes* (infrequently *Staph. aureus*) are the bacterial pathogens responsible for neonatal sepsis.

2. The **history** should include a maternal history for pregnancy, labor or delivery complications, evidence of genitourinary infections, and the pres-

ence of maternal fever. **Review of systems** should include birth and subsequent weights, and signs of infection: lethargy, irritability, poor feeding, pallor. Onset and height of fever should be documented.

3. **Physical examination**
   a. **General appearance.** Note evidence of irritability, lethargy, or decreased response to the environment.
   b. **Vital signs.** Document *rectal* temperature. Tachycardia may be due to fever, hypovolemia, or shock. Tachypnea may be caused by fever, pneumonia, or a compensation for acidemia. Hypotension is a late sign of shock.

4. **Laboratory data**
   a. **Culture specimens.** Cultures are obtained from **blood, urine** by suprapubic aspiration or catheterization, and **CSF** by lumbar puncture.
   b. **Hematologic.** CSF cell count may reveal pleocytosis. **CBC** may or may not show leukocytosis, and in early neonates may reveal neutropenia (ANC < 500 mm^3). **Urinalysis** may reveal evidence of infection.
   c. **Chemistry.** CSF protein and glucose and **blood glucose** should be measured.
   d. **Radiography.** Chest x-ray.
   e. **Latex agglutination** assays are available for CSF, urine, and blood for some bacteria (e.g., group B *Streptococcus*).

5. **Therapy** (see also Chaps. 6 and 14)
   a. **Infants 28 days of age and younger.** These infants are hospitalized and treated with intravenous ampicillin (200–400 mg/kg/day) and gentamicin (2.5 mg/kg q8–12h).
   b. **Infants 29–90 days of age**
      (1) Any infant in this age group who is ill-appearing must be hospitalized and treated as above.
      (2) Well-appearing infants in this age group without an identified focus of infection on physical or laboratory examination can be treated as outpatients if good follow-up can be ensured. Ceftriaxone, 50 mg/kg IM, is given after evaluation and then again in 20–28 hours on reexamination.

B. **Evaluation of the febrile child 3–36 months of age.** Fever greater than 39.0°C in this age group without obvious source on physical examination indicates a 3–5 percent risk of bacteremia. *Occult* bacteremia must be investigated so as to minimize the possibility of the sequelae of bacteremia, that is, meningitis, periorbital cellulitis, pneumonia, infectious arthritis, and osteomyelitis.

1. **Etiology.** Viral causes of fever are present in 95–97 percent of cases. The encapsulated organisms, *Strep. pneumoniae, H. influenzae, Neisseria meningitidis,* and *Salmonella* species, are not always well handled by the immune system of the child in this age group, and are responsible for nearly all cases of bacteremia.

2. **History.** Should include a review of all systems that are susceptible to invasion by blood-borne bacteria, as well as nonspecific findings, such as irritability or lethargy, poor feeding, pallor, etc.

3. **Physical examination**
   a. **General appearance.** Children with bacteremia may be well-appearing and active. Fever may be the only sign. Note history of irritability, lethargy, or diminished response to stimuli.
   b. **Vital signs** (see A.3.b)
   c. A careful examination should include noting the presence or absence of meningismus, cough, rales or wheezing, peripheral perfusion and hydration state, abdominal pain, and evidence of bone or joint infections.

4. **Laboratory data**
   a. **Culture specimens.** Blood and urine cultures should be sent. Lumbar puncture should be performed based on clinical impression. **Meningismus is not always present, especially in children less than 18–24 months of age.**

   b. **Hematologic.** CSF cell count, peripheral blood smear, and urinalysis may
      show evidence of infection.
   c. **Chemistry.** CSF protein and glucose should be measured.
   d. **Radiologic.** Chest radiography should be performed if a febrile child in
      this age group is tachypneic, and has cough, rales, and wheezing or other
      respiratory symptoms.
5. **Therapy.** Empiric treatment for bacteremia while awaiting culture results is
   controversial. It has not been proved yet whether early treatment prevents
   the sequelae of bacteremia. Therefore, options exist as to therapy for the
   febrile child without an obvious source of infection. Empiric treatment can be
   amoxicillin, 25 to 40 mg/kg/day, or ceftriaxone, one dose, 50 mg/kg IM,
   pending culture results.
C. **Sudden infant death syndrome (SIDS)** is the leading cause of death in infants
   between 1 week and 1 year of age, with a peak incidence from 2–4 months. In
   the United States the incidence is 2–3 per 1,000 live births.
   1. **Clinical findings.** SIDS is most commonly a quiet death that occurs during
      sleep. The victims are usually previously healthy children.
   2. **Epidemiology**
      a. A higher incidence of SIDS is seen in the winter months, even in cities
         where there is little temperature variation.
      b. Lower socioeconomic groups have a slightly higher incidence.
      c. The incidence is higher in boys and in low-birth-weight infants. Approx-
         imately 20 percent of the infants in two studies had a birth weight below
         2.5 kg.
      d. Incidence is slightly higher in siblings, but there is no predictable genetic
         pattern. Twins are more susceptible than nontwins (3.87/1,000 live
         births), and triplets are probably at greater risk (8.33/1,000).
      e. The least susceptible populations are Orientals (0.51/1,000), followed by
         whites (1.32), Mexican-Americans (1.74), and blacks (2.92). Most vulner-
         able are American Indians (5.93).
   3. **Mechanism.** The mechanism for SIDS is unknown. At present there is a shift
      of attention from the immediate events of death toward a search for chronic
      abnormalities. If high-risk profiles can be developed, some deaths may be
      preventable.
   4. The emergency room treatment of SIDS should include:
      a. A detailed history and physical examination to rule out other causes of
         death
      b. Support of the parents and surviving siblings
      c. Report of the death to the medical examiner
   5. **Apparent life-threatening event (ALTE, previously termed "near-miss
      SIDS").** An ALTE refers to any unexplained, sudden near death of a young
      child. Careful history and physical examination should seek an etiology,
      including hypothermia, sepsis, overwhelming pneumonitis, aspiration,
      trauma or abuse, seizure, adrenal crisis, or toxic ingestion.
      a. A history to elicit any of the above etiologies is imperative. Also, any
         description of the surrounding events or observed episode is important.
         Underlying or chronic illnesses and medications should be discussed.
      b. The **physical examination** should ensure that the infant is in no imminent
         danger and should carefully identify the underlying disorders. Measure-
         ment of vital signs and a respiratory and neurologic examination are
         mandatory.
      c. **Laboratory tests** should include a CBC with differential, electrolytes,
         calcium, BUN, creatinine, blood glucose (and Dextrostix), and urinalysis.
         Evidence of infection or a metabolic abnormality should be reviewed.
         Other tests should reflect specific concerns raised by the history or
         physical findings: an electroencephalogram, lumbar puncture, and radio-
         logic studies to evaluate swallowing and gastroesophageal reflux (see
         Chap. 10, p. 289).
      d. **General management** includes a period of inhospital observation and

monitoring. If sepsis is suspected, antibiotics should be started pending negative cultures (see Chap. 14, p. 368). After initial management is decided, further evaluation, including pneumography, parental education and support, and arrangements for home monitoring when appropriate, should be coordinated with a medical center that has an active program for infants who have an ALTE.

D. Child abuse and neglect

1. Objectives and problems

a. Recognition or suspicion of child abuse should be met by a long-range therapeutic plan, with attention to the establishment of supportive relationships. The goal of the initial process of management is protection of the child while the parents are helped through an acute family crisis.

b. Problems include:

(1) Parental personalities in which denial and projection serve as the principal modes of ego defense

(2) The family's anxious confusion in facing an array of clinical specialty services and social agencies, often working in an uncoordinated manner to protect the child

(3) The exigencies of poverty, including mistrust of community institutions, racism, unemployment, and drugs

(4) The clinical team may be frustrated by missed appointments, angry parental confrontations, time-consuming contacts with outside agencies, and conflicts among the responsible personnel stemming from the emotions brought forth by prolonged contact with disturbed families.

2. Diagnosis

a. Clinical findings. The physical manifestations of child abuse may be present in any body system. A *thorough* physical examination is imperative. Suspect child abuse or neglect whenever a child presents with **any one or a combination** of the following clinical findings:

(1) Fractures that a simple fall would be unlikely to produce
  (a) Different stages of healing in multiple fractures
  (b) Metaphyseal fractures
  (c) Epiphyseal separations
  (d) Subperiosteal calcifications

(2) Subdural hematomas

(3) Multiple ecchymoses that may resemble purpura

(4) Intestinal injuries, ruptured viscera

(5) Burns of any kind, especially in infants

(6) Poor hygiene

(7) Inadequate gain in weight or height

(8) Marked passivity and watchfulness; fearful expression

(9) Bizarre accidents, multiple ingestions

(10) Malnutrition

(11) Developmental retardation

b. Some frequent behavior patterns of abusive or negligent parents. They may:

(1) Use severe punishments

(2) Give a past history of abuse in their own upbringing

(3) Display suspicion and antagonism toward others

(4) Lead isolated lives

(5) Make pleas for help in indirect ways, such as
  (a) Bringing the child to the clinician or emergency room for no specific reason or for repeated minor medical complaints
  (b) Insisting that the child be admitted to the hospital for a minor illness and expressing anxiety if he or she is not

(6) Lean on their children for support, comfort, and reassurance

(7) Sample a variety of health care facilities without establishing a relationship with any one in particular

(8) Display poor impulse control or an openly hostile attitude toward the child

(9) Be unable to carry out consistent discipline, yet threaten or punish the child if he or she does not live up to an expectation or whim

(10) Understand little about normal child development and seem unable to integrate such information

3. Axioms of management

a. Once child abuse or neglect is diagnosed, the child is at great risk of reinjury or continued neglect.

b. Protection of the child must be a principal goal of initial intervention, but this protection must go hand in hand with a program to help the family through its crisis.

c. Traditional social casework cannot in itself protect an abused or neglected child in a dangerous environment. Medical follow-up is also necessary, and day-to-day contact with a child care center may help significantly to encourage the child's healthy development.

d. If a child is reinjured and medical attention is sought anew, the parents are likely to seek care in a facility other than that where the diagnosis was originally made or suspected.

e. Public social service agencies in both urban and rural areas do not have sufficient well-trained personnel, and the quality of administration and supervision in these agencies often is not high. These factors militate against their operating effectively in isolation from other social agencies. Simply reporting a case to the public agency mandated to receive child abuse case reports may not be sufficient to protect an abused or neglected child or to help the family.

f. Early attempts by the hospital staff to identify the agent of an injury or to determine if neglect was "intentional" may be ill advised. There is rarely a need to establish **precisely** who it was who injured or neglected a child and why. Clinical experience has shown that it is more important to establish confidence and trust in the hospital personnel. This may be jeopardized by overly aggressive attempts to ferret out the specific circumstances of the injury. On the other hand, lack of evidence for parental "guilt" is not a criterion for discharge of the patient.

g. If there is evidence that the child is at major risk, hospitalization to allow time for assessment of the home setting is appropriate. Children under the age of 3 are frequent victims; infants under 1 year of age with severe malnutrition or failure to thrive, fractures, burns, or bruises of any kind are especially at risk of reinjury or neglect. Prompt and effective intervention is vital to ensure their survival.

4. Assessment of the child and family

a. An adequate **medical history** and **physical examination** are necessary at the time the child is brought to the clinician. Photographs and a skeletal survey are made when indicated by the child's condition and the clinician's impression.

b. If a social worker is available, he or she is called promptly at the time of the family's visit. The physician should introduce the social worker as someone who is interested and able to help them through this difficult period. After the interview, the physician and social worker should confer.

c. **Interviewing the parents**

(1) In the initial interviews and in subsequent contacts, **no direct or indirect attempt to draw out a confession from the parent is made.** Denial is a prominent ego defense in virtually all abusive parents. Their often bizarre stories of how their child was injured should not be taken as intentional falsifications. These odd accounts frequently indicate parents' profound distress in acknowledging infliction of an injury or failure to protect a child. In the face of such a threatening reality, they repress it and may offer a blatant fabrication that must be accepted for the moment.

(2) A good interview technique allows parent and child to maintain the integrity of ego and family. It is appropriate to emphasize the child's need for hospital care and protection from harm. At this time the clinician should demonstrate concern and the ability to help the **parents'** distress as well.

d. In explaining the legal obligation to report the case, the clinician's compassion and honesty will go far to allay the family's anxiety.

e. The opportunity to observe parent-child interaction and the child's physical and psychological milestones, which might lead to insight into the familial causes of a child's injury or neglect, may not be available to a clinician in an ambulatory setting.

E. Rape and sexual abuse of children are now recognized to be extremely common in the United States, with an estimated one of four adolescent girls victimized before reaching adulthood. Fewer than half of these incidents are reported to medical and legal personnel.

1. Definitions

a. *Rape* is a legal conclusion defined by state law. Most states distinguish between statutory rape and common law rape, the latter being penetration without consent. *Rape* as a term is used to refer to a violent act initiated by an assailant in which a victim is subjected to sexual act(s) performed by force or the threat of force without the victim's consent.

b. *Sexual abuse* refers to sexual activity involving a child that is inappropriate because of the child's age, level of development, or role within the family. Authority and power allow the perpetrator to coerce the child into compliance. Sexual abuse is more chronic than rape and usually involves an acquaintance or a relative of the child.

2. Evaluation

a. The **history** should gather information necessary to assess the need for protective care and support services and the nature of medical therapy. A review of the abuse may be traumatic for the child and family, who should be interviewed together and then separately if possible. Great care and sensitivity must be demonstrated, as with other forms of child abuse (see **B**). The assistance of an experienced social worker, rape counselor, or psychiatrist is helpful.

b. Evaluation should include:

(1) The time of the abuse and the circumstances surrounding it

(2) Identification, when possible, of the perpetrator, to assess the risk involved should the child return home

(3) The nature of the sexual contact—oral, rectal, penile, or vaginal

(4) Vaginal discharge or perineal complaints

(5) Nonspecific complaints that may reflect chronic abuse: abdominal pain, enuresis, encopresis, recent school problems

c. The **physical examination** is directed at careful observation and recording evidence of abuse, associated injuries, the presence of ongoing medical problems, and the emotional status of the child (Table 3-5). In most cases of sexual abuse (especially chronic intrafamily abuse), there are no positive physical findings. Consequently, the likelihood of sexual abuse is best assessed by examining data from the history and psychological data as well as the results of the physical examination. The examination should be done gently and only after careful explanation to the child and the family. Consent forms and standard evidence collection procedures should be explained and utilized in all suspected cases. Some of these cases may well be prosecuted.

A full pediatric examination is required. In addition, special attention should be paid to:

(1) The general emotional state of the child (e.g., anxious, apathetic)

(2) The presence of bruises, abrasions, lacerations, and other cutaneous lesions

Table 3-5. Collection of evidence during the examination for sexual abuse and/or rape

Study	Procedure	Comments
Clothing	If still wearing same clothing, collect in paper bag	Plastic bags may alter evidence
Wood's light examination	Shine Wood's light over scalp, skin, and perineum	Fluorescent areas may indicate semen
Pubic hair	Comb out pubic hairs and collect in envelope	Foreign hairs may be identified
Acid-phosphatase test	Wipe perineum or suspected area with moistened gauze and apply gauze to acid-phosphatase tape	If tape turns purple in <60 seconds, examination is consistent with sperm being present
GC cultures of genital area, throat, rectum	Routine (using cotton swabs and Thayer-Martin media); prepubertal—vaginal, pubertal—cervical, males—urethral	
Chlamydia culture of genital area	Routine (using Dacron swab, culture media, and immunofluorescence kit if available)	Important even for youngest children
Fixed slides	Swab of posterior fornix onto dry slide	For examination of sperm, blood group, acid phosphatase
Urinalysis	Routine	May reveal urologic injuries, and inflammation, and may be useful in ruling out pregnancy at time of examination
Blood sample	Send for VDRL and, if necessary, blood typing and pregnancy test	CBC may also be useful if infection or blood loss is suspected

(3) The presence of significant trauma, including fractures and abdominal injuries

(4) The external genitalia, which should be carefully examined for ecchymoses, edema, lacerations, and erythema. The genital examination can best be visualized by placing the prepubertal child in the frog-leg or knee-chest position. Specula are not needed in prepubertal girls.

(5) An internal vaginal examination must be performed whenever

    (a) A history of vaginal or rectal penetration by a penis, finger, or foreign object is elicited or suspected.

    (b) The history reveals symptoms relating to the vaginal or perineal area (e.g., discharge, dysuria).

    (c) Abnormalities (even minor) are observed on the external genital examination.

    (d) There are questions as to the veracity or completeness of the history regarding the nature and scope of abuse.

    (e) Rape is a crime of violence. More than 80 percent of rape victims suffer from associated injuries. Great care must be taken to rule out vaginal and internal trauma.

  d. Laboratory studies should include examination of vaginal secretions for fungi, *Trichomonas*, *Neisseria gonorrhoeae*, and *Chlamydia*. Rectal and pharyngeal cultures should also be obtained when appropriate. Completion of a standardized specimen kit should be performed in all cases of alleged sexual abuse, misuse, or rape. Urine should be obtained for pregnancy testing when age-appropriate, as well as for serology for syphilis.

3. Therapy consists of management of acute medical conditions, venereal disease prophylaxis, pregnancy prophylaxis when appropriate, psychiatric support, social service management, and medical follow-up.

  a. The therapy of acute medical conditions should be directed by the history and physical findings. Abdominal and vaginal trauma are common in violent assaults.

  b. Venereal disease prophylaxis is recommended for all patients who have had contact with the assailant's genitals. It is often best administered PO, particularly in young children, in the hope of minimizing the pain and emotional upset (injections are often seen by the child as punitive) associated with the assault.

    (1) Oral prophylaxis. Amoxicillin, 50 mg/kg (maximum 3.0 gm) is given in one dose with probenecid, 25 mg/kg (maximum 1.0 gm). **Contraindications** to oral therapy are

      (a) Rectal or oral penetration, because oral medication is ineffective with pharyngeal or rectal gonorrhea

      (b) Uncertainty of follow-up VDRL determinations, as oral therapy does not adequately treat incubating syphilis

    (2) Intramuscular prophylaxis. Give ceftriaxone, 250 mg IM once.

    (3) Chlamydia prophylaxis. Give doxycycline, 100 mg PO twice a day for 7 days. In the younger child at risk for dental staining secondary to tetracyclines, it is often more judicious to wait for culture results before initiating an alternative therapy.

  c. Pregnancy prophylaxis

    (1) Indications. Pregnancy prophylaxis should be considered when the following conditions are met:

      (a) There is documentation or strong suspicion that intercourse has occurred.

      (b) The patient has experienced menarche and is not presently menstruating.

      (c) The time of unprotected intercourse is less than 72 hours before treatment.

      (d) The patient would have an abortion if already pregnant from previous intercourse (because of the risk to the fetus of high-dose estrogens).

    (2) Prophylaxis consists of conjugated estrogens, e.g., Ovral, two tablets stat and two more 12 hours later. This regimen is almost universally associated with nausea and vomiting. Therefore, prochlorperazine, 5–10 mg PO, given 2 hours before estrogen, is usually helpful.

  d. Psychiatric evaluation and support are essential, both for child and family. Victims of sexual abuse, even those who initially display seeming tranquility or aloofness, may suffer from deep emotional disturbances. Rape counselors provide critical support, and many cities maintain excellent rape counseling services that should be utilized.

  e. Social service evaluation is helpful in assessing the circumstances surrounding the abuse and the relative safety of the child if he or she returns home. As in other forms of child abuse, when the safety of the home is uncertain, admission to the hospital or alternative placement is indicated. Sexual abuse is considered a form of child abuse, and state reporting laws will thus apply.

f. Medical follow-up. While the follow-up care is multidisciplinary, it is usually most helpful when one health provider is identified to the child and family and has the responsibility for coordinating the various services and explaining the medical data to the child and family. Medical follow-up should be carefully arranged to encompass the following:

(1) Follow-up examination and assessment of healing injuries

(2) Check of cultures and other laboratory data

(3) Management of adverse effects of prophylactic therapy

(4) Emotional and social service support

F. Psychiatric emergencies

1. Acute psychosis encompasses a group of conditions in which there is a gross impairment in reality testing such that an individual incorrectly evaluates thoughts or perceptions. Direct evidence includes delusions or hallucinations, or behavior so grossly disorganized that disturbed reality testing can be implied. Among other concerns are suicidal or homicidal intentions, medications or hospitalization, and social support services. The assistance of an experienced psychiatrist is usually required.

a. Etiology

(1) Nonorganic psychosis includes the schizophrenic, paranoid, and major affective disorders. Specific organic causes have not been identified.

(2) Organic psychosis includes metabolic, infectious, neoplastic, cardiovascular, and traumatic conditions, as well as drug ingestion (see Table 4-1).

b. Diagnosis

(1) An organic cause should be ruled out first. Clues to an organic cause include:

(a) Clouding of consciousness

(b) Visual hallucinations

(c) An acute mental status change

(d) A family history of nonorganic psychosis

(2) A psychiatric evaluation is necessary to assess the nature and course of the disease.

c. Therapy

(1) Indications for hospitalization include:

(a) Suicidal or homicidal ideation

(b) Confusion severe enough to impair daily self-care or family attempts to provide care

(c) When familial support or understanding of the patient's condition is judged inadequate

(d) When the cause or nature of psychosis remains unclear

(2) Medication. Emergency medication (Table 3-6) is indicated when aggression or agitation is severe and unresponsive to supportive reassurance. Ingestion of an anticholinergic agent should be ruled out before antipsychotic medication is administered because it may mimic psychotic agitation.

2. Suicide. In the United States, suicide represents the third leading cause of

Table 3-6. Medications for the acutely agitated child

Drug	Dose*
Chlorpromazine	0.5 mg/kg IM
Thioridazine	0.5 mg/kg PO
Haloperidol	0.05–0.15 mg/kg/day PO q8–12h

* Medication can be repeated after 1 hr if no improvement is seen.

death in adolescents. Girls attempt suicide more commonly than boys, but boys' attempts are more often successful.

   a. Precipitating factors. Suicide attempts are most commonly related to family problems, depression, school problems, relationship discord, and pregnancy.

   b. Evaluation. All suicide attempts should be taken seriously. Although varying in intent and severity, all suicide attempts imply a significant breakdown of social communication and relationships. The following are relevant to the assessment of suicide risk:

     (1) Depression. Severe guilt, hopelessness, and vegetative signs reflect a serious disturbance and an increased risk of subsequent suicidal behavior.

     (2) Previous thoughts, attempts, and careful planning of attempts usually imply an increased risk of subsequent attempts and a greater requisite intervention.

     (3) Social and family dynamics that precipitated the attempt and show little evidence of potential for rapid amelioration

     (4) Psychosis. Suicidal attempts or ideation secondary to delusions or hallucinations are extremely serious and require hospitalization.

   c. Management

     (1) Hospitalization is indicated if the risk of suicide seems imminent, particularly if the conditions outlined in **b.(1)–(4)** are evident or suspected.

     (2) Home management should be undertaken only after careful psychiatric evaluation and when a sustained follow-up plan can be assured.

       (a) The crucial goal must be to modify the home environment sufficiently to make it tolerable for the child.

       (b) Access to immediate telephone or other personal support or counseling can be an important way to defuse a situation that is potentially intolerable for the patient.

3. The violent patient

   a. Acute and subacute violence. Aggression is common in children and usually takes developmentally appropriate and controllable forms. However, occasionally the clinician is confronted by an acutely violent or threatening patient.

   To prevent harm to the patient and others, rapid and purposeful control of the patient is imperative. There are generally two types of situations that require intervention.

     (1) Acute. An actively combative, dangerous, violent patient whose cooperation is not obtainable

     (2) Subacute. A severely agitated, threatening patient in whom violence appears imminent and whose cooperation is questionable

   b. Management

     (1) Verbal intervention may be useful in younger children in whom violent behavior is part of stereotyped tantrums or rage displays.

     (2) Physical restraint should be instituted as quickly and humanely as possible.

     (3) Medications should be used judiciously. In the actively violent patient, they should be prepared before the patient is restrained.

       (a) Antipsychotics are useful to control agitation or combative behavior. They may enhance the effects of anticholinergic and narcotic agents and may produce hypotension, extrapyramidal reactions, tachycardia, and laryngospasm. **Chlorpromazine** (0.5 mg/kg IM q4–6h) can be used.

       (b) Benzodiazepines are most effective given IV or PO to patients who are severely anxious rather than actively violent. Respiratory depression may occur with large doses and enhancement of the depressant effects of alcohol, monoamine oxidase inhibitors, phenothiazines, tricyclic antidepressants, and barbiturates. Give **diazepam,** 0.1 mg/kg IV or PO (maximum 10 mg).

(4) Continuing care involves appropriate psychiatric placement, social service, and psychiatric evaluation (see Chap. 20).

(5) Ethical considerations. It is **imperative** that the use of restraints or medication meets the needs of patients and not the needs of the treating facility. In addition, it is often difficult to determine which patients are violent because of primary psychiatric conditions or which patients come to violence in response to oppressive social inequities. The potential for the "medicalization" of what are in fact social problems is significant. Strong efforts must be made to prevent the use of psychiatric or medical therapy to subvert the civil rights of patients or undermine the redress of social grievances.

Note: State laws regarding the medicating of patients against their wishes vary. Clinicians should be acquainted with local provisions.

VII. Surgical acute care
A. Appendicitis
  1. Evaluation and diagnosis
    a. History. Establish the time of onset. The appendix commonly perforates within 36 hours after pain begins. The *pain* is periumbilical and is almost always the first symptom. *Vomiting* is present and always follows the onset of pain. After several hours, pain usually shifts to the right lower quadrant. In the infant, decreased appetite, fever, and vomiting are usually present. Diarrhea may be present, especially in retrocecal appendicitis.
    b. Physical examination, when right lower quadrant pain is present, will usually reveal *tenderness, guarding,* and *rebound.* **Rectal examination** is imperative to elicit tenderness.
    c. Laboratory data
      (1) Urinalysis, urine culture, and Gram stain
      (2) The **WBC** usually is elevated, but rarely above 20,000 in a child with a nonperforated appendix.
      (3) Abdominal x-rays will show concave curvature of the spine to the right due to the spasm of right-sided abdominal musculature. An air-fluid level may be seen in the cecum. A fecalith may be seen and increases the likelihood of a perforation. With perforation, decreased bowel gas in the right lower quadrant and free peritoneal fluids can be seen, especially in children under 2 years of age. A chest film may be helpful, since lower-lobe pneumonia may occasionally mimic appendicitis.
  2. Therapy
    a. Appendectomy
    b. When a perforated appendix is suspected, a triple antibiotic regimen (ampicillin, gentamicin, and clindamycin or cefoxitin) is usually given (see Chap. 14).
B. Obstruction
  1. Intussusception
    a. Etiology. Intussusception is usually found in children from 1 month to 2 years of age and occurs when a segment of intestine telescopes into itself, causing obstruction, ischemia, and necrosis. The majority of cases are idiopathic, but a lead point such as Meckel's diverticulum or adenopathy is common. Henoch-Schönlein purpura can be associated with intussusception.
    b. Evaluation and diagnosis
      (1) History
        (a) Intermittent abdominal pain, vomiting, and bloody ("currant-jelly") stools
        (b) Violent episodes of colicky, severe abdominal pain, causing the

child to cry out and draw the legs into flexed position are interspersed with relatively normal periods.

(2) Physical examination

(a) The child may be quiet, listless, irritable, or normal-appearing between episodes of pain.

(b) When the process presents later in the course, the child may show signs of prostration, pallor, and altered mental status. Careful vital sign measurement is essential in this setting.

(c) A vague, sausage-shaped mass is palpable, either abdominally or rectally, in most.

(d) Fever is common, particularly in infants.

(3) Laboratory data

(a) A characteristic filling defect extending from the cecum to distal parts of the colon is observed in the **barium enema.**

(b) Hematocrit

(c) Stools should be tested for occult blood.

c. Therapy

(1) IV fluids resuscitation is always necessary

(2) Barium enema. Most intussusceptions can be reduced by the hydrostatic pressure of the barium during the diagnostic enema. When done in a controlled manner, with close collaboration between the surgeon and radiologist, this procedure is safe and may obviate the need for surgery.

(3) When hydrostatic reduction is unsuccessful, **laparotomy and direct reduction** are required.

2. Malrotation and volvulus

a. Etiology. Congenitally abnormal position of the small bowel and associated abnormal posterior fixation of the mesentery. The most common age of presentation is under 1 month.

b. Evaluation and diagnosis

(1) The **history** almost always includes vomiting, usually bile stained. In older children, a past history of attacks termed *cyclic vomiting* may be elicited.

(2) Physical examination may reveal abdominal distention, jaundice, blood-stained vomitus or stools, and shock.

(3) Laboratory data

(a) Abdominal films may reveal gas in the stomach with a paucity of air in the small intestine.

(b) An **upper GI series and small bowel follow-through** will confirm the diagnosis, defining the positions of the ligament of Treitz and the cecum.

(c) Stool testing positive for blood is a poor prognostic sign, indicating significant bowel ischemia.

c. Therapy

(1) Nasogastric tube

(2) Operative relief of the obstruction should be attempted as rapidly as possible.

(3) IV fluids (see Chap. 7)

3. Pyloric stenosis is a cause of obstruction in the first 8 weeks of life, with a peak in 2–4 weeks. Boys are affected 4 : 1 over girls, and it occurs more frequently in infants with a family history of the condition.

a. The **history** reveals the onset of nonbilious vomiting of feedings, sometimes, but not always, "projectile."

b. Physical examination. The findings will vary with the severity of the obstruction.

(1) Dehydration and weight loss are common.

(2) The classic palpation of an **olive-sized muscular tumor** following vomiting occurs in the majority of cases.

(3) Visible gastric peristaltic waves are also common.

c. **Laboratory data**
   (1) Ultrasonography reveals the hypertrophic pylorus.
   (2) If ultrasonography is not available, roentgenographic studies after a barium meal reveal stenosis ("railroad-track sign").
   (3) Electrolytes, BUN, glucose, pH, and serum bicarbonate should be followed, since significant abnormalities, usually metabolic alkalosis, may accompany the vomiting (see Chap. 7).
d. **Therapy**
   (1) **Nasogastric tube**
   (2) Correction of the dehydration, alkalosis, and electrolyte abnormalities is a critical aspect of initial therapy (see Chap. 7, p. 200).
   (3) Surgical correction should take place as soon as the metabolic abnormalities have been satisfactorily corrected.
C. **Blunt trauma to the abdomen** can be a serious injury, yet may present with subtle symptoms and signs that mimic other causes of abdominal pain. A child with significant internal abdominal injury might present many hours or even days after the traumatic event.
   1. **Evaluation** includes surgical consultation.
      a. A careful history of trauma, from even seemingly minor events, should raise this possibility.
      b. Initially, careful observation for deterioration of vital signs or increasing abdominal tenderness, particularly in the liver or splenic area; abdominal bruises; or hematuria is also suggestive.
      c. **Laboratory studies** should include: CBC, prothrombin time, partial thromboplastin time, platelet count, and clot for type and crossmatch in case blood loss is significant or surgical intervention is required.
   2. **Initial therapy** should be directed at maintaining adequate blood volume. **Two large-bore IVs should be placed if abdominal hemorrhaging is suspected.**
   3. Surgical intervention may be required if bleeding is massive or persistent.
D. **Ectopic pregnancy** has become an important diagnostic consideration in evaluating the acute abdomen in adolescent girls.
   1. **Etiology.** Ninety-eight percent of ectopic pregnancies occur in the fallopian tube.
   2. **Evaluation and diagnosis.** Ectopic pregnancy in an adolescent may present as an abdominal catastrophe or, more subtly, with colicky pain and mild vaginal bleeding.
      a. A **catastrophic** presentation demands a rapid yet careful evaluation.
         (1) The patient usually is in shock, with signs of peritoneal irritation, including tenderness and rigidity but *rarely* fever.
         (2) *Intraperitoneal blood* may be palpated as a doughy mass in the cul-de-sac.
         (3) Although an ultrasound can often be diagnostic, **laparoscopy** is the definitive study.
         (4) **Culdocentesis** can be performed to confirm hemoperitoneum.
         (5) **Laboratory tests** should include preoperative studies and type and crossmatching for at least 4 units of blood.
      b. **Nonacute presentation**
         (1) The history includes vaginal bleeding after a missed period and lower abdominal pain.
         (2) The **physical examination** reveals an adnexal mass by palpation. Extreme sensitivity to cervical motion is an important finding.
         (3) **Laboratory tests** include CBC and erythrocyte sedimentation rate (ESR) with serial hematocrits. Urinalysis should help rule out alternative diagnoses, including urinary tract infection (UTI) and renal calculi.
         (4) A urine pregnancy test is positive in only half of ectopic pregnancies. Serum human chorionic gonadotropin determinations are more reliable indicators of pregnancy.

3. Therapy
a. The catastrophic presentation, with the patient in shock, requires rapid stabilization and transfer to the operating room for definitive **surgery.**
b. In a nonacute presentation, surgery is performed when there is a high index of suspicion of ectopic pregnancy based on procedures that may include culdocentesis, pelvic ultrasound, examination under anesthesia, and laparoscopy.
E. Pelvic inflammatory disease is an important cause of abdominal pain in female adolescents. Its clinical presentation may be similar to that of *appendicitis, ectopic pregnancy,* and *menstrual cramps.* For a discussion of evaluation and therapy, see Chap. 14, p. 414.

VIII. Environmental emergencies
A. Near-drowning implies survival or temporary survival following asphyxia secondary to a submersion episode.
1. Cold versus warm water drowning. Hypothermia associated with cold water drowning may provide protection against CNS hypoxic damage. There are no protective mechanisms in warm water immersions.
2. Freshwater versus saltwater drownings. Both freshwater and saltwater near-drownings damage alveoli, destroy surfactant, and result in pulmonary edema and hypoxia.
a. Freshwater. If a large amount of freshwater is aspirated, hypervolemia and water intoxication can also result.
b. Saltwater. If a large volume of saltwater is aspired, *hypovolemia, hemoconcentration,* and *hypernatremia* can occur. The *pulmonary edema* can be massive.
3. Evaluation of near-drowning victims
a. A **precise history** of the event should be obtained, including:
(1) The **type of water**—whether cold or warm, fresh or salt—and estimation of pollution
(2) Associated injuries
(3) Estimation of the time submerged
(4) Clinical status when rescued. Note if there were any spontaneous respiration or heartbeat.
(5) Type of CPR required and when it was begun
b. A **complete physical examination** should be done, with particular attention given to the cardiovascular, respiratory, and neurologic systems.
(1) Vital signs: blood pressure, pulse, respirations, and temperature
(2) Associated injuries, with particular attention to signs of neck injury and spinal cord injury
c. Laboratory evaluation includes a general screen for hypoxic and hypotensive injury.
(1) Blood studies: ABGs, electrolytes, blood sugar, calcium, CBC, prothrombin time, partial thromboplastin time, liver function tests. A toxic screen may also be indicated.
(2) Chest x-ray and other radiographs (i.e., cervical spine films) as required to rule out associated injury
(3) ECG
(4) Urinalysis, with a flow chart showing the hourly output
4. Treatment
a. All patients who are victims of near-drowning should be admitted for observation. This includes patients who revive spontaneously at the site of the accident.
b. Initial therapy
(1) Early resuscitative measures are the key to reducing morbidity and mortality.
(2) Full CPR may be required. Attention to a patent airway includes suctioning and clearing the airway of water-borne debris. **Immobilizing the cervical spine** is vitally important until injury is

ruled out. Atelectasis and hypoxia are major problems. Positive end-expiratory pressure (PEEP) is indicated.

(3) **Temperature resuscitation must begin immediately** (see sec. **VIII.C**) CPR will often be unsuccessful until the victim's temperature normalizes.

c. **Subsequent therapy.** When initial CPR is successfully completed, the following treatment plan is started:

(1) **Cardiovascular support** is given as required (see sec. **II**).

(2) **Recognition and treatment of increased ICP** if it occurs (see sec. **V.B**)

(3) **Prophylactic antibiotics** and the use of corticosteroids have not been shown to be efficacious.

(4) All associated injuries must be treated.

(5) **Antibiotics** are used for aspiration pneumonitis.

(6) Early and intense **social service intervention** is necessary for the family of the victim.

B. Heat-related injury

1. Burns

a. **Severe burn injuries require immediate management with a team approach.**

b. **Evaluation of the burn patient**

(1) The **history** must include:

(a) The **type of heat exposure** (e.g., an open flame, scald burn, electrical burn, explosion)

(b) How or why the patient was exposed. **Try to assess for inadequate supervision or evidence of child abuse.**

(c) Note if there is any evidence of **associated injuries.**

(d) Assess for the possibility of an **inhalation burn.** The possibility of pulmonary burns is increased in explosion or closed space burn.

(2) The **physical examination** must be complete.

(a) **Immediate attention is directed to the airway.**

(b) **Vital signs** should be obtained quickly in order to guide appropriate resuscitation.

(c) Indications of **inhalation injury** include: **cyanosis,** carbonaceous sputum, carbon deposits in the oropharynx, stridor or hoarseness, facial burns, and singed nasal hairs. If any of these are present, **intubation** should be performed before further physical assessment is completed.

(d) The **surface burn** must be assessed for

(i) Its **surface area.** Charts are available to help estimate the size of the involved area. In children over 12 years of age, the "rule of nines" can be used; in younger patients, burn charts can be used or estimated based on the child's hand as 1 percent body surface area (BSA).

(ii) The **depth of the burn** or level of tissue injury must be evaluated. **Superficial partial-thickness** (first-degree) burns involve the epithelium only. There is vasodilation and little edema. **Partial-thickness** (second-degree) burns involve destruction of the epithelium and part of the corium, with sparing of the dermal appendages. Capillary damage presents with blister formation. **Full-thickness** (third-degree) burns cause destruction of the entire dermis with loss of sensation. Clinically, these burn areas appear white, with no blister formation.

(iii) The **presence of circumferential burns must be noted** and **distal blood flow assessed.**

(e) The remainder of the examination should be devoted to an evaluation of neurologic and cardiovascular status and a search for evidence of **associated injuries.**

(3) The **laboratory examination** includes:
    (a) **Blood studies:** CBC, electrolytes, blood sugar, BUN, creatinine, calcium, prothrombin time, partial thromboplastin time, total protein, carboxyhemoglobin, and, if it is an electrical burn, creatine phosphokinase (CPK)
    (b) Chest x-ray
    (c) Urinalysis
    (d) Radiographs to rule out associated injuries
c. **Therapy.** The general goals of therapy are to support the cardiovascular system in the face of massive volume loss, to maintain adequate ventilation and oxygenation, and to minimize tissue loss with local care and infection control.
    (1) If there is evidence of a pulmonary burn, the patient should be **intubated.** Supplemental **oxygen** should be administered as indicated.
    (2) **Apply cold sterile saline soaks** to the burn to stop any remaining thermal damage.
    (3) **Establish IV access.** If the burn is extensive, a CVP line should be placed.
    (4) **Volume replacement** should be started if the patient has second- or third-degree burns involving more than 10 percent of the BSA. Volume replacement can be calculated as follows (see also Chap. 7):

Volume replacement (ml) = %BSA burn × 4 ml/kg + maintenance fluid requirements

This volume is given as normal saline or lactated Ringer's solution. One half is administered over the first 8 hours and the remainder over the next 16 hours. For this calculation, 50 percent BSA is the maximum percentage that can be used. Although calculations can serve as guidelines, the volume status should be assessed with hourly urine output and CVP measurements.

    (5) A **Foley catheter** is placed to monitor urine output.
    (6) **Sedation** is given for pain control; morphine, 0.1 mg/kg/q3–4h.
    (7) **Tetanus toxoid** (0.5 ml IM) is given if tetanus prophylaxis status is uncertain or if more than 5 years have elapsed since the last booster.
    (8) **Antibiotic coverage is started.** Penicillin, 200,000–400,000 units/kg in divided doses qid, or cephalothin (Keflin), 40–80 mg/kg/day in divided doses qid.
    (9) **Topical care.** Silver sulfadiazine (Silvadene) cream can be used over the entire burn area. Antibiotic-impregnated (Xeroform) gauze can be used as well. Sterile, bulky, dry dressings should then be applied.
    (10) **Early escharotomies or fasciotomies, or both, should be performed in all circumferential burns** if any distal circulatory impairment is present.
d. **Electrical burns: evaluation and treatment**
    (1) The patient should be **examined carefully for** an **entrance** as well as an **exit** wound and any **associated injuries.**
    (2) **Laboratory evaluation** includes CPK and urine for hemoglobin and myoglobin, and an ECG.
    (3) A very common burn injury in pediatrics is an **electrical burn to the mouth.** These patients must be followed closely for a minimum of 3 weeks because of the complications of hemorrhage at the site of the lesion. Surgical intervention for bleeding is often required.
2. **Heat stroke** is a life-threatening syndrome characterized by impaired heat dissipation secondary to high ambient temperature and humidity.
    a. **Characteristic triad in heat stroke**
        (1) **Severe CNS disturbances** manifested by coma, seizures, headache, agitation, or confusion
        (2) **Hyperpyrexia,** or a rectal temperature greater than 41°C (105.8°F)

(3) Hot, dry skin with no evidence of sweating
b. Other clinical symptoms and findings include:
  (1) Tachycardia and hypotension
  (2) Oliguria or anuria with acute tubular necrosis
  (3) Acute changes in the hepatic function
  (4) Rhabdomyolysis, which can complicate and compound renal injury
c. Evaluation
  (1) The history may reveal the following predisposing factors: alcoholism, obesity, heart disease, or fever. A careful history must include the duration of the temperature elevation, the therapeutic maneuvers attempted at home, and a history of oral intake and urine output.
  (2) The physical examination will reveal the findings enumerated in 2.a and b.
  (3) Laboratory evaluation
    (a) Blood studies; electrolytes, blood sugar, serum osmolarity, BUN, creatinine, liver function tests, prothrombin time, partial thromboplastin time, CBC, and CPK
    (b) Urinalysis, urine for myoglobin
d. Therapy
  (1) Assess airway and ventilation; give oxygen for cardiorespiratory or neurologic compromise.
  (2) Rapid cooling. The patient should be cooled by:
    (a) Removing all clothing.
    (b) Placing the patient in an ice bath or using ice bags at the neck and femoral and axillary areas until the rectal temperature is less than 38.5°C (101°F)
    (c) Phenothiazines can be given to decrease shivering (which is a heat-producing process), but be aware that phenothiazines may cause hypotension.
    (d) Keep skin moist; use fans to increase evaporative heat loss.
  (3) Volume replacement and a CVP line are required (see sec. II).
  (4) The renal status is monitored and an accurate record of the intake and output kept.
  (5) If seizures are present, the patient should receive a loading dose of phenytoin, 10 mg/kg IV, or phenobarbital, 10 mg/kg IV (see sec. V.A.3.c).
3. Heat "cramps" are muscle cramps secondary to an acute loss of electrolytes. Treatment includes cooling, and fluid and electrolyte replacement.
4. Heat exhaustion or prostration is a *hypovolemic* state that presents with progressive lassitude, headache, nausea and vomiting, tachycardia, and hypotension. Treatment includes volume resuscitation with close electrolyte monitoring.
C. Cold-related injury
  1. Hypothermia
    a. Definition. Hypothermia, or a core temperature of less than 35°C, can result from any cold exposure, but in pediatrics it is commonly an emergency situation in the near-drowning patient. Hypothermia causes marked depression of all organ systems, but is critical in the cardiovascular system in that it results in a marked decrease in cardiac output with a propensity for malignant arrhythmias. Atrial flutter and atrial fibrillation are noted above 30°C, followed by ventricular ectopy and fibrillation at less than 30°C, and asystole at approximately 26°C.
    b. Evaluation. Careful management of severely hypothermic patients is necessary to avoid precipitation of dysrhythmias in the irritable myocardium.
      (1) A full history should document the patient's symptoms, the duration and type of exposure, and any medical therapy.
      (2) The general physical examination will show profound peripheral vasoconstriction.

(a) The patient should be examined closely for localized tissue damage (frostbite) (see **E.2**) and associated injuries.

(b) **Vital signs. Oral and axillary temperature measurements are inadequate.** Temperature must be obtained rectally or by esophageal catheter with a special "cold" thermometer.

(c) The **cardiovascular system** should be assessed for perfusion and any evidence of arrhythmias.

(d) **Neurologic examination.**

    (i) **Above 35°C.** Alert, conscious, shivering

    (ii) **35–30°C.** Clouded mentation, dilated pupils with lower temperatures, decreased shivering

    (iii) **Below 30°C.** Unconscious, diminished deep tendon reflexes, diminished respirations

    (iv) **26°C and below.** The patient appears dead. Respiration is barely detectable.

(3) **Laboratory studies.** The requirements for laboratory testing increase with the severity of the hypothermia.

(a) Acutely, **ABGs** should be obtained.

(b) Later, the following studies are important: electrolytes, BUN, creatinine, CBC, clotting variables, liver function tests, and a toxic screen as needed.

(c) A **chest x-ray** should be obtained to ascertain if there was any aspiration during the acute event or resuscitation.

c. **Treatment**

(1) **Rewarming should be started immediately.** For patients with a temperature below 32°C, *core rewarming* is necessary. The methods for rewarming are as follows:

(a) **External rewarming.** This has the advantage of ease, but the disadvantages of inefficiency and increased complications of afterdrop and rewarming shock.

    (i) **Passive external rewarming. This method should be used only if the core temperature is greater than 35°C.** Remove all clothing, and place the patient in a warm room under warmed blankets.

    (ii) **Active external rewarming is not to be used if the temperature is less than 32°C.** Heat is applied to the body surfaces: warming blankets, water baths (temperature 37–40°C), and hot water bottles over the femoral and axillary areas. **Caution should be taken to avoid burn injury.**

(b) **Core rewarming.** These methods as a group are more effective and efficient than external rewarming methods. Specific methods include:

    (i) Heating all parenteral infusions in a blood warmer to 40–42°C.

    (ii) Colonic and bladder lavage with warmed saline (40–44°C).

    (iii) **Nasogastric lavage is contraindicated because of the risk of inducing dysrhythmias.**

    (iv) **Airway rewarming.** Inspired gases can be warmed to 42–46°C.

    (v) **Peritoneal dialysis.** The dialysate should be warmed to 45°C. This may require bathing the dialysate bottles in a 54°C bath.

    (vi) **Cardiac bypass** when available

(2) **Cardiac resuscitation must accompany rewarming.** Meticulous CPR is imperative.

(a) **A patient cannot be pronounced dead until he or she remains asystolic after rewarming to a core temperature of 30°C or the patient cannot be rewarmed to 30°C even with invasive measures.**

(b) If the patient has asystole or ventricular fibrillation, continue CPR while rewarming.

(i) **Medications** and **countershock** are ineffective when the temperature is below 30°C.

(ii) **Avoid giving too much NaHCO₃**; alkalosis can precipitate ventricular fibrillation in these patients. Therefore, ABGs must be monitored.

2. **Frostbite and other cold injuries**

a. **Etiology.** Tissue damage from cold exposure is caused by vascular injury. Cold exposures can cause both

(1) **Freezing injuries** (*frostbite*) that result from exposure to freezing temperatures that cause crystallization of the tissue water.

(2) **Nonfreezing injury** (*chilblain, immersion foot, trench foot*). These generally occur after long exposure to temperatures above freezing, usually with very high humidity.

b. **Evaluation and diagnosis** require the following:

(1) The **core temperature must be obtained**, and if hypothermia is present, rewarming should be started immediately (see **1**).

(2) The **level of tissue damage** should be assessed by using the following classification system.

(a) **First-degree injury** presents with hyperemia and edema and is quite painful.

(b) **Second-degree injury** also presents with hyperemia, but has clear vesicle formation. It also is painful.

(c) In **third-degree injury**, necrosis of the cutaneous tissue with dark vesicle formation develops.

(d) **Fourth-degree injury** demonstrates complete necrosis and loss of tissue extending into and below the subcutaneous level. This is a painless lesion.

c. **Therapy.** The goals of therapy are to stop the cold injury and minimize further tissue damage and loss.

(1) The skin should be **rewarmed** by

(a) Removal from the cold

(b) Removal of any restrictive clothing

(c) Topical ointments should be **avoided.**

(d) The patient should not be allowed to smoke cigarettes or drink alcohol, in order to avoid any vascular reactivity.

(e) If the area is still frozen when the patient presents (i.e., no sensation; white, hard, brittle skin), the involved skin should be warmed in a water bath of 40°C. **Warm only until the area is unfrozen. The water bath temperature should not exceed 42°C.**

(2) **Local care** should include only *loose, dry dressings*. Third- or fourth-degree injury blisters should not be broken. First- or second-degree blisters can be broken, followed by application of aloe vera cream to help prevent thrombosis.

(3) **Tetanus toxoid,** 0.5 ml IM, is given unless the patient has received tetanus in the 5 years preceding the cold injury.

(4) **Pain medication** may be required: Morphine, 0.1 mg/kg q4–6h, is adequate.

(5) **Antibiotics** should be given if there is any evidence of infection.

(6) **Physical therapy** is required if there is any tissue damage over a joint.

(7) **Amputation,** if needed, should be delayed until optimal healing has occurred.

IX. **Acute care procedures**

A. **Intubation** (see Chap. 6, p. 142 for newborn)

1. **Indications for tracheal intubation** include:

a. Airway protection

b. Pulmonary toilet

c. Respiratory support

2. **Preparation**

a. **Equipment:** oxygen, suction with "tonsil tip" catheter, breathing system (self-inflating Ambu type or oxygen-inflated Mapleson type), laryngo-scope handles (check batteries and bulbs) and age-appropriate blades; appropriate-sized masks, oral airways, endotracheal tubes, and stylets. **Endotracheal tube** (ETT) size can be estimated as follows:

ETT size = (16 + age in years) divided by 4

For example: if a child is 4 years old:

ETT size = (16 + 4)/4 = 20/4 = 5

For all equipment, always have one size larger and one size smaller immediately available.

  b. Medications. Atropine, methohexital (Brevital), thiopental, or ketamine; succinylcholine, midazolam (Versed), morphine or fentanyl, cocaine, lidocaine (Xylocaine), Cetacaine

3. **Monitoring** will require ECG, pulse oximetry, blood pressure cuff, and stethoscope.

4. **General instructions for intubation**

  a. Assemble all the necessary equipment *within easy reach.*

  b. Pretreat the child with atropine, 0.03 mg/kg IV or IM, to avoid a vagally induced bradycardia.

  c. Preoxygenate the child with 100% oxygen by face mask. *This will delay arterial desaturation if intubation proves difficult and requires more time than anticipated.*

  d. Positioning. The child's head should be in the midline; this position should be maintained by an assistant. Because the child's larynx is more anterior and cephalad than the adult's, head positioning is slightly different. The child should be put in the "sniffing position," which in the infant is provided naturally by the prominent occiput and in older children can be obtained by placing a small blanket, diaper, or towel under the occiput. **Placing a roll under the shoulders may, in fact, obscure the airway.**

  e. Laryngoscopy. The laryngoscope is held in the left hand, while the mouth is opened with the right. The blade of the laryngoscope is placed in the right side of the mouth near the tonsillar pillar and swept to the midline, carrying the tongue to the left side of the mouth and out of the way. When a straight blade (Miller or Wis-Hipple) is used, the tip of the epiglottis is lifted to reveal the larynx. When a curved (Macintosh) blade is used, its tip is placed in the vallecula (above the epiglottis) and lifting exposes the vocal cords. In both cases the blade is moved by *lifting* the laryngoscope handle along its axis. **Tilting the handle does not improve visualization and leads to oral damage.** Occasionally, further positioning of the head, or application of gentle cricoid pressure, may help bring the larynx into better view. Suctioning may be necessary.

  f. Intubation. The endotracheal tube is brought in from the right side of the mouth and placed between the cords under direct visualization. **Passage of the tube directly down the laryngoscope blade obscures the view and causes failure.** With the start of ventilation, position of the tube is confirmed by

  (1) Symmetric chest rise

  (2) Fogging of the endotracheal tube

  (3) Absence of sounds over the stomach

  (4) Clear breath sounds on both sides of the chest. The tube is then secured into place and a confirmational x-ray is obtained.

  g. Postintubation sedation and restraints. The pediatric patient will often attempt to remove the tube; therefore every precaution should be made to protect the airway. This may require sedation (chloral hydrate, 30–50 mg/kg q6h) or morphine (0.1 mg/kg q2–4h) and restraints that can be applied as arm/elbow splints. The feet should also be secured. The need for this should be explained gently to parents.

5. **Sedation and relaxation techniques:** (see also Chap. 1). Awake intubation provides the important advantage of maintaining spontaneous ventilation,

yet is a stressful and often difficult technique. While possible in infancy, in debilitated patients, or in cooperative older children after topical anesthesia and light sedation, it is usually unsuitable for others. When heavy sedation is employed, the risk of apnea is present and, when paralysis is employed, it is essential that the practitioner be skilled in management of the airway.

   a. **Anesthetics and muscle relaxants.** The patient is given an induction of intravenous anesthetic, such as *thiopental* (4–6 mg/kg IV), *methohexital* (1.0–1.5 mg/kg IV), or *ketamine* (1.0–1.5 mg/kg IV). When the stomach is empty, adequacy of the airway is assessed with bag-and-mask ventilation. If the airway can be maintained easily, succinylcholine (1 mg/kg IV) is given for muscle relaxation. When the child is fully relaxed, the intubation is completed. The following *limitations of this technique* must be considered:

   (1) A muscle relaxant should only be given by a person who is competent with intubations, usually an anesthesiologist.

   (2) A child who has an airway obstruction or is known to be difficult to intubate is only managed in the operating room by an anesthesiologist and otolaryngologist. Children with obstructed airways can, as a rule, maintain their own airway better than the physician can with bag-and-mask ventilation.

   (3) A child with hypotension, hypovolemia, or evidence of myocardial compromise should not receive a barbiturate because it can cause cardiovascular collapse. In such children, *ketamine* is a reasonable choice.

   (4) Any child with progressive myopathy, evolving neuromuscular disease, acute major denervation, or burn injury should not receive succinylcholine. In these conditions, succinylcholine may cause profound *hyperkalemia*. **Children who have renal failure and difficulty with high serum potassium levels should not receive succinylcholine. In patients with muscular dystrophy, succinylcholine is associated with malignant hyperthermia.** Alternatives include *pancuronium* (Pavulon) or *vecuronium* (Norcuron), 0.1 mg/kg IV.

   (5) Any child who has a full stomach should be intubated awake or in "rapid-sequence" fashion with cricoid pressure to prevent gastric aspiration. In *rapid sequence technique*, cricoid pressure is applied during preoxygenation and maintained until the endotracheal tube is in place. Medications are given in rapid succession and the patient is not ventilated by mask. Success must be swift and immediate; the technique is contraindicated in patients in whom any potential difficulty with intubation is suspected.

   b. **Benzodiazepines, narcotics, and topical anesthetics** (see also Chap. 1)

   (1) For awake intubations, children can be sedated with *midazolam* (Versed) given in 0.025 mg/kg IV increments and *morphine* (0.05–0.1 mg/kg IV increments) or *fentanyl*, 2 µg/kg IV increments. The oropharynx is sprayed with lidocaine or Cetacaine.

   (2) As a vasoconstrictor and anesthetic, cocaine is ideal for *nasal* topicalization. Alternatively, use a combination of phenylephrine and lidocaine.

   c. **Blind nasotracheal intubations.** In young children, this technique is exceedingly difficult but in the older child and adolescent, it is acceptable. The naso-oral airway is topically anesthetized. Then, with the child in a sitting position with the head forward, the tube is slowly advanced with each inspiration. As the tube approaches the glottis, louder breaths are heard through it.

B. **Ventilators**
   1. **Definition of terms used in mechanical ventilation**
      a. **Controlled ventilation** is complete mechanical ventilation in which the patient does no spontaneous breathing.
      b. **In assisted ventilation** the patient initiates a breath that the ventilator

completes. This is usually combined with an occasional mandatory breath.

c. In **intermittent mandatory ventilation (IMV)**, the patient receives breaths at a preset rate, but can spontaneously generate his or her own respirations at any rate.

d. In **continuous positive airway pressure (CPAP)**, no preset breaths are given, and the patient breathes against a constant distending pressure.

e. In **pressure support ventilation,** patient-initiated breaths are supplemented by a preset pressure supplied to the airway.

f. In **pressure control ventilation,** a preset pressure is maintained throughout inspiration.

2. The **types of ventilators** available are outlined below and compared in Table 3-7. Ventilators are classified by the event that terminates ventilation.

   a. **Time-cycled ventilator.** Inspiration continues for a preset time.

   b. **Volume-cycled ventilator.** Inspiration continues until the preset volume is delivered.

   In both time-cycled and volume-cycled ventilators, pressure limits can be set to avoid the problems of overdistention and barotrauma.

3. **Indications for ventilation therapy.** Mechanical ventilation is used to treat or to prevent respiratory failure, indicated by hypoxia, hypercapnia, and respiratory acidosis. Specific clinical situations include:

Table 3-7. Comparison of time-cycled and volume-cycled ventilators*

	Time-cycled	Volume-cycled
Examples	Baby Bird, Healthdyne, Seachrist, Biomed, BP 200	MAI, MAII, Emerson, Bear II, V, Hamilton
Modes	CPAP, IMV, control, cannot assist	CPAP, IMV, assist, control
Physiology	Tidal volume will change with compliance and resistance changes	In patients weighing over 10 kg, tidal volume is relatively stable despite changes in airway resistance and compliance. In smaller children the compressible volume of the tubing is relatively large in comparison with the set tidal volume, so that with changes in airway resistance or compliance, delivered tidal volume cannot be accurately predicted
Patients	Best used in patients weighing less than 10–15 kg; in larger patients it is difficult to maintain a high enough flow rate to deliver an adequate tidal volume	For the reasons enumerated above, best used in patients weighing more than 10 kg
How to start	Child is ventilated by hand with a manometer in line to predict the pressures necessary for adequate chest movement	Tidal volume is estimated to be 15–20 ml/kg, and a rate is selected between 10–20 cycles/min

* Whenever a patient is started on mechanical ventilation, it is imperative to evaluate the adequacy of oxygenation and ventilation with ABGs.

a. **Apnea**
b. **Fatigue** from increased work of breathing caused by dynamic airway disease, parenchymal disease, or mechanical obstruction inhibiting diaphragmatic movement. In these cases it is important both to assist ventilation and to decrease or prevent atelectasis.
c. **Neuromuscular disease.**
d. **Skeletal problems** producing restrictive lung disease or an unstable thorax.

4. **How to use the ventilator:**
   a. Specific therapy must be tailored to accommodate each clinical situation:
      (1) **CPAP** prevents or reverses small airway closure and alveolar collapse, decreasing the work of breathing and possibly any intrapulmonary right-to-left shunt.
      (2) **IMV, assisted, or controlled ventilation** is used when the physician cannot generate an adequate minute ventilation.
   b. **Sedation** is usually required for the patient to tolerate the endotracheal tube and the ventilatory support (see above and Chap. 1).
   c. **Muscle relaxation** may be required when high inflating pressures are used or when ventilation is difficult because the patient "fights" the ventilator.

5. **Assessment of mechanical ventilation:**
   a. The patient's **tidal volume** should be evaluated by visual auscultation and by measurement of expired volume at the airway. Chosen initial tidal volumes are typically 10–15 ml/kg. Cyanosis, nasal flaring, retractions, and patient discomfort indicate *inadequate* mechanical ventilation.
   b. **When a patient is started on mechanical ventilation, it is imperative to evaluate adequacy of oxygenation and ventilation with ABGs.**
   c. When a patient continues on mechanical ventilation, continual monitoring of gas exchange can be done with pulse oximetry, end-tidal carbon dioxide monitors, and arterial or capillary blood gases.

6. **Complications of positive pressure ventilation:**
   a. Barotrauma from high airway pressures can produce *pneumothoraces, pneumomediastinum, and pneumoperitoneum.*
   b. If CPAP or PEEP is too high or air trapping occurs, there will be overdistention of the alveoli and *carbon dioxide retention.*
   c. Decreased systemic venous return producing a *decrease in cardiac output* can occur in a patient on positive pressure ventilation. This is exaggerated in the patient who is hypovolemic, has poor myocardial function, or has tamponade.
   d. **The most common complication is the selection of inappropriate ventilator settings with inadequate monitoring.**

C. **Central venous pressure (CVP) monitors**
   1. **Definition.** CVP lines are intrathoracic catheters used for the assessment of preload or intravascular volume status.
   2. **Placement is indicated in**
      a. Any situation in which a CVP measurement will help to guide therapy, i.e.,
         (1) Shock
         (2) Anuria or oliguria
         (3) During vasoactive drug therapy
         (4) During therapeutic osmotherapy
         (5) Congestive heart failure
         (6) Situations in which massive fluid shifts are anticipated, i.e., sepsis, burns, major trauma, surgery
      b. Any situation in which secure vascular access is necessary or irritating medications must be given:
         (1) During cardiac arrest
         (2) During chemotherapy
         (3) For infusion of vasoactive medications

(4) For hyperalimentation

(5) For rapid electrolyte repletion

(6) For repeated "mixed-venous" blood sampling

3. **Required equipment** includes:

   a. **Sterile preparations.** Betadine, alcohol, gloves, masks, sterile drapes

   b. Tourniquet, arm board

   c. Long angiocatheters or other catheter

   d. Cutdown tray

   e. Lidocaine 0.5%, without epinephrine

4. **How to place the line**

   a. Technical line placement is similar in the adult and pediatric patient, but the degree of difficulty is usually inversely related to the size of the patient.

   b. **Access sites** include the following:

      (1) The *internal jugular vein* is a preferred site, but access to this vein can be difficult in infants.

      (2) The *external jugular vein* is an excellent access site, but it can be difficult to thread the catheter into the chest.

      (3) The *subclavian vein* is easier to cannulate in the older child than in the infant.

      (4) The *brachial vein* is another preferred site. In an older child, percutaneous cannulation can be done, whereas a cutdown is often required in an infant.

      (5) The *femoral vein* offers an easy site for fast cannulation, particularly when other procedures such as intubation or CPR are in progress. *When properly dressed,* infection rate is similar to that of other sites. **Sites below the diaphragm should not be used in the presence of intraabdominal trauma.**

      (6) The *umbilical vein* offers an easy access route in infants, but it can be difficult to thread the catheter through the liver and into the chest.

   c. **All lines should be placed with sterile procedure.**

   d. Before beginning the cannulation, *estimate the length of catheter* that will be required to reach the right atrium.

   e. Once the vein is entered, the catheter should be advanced until the tip is, ideally, just above (or, for femoral lines, below) the right atrium. The position can be evaluated during the procedure by the transducer wave forms. A chest x-ray should be obtained to ascertain the specific location of the catheter.

   f. Once the line is placed, CVP is most accurately measured with an electrical transducer. A water column can be used, but the normal tachycardia of younger children tends to produce a falsely high CVP reading. Transducers are zeroed at the level of the right atrium and measurements taken at the end of exhalation.

5. **Complications of CVP placement** include:

   a. **Infection.** The line should be handled with sterile procedure at all times.

   b. **Air embolism** can occur. The system should be closed to air at all times.

   c. **Arrhythmias** can occur if the catheter advances into the right ventricle. If a right ventricular tracing is present on the monitor, the line should be pulled back into the correct position.

   d. **Pneumothorax or hemothorax** can result from line placement. The postplacement chest x-ray can rule out this complication.

D. **Arterial lines**

1. **Definition.** An arterial line is a direct cannulation of a peripheral artery for the purpose of continuous pressure monitoring or frequent arterial blood sampling, or both.

2. **Indications for placement**

   a. **Blood pressure monitoring** for any clinical situation characterized by blood pressure lability.

b. Frequent ABG monitoring (e.g., respiratory failure, therapeutic hyperventilation)
  c. Vascular access for frequent **blood sampling**
3. **Equipment.** The general equipment requirements are:
  a. Sterile preparations. Betadine, alcohol, gloves
  b. Tape, arm board, tincture of benzoin
  c. Short Medicuts or angiocatheters (20- or 22-gauge)
  d. A 10-ml syringe with a flush solution of heparinized saline (1 unit heparin/ml)
  e. Pressure monitoring equipment with high pressure tubing
4. **How to place the arterial line:**
  a. Any of the peripheral arteries can be used, but preferred sites include
    (1) Radial artery. The Allen test is often performed to document good ulnar flow.
    (2) Posterior tibial or dorsalis pedis. Both of these arteries can be used. A modified Allen test may be performed to evaluate the adequacy of the artery not being used.
    (3) Axillary artery.
    (4) Use of the temporal artery is discouraged because of the potential for backflow during flushing and reports of associated cerebrovascular accidents.
  b. The extremity should be securely taped to an arm or foot board for support and stabilization. Be certain that the distal toes or fingers are visible, so that blood flow can be constantly evaluated.
  c. Cannulation should be performed under a sterile technique.
  d. Percutaneous cannulation or cutdown procedures are acceptable. Percutaneously, the overlying skin is *anesthetized* with a wheal of 1% lidocaine and the skin broken with a 20-gauge needle. The angiocath is advanced at a shallow angle toward the palpated pulse. Entry of the vessel produces immediate flashback, on which the needle is advanced very slightly and the catheter threaded into the vessel. Alternatively, the artery can be transfixed, the needle removed, and the vessel cannulated by slow withdrawal of the catheter until blood return is seen and it can be advanced directly or over a spring wire.
  e. After the line is placed, it should be secured with tape and tincture of benzoin. The patient should be under constant visual supervision while the line is in place.
  f. NS with 1 unit of heparin/ml is infused at a rate of 1–2 ml per hour. **This line is clearly labeled and is not a medication line.**
5. **Complications of arterial lines**
  a. The main complication is **vascular compromise distal to the site of insertion,** either from spasm or from thromboembolism. If there is any evidence of vascular compromise, the line should be removed.
  b. Massive blood loss can occur if the line becomes disconnected. To prevent this, all lines should be taped securely, the patient kept in a monitored setting, and the site accessible for continuous visual observation at all times.
  c. Infection, although uncommon, is always possible.
E. **Intraosseous** fluid administration
1. **Definition.** An intraosseous line is a direct cannulation of the bone marrow to achieve emergency access when vascular access cannot be obtained after 5–10 minutes of percutaneous attempts.
2. **Indications.** Vascular access for volume and pharmacologic support of a critically ill child. All IV fluids and resuscitation medications can be given via this route.
3. **Equipment.** No. 18–20 gauge spinal needle, bone marrow needle, or commercial intraosseous line kit; sterile preparations
4. **Placement.** The most common site is 1–2 fingerwidths below the tibial

tubercle on the anteromedial aspect of the tibia. **The needle is directed inferiorly to avoid growth plate injury.** Bone is penetrated with continuous pressure and a screwing motion; marrow entry is signified by loss of resistance and confirmed by aspiration. Saline injection is met with mild resistance and gravity flow is less than in the usual IV line.

5. **Stabilization.** Spinal needles can be stabilized with a surgical needle holder clamped at skin level and taped in place.

6. **Complications** include:
   a. Growth plate injury
   b. Infections if this route of access is maintained for over 24 hours
   c. Clysis secondary to improper placement into the soft tissues

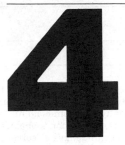

Poisoning

Michael Shannon and
John W. Graef

Ingestion of toxic products by children is a common occurrence. It is estimated that annually about 6,000,000 children ingest a potentially toxic substance. Children under 5 years of age account for 80 percent of recorded cases of poison ingestion. However, the majority of these poisonings results in a low morbidity and mortality. Plants, household products, cosmetics, and over-the-counter medications are the toxic agents most frequently encountered in children less than 5 years old. Although toxic ingestions in children less than 5 are generally of single substances, in adolescents and young adults multiple substances are frequently ingested after a suicide gesture or an attempt to "get high."

I. **Emergency management** (see also Chap. 3)
  A. **Identification of the poison.** Usually, the ingested material can be identified by a careful history.
    1. The **initial history** should include the identification of the product ingested (containers or bottles should be brought to assist identification), the amount taken (a swallow for a 3-year-old child is approximately 5 ml; for a 10-year-old, 10 ml; and for an adolescent, 15 ml), the time of ingestion, and the child's present condition. Pertinent past medical history should be obtained.
    2. In determining therapy, the physician should accept the **largest estimated amount** ingested.
    3. **Physical examination** will often reveal supporting evidence for a particular ingestion. When the nature of the substance ingested is unknown, the list of common signs or symptoms presented in Table 4-1 may be useful.
    4. The specific substance causing a poisoning should be confirmed by **qualitative** analysis performed on blood or urine. Gastric fluid analysis has little utility *unless performed within 2–3 hours of an ingestion.* When possible, a **quantitative** analysis should be performed on blood.
  B. **Supportive therapy.** While allowing normal renal and hepatic processes to remove or detoxify the ingested toxin, general principles of supportive care must be observed. These principles include the following:
    1. **Respiratory support** (see also Chap. 3). Ensure adequate respiratory exchange by maintaining a patent airway and the provision of oxygen, if necessary. Airway protection by endotracheal intubation may be required to prevent aspiration in patients with a depressed or absent gag reflex. Assisted ventilation is often necessary after exposure to central nervous system (CNS) depressants.
    2. **Cardiac support** (see also Chaps. 3 and 9). Correction of hypotension or shock is accomplished initially by intravenous access and administration of crystalloid fluid. Vasopressors may be required after ingestion of myocardial depressants (e.g., tricyclic antidepressants). Cardiac arrhythmias are managed according to advanced cardiac life support algorithms.
    3. **Fluid homeostasis** (see Chap. 7). Replace previous and ongoing fluid losses while correcting electrolyte derangements.
    4. **Hematologic** (see Chaps. 3 and 16). Correction of hemolytic anemias with packed cell transfusions or exchange transfusions.
    5. **Central nervous system** (see Chaps. 3 and 19). Toxicity typically includes CNS depression or seizures, or both.

Table 4-1. Common signs and symptoms of toxic exposures

System involved	Substances involved
Central nervous system	
Depression and coma	Sedative-hypnotics, narcotics, anticonvulsants, tranquilizers, tricyclic antidepressants, phenothiazines, antimuscarinic agents, hypoglycemic agents, alcohols, aromatic hydrocarbons, carbon monoxide, lead, mercury, lithium cyanide, gases, solvents
Stimulation and/or convulsions	Amphetamines, xanthines, sympathomimetic agents, psychotropic drugs (PCP, mescaline), cocaine, nicotine, salicylates, ergot, camphor, lead, strychnine, organophosphate and carbamate, chlorinated insecticides
Hallucinations	Psychotropic drugs, amphetamines, alcohol withdrawal, antihistamines, antimuscarinic agents, cocaine, camphor, tricyclic antidepressants
Hyperpyrexia	Salicylates, atropine
Cardiovascular system	
Arrhythmias	Digitalis, quinidine, tricyclic antidepressants, cocaine
Tachycardia	Amphetamines and sympathomimetic agents, xanthines, cocaine, tricyclic antidepressants
Bradycardia	Beta blockers, cardioglycosides, quinidine, calcium-channel blockers
Hypotension	Narcotics, phenothiazines, antihypertensive agents, tricyclic antidepressants
Hypertension	Cocaine, amphetamines, psychotropic drugs
Gastrointestinal system	
Nausea, vomiting, and diarrhea	Almost any toxic substance can produce these signs or symptoms
Increased salivation	Insecticides, mushrooms
Decreased salivation	Antimuscarinic agents, antihistamines
Respiratory system	
Hypoventilation	CNS-depressant substances
Hyperventilation	Salicylates, cocaine, nicotine, carbon dioxide
Abnormal odors on breath:	
Alcohol	Alcohols, phenols, chloral hydrate
Acetone	Alcohol, acetone, lacquer
Wintergreen	Methyl salicylate
Garlic	Phosphorus and arsenic
Bitter almonds	Cyanide
Pears	Chloral hydrate
Others	Turpentine, camphor
Ocular system	
Mydriasis	Antimuscarinic agents, sympathomimetic agents, psychotropic drugs, cocaine, amphetamines
Miosis	Narcotics, organophosphate insecticides, parasympathomimetic drugs
Blurred vision	Antimuscarinic agents, alcohols
Colored vision	Digitalis, quinine
Scotomas	Quinine, salicylates
Conjunctival infection	Marijuana, ethanol
Auditory system	
Tinnitus	Salicylates, streptomycin, ergot, quinines

Table 4-1 (continued)

System involved	Substances involved
Cutaneous system	
Cyanosis	Nitrites, nitrobenzene, aniline dyes
Jaundice	Carbon tetrachloride, benzene, aniline dyes, chromates, phenothiazines, quinacrine
Staining or coloring	Bismuth black; carbon monoxide and cyanide, pink blood; methemoglobinemia, brown blood; atropine, flushed face
Discoloration of gums	Lead, bismuth, arsenic
Alopecia	Thallium, radium, arsenic, hypervitaminosis A
Abnormal color of urine	
Dark green	Phenol, resorcinol
Yellow	Picric acid

    a. An intravenous benzodiazepine (diazepam or lorazepam), phenytoin, or phenobarbital is the anticonvulsant of choice, although paraldehyde remains a therapeutic option. Under select circumstances (e.g., isoniazid toxicity) a specific agent such as pyridoxine is indicated.

    b. Supportive measures are to be provided for prolonged coma.

  6. Renal insufficiency often accompanies poisoning by ethylene glycol and nonsteroidal antiinflammatory agents. Renal function should be monitored with hemodialysis instituted as needed.

C. Gastrointestinal decontamination. Removal from a toxic exposure includes **flushing** after ocular or cutaneous exposure and **removal to fresh air** after inhalational exposure. After toxic *ingestions,* attention is first directed to means of preventing systemic absorption of the toxin. Such intervention is termed *gastrointestinal decontamination* and has three distinct components: **gastric evacuation,** administration of an **adsorbent** (usually activated charcoal), and administration of a **cathartic** to enhance fecal expulsion of toxin.

  1. Gastric evacuation is the cornerstone of intervention after a toxic ingestion. However, its efficacy falls dramatically when it is instituted more than 1 hour after an ingestion. In such cases, it can be deferred if its use will cause significant treatment delay.

    a. Chemical methods. Ipecac syrup is the only available emetic for gastric emptying.

      (1) Ipecac syrup is the method of choice for gastric emptying when ingestions are promptly recognized because it induces emesis within 15–20 minutes in 85 percent of patients after one dose and within 30–40 minutes in 96 percent of patients after two doses. It removes approximately 30–40 percent of an ingested product when administered within 1 hour of ingestion. It is available without prescription and has a long shelf life, which allows for storage at home for emergency use. It is safe when taken in the recommended dosage.

      (2) For children age **6–12 months,** 10 ml is given once only, followed by clear fluids. **It should be administered under medical supervision.**

      (3) For the child **1–10 years old,** 15 ml (1 tbs) ipecac syrup is given, followed by liberal quantities of clear fluid. If vomiting does not occur within 20 minutes, the same dose can be repeated once.

      (4) For the patient **10 years of age and older,** 30 ml ipecac syrup is given along with clear fluids. If vomiting does not occur in 20 minutes, the dose can be repeated once.

      (5) Ipecac is **contraindicated** in patients who have ingested caustic agents, hydrocarbons, or agents that cause rapid coma (relative contraindication) or in those who are comatose or having seizures.

b. Mechanical methods. Orogastric lavage is as effective as ipecac and may be the preferred means of gastric evacuation in children who arrive at the emergency department without having received ipecac. It offers the advantage of speed and the prompt administration of adsorbent and cathartic. *For the patient with depressed airway reflexes, intubation with an endotracheal tube before passage of a lavage tube is indicated.*

(1) **Equipment.** No. 18–40 French single-lumen lavage tube, 4-oz Asepto syringe

(2) For lavage, place the patient on the left side. A restraining papoose expedites the process.

(3) Use jelly to facilitate insertion of tube.

(4) Measure the distance to the stomach, and ensure entrance into the stomach by injecting air with auscultation over the stomach.

(5) Aspirate the gastric contents before lavage.

(6) Lavage with normal saline, 10–20 ml/kg aliquots.

(7) Perform lavage until the return is clear.

(8) Leave activated charcoal in the stomach on completion, or, if indicated, a specific antidote (e.g., *N*-acetylcysteine [Mucomyst]).

(9) Pinch the tube on removal to prevent aspiration.

2. **Adsorbents**

a. **Activated charcoal,** an odorless, tasteless black powder, is the residue from the distillation of wood pulp. It forms a stable complex with the ingested toxin, thus preventing adsorption.

(1) **It should not be given before ipecac syrup.** Its effectiveness depends on its small particle size and large surface area. It should be used for drugs against which it is known to be effective (Table 4-2). **It is not effective against metals, alcohols, hydrocarbons, or caustics.**

(2) The dose is 1 gm/kg PO in 8 oz water or with cathartic (see **3**). It can be given following induced emesis or via gastric lavage tube.

b. The "universal antidote" (a mixture of charcoal, magnesium hydroxide, and tannic acid) is **ineffective** and is **hepatotoxic. It should not be used.**

3. **Cathartics** hasten intestinal transit of gastrointestinal contents, thus decreasing the opportunity for systemic absorption. Doses of common cathartics are found in Table 4-3. **Sorbitol should be used with caution in children less than 2 years old since it may induce excessive fluid losses and dehydration.** Whole bowel irrigation (WBI) involves the administration of 5–20 liters of an electrolyte balanced solution, e.g., Golytely, until the rectal effluent is clear. It is particularly efficacious for the expulsion of iron tablets and foreign bodies.

4. **Dilution** is a relatively ineffective method of gastrointestinal decontamination. It may be useful in ameliorating the GI upset that accompanies ingestion of gastric irritants.

5. **Neutralization** of ingested bases with acids and ingested acids with bases **is no longer advised.** It is generally instituted too late to be effective, and **the resultant exothermic reaction may cause secondary tissue damage.**

D. **Elimination enhancement.** Methods of enhancing excretion should be used only in **serious poisoning,** because they involve some risk. **Most cases of poisoning are handled conservatively, allowing the patient to excrete or metabolize the ingested drug. Only a small percentage will require the more radical forms of therapy that follow.**

1. **Fluid diuresis** enhances excretion by increasing the rate of glomerular filtration, so that the resorptive sites in the distal tubules have a shorter exposure to the ingested drug. Fluid diuresis will enhance excretion of drugs mainly excreted by the kidneys (e.g., lithium). A sustained diuresis of two to three times normal is recommended.

2. **Ionized diuresis** is based on the principle that excretion is favored when a drug is maintained in its ionized state. Excretion of acidic compounds, such as salicylates and long-acting barbiturates, is enhanced by sustained **alkalinization** of the urine.

Table 4-2. Drugs and chemicals adsorbed by activated charcoal*

Analgesic and antiinflammatory agents
  Acetaminophen
  Aspirin
  Indomethacin
  Mefenamic acid
  Morphine
  Opium
  Propoxyphene
  Phenylbutazone
Anticonvulsants and hypnosedatives
  Barbiturates
  Carbamazepine
  Chlordiazepoxide
  Diazepam
  Glutethimide
  Ethchlorvynol
  Phenytoin
  Sodium valproate
Other drugs and chemicals
  N-Acetylcysteine (Mucomyst)
  Amphetamines
  Atropine
  Camphor
  Chlorpheniramine
  Cocaine
  Colchicine
  Digitalis glycosides
  Iodine
  Ipecac
  Mercuric chloride
  Methylene blue
  Muscarine
  Nicotine
  Oxalates
  Paraquat
  Parathion
  Penicillin
  Phenol
  Phenolphthalein
  Phenylpropanolamine
  Promazine
  Propantheline
  Quinine
  Strychnine
  Tetracycline
  Theophylline
  Tolbutamide
  Tricyclic antidepressants

* Drugs not adsorbed: metals, inorganic salts (lithium, arsenic), alcohols, acids, and alkalis.

    a. Alkalinization is accomplished by the intravenous administration of 1–2
       mg/kg sodium bicarbonate to attain a urine pH > 7.
    b. **The more acidic the toxin, the more effective is alkalinization in
       enhancing excretion.**
  3. **Osmotic diuresis** is based on the principle that an osmotic load will prevent
     the renal resorption of an ingested drug.

Table 4-3. Commonly used cathartics

Agent	Dose	
	Adult	Child
Sorbitol (70% sol.)	50–150 ml	2 ml/kg
Magnesium sulfate (10% sol.)	15–20 gm	250 mg/kg
Magnesium citrate (6% sol.)	300 ml	4 ml/kg
Sodium sulfate (10% sol.)	15–20 gm	250 mg/kg

    a. A diuresis of two to three times the normal excretion is recommended.
    b. Mannitol, 0.5 gm/kg/dose IV of a 25% solution q4–6h, can be used.
    c. Close monitoring of serum and urinary electrolytes, serum osmolality, and central venous pressure (CVP) is indicated.
    d. Contraindications to the procedure are cardiac disease, oliguria or anuria, hypotension, and pulmonary edema.
  4. Diuretics. An output of two to three times normal in a child is sought.
    a. Furosemide (Lasix), 2 mg/kg/dose IM or IV, can be used.
    b. Electrolytes should be closely monitored.
  5. Extracorporeal drug removal. Exchange transfusions, peritoneal dialysis, hemodialysis, and hemoperfusion are **not** part of the usual emergency management of poisoning. Their use is reserved for the most severe cases, with the decision based on the patient's ability to maintain adequate cardiorespiratory function and adequate urinary output, and the inherent toxicity of the ingested drug, but principally on the effectiveness of these methods in removing the toxic substances.
    a. Hemodialysis and **hemoperfusion** are the most effective techniques of toxin removal. *Only substances with a small volume of distribution (< 1 liter/kg), low protein binding, and a small molecular weight will benefit from these methods.* However, hemodialysis offers the advantage of permitting correction of concomitant electrolyte or acid-base disturbances.
    b. Peritoneal dialysis is less effective and should be used only when hemodialysis or hemoperfusion cannot be performed (see Chap. 8, p. 236ff).
    c. Exchange transfusion is usually reserved for young children who cannot undergo hemodialysis or hemoperfusion (see Chap. 6, p. 163).
E. Antidotes. The number of ingestions for which there is a specific antidote is small. The following list includes the drugs or substances for which an antidote is available.
  1. Dimercaprol (British antilewisite [BAL]), for *arsenic, bismuth, chromium, cobalt, copper, iron, lead, magnesium, radium, selenium, and uranium.* The dose is 2–4 mg/kg/dose intramuscularly at intervals of 4–8 hours for 5 days and then 3 mg/kg/dose q12h (see sec. **III.D.1.b**).
  2. Dimercaptosuccinic acid (**DMSA,** Succimer) (see also sec. **III.D.1.d**) for lead. This drug has recently been approved by the Food and Drug Administration for treatment of children below the age of 12 only with lead levels > 45 µg/dl whole blood. The current regimen is 30 µg/kg/day in three divided doses for 5 days followed immediately by 20 µg/kg/day in two divided doses for 14 days. Abnormalities in hepatic enzymes, sometimes marked, have been noted, as well as vomiting and cutaneous reactions in patients receiving repeated courses of therapy. Blood lead values generally "rebound" to approximately 70 percent of their original value following cessation of therapy.
  3. Ethylenediaminetetraacetate (CaNa$_2$EDTA), for *lead, mercury, copper, nickel, zinc, cobalt, beryllium, and manganese.* The dose is 25–50 mg/kg/day

IM in two to four divided doses or IV in continuous infusion for 5 days. Add 0.5% procaine for IM use. **Only the calcium, disodium form, should be used to avoid severe hypocalcemia.**

4. **Penicillamine,** for *lead, copper, and mercury.* The dosage is 15–30 mg/kg/day PO in divided doses. The maximum daily dose is 1 gm (see sec. **III.D.1.c**).

5. **Amyl and sodium nitrite followed by sodium thiosulfate,** for *cyanide.* The dosage is as follows: sodium nitrite, 0.33 ml/kg of a 3% solution IV at a rate of 2.5–5.0 ml/min, followed in 15 minutes by sodium thiosulfate, 1.65 ml/kg of a 25% solution IV at a rate of 2.5–5.0 ml/min.

6. **Naloxone hydrochloride (Narcan),** for *narcotics and propoxyphene.* Give 0.1 mg/kg/dose IV (a 2-mg single dose in adolescents). If there is no response after 2 minutes, give 0.3 mg/kg IV. If there is a response, continue this therapy until a narcotic effect is no longer present.

7. **Vitamin K₁,** for *warfarin and bishydroxycoumarin.* The dose is 2–5 mg/kg IM or IV. Its brief elimination half-life requires its repeated administration.

8. **Desferoxamine,** for *iron.* The dose is 50 mg/kg IM (maximum 1 gm) q4h. For severe intoxication, give IV at a rate **not to exceed** 15 mg/kg/hr. Do not exceed 6 gm in 24 hours.

9. **Ethanol,** for *methanol and ethylene glycol.* The loading dose is 600 mg/kg IV (10% solution) or PO (50% solution), followed by a continuous infusion of 100–120 mg/kg/hr to maintain the blood ethanol level at 100 mg/dl. Higher doses are needed if the patient undergoes hemodialysis.

10. **Atropine sulfate** or **pralidoxime chloride** (Protopam), or both, for *organophosphate insecticides* (cholinesterase inhibitors)
    a. The dose of atropine is 1–4 mg or 0.05 mg/kg IV, with repeat doses of 2 mg at intervals of 2–5 minutes to reverse muscarinic effects until full atropinization is achieved and then as necessary to maintain atropinization.
    b. The dose of pralidoxime is 20–50 mg/kg given slowly IV, followed by a continuous infusion of 10–20 mg/kg/hr to reactivate phosphorylated acetylcholinesterase.

11. **Methylene blue,** for *methemoglobinemia* induced by nitrites, aniline dyes, chlorates, phenacetin, nitrobenzene, sulfonamides, quinones, and dapsone. The dose of methylene blue is 1–2 mg/kg IV as a 1% solution and is repeated in 4 hours if needed. Infants should receive no more than 4 mg/kg/day.

12. **Diphenhydramine (Benadryl),** for *phenothiazine extrapyramidal reactions.* The dose is 1–2 mg/kg IV q6h for four doses (maximum single dose is 50 mg IV). Benztropin (Cogentin) can be used alternatively in a dose of 1–2 mg.

13. **Oxygen** for *carbon monoxide* (100% O_2 for 30 min–4 hr)

14. **N-acetylcysteine,** for *acetaminophen intoxication.* Give 140 mg/kg PO as a loading dose and then 70 mg/kg q4h for 17 doses.

F. **Prevention. No course of therapy, no matter how trivial the ingestion, is complete without a discussion about why the poisoning occurred and a review of ways to ensure that the incident will not be repeated.** Recognition that the agent, an unpredictable child, and an emotionally or socially unstable milieu may play a part in poisoning is essential in such discussions.

II. **Specific ingestions.** Table 4-4 lists certain common substances of low toxicity that either necessitate no treatment when ingested or require only emesis when ingested in large quantities. The specific ingestions listed in this section were chosen because their management remains complex and difficult.

A. **Caustics**
   1. **Etiology.** The severity of the caustic burn is related to the concentration and duration of contact. Following ingestion, a **burn** ensues during the first week, **granulation tissue** during the second week, and **fibrosis** during the third week. Typical **acids** ingested are toilet-bowl cleaners, metal-cleaning fluids, and industrial bleaching products. Typical **alkalis** ingested are powerful detergents, toilet-bowl cleaners, and dishwasher and laundry granules.
   2. **Evaluation and diagnosis**
      a. **Pain** in the mouth and retrosternal area may be experienced. **Oropha-**

Table 4-4. Common ingestions of low toxicity

No treatment required	Removal necessary if large amounts ingested
Ballpoint inks	Aftershave lotion
Bar soap	Body conditioners
Bathtub floating toys	Colognes
Battery (dry cell)	Deodorants
Bubble bath soap	Fabric softeners
Candles	Hair dyes
Chalk	Hair sprays
Clay (modeling)	Hair tonic
Crayons with A.P., C.P., or C.S.	Indelible markers
130–46 designation	Matches (more than 20 wooden
Dehumidifying packets	matches or 2 books of paper matches)
Detergents (anionic)	No Doz
Eye makeup	Oral contraceptives
Fishbowl additives	Perfumes
Golf balls	Suntan preparations
Hand lotion and cream	Toilet water
Ink (blue, black, red)	Toothpaste
Lipstick	
Newspaper	
Pencils (lead and coloring)	
Putty and Silly Putty	
Sachets	
Shampoo	
Shaving cream and shaving lotions	
Shoe polish (occasionally, aniline dyes are present)	
Striking surface materials of matchboxes	
Sweetening agents (saccharin, cyclamate)	
Teething rings	
Thermometers	

ryngeal burns may develop. **The absence of oral burns and symptoms is not sure evidence against esophageal involvement.** Other symptoms include drooling, nausea, vomiting, abdominal pain, and bloody diarrhea.

   b. **Esophageal perforation** with mediastinitis and **gastric perforation** with peritonitis may occur. **Aspiration** may lead to pulmonary necrosis or glottic edema. Bacterial **superinfection** may occur during the first and second weeks, and **esophageal stricture** formation in later weeks.

   c. **Esophagoscopy** is the best way to determine the presence and extent of esophageal injury. If not, a **barium swallow** can sometimes reveal esophageal mucosal injury.

3. **Treatment**

   a. **Emesis and lavage are contraindicated.**

   b. **Neutralization with acids or alkalis is contraindicated.** The caustic should be washed off the esophagus with water or milk.

   c. Perforations, volume losses, and infection should be treated accordingly.

   d. Prophylactic antibiotics are not indicated.

B. **Hydrocarbons**

1. **Etiology**

   a. **Aromatic hydrocarbons** (benzene, toluene, xylene, styrene) affect mainly the CNS and pulmonary systems. The liver, kidney, myocardium, and bone marrow may also be involved. Organ toxicity results from **absorption** (Table 4-5).

  b. Aliphatic hydrocarbons (gasoline, naphtha, kerosene, lighter fluid) produce mainly pulmonary damage. Pulmonary involvement is caused by **aspiration** during ingestion or subsequent vomiting (see Table 4-5).

2. Evaluation

  a. Ingestion of hydrocarbons may induce **mucous membrane irritation,** nausea, vomiting, diarrhea, and perianal excoriation.

  b. Pulmonary involvement may be subclinical or evidenced by coughing, dyspnea, cyanosis, and rales.

   (1) Pneumatocele, pneumothorax, pleural effusion, and **pneumonia** may complicate the pulmonary picture.

   (2) Fever and **leukocytosis** with or without pulmonary involvement are frequently present in the first 48 hours.

   (3) Radiologic findings do not correlate with the clinical picture.

  c. CNS manifestations include restlessness, confusion, drowsiness, and coma.

3. Treatment

  a. Removal of **aromatic hydrocarbons** is indicated if an amount greater than 1 ml/kg has been ingested.

  b. For **aliphatic hydrocarbons,** the danger from aspiration is greater than the risk from GI absorption. Removal is indicated only if large amounts (> 5 ml/kg) have been ingested, or if a more toxic substance is ingested along with the hydrocarbon (metals, pesticides).

  c. In the **alert** patient, lavage may be a safer method than emesis with ipecac syrup. In the **obtunded** patient, protection of the lungs with a cuffed endotracheal tube and subsequent lavage constitute the therapy of choice.

  d. The use of activated charcoal is not indicated.

  e. For pulmonary involvement, oxygen, humidity, and bronchodilators may be necessary. Antibiotics should be reserved for superinfection.

  f. Present evidence does not support the use of corticosteroids.

  g. Infiltrates may take weeks to resolve fully.

  h. Management of CNS, liver, and renal involvement is supportive.

  i. Due to myocardial irritability, **sympathomimetic drugs should be avoided.**

Table 4-5. Petroleum products: Estimation of aspiration hazard versus systemic toxicity

Product	Source(s)	Systemic toxicity	Aspiration hazard*
Toluene, xylene, benzene, or ether	Industrial or rubber solvents	+ + +	+
Gasoline	Fuel	+	+ + +
Naphtha	Solvent, lighter fluid, dry cleaner, thinner	+	+ + +
Kerosene	Fuel, charcoal lighter fluid, thinner, pesticide solvent	+	+ + +
Mineral seal oil	Furniture polish	+	+ + +
Diesel oil	Fuel	+	+ +
Mineral oil		−	+
Lubricating oil	Motor oil, cutting oil, transmission fluid	−	−

+ = low risk; + + = moderate risk; + + + = high risk; − = no risk.
* Formulations with increased viscosity have decreased aspiration hazard.

C. Iron
   1. **Etiology.** Because iron tablets and vitamins with iron are ubiquitous in homes, iron ingestion is common.
   2. **Evaluation and diagnosis**
      a. Symptoms generally occur 30 minutes to 2 hours after ingestion. Early symptoms include vomiting, bloody diarrhea, abdominal cramps, and drowsiness.
      b. After the initial phase (6–24 hr after ingestion), fever, metabolic acidosis, hepatic impairment, restlessness, convulsions, shock, and coma may appear.
      c. **Stricture** of the GI tract is an infrequent and late complication, occurring 3–4 weeks after ingestion.
      d. Initial laboratory studies should include a complete blood count (CBC), glucose, serum electrolytes, serum iron, total iron-binding capacity (TIBC), and an x-ray film of the GI tract to detect the presence of radiopaque iron tablets.
   3. **Treatment**
      a. Early **emesis** with ipecac syrup is indicated if 20 mg/kg or more of elemental iron has been taken.
         (1) A flat plate of the abdomen should be obtained after emesis, to see if all iron tablets have been removed.
         (2) Activated charcoal is not indicated.
         (3) Sodium bicarbonate (50–100 ml of a 1% solution) by mouth may decrease absorption of iron. Hypernatremia may result from excessive amounts of sodium bicarbonate, however.
      b. IV fluids, sodium, bicarbonate, and volume expanders should be used to correct acidosis and fluid loss.
      c. **Deferoxamine**
         (1) **Chelation test**
            (a) **Indications** include:
               (i) History of a large amount ingested, with symptoms other than minimal vomiting and diarrhea *or*
               (ii) Serum iron level exceeding the TIBC *or*
               (iii) A symptomatic patient, with a white blood cell (WBC) count greater than 15,000 or glycemia greater than 150 mg/dl.
            (b) **Administration.** Deferoxamine, 50 mg/kg (maximum 1 gm), is given IM. The urine turns burgundy red (vin rose) when the serum iron level exceeds the TIBC (serum iron > 500 mg/dl).
         (2) **Deferoxamine therapy**
            (a) **Indications** include:
               (i) Coma or shock
               (ii) Serum iron level exceeding the TIBC
               (iii) Positive provocative chelation
            (b) **Administration**
               (i) The parenteral route, whether IM or IV, will depend on the clinical state of the patient and the serum concentration. The IM dose is 50 mg/kg (maximum 1 gm) q4h.
               (ii) In case of coma, hypotension, or acidosis, the IV route should be used. Give 50 mg/kg over 4 hours by slow infusion at a rate not exceeding 15 mg/kg/hr.
               (iii) Cessation of therapy is dictated by improvement in the patient's clinical condition, a serum iron concentration within normal range, and the disappearance of the color in the urine.
         (3) **Dialysis.** Iron is not dialyzable except when bound to deferoxamine. Dialysis is indicated only in the presence of oliguria or anuria.
D. Salicylates are one of the most common drugs encountered in poisonings of children less than 5 years of age.
   1. **Etiology.** Accidental ingestion of excess salicylate used at therapeutic doses

or ingestion of small amounts of oil of wintergreen (methyl salicylate). In general, victims of chronic salicylate poisoning are at higher risk for seizures and metabolic acidosis than those with acute single overdoses.

2. **Evaluation**

   a. Salicylates produce an initial respiratory alkalosis due to hyperventilation secondary to central stimulation. A state of metabolic acidosis, especially in young children, is quickly superimposed. Dehydration and worsening acidosis occur due to hyperventilation, renal solute loss, an increased metabolic rate, and vomiting. Presenting symptoms in the younger child generally include metabolic acidosis and respiratory alkalosis.

   b. The first symptoms seen in both alkalosis and acidosis are deep, rapid respiration, thirst, vomiting, and profuse sweating. In severe intoxication, confusion, delirium, coma, convulsions, circulatory collapse, and oliguria may ensue.

   c. Salicylates increase body metabolism, prolong prothrombin times, cause platelet dysfunction, and may induce either hyperglycemia or hypoglycemia. Peak serum levels occur 2–6 hours after ingestion. Of an ingested load of aspirin, 75 percent is excreted through the kidneys, and 25 percent is handled by hepatic metabolism.

   d. Initial laboratory studies include a CBC, electrolytes, blood gases, serum ketones, blood glucose, prothrombin time, serum salicylate level, urine acetone, pH, protein, and ferric chloride.

3. **Diagnosis.** Ingestion of 150 mg/kg will cause symptoms. A salicylate level of 50 mg/dl causes mild symptoms, 50–80 mg/dl produces symptoms of moderate severity, and 80–100 mg/dl causes severe symptoms. A level of 50 mg/dl or any symptoms (except mild hyperventilation) generally indicate that hospitalization is necessary.

4. **Treatment**

   a. Gastric evacuation is indicated when a toxic dose (> 150 mg/kg) has been ingested.

   b. IV fluids to replace fluid losses (see Chap. 7, p. 204) and adequate glucose to correct hypoglycemia

   c. Lowering of temperature elevation with tepid sponging

   d. Vitamin K can be administered to combat bleeding due to hypoprothrombinemia (although vitamin K–dependent and independent factors as well as platelet dysfunction are involved in coagulopathy).

   e. Alkalinization of the urine (2–3 mEq/kg of $NaHCO_3$ q4–6h) and monitoring of the urinary pH (keeping it above 7.5) will result in enhanced excretion of salicylates, with serum half-lives being lowered from 24–36 hours to 6–8 hours. Generous amounts of potassium (3–5 mEq/kg/day) are necessary to replace potassium loss and *alkalinize the urine*. Systemic pH should be monitored as well.

   f. Potentially fatal serum levels (100–150 mg/dl), oliguria or anuria, and cardiac disease are all indications for hemodialysis. A poor response to $NaHCO_3$, coma, and seizures are *relative* indications for dialysis.

   g. Repeated doses of oral activated charcoal will enhance elimination of activated charcoal via "gastrointestinal dialysis" and are recommended for serum levels > 50 mg/dl.

E. **Acetaminophen**

1. **Etiology.** At present, acetaminophen is used more than aspirin as an analgesic and antipyretic. It is consequently widely available in homes and is thus one of the drugs most frequently ingested by children and adolescents.

2. **Evaluation**

   a. The major target organ of acetaminophen overdose is the liver.

   b. Signs and symptoms within the first 12–24 hours of ingestion include nausea, vomiting, and diaphoresis. Evidence of hepatotoxicity appears 24–36 hours after ingestion and includes hepatic enlargement with tenderness and jaundice, hyperbilirubinemia, hyperammonemia, and prolongation of the prothrombin time. Liver biopsy shows focal hepatocyte cytolysis and centrizonal necrosis. Serum transaminase activity peaks by 3–4 days following ingestion and returns to normal within a week in those who recover.

c. Metabolites of acetaminophen, rather than the parent compound, are hepatotoxic. In overdose, normal metabolic pathways are saturated, and reactive intermediates are consequently formed that bind to liver macromolecules, causing liver necrosis.

d. The consequences of acetaminophen ingestion cannot be anticipated from the initial nonspecific signs. Although the history is often unreliable, a single ingested dose of 3 gm in a 2- or 3-year-old (approximately 150 mg/kg) and a dose greater than 8 gm in an adolescent may result in hepatic damage.

e. *An acetaminophen blood level drawn 4 or more hours following ingestion is the best predictor of subsequent hepatotoxicity.* When interpreted on the Rumack-Mathews nomogram (Fig. 4-1), a plasma concentration greater than 200 μg/ml at 4 hours or 50 μg/ml at 12 hours after ingestion is associated with probable hepatotoxicity (i.e., transaminases exceeding 1,000 IU/liter).

f. Acetaminophen overdose must be distinguished from Reye syndrome, amino acid disorders, and alpha-1-antitrypsin deficiency in the child and from drug abuse (alcohol, heroin, volatile hydrocarbons) and Wilson's disease in the adolescent.

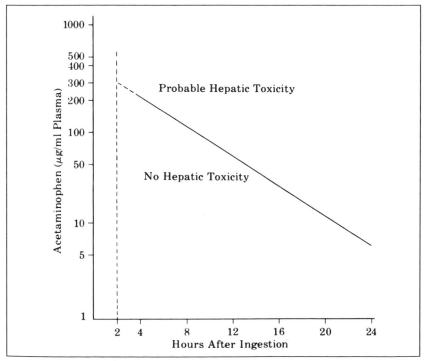

Fig. 4-1. Semilogarithmic plot of plasma acetaminophen concentration versus time based on data from adult patients. Patients with concentrations above the line at the corresponding times after ingestion may develop hepatotoxicity. Patients with concentrations below the line have a low probability of developing hepatotoxicity. (From B. H. Rumack and H. Mathews, *Pediatrics* 55:871, 1975. Copyright © 1975 by the American Academy of Pediatrics.)

3. **Treatment**
   a. Removal of the ingested dose with ipecac syrup or gastric lavage when the patient is seen within 4 hours of ingestion
   b. Activated charcoal will bind acetaminophen and should be administered if the patient presents within 4 hours after ingestion. After this interval, activated charcoal is only warranted if other ingested toxins are suspected. In these cases, activated charcoal can be administered with N-acetylcysteine (Mucomyst) since, despite 10–39 percent adsorption of Mucomyst to activated charcoal, Mucomyst doses are far in excess of those needed for hepatoprotection.
   c. Avoid enzyme inducers such as phenobarbital.
   d. Avoid forcing fluids or ionized diuresis.
   e. When acetaminophen has been taken in high doses, or when acetaminophen levels are in the range that is likely to cause hepatotoxicity, N-acetylcysteine should be administered. The loading dose is 140 mg/kg PO. Maintenance doses of 70 mg/kg q4h should be administered thereafter for 17 doses. Once the need for N-acetylcysteine is determined, *all* doses must be given. N-acetylcysteine should be diluted to a 5% solution before it is administered and repeated if vomiting occurs within 1 hour of administration. Placing the solution on ice with a lidded cup will inhibit the release of nauseating sulfurous fumes. An intravenous form is under investigation.

F. **Theophylline**
   1. **Etiology.** Theophylline is a widely used xanthine bronchodilator.
   2. **Evaluation**
      a. **Signs and symptoms** are widely disparate depending on whether the intoxication is the result of acute or chronic ingestion. In general, those in whom toxicity develops after chronic ingestion have a greater risk of seizures and arrhythmias.
         (1) **GI symptoms** are the most frequent and include nausea, vomiting, and hematemesis.
         (2) **CNS toxicity** includes agitation, restlessness, irritability, or mild obtundation. **Seizures** may occur in severe poisonings.
         (3) **Mild supraventricular tachycardia** is frequent, but life-threatening arrhythmias are less frequent than in adults.
         (4) **Hypokalemia** is common, particularly in acute overdoses.
      b. Therapeutic serum concentrations range between 10 and 20 µg/ml. The severity of the toxicity increases with increasing serum concentrations. Life-threatening arrhythmias and seizures usually occur with serum concentrations greater than 80–100 µg/ml after acute overdose.
      c. **Prolonged absorption** (as long as 17–36 hr) may occur after an overdose, especially with slow-release preparations.
   3. **Treatment**
      a. Remove theophylline by inducing emesis with ipecac syrup or, if necessary, by gastric lavage.
      b. Repeated doses of activated charcoal and ionic cathartics are indicated (see secs. **I.C** and **E**).
      c. Theophylline serum concentrations should be obtained and followed q4h to evaluate the effectiveness of treatment.
      d. Do not induce fluid diuresis.
      e. Diazepam, phenytoin, and/or phenobarbital should be used in the treatment of seizures (see Chap. 3, p. 66).
      f. Monitor for cardiac arrhythmias.
      g. **Hemodialysis or hemoperfusion** should be considered in patients who are unresponsive to adequate supportive care and/or have serum concentrations above 80–100 µg/ml.

G. **Tricyclic antidepressants**
   1. **Etiology.** These drugs are widely prescribed for mood disorders. Overdoses are frequently intentional. Other drugs may be ingested concomitantly.

2. **Evaluation**
   a. Signs or symptoms usually develop within 4 hours of ingestion. Anticholinergic signs, including mydriasis, dry mucous membranes, tachycardia, and decreased peristalsis, are usually the first to appear.
   b. Confusion, agitation, and hallucinations or various stages of coma may be present. Seizures may also occur.
   c. **Sinus tachycardia** is present in virtually every intoxication, but serious cardiac arrhythmias occur in patients with serum concentrations greater than 1,000 ng/ml and/or a prolongation of the QRS complex greater than 100 msec. Ventricular arrhythmias, conduction blocks, and hypotension may occur.
3. **Treatment**
   a. Gastric emptying by gastric lavage is indicated. Ipecac is relatively contraindicated because of the risk of rapid onset of seizures or coma.
   b. Activated charcoal and cathartic should be administered and repeated q4–6h for 24 hours in severe intoxication.
   c. Fluid diuresis, dialysis, or hemoperfusion is **ineffective.**
   d. **Seizures** should be treated with diazepam, followed if necessary by phenytoin or phenobarbital (see Chap. 3, p. 66).
   e. **Cardiac arrhythmias** should be treated with appropriate agents (see Chap. 9, p. 249).
   f. **Hypotension** should be treated with fluid followed by vasopressors (dopamine, dobutamine, or norepinephrine) if necessary.
   g. Continuous cardiac monitoring can be ended when the patient has been completely asymptomatic and the electrocardiogram normal for 24 hours.
H. **Substances of abuse**
   1. **Etiology.** Drugs and chemicals abused by adolescents and young adults depend on age, sex, race, socioeconomic group, and geographic location.
   2. **CNS depressants** include narcotics, hypnotic-sedative agents (barbiturates and nonbarbiturates), benzodiazepines (e.g., diazepam, chlordiazepoxide), and alcohols.
      a. **Evaluation**
         (1) Following an acute overdose, all induce CNS depression (see Table 3-4) and cardiorespiratory depression as well.
         (2) Pupils are usually small, or constricted in the case of narcotics.
         (3) Reflexes are diminished. Seizures are more frequent with propoxyphene, meperidine, and methaqualone.
         (4) In ethanol intoxication there is a correlation between ethanol serum concentration and CNS effects:
            (a) Blood concentrations above 100–150 mg/dl: ataxia and incoordination
            (b) Blood concentrations 150–300 mg/dl: dysarthria, visual disturbances, and somnolence
            (c) Blood concentrations 300–500 mg/dl: coma
            (d) Above 500 mg/dl: potentially lethal
         (5) Hypoglycemia is associated with alcohol intoxication in young children.
         (6) All these substances can produce physical and psychological dependence. Withdrawal symptoms can be expected with their abrupt cessation. However, severe manifestations, such as **seizures, delirium, cardiovascular collapse,** and **possibly death,** are seen only in the case of alcohol and barbiturate withdrawal.
      b. **Therapy**
         (1) **If the patient is comatose,** administer naloxone, 0.1 mg/kg IV. If there is no response within 1 minute, administer 0.3 mg/kg IV. If there is still no response, narcotic overdose is probably **ruled out.** If naloxone is successful in reducing coma, continue to administer it as needed.
         (2) **GI decontamination** should be instituted (see sec. **I.C**). Adequate supportive care (e.g., of respiration, circulation) should be provided.

(3) Hemodialysis should be considered for patients with severe ethanol intoxication that is unresponsive to adequate supportive care and/or with serum ethanol concentrations above 500 mg/dl.

3. **CNS stimulants** include amphetamines and amphetamine-like drugs, caffeine, and cocaine.

a. **Evaluation**

(1) Increased CNS excitation may culminate in seizures.

(2) Pulse rate and blood pressure are increased.

(3) The pupils are dilated and the reflexes hyperactive.

(4) These substances can induce psychological and physical dependence. The withdrawal syndrome is characterized by lack of energy, prolonged periods of sleep, increased appetite, and psychological depression.

b. **Therapy**

(1) Following acute intoxication, GI decontamination measures (see sec. I.C) should be instituted.

(2) Hypertension is usually of short duration and rarely necessitates treatment. If necessary, phentolamine or nitroprusside can be used.

(3) **Amphetamine psychotic reaction** can be treated with chlorpromazine or haloperidol. Diazepam is the drug of choice for the treatment of **hyperactivity** and **seizures.**

(4) Acidification of the urine with ammonium chloride and ascorbic acid can enhance amphetamine elimination, but induces metabolic acidosis and is not recommended.

4. **Substances that modify CNS perception** include the hallucinogens phencyclidine (PCP), lysergic acid diethylamide (LSD), and mescaline; the cannabis group including marijuana and hashish; and volatile inhalants, namely, butyl nitrites and hydrocarbon (sniffing).

a. **Evaluation**

(1) Hallucinogens induce euphoria, anxiety, or panic. The affect is inappropriate; the patient experiences time and visual distortion and visual hallucinations.

(2) PCP overdose produces extreme hyperactivity or cyclic coma, nystagmus, muscle rigidity, seizures, and hypertension. The pupils may be large or small. Flashbacks may occur.

(3) The cannabis group usually induces a state of euphoria and feeling of well-being. Hallucinations are rare. The pupils are unchanged but the conjunctivae are injected.

(4) Transient euphoria can be experienced by volatile inhalant users. Cardiac arrhythmias are the major acute complication. Lead intoxication can occur with gasoline sniffing. Butyl nitrite can produce methemoglobinemia.

(5) Physical dependence on substances that modify CNS perception does not develop. Psychological dependence is possible. No withdrawal syndrome is seen.

b. **Therapy**

(1) The patient with hallucinations or distorted perceptions should be provided a quiet and safe environment.

(2) Physical or chemical restraints should be avoided. If necessary, diazepam can be used (0.1 mg/kg PO or IV [maximum 10–20 mg]).

(3) GI decontamination measures should be reserved for the severely intoxicated (i.e., comatose) patient.

(4) Acidification of the urine may enhance PCP elimination.

III. Lead poisoning

A. **Etiology.** Lead poisoning in childhood results mainly from the ingestion of lead-based paint or plaster, or other materials or objects saturated or coated with lead-based paint (lead content > 0.06%) and from ingesting lead-containing soil (500 ppm) and household dust. Airborne lead contributes to increased lead absorption by ingestion of fallout on soil or dust rather than by direct inhalation. Infants may be at risk when fed formula prepared with lead-contaminated water. Recent studies indicate that blacks have a greater incidence of lead poisoning than whites, irrespective of socioeconomic status, but the reason is obscure. Malnutrition enhances lead absorption and toxicity. The incidence is highest among the urban poor, but cases can be readily found among suburban, middle-class children, particularly when they reside in older homes (pre-1950) where renovation is occurring. Predisposing factors include iron, calcium, and zinc deficiency; conditions of poor, older housing; low socioeconomic status; and pica.

B. **Evaluation**

1. The **history** should emphasize the location, age, and condition of the home or other frequented areas. Although common, the presence of pica is not a sine qua non in lead poisoning. Questions should be asked about the child's appetite, bowel habits, general behavior, and nutrition, as well as about signs of irritability and lethargy.

2. A **complete physical examination** should include a thorough neurologic examination, a developmental assessment and, if possible, a psychometric examination.

3. **Laboratory studies**

a. Blood lead levels should be determined by **venous samples** whenever possible, to avoid the problem of skin contamination by lead-laden soil. If a fingerstick sample is used, the finger should be carefully washed and rinsed. Elevated fingerstick lead levels should be confirmed promptly by follow-up venipuncture before consideration of therapy.

b. Erythrocyte protoporphyrin (EP) reflects lead toxicity when blood lead levels exceed 30 μg/dl, as well as iron deficiency. Since the interpretation of values is complicated by the effect of iron deficiency on EP, **absolute criteria for lead poisoning are difficult to establish.** Normal mean EP levels are 18 μg/dl whole blood. Up to 35 μg/dl whole blood is presently considered acceptable in the absence of anemia. Because EP is insensitive to Pb levels < 25 μg/dl, it is no longer recommended for screening. In the presence of iron deficiency alone, EP values of 50–125 μg/dl whole blood are common. **However, levels of this kind can be due to moderate lead poisoning as well.** In general, values of EP above 100 μg/dl whole blood usually reflect some effect of lead exposure. Other causes of elevated EP include porphyria, sickle cell disease, acute viral illness, and liver disease.

Because 1–3 weeks of lead exposure is required to elevate protoporphyrin levels, it is possible for lead levels to be elevated in the presence of normal EP. For a complete discussion, see the Centers for Disease Control's (CDC's) pamphlet, *Preventing Lead Poisoning in Young Children*, 1991.

c. **Other blood tests.** Blood tests in any child with elevated blood lead, EP, or both should include a CBC, with attention to basophilic stippling of the erythrocyte, iron and iron-binding capacity, serum ferritin, blood urea nitrogen (BUN), and serum creatinine. **Even in the absence** of clinical anemia, elevated levels of EP can be due to lead poisoning, iron deficiency, or both.

d. **X-ray films** of the knees are helpful in detecting widening and increased density of the zones of provisional calcification in the distal femur, proximal tibia, and proximal fibula (chronic ingestion). Anteroposterior views of the abdomen should be obtained for radiopacities (acute ingestion). Knee films in children 18–30 months of age should be interpreted cautiously, since a wide range of normal changes during rapid growth can mimic "lead lines." However, when widening and increased density of the zone of provisional calcification include the proximal fibulas as well as the proximal tibia and distal femur, the likelihood is increased that chronic exposure to a heavy metal, most probably lead, is responsible for the findings. In general, lead lines are associated with prolonged (i.e., > 6 weeks) Pb levels > 50 μg/dl.

e. **If encephalopathy is suspected, a computed tomographic (CT) scan of the skull should be obtained immediately to evaluate the possibility of cerebral edema.**

f. **Lumbar puncture is contraindicated** unless it is certain that cerebrospinal fluid (CSF) pressure is not increased. Lumbar puncture adds little to the evaluation, and the findings do not affect therapy.

g. **Lead mobilization test (provocative chelation)**

(1) In children with only moderate elevations of blood lead (i.e., 35–45 μg/dl) in whom the results of the preceding tests are conflicting or who have already undergone chelation therapy, the lead mobilization test can clarify the size of the **mobilizable** pool of lead. Because this pool has been correlated with indicators of toxicity, a positive lead mobilization test should be considered an indication for therapy.

(2) **Procedure.** 1,000 mg/M^2/24 hr or 35 mg/kg calcium disodium EDTA is administered IM or by IV drip over one hour. The dose can be divided or given in toto in a single dose. Urine is collected quantitatively for up to 24 hours. The test is positive if the 24-hour collection yields more than 1 μg lead/mg EDTA injected. Alternatively, on an outpatient basis, a shorter urine collection (6–8 hr) can be used, with a concomitant reduction in the yield of lead. Because the large bulk of lead is excreted within 6–12 hours following the EDTA dose, an excretion of 0.5–0.7 μg lead/mg EDTA injected is considered positive. Under some conditions, a smaller "yield" could still be considered an indication for chelation therapy, particularly in a very young child or in a child with lingering elevated lead levels. Note that determinations of the urinary **concentration** of lead are **not helpful.** It is the **absolute** excretion of lead per time interval per chelation dose that is measured, requiring good hydration and quantitative urine collections during the test, which is no mean feat in the toddler who is not yet toilet trained.

h. **Nerve conduction times** may be abnormal, particularly in children with sickle cell disease, but have little clinical value.

i. **Routine urinalysis** may show pyuria, casts, glucosuria, or aminoaciduria, particularly when lead levels exceed 100 μg/dl. A Fanconi-type tubular acidosis characterized by aminoaciduria, glucosuria, and hypophosphatemia may be found in such patients.

C. **Diagnosis** (see Table 4-6)

D. **Therapy. At all costs, the source of lead must be identified and removed despite the existence of other problems.**

1. **Commonly used chelating agents** are EDTA, BAL, ᴅ-penicillamine, and DMSA. (For a discussion of the use of chelating agents, see *J. Pediatr.* 73:1, 1968; *J. Pediatr.* 105:523, 1984; and CDC's pamphlet, *Preventing Lead Poisoning in Young Children,* 1991.)

a. **EDTA**

(1) **Mechanism of action.** Urinary lead excretion is increased 20- to 50-fold. Lead is removed from the soft tissues but **not** from red blood cells. Bone pools of lead are reduced after multiple chelations with EDTA. EDTA crosses the blood-brain barrier poorly and enhances removal of other metals, notably zinc.

(2) **Route of administration.** EDTA can be given IV or IM. When it is given IV, a slow drip gives the best results and is safest. In IM administration, EDTA should be given with procaine (0.5–2.0%) in deep injection. To avoid enhanced absorption of lead from the GI tract, **oral EDTA is contraindicated.**

(3) **Dosage.** Under most circumstances, a total daily dose of 1,000 mg/M^2 will provide sufficient lead diuresis. This dose is administered for 3–5 days sequentially and then discontinued for at least 48 hours to permit clearance of the lead-EDTA complexes and permit some reequilibration of lead stores. Under these conditions, as many

Table 4-6. Clinical and laboratory evidence of lead intoxication

Mild	Moderate	Severe
Clinical		
Lead exposure, usually to soil or dust	Probably paint exposure	Pica for paint
Asymptomatic	Predisposing iron deficiency	Secondary iron deficiency
May be predisposing iron deficiency	Positive family history	Abdominal pain, irritability, lethargy, fever, hepatosplenomegaly
Cognitive sequelae	Usually asymptomatic	
	Loss of appetite and behavior changes	Ataxia, seizures, coma, increased ICP, neurologic sequelae
	Behavioral and cognitive sequelae	
Laboratory		
Lead levels in whole blood 25–49 μg/dl	Lead levels 49–70 μg/dl	Lead levels > 70 μg/ml
EP in whole blood 35–125 μg/dl	EP in whole blood 125–250 μg/dl	EP levels > 250 μg/dl
KUB and knee x-rays usually negative	KUB x-rays negative	KUB x-rays positive
Serum iron/iron-binding capacity ≤ 16%	Knee x-rays positive	Knee films positive
Serum ferritin < 40 μg/ml	Serum iron/iron-binding capacity ≤ 16%	Serum iron/iron-binding capacity ≤ 16%
CBC normal	Ferritin < 20 μ/dl	Ferritin < 10 μg/dl
Lead mobilization test: ≤ or ≅ 1 μg Pb/mg EDTA/24 hr	CBC shows mild anemia	CBC shows basophilic stippling, anemia
	Lead mobilization test: ≅ 1 μg Pb/mg EDTA/24 hr	Decreased nerve conduction time
		CT scan shows increased ICP
		Aminoaciduria, glycosuria
		Lead mobilization test: > 1 μg Pb/mg EDTA/24 hr

ICP = intracranial pressure; KUB = kidneys, ureters, bladder.

courses of EDTA as indicated can be administered. As a rule, the longer the hiatus between courses of EDTA, the lower the risk of toxicity. In severe lead poisoning (blood lead ≥ 80 μg/dl or symptoms present), EDTA should only be used in conjunction with BAL. In this case, the dose can be increased to 1,500 mg/M², **although the risk of renal toxicity is thereby also increased.**

    (4) Toxicity. The kidney is the principal site of toxicity, with renal effects seen at doses as low as 65 mg/kg/24 hr. The risk of toxicity is increased in patients with very high lead burdens. During chelation, daily urinalyses and careful monitoring of BUN, creatinine, and calcium should be done. Although hypocalcemia is avoided by the use of the calcium salt of EDTA, **hyper**calcemia, usually mild, can be seen with prolonged therapy. **Recent animal studies have suggested that single doses of EDTA may actually increase brain lead, albeit transiently. However, the doses used range from 75–150 mg/kg and no long-term follow-up was reported. Therefore, application of these data to human use at the doses recommended remains doubtful. Other toxic effects** include removal of zinc and other metals. When chelation therapy is completed, replacement of iron and, if indicated, zinc should be undertaken.

    b. BAL

      (1) Mechanism of action. Two molecules of BAL combine with one of heavy metal to form a stable complex. Fecal as well as urinary excretion of lead is enhanced. In addition, BAL diffuses well into erythrocytes. It can be administered in the presence of renal impairment because it is predominantly excreted in bile.

(2) **Route of administration.** BAL is available only for IM administration in, of all things, peanut oil.

(3) **Dosage.** The usual dosage is 300 mg/M^2/day (up to 600 mg/M^2/day in severe cases) in three to six divided doses. Since BAL is mainly used to lower the blood lead rapidly, it need not be given for a full 5 days with EDTA (see **E.2.d**); 48–72 hours may suffice, **provided EDTA is continued.**

(4) **Toxicity.** Toxic reactions may occur in as many as 50 percent of patients. A febrile reaction peculiar to children occurs in 30 percent, which may lead to the erroneous conclusion that infection is present. The presence of a transient granulocytopenia may further confuse the observer. In both adults and children, other reactions include transient hypertension, nausea, headache, burning sensation of the oropharynx, conjunctivitis, rhinorrhea and excessive salivation, paresthesias, a burning sensation in the penis, sweating, abdominal pain, and occasional sterile abscesses. Such reactions are most likely with the inappropriate use of BAL, i.e., when heavy metal concentration is relatively low. It is **contraindicated in patients who are sensitive to peanuts.**

c. **D-Penicillamine,** an oral chelating agent, is particularly useful in the treatment of low-level lead poisoning (i.e., blood Pb 20–35 µg/dl).

(1) **Mechanism of action.** D-Penicillamine enhances the urinary excretion of lead. Lead is not removed from erythrocytes but may be from bone. Excreted lead is not necessarily in the form of chelated complexes, and the specific mechanism is not well understood.

(2) **Route of administration.** The D-isomer is administered PO. It is currently available as both 125- and 250-mg capsules and scored 250-mg tablets. The capsules can be opened or the tablets crushed and suspended in liquid, if necessary. Strong fruit flavor masks the bitter taste. It should not be given with dairy products or iron.

(3) The usual **oral dose** is 20–40 mg/kg (600–1,200 mg/M^2). Side effects can be minimized by initiating therapy with small doses; e.g., 25 percent of the expected dose, increasing after 1 week to 50 percent, and again after 1 week to the full dose, as well as by monitoring for toxicity.

(4) **Toxicity and side effects.** The D-isomer of penicillamine is relatively nontoxic. However, in our experience as many as 30 percent of patients receiving the drug will experience some form of mild toxicity, usually reactions resembling those of penicillin sensitivity, including rashes, transient leukopenia and/or thrombocytopenia, and eosinophilia. Anorexia, nausea, and vomiting are infrequent. Of most concern, however, are isolated reports of nephrotoxicity, possibly from hypersensitivity reactions. We have noted reversible hematuria, frequency, and enuresis in a few patients. Toxicity may be reduced by concurrent administration of pyridoxine, although no controlled studies of this effect are available. **D-Penicillamine should not be administered to patients with known penicillin allergy.**

d. **Dimercaptosuccinic acid (DMSA, Succimer)** is an oral, water-soluble, congener of BAL. Recently approved by the FDA for use in children under 12 (it is the *only* drug in the USP licensed for use exclusively in children), it is indicated for treatment when lead levels exceed 45 µg/dl. Because children with Pb levels this high are more likely to have pica for paint chips, it is doubly important that the clinician ascertain that patients have been removed from the lead hazard *before* oral therapy with DMSA is instituted. This may and often does require hospitalization for the child's protection. DMSA is presently undergoing clinical trials for treatment of children with lead levels > 25 µg/dl.

(1) Mechanisms of action. DMSA dramatically lowers blood lead, but its effect on soft tissue lead burden has, in our experience, been disappointing, requiring several courses of therapy to adequately deplete the body burden of lead. It is specific for removing lead alone, in contrast to other chelators. Iron can be given concurrently. DMSA should not be used in symptomatic patients.

(2) Route of administration. DMSA is administered PO. It is presently available in 100-mg pelletized capsules that can be opened and sprinkled on food or in juice.

(3) The usual oral dosage is 30 mg/kg/day in three divided doses (q8h) for 5 days followed by 20 mg/kg/day in two divided doses (q12h) for 14 days. Although blood lead is initially lowered dramatically, "rebound" values 1–2 weeks following completion of a course of therapy reach 70 percent of the original value or even higher. Thus, multiple courses of therapy will be needed to reach steady-state blood levels < 15 µg/dl.

(4) Toxicity and side effects. The principal toxicity is to the liver, producing mild and apparently transient elevations of AST, ALT, and lactic acid dehydrogenase (LDH). However, marked changes in alkaline phosphatase may occur. Experience with this drug is too limited to date to estimate the long-term significance of this hepatotoxicity. Cutaneous urticaria-like reactions have been reported in patients receiving multiple courses of DMSA. Vomiting is a common side effect. Although DMSA is an oxidizing agent, there have been no reports of hemolysis in the presence of glucose 6-phosphate dehydrogenase (G-6-PD) deficiency. Nonetheless, it is prudent to establish the patient's G-6-PD status either before or during therapy lest hemolysis unexpectedly appear.

2. Monitoring chelation therapy. If needed, 24-hour quantitative urinary lead excretion can be used to monitor the effectiveness of chelation therapy, since the blood lead can be misleadingly low in the presence of chelating agents. However, blood Pb should be followed closely during therapy (q48–72h for inpatients and q2–4 weeks for outpatients).

a. During chelation therapy with EDTA, serum calcium, BUN, and lead in the blood and urine, as well as urinalyses, are monitored for evidence of hypocalcemia or renal toxicity. If such evidence is present, EDTA can be reduced or discontinued, and renal function usually returns to normal.

b. In encephalopathic patients, symptoms may worsen during therapy. Removal of lead with BAL should continue, with attention to CNS changes suggestive of cerebral edema (see **E.3**). It may be wise to discontinue EDTA temporarily in such situations to reduce fluid requirements.

c. Patients receiving DMSA should have baseline liver function tests as well as BUN and creatinine. These should be repeated q5–7 days during therapy.

d. EDTA is administered for 3–5 days at a time. In general, urinary lead excretion tends to fall off after the fourth day regardless of the lead burden, while the risk of EDTA nephrotoxicity increases after the fifth day. For this reason, EDTA chelation is interrupted after 5 days, and a "rest period" of at least 48–72 hours is initiated. If the initial lead burden is very high, chelation is again begun after 48–72 hours, and a new 24-hour urine lead is obtained for comparison. In this manner, as many EDTA chelations as are indicated by the lead burden can be undertaken without significant risk until such time as the initial 24-hour urine lead excretion fails to yield ≥ 1 µg lead/mg EDTA. Therapy is then discontinued and long-term follow-up begun. Subsequent chelation may well be necessary, but a longer hiatus between chelations can now ensue.

e. Because of the "rebound" phenomenon during reequilibration of body lead stores, blood lead and EP levels immediately following chelation tend to be misleading and are best obtained 1–2 weeks following therapy.

    f. The goal of therapy is to reduce body lead burden to safe levels (i.e., blood lead < 15 μg/dl) and EP to normal (i.e., < 35 μg/dl). Because chelation therapy tends to be less efficient as the body burden is lowered, the clinician must exercise judgment to decide when enough therapy has been administered. Such factors as the child's age, degree of exposure, likelihood of continued exposure, discomfort, and side effects of chelation must be weighed. In general, the most complete therapy should be applied to children under 3 years of age.

E. Management of plumbism. The criteria for chelation therapy proposed in Table 4-7 are intended as guidelines. Each child is different. Important variables include age, duration of exposure, and risk factors such as iron deficiency, sickle cell disease, and developmental levels.

    1. Mild lead poisoning (Pb < 5–34 μg/dl)

        a. Identify and remove the **lead source.** Parents can help by vacuuming and wet-mopping the home to reduce lead dust.

        b. Administer **oral iron** (6 mg/kg elemental iron/24 hr) to correct iron deficiency and reduce further lead absorption.

        c. Repeat lead and EP determination monthly or more frequently. If values remain > 20 μg/dl longer than 2 months, consider D-penicillamine.

        d. D-Penicillamine (900 mg/M²/24 hr in two divided doses PO) may be useful in reducing an intractable low-level lead burden. The possibility of continued lead exposure, although not desirable, is not a contraindication to the use of D-penicillamine. Oral iron therapy should be discontinued in this situation.

    2. Moderate lead poisoning (35–59 μg/dl)

        a. Identify and remove the **lead source.** If "deleading" is undertaken, remove the child **completely** from the home during the process and until a thorough cleanup is completed. **Permitting children to return home at night during the deleading of a home risks further serious exposure.**

        b. Administer oral iron (see **1.b**) for 1 month or until EP stabilizes.

        c. If the lead level is 35–45 μg/dl, administer a lead mobilization test.

        d. If the lead mobilization test is **positive,** begin chelation therapy by administration of calcium disodium EDTA (Versenate) for 3–5 consecutive days, giving 1,000 mg/M²/day IM in single doses with procaine. Hospitalization is not necessary unless daily clinic or office visits are not feasible.

        e. Daily urinalyses, BUN, creatinine, and lead and iron studies should be obtained on the first and fifth days of treatment.

        f. If further chelation therapy is warranted, provide a hiatus of at least 48–72 hours between courses of treatment.

        g. After chelation therapy is completed, restart iron therapy until both lead and EP values have returned to normal.

        h. It is likely that more than one course of chelation therapy will be needed. Parents should be informed of this as early as possible to enlist their cooperation in the treatment process.

        i. Mild, transient elevations of blood lead following chelation therapy are commonly due to "rebound" (reequilibration of residual body stores of

Table 4-7. Indications for chelation therapy

1. Venous blood lead ≥ 50 μg/dl on two successive occasions, *or*
2. Venous blood lead ≥ 25–49 μg/dl and EP ≥ 125 μg/dl *or*
3. Positive lead mobilization test

Factors contributing to indications
    Age, degree of exposure, underlying developmental level, iron deficiency

lead) rather than reexposure. However, reexposure can and does occur, and is usually accompanied by significant increases in EP values shortly afterward.

j. If the lead level is > 45 μg/dl *and* the lead source has been identified *and* the child is in safe housing, begin a course of DMSA as described on p. 117.

k. Iron therapy can be continued *during* therapy with DMSA.

l. Monitor Pb, CBC, LFTs, BUN, and creatine and urine sediment on day 5–7, day 14, and day 21.

m. Check for rebound at 14 days and 28 days postchelation.

3. **Severe lead poisoning without encephalopathy**
   a. **Identify and remove the lead source.**
   b. **Hospitalize** the child.
   c. Give 1.5 times the usual **maintenance fluids** (see Chap. 7, p. 201).
   d. If the blood lead level exceeds 80 μg/dl, begin BAL IM in three divided doses of 300 mg/M^2/24 hr or 48–72 hours.
   e. Administer EDTA IV if possible in continuous infusion or IM if necessary (1,500 mg/M^2 daily in three divided doses). If the IM route is chosen, the dose can be given bid or even in a single injection *or:*
   f. If the blood lead < 80 μg/dl, a course of DMSA can be begun, provided the child is in the hospital. After 5 days of therapy, *if safe housing has been found*, the child can be discharged to receive the remaining 2 weeks of therapy on an ambulatory basis.
   g. Monitor BUN, blood, 24-hour urine lead (EDTA), LFTs (DMSA), and urinalyses.
   h. After chelation is completed, administer iron (see **1.b**) if it was not already given.

4. **Severe lead intoxication with encephalopathy**
   a. **This is a medical emergency.** Treatment should be administered in an intensive care unit, if possible.
   b. Give maintenance fluids.
   c. Begin BAL IM, 600 mg/M^2/day in six divided doses.
   d. Begin EDTA IV, 1,500 mg/M^2/day in three divided doses by slow drip.
   e. Treat cerebral edema with mannitol and dexamethasone (Decadron) (see Chap. 3, p. 71).
   f. **Continue chelation therapy at all costs, because cerebral edema will not respond to therapy until the lead burden is reduced.**
   g. Treat seizures with anticonvulsants (see Table 19-3).
   h. After 5 days, discontinue therapy for 48 hours and restart.
   i. Monitor BUN, calcium, electroencephalograms, urinalysis findings, and blood and 24-hour urine lead.
   j. Several courses of chelation will be needed.

5. **Sequelae.** Both symptomatic **and** asymptomatic lead poisoning produce sequelae. Gross screening tests are generally not sensitive enough to distinguish subtle deficits and are frequently performed in children too young to provide reproducible results.

   All children with histories of increased lead burden should undergo thorough neuropsychological evaluation before entering school, ideally at ages 5–6. At a minimum, this should include evaluation of visual-motor skills, expressive and receptive language skills, visual and auditory perceptual skills, and fine and gross motor skills. IQ testing may be misleading because it fails to reflect specific functional deficits. The clinician can alert the school to a child's deficits and recommend remedial or special education. Conversely, when no deficit is found, the family and school authorities can be appropriately reassured. Behavior problems related to lead poisoning, such as hyperactivity, may respond to pharmacologic therapy (see Chap. 20).

F. **Prevention. Lead poisoning is a preventable disease.** Federal law prohibits the sale of leaded paint. Many states now have strong penalties for nonremoval of lead from houses in cases of plumbism. **Proper precautions are needed** during deleading and renovation of old housing lest incidental exposure occur. Children should be removed completely from such homes while such work is going on. Heating and sanding of lead paint are particularly dangerous and should be avoided and scraping or chemical stripping used. Intensive screening of children to identify those at risk, widespread inspection of housing, and stringent enforcement of sanitary and housing codes can reduce morbidity in this disease.

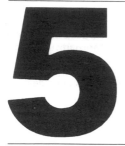

Management of the Normal Newborn

DeWayne M. Pursley and
Douglas K. Richardson

I. **Anticipation of high-risk delivery.** The majority of deliveries results in healthy newborns. However, it is essential to identify maternal, fetal, perinatal, and neonatal conditions associated with newborns at high risk for development of significant illness. If possible, infants under 32 weeks' gestation and those with known anomalies should be delivered in a hospital with an intensive care nursery. Intensive perinatal management (tocolytics, steroids, and fetal monitoring) can minimize asphyxia and delay delivery to allow for greater fetal lung maturation.

A. **General antenatal assessment.** Clinical, behavioral, and demographic factors associated with high-risk pregnancy are listed in Table 5-1. The important information to obtain in a high-risk pregnancy is gestational age, maturity of specific organ systems, fetal size and rate of growth, and evidence of fetal/placental health. Obstetric dating should supersede pediatric estimates unless there is a major discrepancy (> 2 weeks).

1. **Gestational age** is a composite estimate based on any or all of the following:
   a. **Date of the last menstrual period.** The estimated date of confinement (EDC) can be quickly estimated by McDonald's rule: add 7 days and subtract 3 months.
   b. **Date of first reported fetal activity.** "Quickening" is first felt at approximately 16–18 weeks.
   c. **Date of first recorded fetal heart sounds.** These are first detected at approximately 10–12 weeks by ultrasonic Doppler and by about 20 weeks by fetoscope.
   d. **Pregnancy tests** (quantitative)
   e. **Size of the uterus.** This is an accurate predictor in the absence of multiple gestation, pregnancy, and structural abnormalities.
   f. **Early ultrasonographic findings.** Dating by ultrasound is most accurate in the first trimester (± 1 week), less accurate in the second trimester (± 2 weeks), and becomes only an adjunct to estimating dates during the third trimester (± 3 weeks).
   g. **Timed fertility procedure.** A number of new fertility procedures will result in exact dating of conception.
2. **Maturity of specific organ systems.** Pulmonary maturation is determined by measurement of amniotic fluid (AF) phospholipids (see Chap. 6).
3. **Real-time ultrasonography for the identification of**
   a. **Malformations** (e.g., anencephaly; meningocele; cardiac, renal, and GI anomalies)
   b. Fetal position
   c. Multiple gestation
   d. Abnormalities of fetal growth
   e. Ascites and hydrops
   f. Other conditions through its use in procedures such as amniocentesis and fetal blood and tissue sampling
4. **Fetal size and rate of growth** are determined by uterine size and by ultrasonographic estimates based on biparietal diameter, femur length, and abdominal circumference.
5. **Fetal well-being.** When fetuses are at serious risk for intrapartum asphyxia,

Table 5-1. Perinatal risk factors associated with an increased risk to the newborn

Condition	Risk to newborn
Maternal condition	
Maternal age over 35	Chromosomal abnormalities, SGA
Maternal age under 16	Prematurity
Poverty	Prematurity, infection, SGA
Infertility	Low birth weight, congenital anomalies, increased prenatal mortality
Smoking	SGA, increased perinatal mortality
Drug or alcohol abuse	SGA, fetal alcohol syndrome, withdrawal syndrome, sudden infant death
Diabetes	Stillbirth, hyaline membrane disease, congenital anomalies
Thyroid disease	Goiter, hypothyroidism, hyperthyroidism
Renal disease	SGA, stillbirth
Heart or lung disease	SGA, stillbirth, prematurity
Hypertension, chronic or preeclampsia	SGA, asphyxia, stillbirth
Anemia	SGA, asphyxia, stillbirth
Isoimmunization (red cell antigens)	Stillbirth, anemia, jaundice
Isoimmunization (platelets)	Stillbirth, bleeding
Thrombocytopenia	Stillbirth, bleeding
Polyhydramnios	Anomalies (anencephaly, GI obstruction, renal disease, goiter)
Low urinary estriols	SGA, stillbirth
Bleeding in early pregnancy	Prematurity, stillbirth
Bleeding in third trimester	Anemia, stillbirth
Premature rupture of membranes, fever, infection	Infection
TORCH infections	See TORCH infections, p. 175
Past history of infant with jaundice, respiratory distress syndrome, or anomalies	Increased risk of recurrence in neonate
Maternal medications, corticosteroids, antimetabolites, antithyroid medications, reserpine, salicylates, etc.	See individual package inserts, see also J. P. Cloherty and A. R. Stark (Eds.), *Manual of Neonatal Care.* Boston: Little, Brown, 1991.
Fetal conditions	
Multiple birth	Prematurity, twin transfusion syndrome, asphyxia
Poor fetal growth	Asphyxia, stillbirth, congenital anomalies
Abnormal fetal position	Trauma, hemorrhage, deformities
Abnormality of fetal heart rate or rhythm	Asphyxia, heart failure, heart block
Acidosis	Asphyxia, respiratory distress syndrome
Condition of labor or delivery	
Premature labor	Respiratory distress, asphyxia
Labor occurring 2 weeks or more after term	Stillbirth, asphyxia, meconium aspiration
Long labor	Asphyxia, stillbirth
Meconium-stained amniotic fluid	Asphyxia, meconium aspiration syndrome, stillbirth

Table 5-1 (continued)

Condition	Risk to newborn
Prolapsed cord	Asphyxia
Maternal hypotension	Asphyxia, stillbirth
Rapid labor	Trauma
Analgesia and anesthesia	Respiratory depression, hypotension
Neonatal condition	
Low Apgar score	Intracranial hemorrhage, respiratory distress, anoxic-ischemic encephalopathy
Foul smell of baby, amniotic fluid, or membranes	Infection
Placental anomalies	
Small placenta	SGA
Large placenta	Hydrops, heart failure
Torn placenta	Blood loss
Vasa previa	Blood loss

SGA = small for gestational age; TORCH = toxoplasmosis, rubella, cytomegalic inclusion disease, and herpes simplex.

the pediatrician should be prepared for urgent delivery newborn resuscitation. Tests of fetal well-being include
   a. **Nonstress monitoring**
   b. **Oxytocin challenge test**
   c. **Ultrasound biophysical profile (BPP)**
      (1) 10-point scale, similar to Apgar score
      (2) Two points each for fetal breathing, fetal tone, fetal activity, fetal heart rate (nonstress test), amniotic fluid volume
      (3) Interpretation ≤ 3: intervene; 4–7: retest/suspect; ≥ 8: normal
   d. **Amniocentesis** for meconium or evidence of infection (white cells or bacteria)
   e. Intrapartum fetal heart rate monitoring
   f. **Fetal scalp pH**
   g. **Percutaneous umbilical blood sampling** (see below)
   B. **Identified fetal risks.** Pregnancies at high risk or fetuses with known problems should be referred to a high-risk perinatal center for thorough evaluation.
      1. **Maternal medical problems.** Women with a variety of serious maternal conditions should be sent for evaluation and/or subsequent delivery at a tertiary center.
      2. **Maternal infection.** During routine antenatal care, women are screened for rubella, hepatitis B (HBsAg), and syphilis exposure (nonspecific screening–RPR). Many obstetric providers also screen for group B *Streptococcus* colonization. High-risk populations are screened for tuberculosis. The pediatrician should be aware of any positive antenatal screens for infection.
      3. **Genetics.** Fetal chromosome analysis and DNA probes can identify affected fetuses in utero.
      4. **Identified anomalies.** Ultrasonic prenatal identification of major anomalies permits the pediatrician to develop management plans.
II. **General assessment and management of the healthy newborn**
   A. **Physical examination of the newborn.** *At no other time than at birth is more information obtained from the general overall visual and auditory appraisal of a naked infant and less information obtained from an exhaustive system-by-system examination.*
      On initial examination, four categories are of the utmost importance: **cardiorespiratory status**; the **presence of congenital anomalies**; the **effects of gestation, labor, delivery, and maternal medications**; and **signs of infection or**

other systemic disease. A fretful infant should be quieted with a nipple. The usual order of examination is as follows:

1. **Respiratory**
   a. Evaluation of respiratory status includes color, presence of acrocyanosis (quite common in the first 24–48 hours of life), and respiratory rate (normal 40–60 and often periodic), including the presence of apnea.
   b. Rales and questionable breath sounds are usually insignificant if the infant is otherwise well.
   c. Retractions, nasal flaring, and respiratory grunting are significant in the absence of crying.
   d. Percussion has little value.
2. **Cardiac**
   a. Evaluation of the heart includes the position of maximal impulse, palpation of femoral or dorsalis pedis pulses and auscultation of the heart for rate (generally 120–160 beats per minute; occasionally < 100 in term or postterm infants at rest), rhythm, and presence of murmurs.
   b. Because of rapid alterations in systemic and pulmonary pressures, *murmurs,* especially in the first 24 hours of life, usually do not reflect the presence of significant heart disease.
   c. Distant heart sounds, especially if accompanied by respiratory symptoms, may be secondary to pneumomediastinum or pneumothorax.
3. **Abdomen**
   a. Observation for asymmetry (including the musculature), masses, and fullness is critical.
   b. Bowel sounds may or may not be present initially.
   c. Palpate with gentle pressure to determine the size of the liver (may extend 2.5 cm below the right costal margin) or spleen (generally, at most, a tip may be palpable). Palpate *deeply* for both kidneys.
4. **Genitalia and rectum**
   a. In boys, observe for presence of both testes, and normal placement and patency of the urethral orifice and anus. The testes should be similar in size and should not appear blue through the scrotum (a sign of torsion). Hydroceles are common.
   b. In girls, in addition to observing for anal patency, one should search for interlabial masses, although a mucosal tag from the vagina is occasionally noted. A *mucoid vaginal discharge* (occasionally blood streaked) is often noted.
5. **Skin**
   a. Jaundice in the first day of life is abnormal and an investigation for the cause should ensue (see Chap. 6). Mild jaundice on subsequent days is common.
   b. Common findings are
      (1) Milia (tiny yellow papules, representing blocked sebaceous glands, usually found on the nose and cheeks)
      (2) Mongolian spots (bluish, often large, patches most commonly found on back, buttocks, or thighs of infants of Asian or African background)
      (3) Erythema toxicum (papular or vesicular lesions on an erythematous base, seen on the torso and limbs)
      (4) Pustular melanosis (small, superficial pustules that easily rupture leaving hyperpigmented macules and seen most commonly in black infants)
6. **Extremities, spine, and joints**
   a. Observe for anomalies of the digits, hand creases, structural abnormalities (especially in the sacral area), hip dislocation, and positional deformities.
   b. The clavicles should be palpated to detect fracture.
7. **Head, neck, and mouth**
   a. Inspect for cuts, bruises, caput, cephalohematoma, mobility of suture lines, and skull molding.

b. Measure the head circumference from occiput to midbrow—generally 31–36 cm at term (Fig. 5-1).

c. Observe for neck flexibility and asymmetry.

d. Inspect for cleft palate.

8. **Neurologic examination.** Observations for neurologic status can usually be made concurrently while handling the baby for the preceding examinations. Observe for tone, activity, symmetry of the extremities and facial movements, alertness, consolability, and reflexes, including the Moro, suck, root, grasp, and plantar reflexes.

9. **Eye examination.** (Periorbital edema in first few days of life may interfere.)

a. Usually, the presence of cataracts and tumors can be largely ruled out by elicitation of the red reflex.

b. Scleral hemorrhage (very common) and pupillary size and shape can be assessed.

c. All infants should have received prophylaxis for bacterial conjunctivitis with topical ophthalmic ointments—tetracycline 1%, erythromycin 1%, or silver nitrate 1%.

10. The **discharge examination** should include attention to overall appearance, cardiac status (cyanosis, congestive heart failure, or new murmur), abdomen (masses), skin (jaundice, pustules), cord (infection), and circumcision wound. Additionally, feeding, amount of weight loss, and stool/urine output should

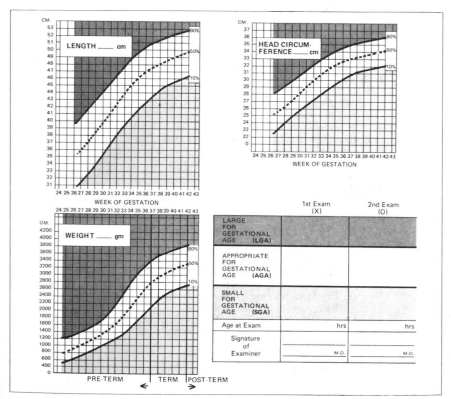

Fig. 5-1. Classification of newborns based on maturity and intrauterine growth. (Adapted from L. C. Lubchenco, C. Hansman, and E. Boyd, *Pediatrics* 37:403, 1966; and F. C. Battaglia and L. C. Lubchenco. *J. Pediatr.* 71:159, 1967. Copyright © 1978, Mead Johnson & Co., Evansville, IN)

be reviewed. Maternal preparation should be assessed and medical follow-up established.

B. Nursery care

1. **Temperature control.** Heat loss may be minimized by placing an infant in a neutral thermal environment, the thermal condition at which heat production is minimal yet core temperature is within normal range (Table 5-2). **Hypothermia can produce apnea, hypoxemia, hypoglycemia, and acidosis.**

   a. **Healthy infant.** The skin should be dried, wet towels removed, and the infant wrapped. Examination in the delivery room should be performed under a radiant warmer with a skin probe, keeping the skin temperature at 36.5°C (97.7°F).

   b. **Sick infant**

   (1) The skin should be dried and the infant wrapped and transported in a heated incubator. A radiant warmer with a servocontrol is used for procedures.

   (2) Very sick neonates, to whom access is important, can be kept in an open radiant warmer with servocontrol of skin temperature; a small, clear-plastic heat shield or Saran blanket, which prevents heat loss by convection and radiation, should be used.

2. **Feeding and nutrition.** Growth requirements for full-term neonates are 90–120 kcal/kg/day. The protein requirement is 2–3 gm/kg/day. Fat should make up 30–50 percent of caloric intake, protein 7–15 percent, and carbohydrate 30–65 percent.

   a. **Breast feeding**

   (1) Breast milk is of proved nutritional, immunologic, and emotional value for the feeding of the full-term and preterm infant, and should be encouraged for all full-term and most preterm infants.

   (2) Whether breast milk alone is nutritionally adequate for all premature infants is disputed. The protein in breast milk is 60 percent whey (beta-lactoglobulin and lactalbumin) and 40 percent casein and relatively digestible by the premature. However, the low *total* protein content of the breast milk may not be adequate to support optimal growth in some premature infants. Premature infants who are *not growing adequately* on breast milk may therefore require protein supplementation (up to 2 gm/day) (Tables 5-3 and 5-4). Some prematures may also have a transient lactase deficiency that requires a lactose-free formula.

   (3) Human milk contains antimicrobial components not found in infant formulas: immunoglobulins, leukocytes, lactoferrin, the third component of complement in colostrum, and lysozymes. **In areas where**

Table 5-2. Neutral thermal environmental temperatures

Birth weight		Incubator air temperature (°C)	First 24 hours (°F)
kg	lb		
	2	35.0	95.0
1		34.9	94.9
	3	34.2	93.6
1.5		34.0	93.2
	4	33.7	92.7
2		33.5	92.3
	5	33.3	92.0
2.5		33.2	91.8
	6	33.1	91.6
3		33.0	91.4

Table 5-3. Oral dietary supplements

	Supplements		Human milk (dl)* (approximate value)	
Nutrient	Enfamil Human Milk Fortifier (Mead Johnson) per 4 packets	Similac Natural Care (Ross) per dl	Plus 4 packets Enfamil HMF (Mead Johnson) per dl	Diluted 1 : 1 with Natural Care (Ross) per dl
Energy (kcal)	14	81	81	77
Protein (gm)	0.7	2.2	1.73	1.6
Fat (gm)	< 0.1	4.4	4.0	4.2
Carbohydrate (gm)	2.7	8.6	9.9	7.9
Minerals				
Calcium (mg)	90	171	118	100
Phosphorus (mg)	45	85	59	50
Magnesium (mg)	—	10	3.5	6.8
Sodium (mEq)	0.3	1.5	1.1	1.1
Potassium (mEq)	0.4	2.7	1.8	2.0
Chloride (mEq)	0.5	1.1	1.7	1.5
Zinc (mg)	0.71	1.9	0.83	0.7
Copper (μg)	80	203	105	114
Manganese (μg)	9	10	9.4	5.3
Vitamins				
A (IU)	780	552	1,003	388
D (IU)	210	122	212	62
E (IU)	3.4	3.2	3.6	1.7
K (IU)	9.1	10	9.3	5.1
Thiamine (μg)	187	203	208	112
Riboflavin (μg)	250	503	285	269
Niacin (μg)	3,100	4,060	3,220	2,105
Pantothenate (μg)	790	1,543	970	862
Pyridoxine (μg)	193	203	213	112
Biotin (μg)	0.81	30	1.2	15.2
Vitamin B$_{12}$ (μg)	0.21	0.45	0.25	0.25
Vitamin C (mg)	24	30	28	17
Folate (μg)	23	30	28	18

* Milk-based and soy-based infant formulas for feeding infants in the hospital. Ross Laboratories, Columbus, OH, 1989.
Source: J. P. Cloherty and A. R. Stark (Eds.), *Manual of Neonatal Care* (3rd ed.). Boston: Little, Brown, 1991. P. 540.

Table 5-4. Oral dietary supplements available for use in infants

Nutrient	Product	Source	Energy content
Fat	MCT oil (Mead Johnson)	Medium-chain triglycerides	8.3 kcal/gm 7.7 kcal/ml
	Corn oil	Long-chain triglycerides	9 kcal/gm 8.4 kcal/ml
Carbohydrate	Polycose (Ross)	Glucose polymers	4 kcal/gm 8 kcal/tsp (powder) 2 kcal/ml (liquid)
Protein	Casec (Mead Johnson)	Calcium caseinate	3.7 kcal/gm 5.8 kcal/tsp
	Promod (Ross)	Whey concentrate	4.2 kcal/gm 5.7 kcal/tsp

Source: J. P. Cloherty and A. R. Stark (Eds.), *Manual of Neonatal Care* (3rd ed.). Boston: Little, Brown, 1991. P. 543.

sanitation is poor, the use of nonhuman milk formulas has been clearly associated with increased infant mortality from infection.

    (4) Fostering successful breast feeding

      (a) Both the obstetrician and the pediatrician should discuss and encourage nursing prenatally with the mother.

      (b) Experienced nursing mothers should be available to discuss the satisfaction and techniques of breast feeding with expectant mothers.

      (c) Obstetric ward and neonatal unit practices should foster successful nursing including:

        (i) Decreasing the amount of sedation or anesthesia given to mothers

        (ii) Encouraging the mother to nurse the infant immediately after delivery, if possible

        (iii) Encouraging "rooming in" to avoid separation of mother and infant

        (iv) Having infants fed on demand rather than on a rigid schedule

        (v) Seeing that personnel caring for new mothers are actively supportive of breast feeding

        (vi) Discouraging the routine use of "supplemental" water or formula by nursery personnel, unless absolutely necessary

    (5) Breast-feeding techniques (see Chap. 2, p. 26).

    (6) Contraindications (see Chap. 2, p. 30, Tables 2-8 and 2-9) Should include active Tb and HIV infection

  b. Formula feeding for full-term infants. A number of commercially available formulas are adequate (Table 5-5). Those based on cow's milk (e.g., SMA, Similac, Enfamil) are the usual formulas for full-term infants under most circumstances. For special circumstances other formulas may be needed:

    (1) Modified formulas are recommended for premature infants in the first weeks of life because of the whey-casein and calcium-phosphorus ratios (see below).

    (2) Soy-based formulas should be reserved for special situations, such as a strong history of cow's milk intolerance.

    (3) For most industrialized countries, the practice of boiling water for preparation of powdered or concentrated infant formula is not necessary and may inadvertently concentrate nonbiologic impurities from the cooking vessel itself.

  c. Supplements (vitamins, iron) for full-term infants. All newborns should

Table 5-5. Human milk and formula composition

Formula (distributor)	kcal/30 ml	Protein, gm/dl	Fat, gm/dl	Carbohydrate, gm/dl	Minerals, mg/dl			Electrolytes, mEq/dl			Vitamins, IU/dl			Folate, mg/dl	Osmolality, mOsmol/kg	Renal solute load, mOsmol/liter[b]
					Ca	P	Fe[a]	Na$^+$	K$^+$	Cl$^-$	A	D	E			
Breast milk (composition varies)	20–22	1.1	4.5	7.1	33	15	0.03	0.8	1.4	1.1	250	2.2	0.18	5.0	290–300	75
Standard cow's milk–based formulas																
Similac 20 (Ross)	20	1.5	3.6	7.2	51	39	0.15 (1.2)	0.8	1.9	1.3	203	41	2.0	10	300	100
Enfamil (Mead Johnson)	20	1.5	3.8	6.9	46	32	0.11 (1.3)	0.8	1.8	1.2	210	41.5	2.1	10.5	300	98
SMA (Wyeth)	20	1.5	3.6	7.2	42	28	0.15 (1.2)	0.7	1.4	1.2	200	40	0.95	5.0	300	91
Similac 24 (Ross)	24	2.2	4.3	8.5	73	56	0.18 (1.5)	1.2	2.7	1.9	244	49	2.4	12	380	146
Enfamil 24 (Mead Johnson)	24	1.8	4.5	8.3	56	38	0.13 (1.5)	1.0	2.2	1.4	251	50	2.5	13	360	117
SMA 24 (Wyeth)	24	1.8	4.3	8.6	50.5	33.5	0.18 (1.4)	0.8	1.7	1.3	240	48	1.1	6.0	364	110
Soy formulas																
Isomil (Ross)	20	1.8	3.7	6.8	71	51	1.2	1.4	1.9	1.2	203	41	2.0	10.0	240	116
Prosobee (Mead Johnson)	20	2.0	3.6	6.8	63	50	1.3	1.0	2.1	1.6	208	41.5	2.1	10.5	200	127
Nursoy (Wyeth)	20	2.1	3.6	6.9	60	42	1.2	0.9	1.8	1.1	200	40	1.0	5.0	296	122

Preterm formulas[c]																
Similac Special Care (Ross)	24	2.2	4.4	8.6	146	73	0.3 (1.5)	1.5	2.7	1.9	552	122	3.2	30	300	149
Enfamil Premature (Mead Johnson)	24	2.4	4.1	8.9	134	68	0.2	1.4	2.3	2.0	970	220	3.7	29	300	153
SMA "Preemie" (Wyeth)	24	2.0	4.4	8.6	75	40	0.3	1.4	1.9	1.5	240	48	1.5	10	280	128
Specialized formulas																
Pregestimil (Mead Johnson)	20	1.9	3.8	6.9	63	42	1.3	1.4	1.9	1.6	250	51	2.5	10.5	320	125
Nutramigen (Mead Johnson)	20	1.9	2.6	9.1	63	42	1.3	1.4	1.9	1.6	208	42	2.1	10.5	320	125
Portagen (Mead Johnson)	20	2.4	3.2	7.8	63	48	1.3	1.6	2.2	1.6	530	53	2.1	10.5	220	152
Similac PM 60/40 (Ross)	20	1.6	3.8	6.9	38	19	0.15	0.7	15	1.1	203	41	2.0	10.0	280	96
Similac 27 (Ross)	27	2.5	4.8	9.6	82	64	0.2	1.4	3.1	2.1	274	55	2.7	14.0	430	164
SMA 27 (Wyeth)	27	2.0	4.9	9.7	57	38	0.2	0.9	1.9	1.4	270	54	1.3	7.0	416	123

Key: Ca = calcium; P = phosphorus; Fe = iron, Na$^+$ = sodium; K$^+$ = potassium; Cl$^-$ = chloride.
[a] In instances in which high and low Fe formulations are available, the low Fe value appears.
[b] Estimated renal solute load = [Protein (gm) × 4] + [Na(mEq) + K(mEq) + Cl(mEq)].
[c] 20 kcal/30 ml formulations are also available.
Source: J. P. Cloherty and A. R. Stark (Eds.), *Manual of Neonatal Care* (3rd ed.). Boston: Little, Brown, 1991. Pp. 538–539.

receive vitamin K (vitamin K oxide, 1.0 mg IM; 0.5 mg IM if < 1,500 gm) at birth.

(1) Breast-fed infants

(a) There is no conclusive evidence that healthy, breast-fed infants of well-nourished mothers require vitamin supplementation provided that sunlight exposure is adequate for vitamin D synthesis.

(b) The use of iron supplements in breast-fed infants is controversial (see *Pediatrics* 63:52, 1979). Some have suggested a dose of 2 mg/kg/day elemental iron, particularly in areas where the risk of lead exposure is high.

(c) If infants are fully breast fed, they should receive fluoride supplementation (0.25 mg/day) *if* the mother drinks spring or well water *or* when the community water supply contains less than 0.3 ppm fluoride.

(2) Formula-fed infants

(a) Formulas usually contain adequate vitamins (1 qt formula/day), though iron-fortified formula or iron supplementation after 6–8 weeks of age may be necessary (2 mg/kg/day elemental iron).

(b) Fluoride supplementation is recommended if babies are receiving formula diluted with nonfluoridated water (0.25 mg/day up to age 2).

d. Special nutritional needs of the low-birth-weight infant

(1) Nutritional requirements. Daily caloric requirements for premature infants are 50–100 kcal/kg/day by 3 days of age and 110–150 kcal/day during later growth.

(2) Formulas for premature infants. The caloric, protein, and calcium requirements for prematures are somewhat higher than those for term infants.

(a) Breast milk. Premature infants should receive breast milk whenever possible. Appropriate supplementation can be provided by adding milk fortification (HMF or Natural Care, see Table 5-3) to adjust caloric density to 24 kcal/oz.

(b) Formula feeding. Modified formulas (e.g., Special Care or Enfamil Premature) are acceptable alternatives to breast milk. These have higher whey-casein and calcium-phosphorus ratios, and are supplied in kcal/oz concentrations (see Table 5-5). Increased caloric content may be achieved by carbohydrate or fat supplements (see Table 5-4).

(3) Fluid requirements of premature infants. Fluid intake of low-birth-weight infants should increase from 75 ml/kg/day on day 1 to approximately 150 ml/kg/day after day 5 (see Chap. 7).

(4) Feeding techniques. Coordinated sucking and swallowing may not mature until 34–35 weeks' gestational age. Direct breast feeding can be attempted but may not be successful. Such infants can be fed using smaller/softer nipples.

(a) Gavage feeding. For infants who are too immature for oral feedings, enteral feedings can be administered by gavage. See Table 5-6 for recommended schedule.

(b) IV supplementation

(i) If the infant is under 1,500 gm, start an IV line with 10% dextrose in water (D/W) at 75–100 ml/kg/day. Decrease this IV fluid supplement as gavage volume increases until gavage feedings exceed 100 ml/kg/day.

(ii) Electrolyte supplementation may be necessary if IV support is required beyond the first day.

(5) Keep gastric intake below 200 ml/kg/day to avoid aspiration. Infants who need to suck in excess of their appetite can be appeased with pacifiers, which also appear to improve gastric motility.

(6) Close monitoring

Table 5-6. Schedule of gavage feeding

Weight (gm)	Age (hr)	Size of feeding (ml)	Interval	Content of feeding
Less than 1,200 (expected gastric residual* is 1–2 ml)	4–12	1–2	q2h	Sterile water, then 5% dextrose in water (D/W)
	12–24	2–4	q2h	5% D/W
	24–48	3–6	q2h	Equal parts of formula and 5% D/W
	48–72	4–8	q2h	Equal parts of formula and 5% D/W
	>72	5–10	q2h	Full-strength formula
1,200–1,500 (expected gastric residual* is 2 ml)	4–12	2–3	q2–3h	Sterile water, then 5% D/W
	12–24	4–6	q2–3h	Equal parts of 5% D/W and formula
	24–48	6–9	q2–3h	Equal parts of 5% D/W and formula
	48–72	8–12	q2–3h	Equal parts of 5% D/W and formula or full-strength formula
	>72	10–15	q2–3h	Full-strength formula
1,500–2,000 (expected gastric residual* is 3 ml)	4–12	5–15	q3–4h	Sterile water, then 5% D/W
	12–24	5–15	q3–4h	Equal parts of 5% D/W and formula
	24–48	10–25	q3–4h	Equal parts of 5% D/W and formula or full-strength formula
	48–72	15–35	q3–4h	Full-strength formula
	>72	20–45	q3–4h	Full-strength formula

* For intermittent gavage feeding, if the prefeeding residual is more than 25% of the amount of the feeding, the volume of the feeding should be reduced or alternative feeding methods considered.
Note: After 72 hr, the amount of each feeding should be increased each day by 1–2 ml in babies weighing less than 1,200 gm, 2–3 ml in babies weighing 1,200–1,500 gm, and 5–15 ml in babies weighing 1,500–2,000 gm, up to a volume of 150–175 ml/kg/24 hr.
Source: J. P. Cloherty and A. R. Stark (Eds.), *Manual of Neonatal Care.* Boston: Little, Brown, 1985.

- **(a)** Follow serum glucose carefully, starting at birth, 1 and 2 hours of age, and then before feeds until stable. Infants can become hypoglycemic if the IV supplement stops abruptly.
- **(b)** Monitor urine specific gravity, skin turgor, body weight, serum and urine osmolarity, and electrolyte concentrations as necessary. **Scrupulous attention to this is vital in very immature infants** (see Chap. 7).
- **(7) Supplements**
  - **(a) Calories.** Caloric concentration of formula should not exceed 30 calories/oz. A caloric concentration of 24 calories/oz is usually sufficient (see Tables 5-4 and 5-5).
    - **(i) Carbohydrates.** Glucose polymer (Polycose) provides 8 kcal/tsp (powder) or 2 kcal/ml (liquid).
    - **(ii) Fat.** MCT oil provides 7.7 calories/ml.

(b) Vitamins. Vitamin supplementation is begun as soon as the infant is receiving full volume feedings. A typical supplementation schedule, which assumes a formula intake of 150 ml/kg/day, is shown (Table 5-7).

(i) Vitamin supplementation is needed for preterm babies in order to meet recommended intakes, particularly with respect to vitamin D (400 IU per day) and folate (50–65 µg per day).

(ii) Liquid drop preparations currently available in the United States for infants contain either vitamins A, C, and D or vitamins A, C, D, thiamine, riboflavin, niacin, B_6, B_{12}, and E. Folate is not included because it is relatively unstable in solutions.

(c) Calcium. Supplemental calcium (150 mg/kg/day elemental calcium is the recommended total daily consumption) may be necessary because formulas commonly used for full-term infants contain approximately 44–53 mg/dl calcium. The special premature infant formulas (see Table 5-5) contain sufficient calcium such that supplementation is rarely necessary.

(8) Infants who are unable to tolerate oral gavage feedings need parenteral nutrition (see Chap. 10).

(a) Fluid needs are described in Chap. 10, but they may vary, depending on the need to restrict fluid (e.g., as in hyaline membrane disease) or the need to give extra fluid (e.g., in small premature infants with large insensible water losses, who may have fluid requirements up to 200 ml/kg/day or more).

(b) On day 2, 3 mEq/kg/day **sodium** and 2 mEq/kg/day **potassium** are required. Small premature infants may need 4–8 mEq/kg/day sodium to prevent hyponatremia due to obligate renal sodium loss.

(c) Caloric requirements are initially provided as 10% **dextrose** (3.4 kcal/gm) as tolerated and as **protein** (4 kcal/gm) as protein hydrolysates in gradually increasing dosage from 1 gm/kg/day on day 2 to 2.2 gm/kg/day (term) or 3.5 gm/kg/day (preterm) on days 4–7.

(d) Fat (9 kcal/gm) is given as 10 or 20% soy oil emulsion. **Lipids** can be used to provide additional calories without excessive fluid intake if the infant is receiving inadequate calories.

III. Anticipation of common problems (see also Chap. 6)

A. Premature infants (under 37 weeks' gestation)

1. Thermal regulation. Particular care should be directed toward **temperature**

Table 5-7. Typical vitamin supplementation schedule for preterm babies*

Food source	Body weight	Polyvisol (ml/day)	Folate (µg/day)
Human milk + 4 pks HMF/dl	< 1,000 gm	0.5	25
Human milk alone	All preterm infants	1.0	50
Enfamil Premature 24	< 1,000 gm	0.5	25
Similac Special Care 24	< 1,000 gm	1.0	25
	1,000–2,500 gm	0.5	0
Nonpreterm formulas	All preterm infants, term infants at nutritional risk	1.0	25

* Goal: 200 mg/kg/day calcium; 100 to 200 mg/kg/day phosphorus.
Source: J. P. Cloherty and A. R. Stark (Eds.), *Manual of Neonatal Care* (3rd ed.). Boston: Little, Brown, 1991. P. 544.

controls for premature infants because of their more rapid heat loss. This usually requires an overhead radiant warmer or a closed incubator for infants < 1,800 gm.

2. **Respiration.** Many healthy premature infants have **transient tachypnea** from delayed resorption of fetal lung fluid. This may be distinguished from hyaline membrane disease or pneumonia, which would require immediate aggressive treatment (see Chap. 6).

3. **Apnea.** Significant **apnea** will occur in 5–10 percent of 33- to 34-week-old infants. The rate is higher for less mature prematures. All infants < 34–35 weeks old should receive apnea monitoring until they are documented apnea free (minimum 5 days).

4. **Cardiovascular.** Careful computation of fluids is essential. Inadvertent fluid overload can easily lead to patent ductus arteriosus.

5. **Hematologic.** Anemia is common, both iatrogenic and physiologic (nadir at 4–6 weeks). This should be monitored. Treatment is described in Chap. 6.

6. **Hyperbilirubinemia,** hypoglycemia, hypocalcemia, and hyponatremia are common.

B. **Small-for-gestational-age (SGA) infants** (birth weight below the 10th percentile for gestational age). Conditions associated with SGA infants are listed in Table 5-8.

1. During **pregnancy,** identification, evaluation, and monitoring of fetal growth and well-being are essential. The cause of intrauterine growth retardation should be investigated. A standard workup includes a review of obstetric causes, examination for identifiable syndromes, and laboratory evaluation for congenital infection (particularly cytomegalovirus). Examination of the placenta is frequently useful.

2. At delivery, **anticipate fetal distress, perinatal depression, meconium aspiration, hypoxia, and heat loss.**

3. In the newborn, monitor for hypothermia, polycythemia, hypoglycemia, and hypocalcemia.

4. Leukopenia, neutropenia, and thrombocytopenia are often seen in infants born to *hypertensive* mothers.

5. SGA infants should receive early feeds.

C. **Large-for-gestational-age (LGA) infants** (birth weight over the 90th percentile for gestational age). Conditions associated with LGA infants are listed in Table 5-8. These infants are at high risk of **birth trauma,** including clavicular fractures, brachial plexus injuries, and perinatal depression. **Hypoglycemia** and **polycythemia** should be anticipated.

D. **Postmature infants** (gestation over 42 weeks). These infants are unusually susceptible to **placental insufficiency.** As a result, fetal distress, meconium aspiration, and neonatal hypoglycemia occur more frequently.

1. Management during pregnancy includes careful estimation of fetal gesta-

---

Table 5-8. Factors associated with gestational age disparities

Infants large for gestational age	Infants small for gestational age	
Constitutionally large infants	Sociodemographic factors: age, parity, income, race, marital status, obstetric history	Sickle cell disease
Infants of diabetic mothers		Chronic disease
Postmaturity		Smoking
Transposition of the great vessels	Drug abuse	Multiple fetuses
	Maternal heart or renal disease	Placental lesions
Erythroblastosis fetalis		Congenital anomaly
Beckwith syndrome	Toxemia	Chromosomal anomaly
Parabiotic syndrome	Chronic hypertension	Congenital infections
		Uterine anomalies

tional age by dates and ultrasound. Monitoring of fetal well-being should start at 41 weeks and especially during labor.

2. Affected infants should receive early feeds and monitoring for hypoglycemia and polycythemia.

E. **Common signs and symptoms.** Newborns manifest illness in a limited number of signs and symptoms. These should prompt evaluation for specific illnesses detailed in Chap. 6.

1. **Respiratory distress.** Most infants have some tachypnea during the first minutes of life. Infants with sustained tachypnea, audible grunting, retracting, or flaring should be evaluated. Common causes are:
   a. Retained fetal lung fluid
   b. Aspiration of amniotic contents (fluid, blood, meconium)
   c. Pneumonia
   d. Hyaline membrane disease
   e. Pneumothorax
   f. Congenital anomalies (lungs, airway, heart)

2. **Cyanosis. Cyanosis in the context of respiratory distress is an emergency.** Other causes of cyanosis are:
   a. Polycythemia
   b. Hypothermia
   c. Apnea, choking, or airway obstruction
   d. Cyanotic congenital heart disease

3. **Apnea.** Apnea in term infants is a serious symptom. Apnea in prematures is common but should be evaluated with the first episode. Causes include:
   a. Infection (systemic or meningitis)
   b. Central nervous system (malformation, bleed, or infection)
   c. Respiratory obstruction (aspiration, anatomic)

4. **Lethargy.** Sleepiness in newborns is common, but marked lethargy should prompt evaluation for:
   a. Sepsis or meningitis
   b. Metabolic disturbances
   c. Neurologic insults

Management of the Sick Newborn

DeWayne M. Pursley and
Douglas K. Richardson

I. Care of the newborn in the delivery room

A. Preparation

1. A thorough knowledge of the maternal and fetal history is essential (see Chap. 5).

2. The factors associated with increased risk to the newborn are listed in Table 5-1. Two clinicians skilled in the resuscitation of the newborn should be present at the delivery of a high-risk infant. One clinician must be skilled in intubation.

3. Before the delivery of a high-risk infant, the pediatric clinicians should discuss with the parents their plans for the care of the infant in the delivery room and nursery.

4. **Equipment** *should be examined and tested before delivery.*

   a. Radiant warmer **bed, blankets** (prewarmed), and **towels.** Turn on radiant warmer before delivery.

   b. Cord-cutting materials and clamp

   c. **Suction** with manometer. Test suction before delivery.

   d. Infant suction bulb, mechanical suction device, and DeLee suction catheter

   e. **Oxygen** source with flow meter and a flow-through **anesthesia bag** or self-inflating bag with a reservoir capable of delivering 100% oxygen. The bag should have an adjustable valve or "pop-off" control and be fitted with an in-line manometer for observing airway pressure should assisted ventilation be required. Turn on O_2 to 5–8 liters per minute before delivery and test bag.

   f. Infant **face masks** of various sizes. An appropriate-sized mask is large enough to cover the mouth and nose without covering the eyes.

   g. **Infant stethoscope**

   h. Laryngoscope with size 0 and 1 blades, fresh batteries, and **bulbs**

   i. Uniform-diameter **endotracheal tubes** with 2.5-, 3.0-, and 3.5-mm internal diameters (two of each) and stylets

   j. **Feeding tube** (No. 8 French), 20-ml syringe, and adhesive tape

   k. **Drugs. Epinephrine,** 1 : 10,000; **NaHCO$_3$,** 0.5 mEq/ml (4.2%); **naloxone** (Narcan), 0.4 or 1.0 mg/ml; saline; and albumin (5%)

   l. **Umbilical catheterization tray** with 3.5F and 5F catheters, three-way stopcock, and 10- and 20-ml syringes

   m. A prewarmed transport **isolette** with portable oxygen supply

   n. Caps, masks, goggles or face shield, gloves, and gown should be worn routinely to avoid infectious exposure.

B. Delivery (Fig. 6-1)

1. Place the infant on a warming table.

2. Dry the infant and remove wet linen from contact with infant.

3. Position the infant in slight Trendelenburg position with the neck slightly extended.

For a more comprehensive discussion of newborn management, consult J. P. Cloherty and A. R. Stark (Eds.), *Manual of Neonatal Care* (3rd ed.). Boston: Little, Brown, 1991.

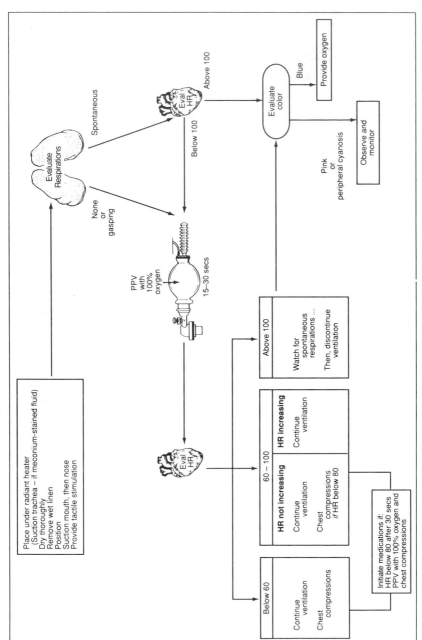

Fig. 6-1. Overview of resuscitation in the delivery room.

4. If thick meconium is present, the obstetrician should suction the *oropharynx* before the shoulders are delivered. Intubate and suction the trachea before the onset of breathing. This is recommended before drying and suctioning.
5. Bulb suction the mouth first, then the nose. **Gastric aspiration and deep suctioning in the first 5 minutes of life may produce bradycardia and should not be done routinely.**
6. If effective respirations have not been established, *stimulate* the infant by briefly vigorously rubbing the back or flicking/slapping the soles.
7. **Evaluate the infant's respirations.**
   a. If respirations are spontaneous and effective, evaluate heart rate.
   b. If infant is apneic, or respirations are ineffective, proceed with positive pressure ventilation (PPV) (see **B.10**).
8. **Evaluate the heart rate.**
   a. If heart rate (HR) > 100, check skin color.
   b. If heart rate < 100, proceed with PPV (see **B.10**).
9. **Evaluate skin color.**
   a. If no central cyanosis is present, observe.
   b. If central cyanosis is present, administer free-flow oxygen at 5–8 liters per minute with tubing held steadily 1 cm from nares or with firmly applied oxygen mask. Slowly withdraw while assuring that infant remains pink.
10. **Positive pressure ventilation** should be administered with 100% oxygen. Ventilate at rate of 40–60 per minute.
    a. The following pressures are recommended:
       (1) First breath: 30–40 cm H_2O
       (2) Succeeding breaths: 15–20 cm H_2O is often adequate.
       (3) Pulmonary disease: 20–40 cm H_2O may be required.
    b. The following steps should be taken if there is inadequate chest movement with PPV:
       (1) Reapply mask to face (for inadequate seal).
       (2) Reposition the head (for blocked airway).
       (3) Suction secretions, if present (for blocked airway).
       (4) Ventilate the infant's mouth slightly open (for blocked airway).
       (5) Increase pressure to 20–40 cm H_2O (for inadequate pressure).
    c. After 15–30 seconds, the heart rate should be rechecked.
       (1) If the heart rate > 100, and spontaneous respirations are observed, free-flow oxygen is applied and withdrawn as above.
       (2) If the heart rate is 60–100 and increasing, PPV is continued, then rechecked after another 15–30 seconds.
       (3) If the heart rate is 60–100 and not increasing, PPV is continued. Chest compressions should be administered if HR < 80.
       (4) If heart rate < 60, PPV is continued, and chest compressions are begun.
11. An orogastric catheter should be inserted and left in place if bag-and-mask ventilation is required for more than 2 minutes. The length of the inserted catheter should be equal to the distance from the bridge of the nose to the earlobe to the xiphoid. A 20-ml syringe is used to remove the gastric contents before it is removed. The catheter is taped to the infant's cheek.
12. **Chest compressions** should be performed by depressing the lower third of the sternum (below a line between the nipples and above the xiphoid) with two thumbs (with the hands encircling the torso) or the index and middle fingers. The sternum should be depressed ½–¾ in. 120 times per minute.
13. **Endotracheal intubation** is necessary in the following situations (see sec. **II.A.3**):
    a. When prolonged positive pressure ventilation is required
    b. When bag-and-mask ventilation is ineffective
    c. When tracheal suctioning is required
    d. When diaphragmatic hernia is suspected (see also sec. **XII.D.3**)
14. **Medications** (see Table 6-1 and Fig. 6-2)

Table 6-1. Medications for neonatal resuscitation

Medication	Concentration to administer	Preparation	Dosage/route	Total dose/infant	Rate/precautions
Epinephrine	1 : 10,000	1 ml	0.1–0.3 ml/kg IV or ET	Weight (kg): 1, 2, 3, 4 — Total ml: 0.1–0.3, 0.2–0.6, 0.3–0.9, 0.4–1.2	Give rapidly
Volume expanders	Whole blood, 5% albumin, Normal saline, Ringer's lactate	40 ml	10 ml/kg IV	Weight (kg): 1, 2, 3, 4 — Total ml: 10, 20, 30, 40	Give over 5–10 min
Sodium bicarbonate	0.5 mEq/ml (4.2% solution)	20 ml or two 10-ml prefilled syringes	2 mEq/kg IV	Weight (kg): 1, 2, 3, 4 — Total dose: 2 mEq, 4 mEq, 6 mEq, 8 mEq — Total ml: 4, 8, 12, 16	Give *slowly*, over at least 2 min. Give only if infant is being effectively ventilated
Naloxone	0.4 mg/ml	1 ml	0.1 mg/kg (0.25 ml/kg) IV, ET, IM, SQ	Weight (kg): 1, 2, 3, 4 — Total dose: 0.1 mg, 0.2 mg, 0.3 mg, 0.4 mg — Total ml: 0.25, 0.50, 0.75, 1.00	Give rapidly, IV, ET preferred; IM, SQ acceptable
Dopamine	$6 \times \dfrac{\text{weight (kg)} \times \text{desired dose } (\mu g/kg/min)}{\text{Desired fluid (ml/hr)}} = $ mg dopamine per 100 ml solution		Begin at 5 μg/kg/min (may increase to 20 μg/kg/min if necessary) IV	Weight (kg): 1, 2, 3, 4 — Total μg/min: 5–20, 10–40, 15–60, 20–80	Give as a continuous infusion using an infusion pump. Monitor HR and BP closely. Seek consultation

IM = intramuscular; ET = endotracheal; IV = intravenous; SQ = subcutaneous.

Source: R. S. Bloom and C. Cropley, *Textbook of Neonatal Resuscitation.* American Heart Association and American Academy of Pediatrics. Dallas: American Heart Association, 1987.

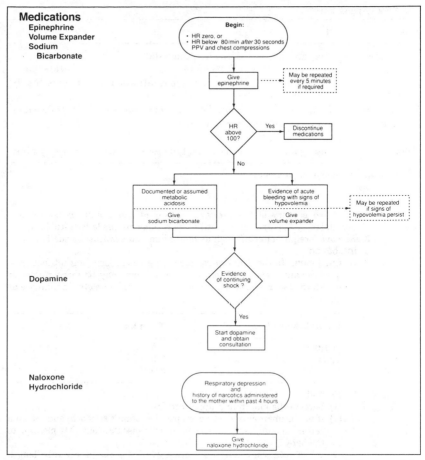

Fig. 6-2. This summary contains key points related to the use of medications during neonatal resuscitation.

    a. Indications
       (1) The infant's heart rate remains below 80 despite adequate ventilation (with 100% oxygen) and chest compressions for a minimum of 30 seconds, or
       (2) The heart rate is zero
    b. Common sites of drug administration
       (1) Endotracheal instillation can be utilized for administering epinephrine or naloxone.
       (2) An **umbilical venous catheter** can be inserted into the vein of the umbilical stump until the tip of the saline-flush catheter is just below the skin level and free flow of blood is present.
  15. All infants should have a brief examination for anomalies.
  16. If the mother is awake, keep her informed. If the infant appears well, encourage her to hold the infant as soon as she wishes.
  17. Apgar scores are assigned to describe the infant's condition (and response to intervention) at 1 and 5 minutes (Table 6-2).
II. Intensive care of the newborn
  A. Management of respiratory complications

Table 6-2. Apgar score*

Sign	0	1	2
Heart rate	Absent	Slow, less than 100 beats/min	Over 100 beats/min
Respiratory effort	Absent	Weak cry, hypoventilation	Crying lustily
Muscle tone	Limp	Some flexion of extremities	Well flexed
Reflex irritability	No response	Some motion	Crying
Color	Blue, pale	Pink body, blue extremities	Entirely pink

* Score infant at 1 and 5 minutes of age.

1. Establish patency of the airway. The infant can usually be adequately ventilated by bag and mask until preparations are made for intubation.
2. Remove foreign material, such as meconium and vomitus, by suction.
3. **Intubation**
   a. **Equipment.** In the delivery room or in an emergency, *oral* intubation is quickest and easiest. *Nasotracheal* placement may be more stable for long-term use. Endotracheal tube sizes (internal diameter in mm) are as follows:

Infant Weight (gm)	Tube size
< 1,000	2.5
1,000–2,000	3.0
> 2,000	3.5

   b. **Method**
   (1) Suction the mouth and upper airway.
   (2) If the intubation is elective, empty the infant's stomach, and attach a cardiac monitor and an oximeter or transcutaneous PO_2 monitor to the baby.
   (3) When vocal cord markers are not available, the proper tube length should be determined **before intubation.** For nasotracheal intubation, see Fig. 6-3. For orotracheal intubation, the mnemonic is "1-2-3 kg, 7-8-9 cm, tip to lip" (Fig. 6-4).
   (4) The baby should be ventilated with a bag and mask just before intubation.
   (5) The infant's head should be in the neutral position, *avoiding excessive extension of the neck.* The laryngoscope is held between the thumb and first finger of the left hand, with the second and third fingers holding the chin and stabilizing the head. Pushing down on the larynx with the fifth finger of the left hand (or having an assistant do it) and keeping the infant's head straight may help to visualize the vocal cords (trachea). The laryngoscope is passed into the right side of the mouth and then to the midline, sweeping the tongue out of the way.
   (6) The endotracheal tube is held with the right hand and inserted directly between the vocal cords to about 2 cm below the glottis. Most commercial tubes are marked with a ring, which should come to rest at the vocal cords. During nasotracheal intubation, Magill forceps are usually necessary to guide the tube between the cords. If the fifth finger is pressing on the trachea, the tube can be felt as it slips into place.
   (7) Check the tube position by auscultation to ensure equal aeration of both lungs. If air entry is poor over the left chest, pull back the

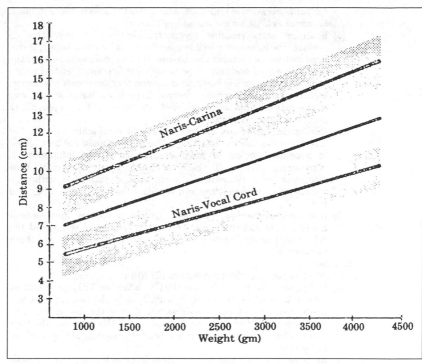

Fig. 6-3. Relation of naris-carina and naris-glottis distance to body weight. (From J. Coldiron, *Pediatrics* 41:823, 1968. Copyright 1968, American Academy of Pediatrics.)

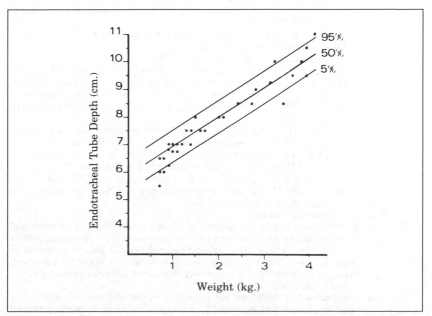

Fig. 6-4. Oral endotracheal tube depth by birth weight. Mnemonic approximation is "1-2-3 kg, 7-8-9 cm, tip to lip." (From M. L. Tochen, *J. Pediatr.* 95:1050, 1979.)

tube until aeration is improved. Auscultate the area over the stomach to ensure against an esophageal intubation.

(8) If an air entry remains asymmetric despite tube repositioning, evaluate the infant for possible pneumothorax by auscultation, transillumination, or portable chest x-ray. If chest movement is poor, the tube is in a good position, no pneumothorax is present, and adequate ventilatory pressure is being used, anatomic or developmental abnormalities (e.g., diaphragmatic hernia, hypoplastic lungs, severe lung immaturity) should be considered and ruled out by appropriate clinical or x-ray examinations.

(9) During the procedure, one person should continually observe the infant and monitor the heart rate. **The infant should not be allowed to become hypoxic or have bradycardia during intubation.** If bradycardia occurs, if there is doubt about successful tube placement, or if intubation has not been accomplished within 20 seconds, stop the procedure and ventilate the infant with a bag and mask.

(10) Intubation in the delivery room is usually temporary, and the tube can be held in place by hand. If prolonged ventilation is required, the tube should be secured by paper tape, and an x-ray obtained to check its position.

4. Ventilation
  a. Continuous positive airway pressure (CPAP) is indicated:
  (1) In hyaline membrane disease (HMD), when an F_IO_2 greater than 0.4–0.6 is required to maintain a PaO_2 of 50–70 mm Hg, or when there is significant clinical worsening during the first day of life, application of CPAP early in the course of HMD decreases the time spent in high oxygen concentrations and lessens the need for mechanical ventilation.
  (2) In apnea that is unresponsive to other forms of therapy (see sec. **III.D**)
  (3) During weaning after extubation
  b. Intermittent positive pressure ventilation (IPPV) is indicated:
  (1) In HMD, when the PaO_2 is less than 60 mm Hg at an F_IO_2 of 0.4–0.6 on adequate CPAP, for the purpose of surfactant administration (see sec. **III.A.4.c**)
  (2) When PCO_2 is over 60–70 mm Hg from any cause
  (3) In persistent respiratory acidosis
  (4) In apnea that is unresponsive to CPAP
  c. The actual levels of PaO_2 and $PaCO_2$ selected for intervention depend on the disease course. Respiratory support is adjusted so that PaO_2 = 50–70 mm Hg, $PaCO_2$ = 45–55 mm Hg, and pH = 7.30–7.40. These values are optimal in HMD and differ for certain diseases (e.g., persistent pulmonary hypertension).
  d. Methods. For a detailed discussion of the methods used in providing CPAP or IPPV and recommendations for ventilation and care of the infant on the respirator, consult J. P. Cloherty and A. R. Stark (Eds.), *Manual of Neonatal Care* (3rd ed.). Boston: Little, Brown, 1991.

B. Shock. See Chap. 3 for a discussion of the causes and therapy of shock. Figure 6-5 shows the normal blood pressure in healthy newborn infants of various birth weights during the first 12 hours of life.

C. Other emergency procedures
  1. Blood gases. Samples can be obtained from a warmed heel in a heparinized Natelson tube by heel stick or by direct puncture of the radial, temporal, or posterior tibial artery. Brachial and femoral arterial punctures should be avoided. If the infant's condition is unstable, cannulation of the umbilical, radial, or posterior tibial arteries may be necessary. Catheters should not be placed in the temporal arteries.
  2. Umbilical artery catheters aid greatly in parenteral therapy, monitoring blood gases, and withdrawing blood samples. However, **indwelling arterial**

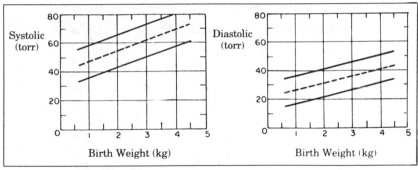

Fig. 6-5. Linear regressions (*broken lines*) and 95 percent confidence limits (*solid lines*) of systolic (*left*) and diastolic (*right*) aortic blood pressures on birth weight in 61 healthy newborn infants during the first 12 hours after birth. (From H. T. Versmold et al., *Pediatrics* 67:607, 1981. Copyright 1981, American Academy of Pediatrics.)

catheters carry great potential dangers, including life-threatening infection and thromboembolism.

   a. **Indications.** Umbilical artery catheters **should not be used** unless the infants under care are considered to have a high risk of death from their primary disease (e.g., extreme prematurity, birth weight < 1,000 gm, HMD, persistent pulmonary hypertension, severe aspiration pneumonia, shock).

   b. **Methods**

     (1) Complete sterility is required, including gloves, gown, and mask.

     (2) The cord and the surrounding area are washed carefully with povidone-iodine (Betadine) and alcohol, and the infant's abdomen is draped with sterile towels.

     (3) Cut the cord 1.0 cm from the skin. Tie the base with a cord tie.

     (4) Identify the arteries. Gently insert the tip of an iris forceps into the lumen of one artery. Allow the forceps to expand and dilate the artery while the cord stump is held between the thumb and forefinger.

     (5) Insert a saline-filled catheter (5F for infants weighing over 1,250 gm and 3.5F for infants weighing under 1,250 gm) into the artery for the appropriate distance. Insertion depth can be estimated using one of the following formulas:

       (a) Shoulder–umbilical cord distance + 2 cm, or

       (b) 3(birth weight in kg) + 9 for high lines, or by chart (Fig. 6-6).

     (6) X-ray films should be taken after placement of all umbilical catheters. The tip should be either at or below the level of L3–L4 or just above the diaphragm (T6–T10).

     (7) When adequate placement is assured, the catheter should be secured by a suture as well as by adhesive tape.

     (8) The infusion solution should contain 0.5–1.0 U heparin/ml infusate.

     (9) Arterial catheters should be removed as soon as possible. Use of the transcutaneous PO_2 monitor or pulse oximeter and blood gas determinations will permit this.

  3. **Peripheral arterial catheters** (see Chap. 3, p. 97 for a discussion of the method of peripheral arterial line placement).

  4. **Umbilical vein catheters**

   a. **Indications.** Umbilical vein catheters are used for emergency access to the circulation, for exchange transfusion, and for access in very sick or very small (< 750 gm) infants. In the latter case, it must be verified by x-ray that the catheter is in the vena cava or low in the right atrium before hypertonic infusions are begun.

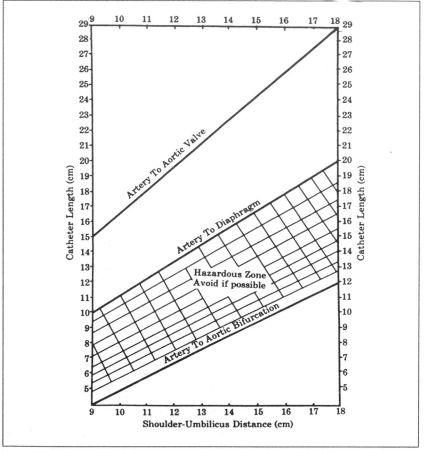

Fig. 6-6. Shoulder-umbilical distance measured above lateral end of clavicle to umbilicus versus length of umbilical artery catheter needed to reach designated level. (From P. M. Dunn, *Arch. Dis. Child.* 41:69, 1966.) Alternative calculation by weight is: Catheter length (in cm) = 3(birth weight in kg) + 9. (From H. Shukla, *Am. J. Dis. Child.* 140:786, 1986. Copyright 1986, American Medical Association.)

b. Methods

(1) Prepare as for umbilical artery catheterization.

(2) Identify the vein, remove visible clots, and dilate with an iris forceps.

(3) Insert a saline-filled 5F catheter. A multiholed catheter is used for exchange transfusions, a single-holed catheter for long-term placement. Insertion depth can be estimated by the formulas:

  (a) ⅔ of shoulder–umbilical cord distance, or

  (b) ½ (UA line calculation) − 1 (see **2.b.(5)**) or by chart (Fig. 6-7).

(4) When free blood flow is achieved (usually at a distance of 5–7 cm), the catheter is adequately placed for exchange transfusion.

(5) Keep the catheter and surrounding area sterile during exchange transfusion. In general, conditions as close to sterile as possible should be maintained in long-term placement as well.

(6) Following exchange, place a purse-string silk suture around the vein before removing the catheter. For subsequent exchanges the cord

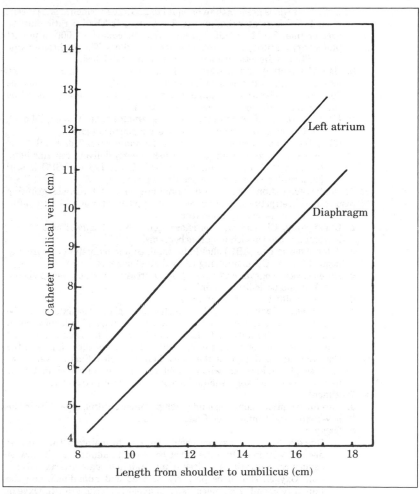

Fig. 6-7. Length from shoulder to umbilicus versus length of umbilical vein catheter. (From P. M. Dunn, *Arch. Dis. Child.* 41:69, 1966.) Alternative calculation by weight is: Catheter length (in cm) = ½(UA catheter length) + 1 (see legend Fig. 6-6). (From H. Shukla, *Am. J. Dis. Child.* 140:786, 1986. Copyright 1986, American Medical Association.)

should be soaked with warm saline until it is soft. The suture will assist in identification of the vein and reinsertion of the catheter.

III. Respiratory diseases
  A. Hyaline membrane disease
    1. Etiology. The cause of HMD is an absence or deficiency of surfactant, a phospholipid that normally lines alveoli. The disease is associated with prematurity and factors that affect lung maturation and surfactant production.
    2. Prenatal evaluation
      a. Measurement of the lecithin-sphingomyelin (L/S) ratio or disaturated phosphatidylcholine (DSPC) concentration in amniotic fluid is a reliable index of fetal lung development in pregnancies that are not complicated by maternal diabetes or Rh sensitization. Alternative tests such as the TD_x-FLM are also in wide use. The incidence of HMD is under 5 percent

if the L/S ratio is greater than or equal to 2 : 1. The incidence is 1 percent if the DSPC is greater than or equal to 500 μg/dl. The L/S ratio must be greater than 3.5 : 1 or DSPC greater than or equal to 1,000 to predict pulmonary maturity in infants of diabetic mothers. The predictive value of the FLM in diabetic women has not been established.

   b. Use of maternal corticosteroids. If an infant of less than 33 weeks' gestation with evidence of pulmonary immaturity (L/S < 2 : 1) must be delivered, acceleration of pulmonary maturity may be accomplished by the administration of glucocorticoids to the mother.

   (1) A full course of **betamethasone** or **dexamethasone,** 12.5 mg IM q24h for 48 hours, must be given to ensure a beneficial effect.

   (2) If the infant remains undelivered for more than 7 days after the course of glucocorticoids and the risk of early delivery remains high, the amniotic fluid should be retested. If the L/S or DSPC is still immature, a repeat course should be given.

3. **Postnatal evaluation.** Signs and symptoms of HMD include grunting respirations, retractions, tachypnea, and hypoxia starting shortly after birth. The infant is usually premature.

   a. Chest x-ray. Classically, this shows generalized haziness or a reticulogranular pattern with air bronchograms.

   b. Arterial blood gas (ABG) should be obtained and oximeter or transcutaneous PO_2 ($TcPO_2$) monitoring (if available) begun.

   c. An electrocardiogram and several blood pressure measurements should be taken and periodically monitored.

   d. A **blood culture** should be obtained.

   e. A **complete blood count (CBC),** including a platelet count, should be obtained. Hematocrit, electrolytes, glucose, calcium, and bilirubin should be determined initially at 6–12 hours of age and followed every 6–24 hours thereafter, depending on the clinical status of the infant and the observed rate of change of the individual variables. Smaller very low-birth-weight infants, in whom rapid changes in fluid and metabolic balance are more likely, should be monitored more frequently.

4. **Treatment**

   a. Careful attention should be paid to **temperature control,** especially in the low-birth-weight infant (see Chap. 5, p. 134).

   b. Oxygen

   (1) Dosage. Sufficient oxygen should be used to maintain the PaO_2 at about 60–70 mm Hg. Care must be taken to administer the lowest oxygen concentration required to maintain adequate arterial saturation. Oxygen should be properly warmed and humidified, and the humidity chamber changed daily to avoid bacterial growth. Oxygen should be administered via oxygen–air blenders that allow precise control over the concentration of administered oxygen. **The oxygen concentrations being administered should be checked at least every hour.** If an infant requires intermittent assisted ventilation with a Mapleson bag, the oxygen concentration administered via the bag should be similar to that usually required by the infant. When supplemental oxygen is used, PaO_2 should initially be checked no less than every 4–6 hours—more frequently if the status of the infant is changing rapidly. Blood gases should be obtained 15–20 minutes after a change in respiratory therapy. The use of a $TcPO_2$ monitor or pulse oximeter allows the continuous assessment of the infant's oxygenation and decreases the need for frequent arterial or capillary blood gas monitoring.

   (2) Toxicity. Arterial oxygen concentration (PaO_2) over 100 mm Hg may be hazardous to the retina in infants less than 1,500 gm.

   (3) Delivery of oxygen. If the infant's oxygen requirement exceeds that which can be delivered by hood (PaO_2 < 50 mm Hg and FiO_2 > 0.6), or if hypercapnia ($PaCO_2$ > 60 mm Hg) or apnea uncontrolled by other therapies is present, the use of CPAP or mechanical ventilation is indicated (see sec. II.A.4).

c. **Surfactant replacement therapy** has been shown to be effective in ameliorating HMD. Surfactant can be administered through an endotracheal tube soon after birth (prevention) or after signs of HMD are present ("rescue"). Generally, two to three doses are administered. Careful monitoring is necessary during treatment since desaturation and bradycardia are frequent adverse effects. Some infants will respond rapidly and dramatically after receiving surfactant, and careful adjustment of ventilator settings is necessary to prevent pneumothorax resulting from sudden improvement in lung compliance. Two surfactant preparations are commercially available in the United States. Dose and method of administration differ in the two preparations.

d. Normal **fluid and electrolyte requirements** should be provided (see sec. VIII). Careful monitoring of electrolytes, calcium, glucose, bilirubin, and hydration status is essential, especially in the very low-birth-weight infant.

e. Severe **metabolic acidosis** should be corrected with bicarbonate infusion. **Always be sure that the infant is adequately ventilated before administering NaHCO₃.**

   (1) In profound metabolic acidosis, treat by infusing a solution of 0.25–0.5 mEq NaHCO$_3$/ml to correct the calculated base deficit (mEq = 0.3 × kg × base deficit) at a rate no faster than 1 mEq/kg/min.

   (2) If the acidosis is less severe (pH 7.10), correct by slow infusion over several hours of an NaHCO$_3$-dextrose solution to replace the calculated deficit. A solution of 15 mEq NaHCO$_3$/dl of 5 or 10% dextrose in water (D/W) will provide adequate treatment of the acidosis while avoiding the use of hyperosmolar solutions, which have been associated with intraventricular hemorrhage in the premature neonate.

f. Follow the **blood pressure** carefully (see Fig. 6-5). If the infant is hypovolemic, maintain intravascular volume with infusions of normal saline, 5% albumin, or packed red blood cells (RBC) as appropriate, depending on the infant's hematocrit and clinical status.

g. Maintain adequate **blood volume** and **oxygen-carrying capacity** by transfusion with packed RBCs. Monitor blood glucose frequently during transfusions to avoid hypoglycemia secondary to the interruption of the intravenous dextrose infusion.

h. **Antibiotic coverage** (ampicillin and an aminoglycoside) should be considered after appropriate cultures have been obtained, because pneumonia can mimic the symptoms and radiographic picture of HMD. If clinical and laboratory evaluation make infection unlikely and cultures are negative, antibiotics can be discontinued after 48–72 hours.

i. **Hypocalcemia and hyperbilirubinemia** should be corrected as described in secs. VI.D.3 and V.A.3.

j. **Nutritional requirements** should be provided. If the course of the illness is relatively mild, feedings can often be begun by the third or fourth day. In more severe illnesses, however, this may not be possible, and IV hyperalimentation can be used to provide additional calories (see Chap. 10, p. 264).

k. The infant should be observed closely for the development of complications, such as intraventricular hemorrhage, patent ductus arteriosus, pneumothorax, retinopathy of prematurity, nosocomial infection, and bronchopulmonary dysplasia.

B. **Meconium aspiration** before or during birth can obstruct airways, interfere with gas exchange, increase pulmonary vascular resistance, and cause severe respiratory distress.

1. **Etiology.** Passage of meconium in utero often results from hypoxic stress. Such infants are at risk of fetal distress and neonatal depression.

   a. **Prevention of passage of meconium in utero.** Tests of fetal well-being, such as nonstress testing, fetal monitoring, and scalp pH sampling, can be done in pregnancies with evidence of uteroplacental insufficiency. The risk of meconium aspiration is markedly increased in postdate (> 42 weeks) pregnancies.

b. **Prevention of meconium aspiration**
   (1) When thick particulate or "pea-soup" meconium is present, the obstetrician should extensively suction the infant's nose and oropharynx before the chest is delivered. This should be done with a 10F catheter.
   (2) When the birth is completed, the infant should be passed to a clinician capable of intubation, who should suction the trachea with a 3.0-mm endotracheal tube. The tube should be introduced **into the trachea** under direct laryngoscopy. Wall suction (set at 100 mm Hg) should be used. One intubation is usually sufficient.
   (3) Oxygen by mask should be administered as soon as the trachea has been cleared.
   (4) The airway should be cleared and ventilation initiated before significant bradycardia occurs.
   (5) It is not necessary to suction the trachea of infants born through thin meconium who have effective respirations at the time of delivery.

2. **Evaluation and diagnosis**
   a. The severity of the disease is related to the thickness of the meconium and the amount the infant has already aspirated.
   b. If tachypnea or respiratory distress increases, evaluation should include:
   (1) **ABG determination.** Unlike HMD, in meconium aspiration arterial desaturation due to right-to-left shunting is likely to be more of a problem than is hypercarbia.
   (2) **Chest x-rays** of infants with meconium aspiration show coarse, irregular pulmonary densities. Also, 10–20 percent of infants may have associated pneumothorax or pneumomediastinum.
   (3) A CBC and blood culture are indicated because meconium enhances the growth of bacteria, and pneumonia may be present.
   (4) Glucose and calcium monitoring

3. **Therapy**
   a. Infants with significant aspiration often have severe problems.
   (1) **Respiratory physiotherapy** and **oropharyngeal suction** should be done every 30 minutes for the first 2 hours and every hour for the next 8 hours. The trachea should be suctioned if a tube is in place.
   (2) **Hypoxia** should be eliminated by increasing the inspired oxygen concentration, and severe metabolic acidosis should be corrected with a bicarbonate infusion (see **A.4.e**). Careful monitoring of blood gases is essential, and the placement of an indwelling arterial catheter for blood sampling and infusion is usually required. For persistent hypoxia ($PaO_2 < 50$ mm Hg) or for severe hypercapnia ($PaCO_2 > 60$ mm Hg), intubation and mechanical ventilation are indicated (see sec. **II.A.3** and **4**).
   (3) **Maintenance fluid and electrolyte requirements** should be provided. Hematocrit, electrolytes, calcium, and glucose should be monitored carefully.
   (4) The use of **antibiotics** is individualized but, in general, if an infiltrate is seen on chest x-ray, broad-spectrum antibiotics are used after cultures have been obtained.
   (5) Hypoxia and acidosis may contribute to **persistent pulmonary artery hypertension** with continued severe hypoxia and right-to-left shunting of blood via the patent ductus arteriosus or foramen ovale. (For a full discussion of the evaluation and management of persistent pulmonary hypertension, see J. P. Cloherty and A. R. Stark [Eds.], *Manual of Neonatal Care* [3rd ed.]. Boston: Little, Brown, 1991.) Both high-frequency ventilation and extracorporeal membrane oxygenation (ECMO) have been shown to be highly effective in the management of this condition.

(6) Pneumothorax or pneumomediastinum develops in approximately 10–20 percent of infants with meconium aspiration (see **C**).

C. Air leak

1. **Etiology.** Air leak in the newborn infant results from alveolar rupture or dissection of air into the pulmonary parenchyma outside the bronchial tree. Infants who have HMD or pneumonia, who have required resuscitation, or who have meconium aspiration syndrome are at increased risk of pneumothorax.

2. **Evaluation and diagnosis**
   a. Clinical signs of **pneumothorax** develop rapidly and include moderate to severe respiratory distress, cyanosis, chest asymmetry, a shift of the apical beat, a change in breath sounds, a drop in blood pressure, and decreased perfusion.
   b. **Pneumomediastinum** may be manifested by distant heart sounds. It is most reliably diagnosed by lateral chest radiograph. It is generally not clinically significant except for its association with other air leak.
   c. **Pneumopericardium** will cause an immediate deterioration in blood pressure, heart rate, and arterial oxygen. This problem should be considered in the presence of pneumomediastinum and pneumothorax. It will lead to death unless it is diagnosed and treated quickly.
   d. Anteroposterior and cross-table lateral x-rays will help differentiate pneumothorax and pneumomediastinum from other causes of respiratory distress.
   e. For acute evaluation of an infant whose condition deteriorates dramatically, the **fiberoptic transilluminator** can be used to diagnose pneumothorax. The room must be sufficiently dark for effective transillumination.
   f. If the infant continues to deteriorate while awaiting x-ray confirmation, needle aspiration should be done as a lifesaving diagnostic-therapeutic procedure (see below).

3. **Treatment**
   a. **Pneumothorax**
      (1) Uncomplicated pneumothorax. In infants with no underlying pulmonary disease or complicating therapy (ventilation or CPAP) and who are not in distress, conservative management may be adequate. This consists of close observation, frequent small feedings to minimize crying, and a follow-up x-ray. The extrapulmonary air will usually resolve in 24–48 hours.
      The use of 100% oxygen, while effective in speeding the resolution of pneumothorax, **is not recommended** in premature infants because of the danger of retinopathy of prematurity and possible pulmonary toxicity.
      (2) Needle aspiration is a useful therapeutic and diagnostic procedure in the critically ill infant with respiratory or hemodynamic compromise, or both, due to pneumothorax. It is also helpful in the occasional infant who has no underlying pulmonary problem or continuing air leak, but **who is in distress** from the pneumothorax.
      (a) Place the infant in a supine position.
      (b) Attach a 23- or 25-gauge "butterfly" needle to a large syringe via a three-way stopcock.
      (c) The needle should enter through the second intercostal space in the midclavicular line. Hit the rib with the needle and slide it over the top to minimize the chance of bleeding from the intercostal artery.
      (d) Apply continuous suction with the syringe as the needle is inserted. A rapid flow of air will occur when the pleural air space is entered.
      (e) If air continues to leak, a chest tube must be inserted. Because the needle can puncture the lung parenchyma (with a small chance of

bronchopleural fistula), it is prudent to remove the needle as soon as possible.

(3) **Chest tube placement.** Infants with a continuing air leak, who have underlying pulmonary disease causing continued distress, or who are on mechanical ventilation or CPAP require **chest tube placement** and suction for drainage of pneumothorax. This should be performed or supervised by experienced nursery personnel or a surgeon.

(4) **Persistent pneumothorax.** Occasionally, more than one chest tube may be required. Selected occlusion of the leaking lung has also proved effective in some cases. The procedure should be undertaken with great caution, as it may cause respiratory decompensation. Selective intubation of the right main-stem bronchus occludes the left, and a small (3–4F) Fogarty catheter can be used to occlude the right.

(5) **High-frequency ventilation.** This modality has been shown to be quite effective for infants with persistent air leak who require mechanical ventilation.

b. **Pneumomediastinum.** Chest tubes are not placed in infants with pneumomediastinum alone.

c. **Pneumoperitoneum.** Air can dissect into the abdomen through the posterior mediastinum. Although this is rarely a cause of significant compromise, such free air raises the question of a gastrointestinal perforation. Differentiation of the two is based on the clinical setting.

d. **Pneumopericardium**

(1) Symptomatic pneumopericardium can be drained using a 20-gauge, 1-in. needle attached via a three-way stopcock to a 10- to 20-ml syringe.

(a) Following surgical preparation, insert a needle at the subxiphoid region, aiming for the posterior left shoulder, and, with suction on the syringe, advance the needle until air appears.

(b) When the air stops flowing, withdraw the needle.

(2) Often, a single aspiration results in clinical improvement. About 25–40 percent of all patients will have a recurrent symptomatic pneumopericardium, which can be treated as just described.

(3) Infrequently, the pneumopericardium will act as if constant air drainage into the pericardial space has occurred. Placement of a 16-gauge Intracath or surgical placement of a pericardial tube into the pericardial space is appropriate in this situation.

D. **Apnea.** In apnea spells, breathing is absent for a defined period of time (i.e., 20–30 sec) or ineffective, after which bradycardia, cyanosis, pallor, hypotonia, or metabolic acidosis is seen. The majority of very small premature infants (under 30 weeks' gestational age) have occasional apneic spells. As many as 25 percent of all premature infants weighing under 1,800 gm (about 33 weeks) will have at least one apneic episode. These spells generally begin at 1–2 days of age and may recur for 2–3 weeks postnatally, although most occur within the first 10 days of life.

Prolonged apnea is apnea lasting over 16 seconds in a full-term infant and over 20 seconds in preterm infants. **Periodic breathing** is defined as pauses in breathing of 3 seconds or longer, interrupted by respirations for less than 20 seconds. **Disorganized breathing** is irregular breathing with short apnea and bradycardia.

Bradycardia and *cyanosis* are usually present after 20 seconds of apnea, although they may occur more rapidly in the small premature infant. After 30–40 seconds, *pallor* and *hypotonia* are seen, and the infant may be unresponsive to tactile stimulation.

1. **Etiology**

a. **Hypoxemia** or diaphragmatic fatigue from respiratory disease (HMD, pneumonia). Anemia, hypovolemia, and congenital heart disease can also result in apnea because of decreased oxygen content.

b. **Respiratory center depression** due to hypoglycemia, hypocalcemia, electrolyte disorders, sepsis, drugs, or intracranial disorders

c. **Abnormal or hyperactive reflexes** due to suction or stimulation of the pharynx, fluid in the airway or pharynx from feeding or gastroesophageal reflux, and paradoxical apnea after lung inflation

d. **Airway obstruction** due to passive neck flexion, pressure on the lower rim of a face mask, submental pressure, and supine position are all encountered during nursery procedures. Spontaneously occurring airway obstruction, which tends to occur when preterm infants assume a position of neck flexion, may contribute to the **prolongation** of apneic spells.

e. **Temperature.** Apnea is more frequent in the absence of a skin–core temperature gradient. Infants in isolettes servocontrolled to maintain skin temperatures at 36.8°C (98.2°F) have more frequent spells than do those maintained at 36.0°C (96.8°F). Sudden increases in incubator temperature increase the frequency of apneic spells.

f. **Apnea of prematurity** is recurrent apnea in the absence of any of the preceding conditions. It may be related to decreased CO_2 sensitivity or to decreased afferent stimulation from peripheral receptors.

2. **Monitoring and evaluation**
   a. All infants of less than 34 weeks' gestational age or weighing under 1,800 gm should be placed on heart rate monitors for at least 5–7 days. Because impedance apnea monitors may not distinguish respiratory efforts during airway obstruction from normal breaths, the **heart rate** should be monitored.
   b. When a monitor alarm sounds, the clinician should respond to the **infant,** not the monitor. Check for bradycardia, cyanosis, and airway obstruction.
   c. Following the first apneic spell, the infant should be evaluated for a possible underlying cause, and specific treatment should be initiated. A precipitating cause is more likely in infants of more than 33–34 weeks' gestational age. Treatable causes should be considered first.
   d. A bag and mask should be available near every infant who is being monitored for apnea. The oxygen concentration should be similar to that which the infant has been breathing. Equipment for intubation and full resuscitation should be present.

3. **Treatment**
   a. Individual spells that do not immediately self-resolve are treated with gentle shaking. Infants who fail to respond should be ventilated during the spell with bag and mask, generally with an FiO_2 equal to that before the spell, to avoid marked elevations in arterial PO_2.
   b. For repeated prolonged spells, i.e., more than two to three per hour or spells requiring frequent bagging, treatment should be initiated in the order of increasing invasiveness and risk. The number of spells may be reduced by:
      (1) Decreasing environmental temperature to the low end of the neutral thermal environment range. Placing a heat shield around a small premature infant may prevent swings in temperature.
      (2) Avoiding stimuli that may trigger apnea. These may be suctioning, nipple feeding, and cold or warm stimulation of the trigeminal area of the face.
      (3) **Theophylline** (2.0–6.5 mg/kg/day PO) or aminophylline (2.5–8.0 mg/kg/day IV) in divided doses q4–12h should be started if the preceding measures fail.
         (a) If the neonate has severe apneic spells and more rapid action is desired, a loading dose of aminophylline, 7–8 mg/kg (equal to 6.9 mg/kg theophylline) IV over 15–20 minutes, can be given. The usual maintenance doses can be given after 6 hours.
         (b) Serum levels should be obtained during therapy, and the dosage should be adjusted to maintain the theophylline concentration in the range of 4–15 µg/ml. The dosage should be reduced if tachycardia or GI toxicity becomes evident.
         (c) The maximum response may take from 3–4 days.

(4) **Caffeine citrate,** a related xanthine stimulant, may also decrease the frequency of apneic spells. As with theophylline, the acute and long-term toxicity of caffeine in newborn infants is not well established, although the therapeutic range is broader and therefore probably safer. Some studies suggest it may be effective when theophylline has failed. A suggested **dosage schedule** for caffeine citrate is a loading dose of 10–20 mg/kg PO or IV, followed by a maintenance dose of 5–10 mg/kg daily in a single dose. When serum concentrations are monitored, optimal levels are 5–20 μg/ml.

(5) **Doxapram,** another analeptic drug, has been reported to be successful in apnea that is unresponsive to theophylline. It can only be administered as a continuous infusion. The suggested dose starts at a rate of 1.0–1.5 mg/kg/hr and increases to 2.5 mg/kg/hr as needed to control apnea. Signs of toxicity include hypothermia, salivation, lacrimation, tremors, jitteriness, hyperactivity, hyperglycemia, and mild liver dysfunction. The infusion is decreased once control is obtained.

(6) Small increases in FiO_2 (0.25–0.26) may reduce the frequency of apneic spells. However, for small infants, without continuous monitoring of arterial oxygenation, the **risk of retinopathy of prematurity** makes this intervention relatively hazardous.

(7) In some infants, CPAP at low pressures (3–5 cm H_2O) is effective.

(8) If all these interventions fail, **mechanical ventilation** may be required until the infant matures.

(9) Most neonates with apnea of prematurity will not require therapy or monitoring by the time they are ready for discharge from the hospital. If infants are free of apnea for 10–14 days while being monitored in the hospital, their medication can be stopped. If they are free of apnea, are off medication for 5–7 days while being monitored in the hospital, and are 34–35 weeks post-last menstrual period, it is usually safe to discharge them.

(10) If there is any concern about the possibility of recurrence of apnea, a *pneumogram* to assess breathing patterns, obstructive apnea, and bradycardia may be useful (the use of the pneumogram to predict apnea is controversial). If there is a documented need for medication (abnormal pneumogram or clinical apnea off medication), the pneumogram must be repeated with the infant on medication. If the infant is normal, he or she can be discharged home, without monitor, on the same daily dose per kilogram and the blood level that was associated with a normal pneumogram.

(11) Subsequent discontinuation of theophylline can be accomplished by a monitored evaluation either at home or in the hospital.

(12) If pneumograms are abnormal or clinical apnea occurs at theophylline levels of 12–15 μg/ml, home monitoring may be required. Each hospital should have its own guidelines for both hospital and home management of apnea of prematurity.

IV. **Cardiac disease in the newborn.** Severe congenital heart disease is seen in approximately 1 of 400 infants. Because many benign murmurs occur in the neonatal period, stable, asymptomatic infants can be followed clinically. Symptomatic infants will usually present in one or more of three ways: congestive failure, cyanosis, or arrhythmia.

A. **Congestive heart failure (CHF)**

1. **Etiology.** CHF can result from anatomic defects or, less frequently, from functional failure. Patent ductus arteriosus (PDA) in premature infants is the most common cause of CHF in the newborn period. Other anatomic causes are large ventricular septal defect (VSD), endocardial cushion defect, left-sided obstructive lesions such as hypoplastic left heart syndrome, and coarctation of the aorta and other complex lesions. Functional cardiac failure may result from myocardiopathies (asphyxial, diabetic, or viral), arteriovenous fistulas, and paroxysmal tachycardias.

2. Evaluation
   a. Common signs of heart failure in the newborn are tachycardia, tachypnea, hepatomegaly, cardiomegaly, and diaphoresis. Murmurs may be present.
   b. ABGs, chest x-rays, four extremity blood pressures, and an ECG are the basics. An ill infant suspected of serious cardiac disease should be transferred immediately to a regional neonatal intensive care unit where echocardiography, cardiac catheterization, and subspecialty evaluation are available.
3. Diagnosis
   a. PDA. Most premature infants with PDA do not require cardiac catheterization, because PDA is usually evident by clinical examination, and its hemodynamic significance can be quantitated by noninvasive tests.
      (1) For signs and symptoms see Table 6-3.
      (2) The diagnosis of a PDA can be confirmed and the amount of the left-to-right shunt quantitated by two-dimensional echocardiography.
   b. The diagnoses of other acyanotic cardiac lesions that may result in CHF are given in Table 6-3.
4. Treatment
   a. Except for rhythm disturbances, **general medical treatment** is directed toward decreasing the workload on the heart.
      (1) Therapeutic measures include diuretics, fluid restriction below 120–150 ml/kg/day, maintenance of a neutral thermal environment (see Chap. 5, p. 134), and decreasing the work of feeding, e.g., gavage rather than nipple feedings.
      (2) For adequate myocardial oxygenation
         (a) Maintain the hematocrit at over 40% (use packed red blood cells, 5 ml/kg, given over 2–4 hr and repeated as necessary) and
         (b) Increase FiO_2 as necessary to maintain the PaO_2 at 60–80 mm Hg
         (c) Digoxin remains the cornerstone of CHF management in the neonate, but may be of little benefit to the very immature preterm infant with CHF secondary to PDA.
   b. Cardiotonic drugs are the cornerstone of CHF treatment.
      (1) For specific recommendations regarding **digoxin** and **diuretics,** see Chap. 9, p. 246.
      (2) Dopamine has been used in the newborn for inotropy and the treatment of severe hypotension.
   c. Indomethacin trial is warranted if the cardiac failure caused by the PDA is not adequately controlled by other medical treatments. (See J. P. Cloherty and A. R. Stark [Eds.], *Manual of Neonatal Care* [3rd ed.]. Boston: Little, Brown, 1991, for a discussion of evaluation, dosage, potential side effects, and contraindications to the use of indomethacin.) If it is contraindicated, or it fails to be effective, surgical ligation of the ductus may be indicated.
B. Cyanosis can indicate life-threatening congenital heart disease.
   1. Etiology
      a. The major cardiac causes of cyanosis in the newborn are transposition of the great arteries, critical pulmonary stenosis or atresia, tetralogy of Fallot, tricuspid atresia, anomalous pulmonary veins, and Ebstein's anomaly. See Table 6-4 for a list of cardiac lesions that may present with cyanosis.
      b. Major pulmonary causes are HMD, meconium aspiration, pneumothorax, and persistent fetal circulation.
   2. Evaluation
      a. These infants must be evaluated rapidly by ECG, chest x-ray, right radial (i.e., preductal) ABGs in room air and 100% oxygen, and an echocardiogram. A cardiologist should be promptly consulted.
      b. Early measurement of PaO_2 in 100% oxygen in a child with developing pulmonary disease can be helpful when cyanotic congenital heart disease is being considered later in the infant's course. Many infants with HMD

Table 6-3. Acyanotic cardiac lesions that may result in congestive heart failure

Diagnosis	Physical findings	Onset of heart murmur	Onset of CHF	ECG findings	CXR findings	Associated pathology
Severe AS	SEM and SEC	Birth onward	3 days onward	Usually LVH; RVH if hypoplastic LV	CE with PV congestion	EFE, MS, or MR
Severe coarctation	Decreased femoral pulses; differential cyanosis	Variable	First month	Usually RVH	CE with PV congestion	Bicuspid AoV, VSD, AS, AR
IAA	Decreased femoral pulses; differential cyanosis	Variable	4 days onward	Usually RVH	CE with PV congestion	VSD, PDA, complex CHD, DiGeorge's syndrome
VSD	SRM; MDR	2–3 days onward	Usually 3–6 weeks	RVH or BVH	CE with ↑ PBF	Prematurity; chromosomal anomalies
CAVC	SRM	Birth onward	Usually 3–6 weeks	Superior axis with CCWL, RVH, or BVH	CE with ↑ PBF	Down syndrome; heterotaxy

PDA	Continuous murmur; bounding pulses; hyperdynamic precordium	2–3 days onward	First week onward	RVH normal for age	CE with ↑ PBF	Prematurity
Transient myocardial ischemia	Transient SRM; quiet precordium	Birth	Birth	NSSTTWA	CE with PV congestion	Perinatal asphyxia
Myocarditis	Other signs of infection (e.g., seizures)	Variable	Birth onward	NSSTTWA; arrhythmia (20%)	CE with PV congestion	Perinatal infection
EFE	Muffled heart sounds; gallop rhythm	Variable	Usually in first 6 months	RVH in newborns; LVH in infants	CE with PV congestion	
Pompe's disease (acid maltase deficiency)	Hypotonia and weak cry; protruding tongue	Variable	Usually within 2 months	LAD with LVH; deep q waves; PR < 0.09 seconds	CE	

Key: CHF = congestive heart failure; ECG = electrocardiogram; CXR = chest x-ray; AS = aortic stenosis; SEM = systolic ejection murmur; SEC = systolic ejection click; LVH = left ventricular hypertrophy; RVH = right ventricular hypertrophy; LV = left ventricle; CE = cardiac enlargement; PV = pulmonary venous; EFE = endocardial fibroelastosis; MS = mitral stenosis; MR = mitral regurgitation; AoV = aortic valve; VSD = ventricular septal defect; AR = aortic regurgitation; IAA = interrupted aortic arch; PDA = patent ductus arteriosus; CHD = congenital heart disease; SRM = systolic regurgitant murmur; MDR = middiastolic murmur; BVH = biventricular hypertrophy; PBF = pulmonary blood flow; CAVC = common atrioventricular canal defect; CCWL = counterclockwise vector loop; NSSTTWA = nonspecific ST-T wave abnormalities; LAD = left axis deviation.
Source: J. P. Cloherty and A. R. Stark [Eds.], *Manual of Neonatal Care* (3rd ed.). Boston: Little, Brown, 1991. Pp. 258–259.

Table 6-4. Cyanotic congenital heart disease presenting with PaO_2 less than 50 mm Hg

Diagnosis	Heart murmur	ECG findings	CXR findings
D-TGA with IVS	None	RVH normal for age	No CE with ↑ PBF
TAPVR with PV obstruction	None	RVH	PV congestion
Ebstein's anomaly	± TR murmur	RAE, RBBB, WPW	Massive CE; normal or ↓ PBF
Tricuspid atresia with PS or PA	± PS murmur	Superior axis, LVH	No CE with ↓ PBF
PA with IVS	± TR murmur, ± continuous murmur	LVH, QRS axis 0–90 degrees	± CE with ↓ PBF
Severe PS	PS murmur	RVH, QRS axis 0–90 degrees	± CE with ↓ PBF
Severe TOF	PS murmur	RVH	No CE with ↓ PBF
TOF with PA	± Continuous murmur	RVH	No CE with ↓ PBF

Key: ECG = electrocardiogram; CXR = chest x-ray, D-TGA = D-transposition of the great arteries; IVS = intact ventricular septum; RVH = right ventricular hypertrophy; CE = cardiac enlargement; PBF = pulmonary blood flow; TAPVR = total anomalous pulmonary venous return; PV = pulmonary venous; TR = tricuspid regurgitation; LVH = left ventricular hypertrophy; RAE = right atrial enlargement; RBBB = right bundle branch block; WPW = Wolff-Parkinson-White syndrome; PS = pulmonary stenosis; PA = pulmonary atresia; TOF = tetralogy of Fallot; ↑ = increased; ↓ = decreased; ± = present or absent.
Source: Adapted from M. D. Freed, Congenital Cardiac Malformations. In M. E. Avery and H. W. Taeusch (Eds.), *Schaffer's Diseases of the Newborn* (5th ed.). Philadelphia: Saunders, 1984. Reprinted from J. P. Cloherty and A. R. Stark [Eds.], *Manual of Neonatal Care* (3rd ed.). Boston: Little, Brown, 1991. P. 262.

may have a PaO_2 greater than 100 mm Hg in 100% oxygen early in their disease, but not by day 2 or 3. A PaO_2 over 150 in an adequately ventilated infant will exclude most significant cyanotic heart disease.

3. **Treatment** of cardiac causes of cyanosis is a **medical emergency.** Newborns with lesions resulting in decreased pulmonary blood flow (e.g., pulmonary or tricuspid atresia), poor mixing (e.g., transposition), or left-sided obstruction may require prostaglandin E_1 (PGE_1) infusion to maintain patency of the ductus arteriosus until definitive surgical therapy. (See J. P. Cloherty and A. R. Stark [Eds.], *Manual of Neonatal Care* [3rd ed.]. Boston: Little, Brown, 1991, for a discussion of evaluation, dosage, potential side effects, and contraindications to the use of PGE_1.)

C. **Rhythm disturbances** (see also Chap. 9, p. 249)
   1. **Bradycardia.** Both sinus bradycardia and that due to congenital heart block are rare.
      a. **Etiology.** Elevated intracranial pressure, hypertension, potassium intoxication, hypothyroidism, and congenital heart disease are among the causes. Congenital heart block may be secondary to maternal collagen vascular disease. Occasionally, postmature infants may show a benign low resting heart rate (90–100 beats/min).
      b. **Treatment.** In general, infants with a heart rate between 50 and 70 beats per minute may be asymptomatic and need no treatment if they remain well for over 72 hours with a normal QRS complex on the ECG.
         (1) Treat the underlying cause if possible. If the low heart rate persists after treatment but there is no evidence of cardiovascular compromise, observation without treatment is a wise course.
         (2) In infants with a heart rate under 50, respiratory distress, cyanosis,

and CHF are frequent. Treatment consists of the use of a chronotropic agent such as isoproterenol to raise the heart rate acutely. If symptomatic bradycardia persists when medication is begun or withdrawn, insertion of a pacemaker may be necessary.

(3) When fetal heart rate monitoring indicates a persistent fetal bradycardia, a cardiologic consultation should be made before delivery.

2. **Supraventricular tachycardia (SVT)** is relatively common.

a. **Etiology.** Congenital SVT may be associated with Wolff-Parkinson-White syndrome, structural congenital heart disease, or no evident cardiac abnormality.

b. **Evaluation**

(1) The heart rate is 200–300 beats per minute; P waves are rarely seen, and the QRS complex may be normal or abnormal.

(2) If the SVT is present prenatally, it carries a risk of CHF in utero, with the possibility of fetal hydrops or stillbirth, or both. Careful ultrasonic monitoring is essential. In utero treatment of the fetus may be accomplished by treatment of the mother with antiarrhythmic drugs that cross the placenta. In situations in which the fetus does not respond to maternal treatment, early delivery should be planned based on pulmonary maturity and signs of hydrops.

c. **Treatment** consists of attempts to convert to sinus rhythm. Infants in good condition at delivery can usually tolerate up to 24 hours of tachycardia without CHF.

(1) Occasionally, infants respond to vagal stimulation (e.g., suctioning, ice applied to the malar area, or pressure applied to the fontanel).

(2) Adenosine therapy has shown great promise in treating neonatal SVT. The starting dose is 50 µg/kg by rapid (1–2 seconds) IV push. It should be infused as close to the IV site as possible and the IV flushed immediately with saline. The dose can be increased in 50-µg/kg increments (up to a maximum of 250 µg/kg) q2min until the return of sinus rhythm.

(3) Intraesophageal pacing has also been used successfully by pediatric cardiologists.

(4) Treatment with digoxin for infants with SVT should be considered whether or not they are responsive to vagal stimulation (see Chap. 9, p. 251).

(5) If the infant's clinical state deteriorates, cardioversion may be necessary.

V. **Hematologic problems**

A. **Jaundice** (including erythroblastosis)

1. **Etiology**

a. **Physiologic hyperbilirubinemia** in full-term infants is defined as unconjugated hyperbilirubinemia (total serum bilirubin < 12 mg/dl, direct fraction < 15% of the total) that appears on or after the third day of life and resolves before 10 days. It is caused by an increased bilirubin load and poor hepatic uptake, conjugation, and excretion of bilirubin. The immature liver of the premature infant may cause the bilirubin to go higher. Breast-fed infants invariably have higher peaks and slower resolution.

b. **Nonphysiologic jaundice** is jaundice due to an abnormality of bilirubin production, metabolism, or excretion. It is manifested by clinical jaundice in the first 36 hours of life, serum bilirubin concentration increasing by more than 5 mg/dl per day, a total bilirubin over 15 mg/dl in a formula-fed full-term infant or over 15 in a premature infant, a total bilirubin over 17 mg/dl in a breast-fed term infant, or clinical jaundice beyond 8 days in a full-term infant or beyond 2 weeks in a premature infant.

(1) **Indirect hyperbilirubinemia.** Direct bilirubin is less than 15 percent of the total bilirubin. The causes of nonphysiologic hyperbilirubinemia in the neonate are as follows:

(a) *Excess bilirubin production* due to

    (i) Maternal-fetal blood group incompatibility
    (ii) Hereditary hemolytic anemia: red cell membrane defects, enzyme defects, hemoglobinopathies
    (iii) Acquired hemolytic anemia: infection, drugs, disseminated intravascular coagulation (DIC)
    (iv) Extravascular extravasation of blood
    (v) Polycythemia
    (vi) Swallowed blood
    (vii) Increased enterohepatic circulation of bilirubin as in pyloric stenosis, delayed emptying of the intestine, bowel surgery, and poor fluid intake
    (viii) Genetic and ethnic factors
  (b) *Decreased clearance of bilirubin* due to
    (i) Errors of metabolism, including familial nonhemolytic jaundice types I and II (Crigler-Najjar syndrome), Gilbert syndrome, Dubin-Johnson syndrome, Rotor syndrome, galactosemia, tyrosinosis, and hypermethionemia
    (ii) Prematurity
    (iii) Hypothyroidism and hypopituitarism; infants of diabetic mothers
    (iv) Poor perfusion of the liver
  (2) **Direct hyperbilirubinemia** (direct bilirubin > 15% of the total bilirubin). Causes of direct hyperbilirubinemia are sepsis, intrauterine viral infections, neonatal hepatitis, intrahepatic and extrahepatic biliary atresia, biliary tract obstruction (by a choledochal cyst, an abdominal mass, or annular pancreas), trisomy 18, galactosemia, tyrosinemia, Rotor syndrome, Dubin-Johnson syndrome, hypermethionemia, alpha-1-antitrypsin deficiency, cystic fibrosis, posthemolytic disease of the newborn syndrome (inspissated bile syndrome), hypopituitarism, hypothyroidism, and prolonged total parenteral nutrition.

2. **Evaluation and diagnosis.** Infants begin to appear jaundiced at serum bilirubin levels greater than 6 mg/dl. A full-term infant whose bilirubin is over 5 mg/dl within the first 24 hours of life, over 10 mg/dl within the first 48 hours, or over 13 mg/dl after 72 hours requires investigation. Premature or sick infants should have daily serum bilirubin measurements until they are past the danger of hyperbilirubinemia. In infants known to be at risk of hyperbilirubinemia, such as infants born to Rh-sensitized mothers, cord blood bilirubin should be measured.

  a. **Laboratory tests** to evaluate jaundice include direct and indirect bilirubin, the blood groups of mother and infant, a direct Coombs test and identification of the antibody if it is positive, a hematocrit, a blood smear for red cell morphologic study, and a reticulocyte count.

  b. In persistent jaundice or direct hyperbilirubinemia, tests of liver function and thyroid function, tests for viral or bacterial infection, and tests for galactosemia may be indicated.

  c. Although tests to assess bilirubin binding may help predict whether the infant is at increased or decreased risk, none is reliable enough to predict the absolute safety or danger of any bilirubin level.

  d. **Kernicterus** is a toxic effect of non–albumin-bound, unconjugated bilirubin on the central nervous system (CNS). Susceptibility to kernicterus is increased by factors that decrease albumin binding (hypoalbuminemia, elevated free fatty acids, lipid infusion or sepsis with catecholamine-stimulated lipolysis, acidosis, hypoglycemia, sulfonamides, organic anions) and factors that increase diffusion of free bilirubin into the brain (increased concentration of bilirubin and/or increased duration of exposure to elevated levels of bilirubin; anoxic-ischemic encephalopathy).

3. **Treatment**
  a. The goal of treatment is to avoid kernicterus or sublethal bilirubin encephalopathy.

(1) In *full-term infants,* kernicterus is unlikely to occur if indirect bilirubin concentrations are kept under 20 mg/dl, provided there are no factors disturbing the blood–brain barrier or interfering with the binding of bilirubin to albumin. **There are no data to show any ill effect from bilirubin concentrations under 25 mg/dl in well full-term infants without hemolytic disease.**

(2) Kernicterus has been described at autopsy in *premature* infants whose bilirubin levels never exceeded 10 mg/dl. However, there is no consistent relationship between subsequent neurologic development and bilirubin levels in low-birth-weight infants if bilirubin levels stay under 20 mg/dl. The bilirubin encephalopathy seen in low-birth-weight infants may be related more to alterations in the blood-brain barrier caused by anoxia, ischemia, or hyperosmolarity than to the actual bilirubin level.

b. The general guidelines used for treatment are in Tables 6-5 and 6-6. (For a discussion of new perspectives on the less aggressive management of jaundice in the full-term, otherwise healthy newborn, see *Pediatrics* 89:809–833, 1992.)

(1) Establish that the baby has adequate fluid intake. In breast-fed infants, supplement the diet with 5% D/W or formula if indicated. Give IV fluids if indicated.

(2) Correct asphyxia, hypotension, hypoxia, hypothermia, and hypoglycemia. Avoid drugs that may interfere with the binding of bilirubin to albumin (e.g., sulfonamides, moxalactam, aspirin, tolbutamide, fusidic acid, apazone, rapid infusions of ampicillin, long-chain free fatty acids) and avoid factors that may disturb the blood-brain barrier.

c. Phototherapy

(1) Indications

(a) Phototherapy should be instituted if there is a risk that unconjugated bilirubin will rise to levels that might saturate albumin-binding sites or that would possibly result in the need for an exchange transfusion.

(b) Prophylactic phototherapy may be indicated in special circumstances (i.e., in tiny infants in whom dangerous levels of bilirubin are likely to develop, in severely bruised premature infants, in hemolytic disease while awaiting exchange transfusion). In hemolytic disease, phototherapy is used as an adjunct to exchange transfusion.

(c) Effectiveness. The amount of skin exposure and radiant energy impinging on the skin is of primary importance for effective

Table 6-5. Serum bilirubin level (mg/dl) as a criterion for exchange transfusion*

	Birth weight (gm)				
	< 1,250	1,250–1,499	1,500–1,999	2,000–2,499	≥ 2,500
Standard risk	13	15	17	18	20
High risk†	10	13	15	17	18

* Both treated and untreated infants received an exchange transfusion if bilirubin levels exceeded these values in each weight category.† High-risk criteria are met when one or more of the following apply: birth weight < 1,000 gm, 5-minute Apgar score of 3, PaO_2 < 40 mm Hg for > 2 hours, pH < 7.15 for > 1 hour, rectal temperature < 35°C for > 4 hours, serum total protein value < 4 gm/dl × 2, serum albumin level < 2.5 gm/dl × 2, hemolysis, or clinical deterioration. Source: From W. J. Keenan, K. K. Novak, J. M. Sutherland, D. A. Bryla, and K. L. Fetterly, Morbidity and mortality associated with exchange transfusion. *Pediatrics* 75(Suppl.): 417, 1985; and J. P. Cloherty and A. R. Stark [Eds.], *Manual of Neonatal Care* (3rd ed.). Boston: Little, Brown, 1991.

Table 6-6. Management of jaundice in low-birth-weight infants

Birth weight (gm)	Indirect bilirubin concentrations					
	5–6 mg/dl	7–9 mg/dl	10–12 mg/dl	12–15 mg/dl	15–20 mg/dl	>20 mg/dl
≤1,000	Phototherapy ——————————→ Exchange transfusion ——————————————————————————————————————→					
1,000–1,500	Observe and repeat BR	Phototherapy ——————→	Exchange transfusion —————————————————————————→			
1,500–2,000	Observe and repeat BR		Phototherapy ———————————————→		Exchange transfusion ——→	
>2,000	Observe	Observe and repeat BR	Phototherapy (<2,500 gm)	Phototherapy (>2,500 gm)	———————→ Exchange transfusion ——→	

Key: BR = bilirubin determination.
Source: From W. J. Cashore and L. Stern, The management of hyperbilirubinemia. *Clin. Perinatol.* 11:339, 1984; and J. P. Cloherty and A. R. Stark [Eds.], *Manual of Neonatal Care* (3rd ed.). Boston: Little, Brown, 1991.

phototherapy. Blue light (wavelength 450–500 nm) is more effective in lowering bilirubin, but cool white light provides better visualization of cyanosis in the infant. We use light banks that have alternating blue and white lights.

(2) Technique of phototherapy

(a) Shield the infant's eyes. Observe the infant for nasal obstruction from the eye shields.

(b) Be certain all electrical outlets are properly grounded.

(c) Use a Plexiglas cover or shield to prevent harm to the infant in case of lamp breakage and to screen out wavelengths below 300 nm, thus protecting the infant from ultraviolet light.

(d) Placing lights over, beside, and under the baby will increase the exposure. Lights can be placed under the baby by using a transparent plastic crib and placing the baby on a plastic air bubble mattress. Phototherapy blankets have been quite helpful in the NICU and can also be used for home phototherapy.

(e) Monitor the temperate q2h to prevent hypothermia or hyperthermia. Use a control alarm if possible and a servocontrolled incubator if necessary.

(f) Weigh the infant daily or, if the infant is small, twice daily and provide extra fluid as necessary.

(g) Do not use skin color as a guide to hyperbilirubinemia in infants under phototherapy. Instead, monitor bilirubin at least q12–24h.

(h) Change the lamps q2,000h of use (alternatively, change them all every 3 months). Monitoring the energy output in the range of 425–475 nm will give more precise information on energy output.

(3) Side effects include:

(a) Increased insensible water loss, which may require a 10–20 percent increase in fluid intake

(b) Transient rashes

(c) Diarrhea

(d) Bronze baby syndrome, a rare complication usually seen in infants with parenchymal hepatic disease who are treated with phototherapy. **Do not use phototherapy in infants with liver disease or obstructive jaundice.**

(e) **Toxicity.** No significant long-term toxicity has been described. However, phototherapy should be used with the same caution as with any other treatment.

d. Exchange transfusion

(1) Indications

(a) Exchange transfusion should be instituted to correct severe anemia or if evaluation of bilirubin levels indicates any potential that free (unbound to albumin) unconjugated bilirubin could be present or that the infant is at risk of bilirubin encephalopathy (see **A.2**; Tables 6-5 and 6-6). The level of bilirubin at which exchange transfusion is recommended for low-birth-weight infants is controversial. There are no studies that permit recommendations to be made for the treatment of low-birth-weight infants with bilirubins under 20 mg/dl. Current recommendations from the American Academy of Pediatrics (*Guidelines for Perinatal Care,* 1992) state:

Some pediatricians use guidelines that recommend aggressive treatment of jaundice in low-birth-weight neonates, initiating phototherapy early and performing exchange transfusions in certain neonates with very low bilirubin concentrations (<10 mg/dl). However, this approach will not prevent kernicterus consistently. Some pediatricians prefer to adopt a less aggressive therapeutic stance and allow serum bilirubin concentrations in low-birth-weight neonates to approach 15–20 mg/dl (257–342 μmol/liter) before considering exchange transfusions. At present, both of these approaches to treatment should be considered reasonable. In either case, the finding of low bilirubin kernicterus at autopsy in certain low-birth-weight neonates cannot necessarily be interpreted as a therapeutic failure or equivalent to bilirubin encephalopathy. Like retinopathy of prematurity, kernicterus is a condition that cannot be prevented in certain neonates, given the current state of knowledge.

(b) Failure of phototherapy to control bilirubin levels in hemolytic disease is a frequent indication.

(c) Early exchange transfusion is often indicated in the presence of hydrops, in a known sensitized infant, or in an infant with splenomegaly or anemia.

(d) The indications for immediate (at birth) exchange transfusion are hydrops or severe anemia. When a hydropic baby is expected, preparation for exchange should begin by alerting blood bank personnel before delivery, thus avoiding unnecessary delay.

(e) A cord hemoglobin <11 mg/dl and a cord indirect bilirubin >4.5 mg/dl are usually indications for exchange transfusion, but the rate of rise of the indirect serum bilirubin is the best indication. A bilirubin rise of over 1.0 mg/dl/hr or a rise of 0.5 mg/dl/hr with a hemoglobin concentration between 11 and 13 gm/dl despite phototherapy usually signifies a need for exchange transfusion.

(f) Late exchange transfusion in hemolytic disease is usually indicated when the bilirubin in full-term infants is 20 mg/dl or it appears that it will reach 20 mg/dl at the rate it is rising.

(2) Blood preparations for exchange transfusions (see also Chap. 16)

(a) **Fresh** (under 24 hr old) **whole blood** should be used in sick infants. In other cases, blood under 72 hours old should be used to prevent problems with hyperkalemia and acidosis.

(b) **Irradiated blood** should be used if the infant has received intrauterine exchange transfusions, is neutropenic, or weighs less than 1,200 gm.

(c) **Viral screening.** Donor blood is tested for the acquired immunodeficiency syndrome (AIDS) virus (human immunodeficiency virus), in addition to hepatitis B, hepatitis C, and syphilis. Ideally, all neonatal blood products should be tested for cytomegalovirus (CMV), frozen and washed, or white cell filtered.

(d) **Citrate-phosphate-dextrose (CPD) blood** has the *advantage* that it can be used up to 72 hours after drawing and that there is no rise in nonesterified free fatty acids in recipients. The *disadvantages* are as follows: low pH (6.9–7.0), which may not be tolerated by sick infants; hypernatremia; high glucose content, which may cause late hypoglycemia in hyperinsulinemic infants with erythroblastosis; and binding of calcium and magnesium. Sodium, potassium, and the pH of blood should be checked if the blood is over 48 hours old.

(e) Fresh (<24 hr old) CPD blood should be used in hydropic or otherwise compromised newborns. Blood should be compatible with the mother's, with a low titer of anti-A and anti-B. Subsequent transfusions should be done with blood compatible with that of the mother *and* infant.

(f) Acid-base problems, hyperkalemia, and hypernatremia can be avoided by using centrifuged packed red cells under 72 hours old resuspended in thawed fresh-frozen AB plasma just before exchange.

(g) All blood over 4 hours old has defects in platelet function.

(3) Technique of exchange transfusion. Asphyxia, hypoglycemia, acidosis, and temperature problems should all be corrected before exchange transfusion is performed.

(a) In all infants, exchange should be done under a *radiant heater,* servocontrolled to the infant. A cardiac monitor should be in place, as should a reliable peripheral IV line to maintain glucose control during and after the exchange.

(b) The *umbilical vein* should be used if possible. If the umbilical vein cannot be entered (rare, when the cord is soaked in saline for 30–60 minutes), the safest route is through a *central venous line* (CVL). This line can be left in place for future exchanges. Alternatively, a peripheral intravenous line and peripheral arterial line can be used.

(c) In sick, hydropic infants, exchange is best performed through umbilical arterial *and* venous catheters, so that blood can be removed and replaced simultaneously.

(d) In sick infants who are anemic (hematocrit under 35%), a partial exchange transfusion can be given with packed red blood cells (25–80 ml/kg) to raise the hematocrit to 40%. After stabilization, more exchange transfusions can be performed for hyperbilirubinemia. The blood for these exchanges should be set up before delivery and packed with the plasma separated into a side bag, so that it can be remixed if a packed cell exchange is unnecessary.

(e) Albumin (salt-poor albumin, 1 gm/kg 1–2 hr before exchange) increases the amount of bilirubin removed by the exchange. Albumin is **contraindicated** in CHF or severe anemia and is not usually used in early exchanges, in which the goal is to remove sensitized red cells rather than bilirubin.

(f) An infant's blood volume is usually about 80 ml/kg, and exchange transfusion should be done using double the infant's blood volume (160 ml/kg), in aliquots of 5–20 ml, depending on the infant's tolerance for the procedure. (An aliquot should never exceed 10% of the infant's estimated blood volume.) A useful approach is to start with 10-ml aliquots, increasing to 20-ml aliquots in infants weighing over 2 kg if all goes well. A two-volume exchange removes 87 percent of the infant's red blood cells.

(g) The rate of exchange has little effect on the amount of bilirubin removed; however, small aliquots and a slower rate reduce the stress on cardiovascular adaptation. The recommended time for an exchange in a full-term infant is 1 hour.

(h) Blood should be kept at 37°C by a temperature-controlled water bath that has an alarm to signal overheating.

(i) Blood should be gently shaken often, since the RBCs will settle rapidly, and the settling can lead to an exchange, with relatively anemic blood at the end of the exchange.

(j) If heparinized blood is used, a Dextrostix blood sugar should be obtained from the blood and from the baby during the exchange; 10 ml of 5% dextrose can be given as an umbilical vein push after each 100 ml blood if necessary. If the catheter tip rests above the liver, a more concentrated sugar solution can be used. When citrated blood is used, the infant's blood sugar should be checked for several hours after the exchange, and oral feedings or parenteral glucose should be given.

(k) When using CPD, most infants will not require additional calcium; following cessation of exchange transfusion, the Ca^{2+} level rapidly returns to normal. If needed, 0.5–2.0 ml of 10% calcium gluconate can be given following each 100 ml of exchange blood. However, this measure increases the ionized calcium fraction only temporarily. **There is a risk of severe bradycardia unless calcium is given very slowly.**

    (l) When the transfusion is finished, place a silk purse-string suture around the vein and leave a "tail" so that it will be easy to find the vein for the next exchange.

    (m) When the catheter is removed, the cord tie is "snugged up" for an hour. If it is not removed, skin necrosis may occur.

    (n) The venous catheter should be removed by pulling all the way out quickly.

    (o) Although their use is controversial, prophylactic antibiotics are recommended if a catheter was passed through an old, dirty cord; if there is great difficulty in passing the catheter; or if there are multiple exchanges.

    (p) Subsequent exchange is indicated when bilirubin levels suggest that unbound bilirubin is potentially present (see Tables 6-5 and 6-6).

  (4) Complications of exchange transfusions

    (a) Vascular. Embolization with air or clots, and thrombosis

    (b) Cardiac. Arrhythmias, volume overload, and arrest

    (c) Electrolytes. Hyperkalemia, hypernatremia, hypocalcemia, and acidosis

    (d) Clotting. Overheparinization and thrombocytopenia

    (e) Infections. Bacteremia, hepatitis, cytomegalovirus, HIV

    (f) Miscellaneous. Mechanical injury to donor cells, perforation of vessels, hypothermia, hypoglycemia, and possibly necrotizing enterocolitis.

  e. Phenobarbital, 5–8 mg/kg/day, will increase bilirubin conjugation and excretion. It may take 3–7 days to be effective. It is most useful in Crigler-Najjar syndrome type II and many cases of direct hyperbilirubinemia.

B. Anemia (see also Chap. 16)

  1. The **causes** of anemia include blood loss, hemolysis, decreased production, and physiologic decreased erythropoiesis.

  a. Blood loss

    (1) Etiology. The causes of blood loss are hemorrhage from the fetal to the maternal circulation, twin-twin transfusion, placenta previa, placental abruption, umbilical cord rupture or hematoma, incision of the placenta or cord, traumatic amniocentesis, rupture of anomalous placental vessels, intracranial bleeding, rupture of the liver or spleen, and GI bleeding due to ulcer, enterocolitis, or thrombosis. Iatrogenic anemia due to inadequate replacement of blood drawn for studies is a frequent cause of anemia in the neonate.

    (2) Evaluation. If blood loss is **acute**, the manifestations are shock, tachypnea, tachycardia, low venous pressure, weak pulses, and pallor. The hematocrit may initially be normal. **Chronic** blood loss is manifested by extreme pallor and a low hematocrit, with less distress than one would expect given the low hematocrit. These infants may be normovolemic. They may have CHF or hydrops.

    (3) Laboratory evaluation

      (a) A Kleihauer-Betke smear of maternal blood to detect fetal red cells in the maternal circulation

      (b) The Apt test for fetal hemoglobin in gastric aspirate or stool

      (c) Intracranial and abdominal ultrasound if symptoms indicate

      (d) Careful examination of the placenta and its vessels

  b. Hemolysis

    (1) Etiology. The causes of hemolysis include:

      (a) The isoimmune anemias: Rh incompatibility, ABO incompatibility, minor blood group incompatibility (e.g., Kell, "e," "c," "E")

      (b) The acquired hemolytic anemias: infection, DIC, vitamin E deficiency, and drug reactions

      (c) The hereditary hemolytic anemias: red cell membrane defects (spherocytosis); enzyme defects (pyruvate kinase [PK] and glucose 6-phosphate deficiency [G-6-PD])

   (d) The thalassemia syndromes

   (2) **Evaluation.** Manifestations may include jaundice, hepatospleno-megaly, pallor, and hydrops.

   (3) **Laboratory evaluations** include hematocrit, serum bilirubin, and reticulocyte count; examination of a peripheral blood smear for red blood cell morphology; direct Coombs test on an infant's red cells, with identification of the antibody if positive; antibody screen of maternal serum; enzyme screen of infant's or parents' red cells (G-6-PD or PK deficiency); and screening for infection.

   c. **Decreased production.** The causes of decreased production include Blackfan-Diamond syndrome, Fanconi's anemia, hemoglobinopathies such as thalassemia, reactions to drugs, infections, and infiltrative diseases such as leukemia, neuroblastoma, and storage diseases.

   d. **Physiologic anemia of full-term and premature infants** is due to physio-logic decreased erythropoieses.

   (1) Full-term infants have a nadir of the hemoglobin level at 9.5–11.0 gm/dl at 6–12 weeks; premature infants (body weight 1,200–2,400 gm) have a nadir of 8–10 gm/dl at 5–10 weeks; and small prematures (body weight under 1,200 gm) have a nadir of 6.5–9.0 gm/dl at 4–8 weeks.

   (2) The laboratory manifestations of physiologic anemia are a decreased hematocrit and a low reticulocyte count. When the infant's oxygen demand increases, erythropoietin will increase, and if iron stores are adequate, the reticulocyte count will increase, and the hemoglobin level will rise.

2. **Transfusion therapy**

   a. If an infant appears to have had **acute blood loss** at birth, immediate **access** should be obtained. Blood should be drawn for studies and crossmatching.

   b. If hypovolemic shock is present (decreased venous pressure, pallor, tachy-cardia), 20 ml/kg of a **volume expander** should be given. Unmatched type O, Rh-negative blood should be kept available for this purpose. Albumin (5%), plasma, and normal saline are the secondary choices, in that order.

   c. If blood loss was acute and not continuing, as in a fetal-maternal hemorrhage, there will be immediate dramatic improvement. If there is continuing internal hemorrhage, the improvement will be less. Infants in shock from asphyxia will have little response.

   d. A repeat transfusion of 10–20 ml/kg can be given if there are signs that the first transfusion was inadequate (decreased venous pressure, tachy-pnea, tachycardia, and shock). If plasma or albumin was given initially, packed red cells are given in the second transfusion.

   e. In **chronic** fetal blood loss (low hematocrit without evidence of hypo-volemia), packed red cells (10–15 ml/kg) are given if the hematocrit is under 30. If the hematocrit is under 25 in a normovolemic or hyper-volemic infant who may be in failure, a partial exchange transfusion with packed RBCs may be indicated.

   f. Premature infants may be comfortable with a hemoglobin concentration in the range of 6.5–8.0 gm/dl. The level itself is **not** an indication for transfusion. However, if any other condition (e.g., sepsis, apnea, pneumo-nia, bronchopulmonary dysplasia) requires increased oxygen-carrying capacity, transfusion is indicated.

   g. When multiple samples are being drawn from sick infants, a careful record must be kept of the amount drawn. Blood replacement as packed red cells should be considered when 10 percent of the volume has been removed. (Average blood volume in a neonate is 80 ml/kg.)

   h. The hematocrit in infants with cardiac or respiratory diseases should be kept above 35–40 with transfusions of packed red blood cells (10 ml/kg).

i. **Transfusion volume** to replace red blood cells with packed RBCs (PRBCs) is calculated with the formula:

$$\begin{matrix} \text{PRBC volume} \\ \text{to be} \\ \text{transfused} \end{matrix} = \frac{(\text{Hct desired} - \text{Hct observed})}{(\text{Hct of PRBCs})} \times \text{weight (kg)} \times \frac{80 \text{ ml}}{\text{kg}}$$

(The average hematocrit of packed red cells is 70.) In most circumstances, the volume to be transfused is about 10 ml/kg, usually given over 1–3 hours. Infants should be monitored during transfusion.

3. **Prevention or amelioration of the anemia of prematurity**
   a. Premature infants are given 25 IU water-soluble vitamin E daily as supplement or in premature formula until they are 2–3 months of age.
   b. Formulas similar to mother's milk, in that they are low in linoleic acid, are used to maintain a low content of red blood cell polyunsaturated fatty acids.
   c. The use of iron in infants less than 2 months old is controversial.
   d. After 8 weeks, iron supplements (2 mg/kg/day) as fortified formula or therapeutic iron are used to decrease the late anemia of prematurity.

C. **Bleeding disorders**
   1. **Etiology** (see Chap. 16, p. 473ff)
   2. **Evaluation and diagnosis** (see Chap. 16, p. 473ff)
   3. **Treatment** (see also **B**)
      a. Any underlying disease, such as shock, asphyxia, or infection, must be treated.
      b. A reliable IV line must be placed.
      c. After blood is drawn for studies, 1.0 mg vitamin K_1 oxide (AquaMEPHYTON) should be given IV over 2–3 minutes. The onset of action may be 2–3 hours. If liver disease is present, the onset of action may be longer.
      d. Fresh-frozen plasma, 10 ml/kg IV q8–12h, provides immediate replacement of clotting factors.
      e. If thrombocytopenia (platelet count < 20,000; < 50,000 if bleeding) is present, give 1 unit of irradiated platelets (platelets from 1 pt of blood concentrated to a volume of 15–20 ml) IV. **Platelets must not be given through an arterial line.** This should elevate the platelet count to 100,000 unless platelet destruction is continuing. In isoimmune thrombocytopenia, platelets from the mother or compatible with the mother are given if bleeding occurs.
      f. Packed red cells, plasma, and platelets are usually used. However, fresh whole blood will replace platelets and clotting factors and provide red blood cells. The amount used is initially 10 ml/kg. This is repeated as needed to replace blood lost.
      g. Clotting factor concentrates are used if a known factor deficiency is present.
      h. **Disseminated intravascular coagulation** should be treated by treating the underlying cause (sepsis, necrotizing enterocolitis) and giving fresh-frozen plasma and platelets to keep the platelet count at about 50,000. If bleeding continues, an exchange transfusion with fresh citrated blood may be helpful. If DIC is associated with gangrenous thrombosis of the large vessels, heparin is given as a bolus of 25–35 units/kg, followed by 10–15 units/kg/hr as a continuous infusion. The aim of heparin treatment is to keep the partial thromboplastin time (PTT) at 1.5 to 2 times normal.

   4. **Prevention**
      a. Infants should be given vitamin K_1, 1 mg intramuscularly, at birth.
      b. Mothers taking phenytoin should be given 10 mg vitamin K_1 IM 24 hours before delivery. These newborns should have prothrombin time, PTT, and platelet counts monitored if any signs of bleeding occur. If these levels are prolonged, the infants should be given fresh-frozen plasma, 20 ml/kg. The

usual dose of vitamin K_1 (1 mg) should be given to the baby postpartum and repeated in 24 hours.
   c. Mothers should refrain from taking aspirin for 1 week before delivery.
D. Polycythemia
   1. Etiology
      a. Placental overtransfusion
      b. Placental insufficiency
      c. Other causes include maternal diabetes, congenital adrenal hyperplasia, Beckwith syndrome, neonatal thyrotoxicosis, congenital hypothyroidism, Down syndrome, trisomy 18, and trisomy 13.
   2. Evaluation and diagnosis
      a. Most infants with polycythemia are asymptomatic.
      b. Suggestive symptoms include cyanosis (due to unsaturated hemoglobin), priapism, hypoglycemia, and jaundice.
      c. *Central* hematocrits should be checked to diagnose or rule out polycythemia.
   3. Treatment
      a. Any central hematocrit above 60 is of concern. Hematocrits peak at 2–3 hours after birth.
      b. Any symptomatic child should have a partial exchange transfusion if the central hematocrit is above 65.
      c. Asymptomatic infants with a central hematocrit of 60–70 can usually be managed by pushing fluids.
      d. Exchange transfusion is probably indicated with a central hematocrit of more than 70 in the absence of symptoms. Exchange is done with 5% albumin to bring hematocrit to 60 by the following calculation:

$$\frac{\text{Volume of exchange}}{\text{(ml)}} = \frac{(\text{Hct observed} - \text{Hct desired})}{(\text{Hct observed})} \times \text{weight (kg)} \times \frac{80\,\text{ml}}{\text{kg}}$$

VI. Metabolic problems
   A. Metabolic disorders. Genetically determined metabolic disorders are seen in 1 of every 200 infants (see Chap. 13).
      1. Etiology (see Chap. 13)
      2. Evaluation and diagnosis (see also Chap. 13)
         a. These disorders should be suspected in the following clinical situations:
            (1) A positive family history of any such disorder
            (2) A history of unexplained neonatal deaths in the family
            (3) Neonatal symptoms and signs, such as poor feeding, lethargy, hypotonia, coma, seizures, vomiting, diarrhea, tachypnea, rashes, coarse facial features, hepatomegaly, jaundice, cataracts, dehydration, constipation, temperature instability, unusual odor of urine or sweat, failure to thrive, and poor progression of development
            (4) Onset of symptoms in an infant who was well at birth
            (5) Onset of symptoms after a change in diet
            (6) Onset and progression of symptoms without evidence of asphyxia, infection, CNS hemorrhage, or other congenital defects
         b. Laboratory signs of these disorders include hypoglycemia, metabolic acidosis, lactic acidosis, ketosis, hyperammonemia, hyperbilirubinemia, abnormal amino acid pattern in the blood, ketonuria, positive ferric chloride test of the urine, and reducing substance in the urine.
         c. For purposes of **genetic counseling,** it is important to make an accurate diagnosis even if the affected infant dies. Infants who die with symptoms that may be caused by a metabolic disorder should be photographed and have full body x-rays and an autopsy. Blood should be saved for chromosomes, and blood and serum saved for analysis. Skin should be saved for fibroblast culture, and rapidly frozen liver and brain tissue should also be saved.
      3. Treatment

    a. If a metabolic disorder is suspected, a metabolic disease center should be contacted. **Rapid transfer to a newborn unit with access to a laboratory capable of performing sophisticated tests should be considered, because many of these disorders are rapidly fatal or cause permanent CNS damage unless they are properly treated.**

    b. Exchange transfusion or peritoneal dialysis should be considered for stabilization while awaiting a specific diagnosis.

    c. An attempt must be made to prevent protein catabolism with possible accumulation of toxic by-products. The infant should be given oral or parenteral glucose. Dextrose polymers (Polycose [Ross Laboratories, Columbus, OH], medium-chain triglycerides, Nil-Priote [product 80056, Mead Johnson]), glucose, emulsifiable fat, minerals, vitamins, and lipids should be considered for use. When a diagnosis is made, specific dietary or vitamin therapy should be started if possible.

  4. Some specific disorders that are lethal in the newborn are outlined here.

    a. Galactosemia

      (1) Signs and symptoms. Jaundice, hepatomegaly, lethargy, weight loss, gram-negative sepsis, cataracts, and hypoglycemia.

      (2) Diagnosis. Reducing substance in the urine (positive Clinitest) with negative urine for glucose (negative glucose oxidase dipstick test); assay of blood for galactase 1-phosphate-uridyltransferase (Beutler test) on filter paper phenylketonuria (PKU) blood specimen; assay of urine for galactose; abnormal liver function tests (SGOT, SGPT, PT, PTT)

      (3) Treatment. Elimination of lactose from the diet

    b. Organic acidemias. Methylmalonic acidemia, propionic acidemia, and isovaleric acidemia

      (1) Signs and symptoms. Poor feeding, vomiting, lethargy, tachypnea, coma, hypotonia, spasticity, and seizures

      (2) Diagnosis. Metabolic acidosis, ketoacidosis, hyperammonemia, hypoglycemia, ammonia odor from sweat or urine, urine methylmalonic acid by paper chromatography, gas layer chromatography, plasma and urine amino acid analysis for increased glycine

      (3) Treatment. Reversal of metabolic acidosis, dietary therapy, and vitamin administration appropriate for the disorder

    c. Hyperammonemia syndromes. These syndromes include urea cycle disorders, the organic acidemias (see above), and rare miscellaneous disorders: carbamyl phosphate synthetase deficiency, ornithine transcarbamylase deficiency, citrullinemia, argininosuccinic acidemia, argininemia, ornithine transaminase deficiency, orotic acidurias, hyperornithinemia, and hyperlysinemia

      (1) Symptoms and signs. Feeding problems, lethargy, irritability, hypertonicity, hypotonicity, tachypnea, coma, and convulsions

      (2) Diagnosis. Metabolic acidosis, hyperammonemia, bacterial inhibition assay, gas layer chromatography, and high-voltage electrophoresis

      (3) Treatment. Control production of ammonia by stopping protein intake and providing sufficient calories to prevent catabolism. Excess ammonia is removed by hemodialysis (ideally), peritoneal dialysis, or exchange transfusion. Alternate pathways for nitrogen excretion are provided by giving sodium benzoate, sodium phenylacetate, or arginine.

B. Infants of diabetic mothers

  1. Pregnancy. Management during the diabetic pregnancy should include:

    a. Close cooperation between obstetrician, pediatrician, and internist

    b. Frequent prenatal visits

    c. Accurate dating of time of conception by menstrual history, early examination, and early ultrasound.

    d. Maintenance of maternal normoglycemia by diet, insulin, or both. Maternal blood sugar should be monitored by frequent blood glucose determinations, by measurement of the daily amount of glycosuria (keep under 20 gm/day), by home glucose monitoring, and by measurement of hemoglobin A_1c. A hemoglobin A_1c greater than 8.5% in the first trimester carries a 22.4 percent risk of major anomalies. Maintenance of normoglycemia in late pregnancy may be associated with a decrease in macrosomia and neonatal hypoglycemia. **Oral hypoglycemic agents should not be used because they cross the placenta and are associated with severe and prolonged neonatal hypoglycemia.**

   e. Fetal ultrasonography should be done in early pregnancy for the detection of congenital anomalies. Maternal alpha fetoprotein should be measured.

   f. As pregnancy progresses into the third trimester, frequent determination of fetal well-being should be made by ultrasonography and nonstress tests (see Chap. 5, p. 122).

   g. When delivery is being considered, amniotic fluid should be obtained for assessment of fetal pulmonary maturity (L/S ratio and phosphatidyl glycerol).

   h. The decision on the timing of delivery is made by a balancing of risks to fetus, mother, and newborn. The risks to the fetus are intrauterine death and growth retardation. The risks to the mother are hypertension, renal failure, retinal hemorrhage, and unmanageable hyperglycemia. The risks to the newborn from early delivery are prematurity and respiratory distress.

2. **Evaluation of the newborn.** Infants of diabetic mothers are subject to the following: perinatal asphyxia, birth trauma, congenital anomalies, hypoglycemia, hypocalcemia, hyperbilirubinemia, respiratory distress syndrome (RDS), polycythemia, feeding problems, and renal vein thrombosis.

3. **Laboratory monitoring**
   a. **Blood sugar** at birth and at 1, 2, 3, 6, 12, 24, and 48 hours (glucose reagent strips and bedside glucometers). It is measured more often if the infant is symptomatic (e.g., lethargic, jittery, in respiratory distress), and has had a low blood glucose level, and to measure the response to therapy.
   b. Calcium if "sick," lethargic, or jittery with normal blood sugar
   c. Hematocrit if signs of polycythemia noted
   d. Bilirubin as needed
   e. Chest x-ray and ABGs as indicated for evaluation of respiratory distress or cyanosis
   f. ECG and cardiac ultrasound for evaluation of cardiac disease as indicated

4. **Therapy**
   a. See treatment of RDS (sec. **III**), cardiac problems (sec. **IV**), hypoglycemia (**C**), hypocalcemia (**D**), polycythemia (sec. **V.D**), and hyperbilirubinemia (sec. **V.A.1.a**).
   b. These infants are given 10% glucose and water or formula by mouth or gavage hourly starting at 1 hour of age until the blood glucose is stabilized. Breast feeding will not supply sufficient glucose. If this is not tolerated, parenteral glucose is given.
   c. If the infant is hypoglycemic and there is difficulty in achieving vascular access, **glucagon** (300 µg/kg SQ, to a maximum dose of 1.0 mg) can be used to raise the blood sugar.
   d. **Rapid infusions of concentrated dextrose solutions may stimulate insulin release in these hyperinsulinemic infants.** Then, if an IV line is suddenly lost, there may be **rebound hypoglycemia** (see below).

C. **Hypoglycemia** in the neonate is defined as any blood sugar less than 30–40 mg/dl in any infant, regardless of gestational age and whether or not it is associated with symptoms. Any blood glucose less than 40 mg/dl should be a cause for concern, and a blood glucose under 30 mg/dl requires treatment.

1. **Etiology** (see Table 6-7)
2. **Evaluation and diagnosis**
   a. **Symptoms** include lethargy, apathy, hypotonia, tremors, apnea, hypothermia, cyanosis, seizures, weak or high-pitched cry, and poor feeding.

Table 6-7. Etiology of neonatal hypoglycemia

Decreased hepatic glucose stores, production, or release
  Prematurity
  Intrauterine growth retardation
  Hypoxia
  Asphyxia
  Hypothermia
  Sepsis
  Congenital heart disease
  Glucagon deficiency
  Glycogen storage disease (type I)
  Galactosemia
  Fructose intolerance
  Adrenal insufficiency
Increased utilization of glucose (hyperinsulinism)
  Infant of diabetic mother
  Erythroblastosis fetalis
  Exchange transfusions (intraexchange hypoglycemia if heparinized blood is
    used, postexchange hypoglycemia if citrated blood is used)
  Beckwith-Wiedemann syndrome
  Nesidioblastosis
  Islet cell adenoma
  Leucine sensitivity
  Maternal chlorpropamide therapy
  Maternal benzothiadiazide therapy
Other causes
  Maternal therapy with beta-sympathomimetics
  Maternal or neonatal salicylate therapy

---

    b. Laboratory data. In the newborn, glucose oxidase methods that measure true glucose should be used rather than those that measure total reducing substances. Glucose reagent strips and bedside glucometers can be useful. Plasma insulin levels should be measured in certain cases of prolonged hypoglycemia.

  3. Treatment. The lower level of blood glucose at which CNS damage occurs in the neonate is not known. We try to keep the blood glucose level over 40 mg/dl.

    a. Anticipation and **prevention** are more important than treatment.

      (1) The blood sugar of well infants who are at high risk of hypoglycemia (e.g., infants with intrauterine malnutrition) should be measured at 3, 6, 12, and 24 hours of age, and they should be given early oral or gavage feedings with formula or 10% glucose and water q2h until the sugar level is stable. At this point, they can be weaned to q3–4h schedules, with continuing attention to their preprandial blood sugars for the first 2 days of life.

      (2) Asphyxiated infants, infants with seizures, and any infant with symptoms that could be due to hypoglycemia should be given parenteral glucose. Parenteral glucose should also usually be given during and after exchange transfusions.

      (3) Infants at high risk of hypoglycemia can be given parenteral glucose at a rate of 4–8 mg glucose/kg/min until feedings are established and the risks of hypoglycemia are gone.

    b. Mild symptomatic hypoglycemia (blood sugar 20–40 mg/dl) in infants >2,000 gm can often be successfully treated with oral glucose and water or formula. Those infants who cannot maintain normoglycemia for 2 hours should then be treated with **parenteral glucose.**

(1) Parenteral glucose can be administered initially as 10% D/W, 2 ml/kg, at a rate of 2 ml per minute.

(2) The glucose should be followed by a continuous infusion of 10% at a rate of 80 ml/kg/day. A constant infusion pump should be used. For most patients, 10% D/W at daily maintenance rates will provide adequate IV glucose.

(3) The concentration of glucose and the rate of infusion are increased as necessary to maintain a normal blood sugar. Dextrose concentrations greater than 12.5% should not be given via a peripheral vein or an umbilical venous line that is not central.

(4) **Glucagon** at a dose of 30 μg/kg IM can be administered to mobilize glucose in infants with adequate glycogen stores. Infants of diabetic mothers will require 300 μg/kg IM (maximum dose 1 mg). This can be used until an IV line is placed.

(5) **Hydrocortisone,** 5 mg/kg/day IM, in two divided doses, can be used in cases that do not respond to glucose infusions.

(6) Epinephrine, diazoxide, and growth hormone are to be used **only with endocrinologic consultation** in special cases of chronic intractable hypoglycemia.

(7) **Phenobarbital** should be used with glucose in the treatment of hypoglycemic seizures.

D. **Hypocalcemia** is defined as a serum total calcium concentration less than 7.0 mg/dl or an ionized calcium concentration below 4.0 mg/dl.

1. **Etiology.** Hypocalcemia usually is related to decreased calcium intake and transient neonatal hypoparathyroidism.

a. **First 3 days**

(1) **Maternal.** Diabetes, toxemia, obstetric complications, severe dietary calcium deficiency, or maternal hyperparathyroidism

(2) **Intrapartum.** Asphyxia, prematurity, or maternal magnesium treatment

(3) **Postnatal.** Hypoxia, shock, asphyxia, poor intake, RDS, or sepsis. A normal serum total calcium and a decreased ionized calcium may be seen in alkalosis caused by treatment with bicarbonate or hyperventilation. The same condition may be seen after exchange transfusion with citrated blood.

b. **After 3 days** (see Chap. 7, p. 197 and Chap. 11, p. 319). Any of the preceding causes and also a high-phosphate diet (milk, cereals), magnesium deficiency, intestinal malabsorption, renal disease, hypoparathyroidism, and vitamin D deficiency or metabolic defect

2. **Evaluation and diagnosis**

a. Signs of hypocalcemia in the newborn are nonspecific, and the classic Chvostek's sign and carpopedal spasm are helpful only if present.

b. Irritability, jitteriness, hypertonia, a high-pitched cry, apnea, and seizures are the most common presenting symptoms.

c. Calcium levels should be measured frequently in infants with the preceding conditions and substantiated if necessary with ECG measurement of the QTc (corrected QT interval) or Q-T interval. Levels should be measured as needed in symptomatic infants of diabetic mothers; at 12, 24, and 48 hours in sick or stressed infants; and at 12 (if ≤ 1,000 gm), 24, and 48 hours of age in premature infants.

d. Ionized calcium, serum phosphorus, magnesium, blood urea nitrogen (BUN), creatinine, parathyroid hormone, and calcitonin can be measured in persistent hypocalcemia. Absence of the thymus on chest film may be associated with hypoparathyroidism (DiGeorge' syndrome).

3. **Prevention and treatment**

a. **Preparations.** It is preferable to use only one calcium salt (gluconate) for either IV or PO administration, e.g., calcium gluconate 10% PO or IV (1 ml of 10% calcium gluconate = 100 mg calcium gluconate = 9 mg elemental calcium or 0.45 mEq/ml).

b. Indications. Infants who are at risk of hypocalcemia because of poor intake or transient hypoparathyroidism (e.g., prematures, infants with RDS) can be monitored carefully or treated as if they were hypocalcemic.

c. Dosage

(1) **For asymptomatic hypocalcemia** (Ca < 7 mg/dl without symptoms), when premature formula is not available, give 5–10 ml/kg/day of 10% calcium gluconate PO or IV. This provides a maintenance calcium (45–90 mg/kg/day elemental calcium). Start with a low dose and increase the dose as needed. The oral dose is mixed in with the total day's feeding. The IV dose is given by slow continuous infusion over 24 hours. If the cause of the hypocalcemia has resolved, the dose can be gradually decreased over 48 hours.

(2) **Acute symptomatic hypocalcemia with significant symptoms such as seizures or cardiac arrhythmias**

(a) Give 1.0–1.5 ml/kg of 10% calcium gluconate IV stat.

(b) The maximum dose is 5 ml for premature and 10 ml for full-term infants. This amount can be given slowly IV (1 ml/min), with careful observation of the heart rate and the vein if a peripheral vein is being used. This dose is conservative and can be repeated in 15 minutes if there is no clinical response.

d. Maintenance

(1) Following the acute dose, maintenance calcium, 45–90 mg/kg/day elemental calcium, should be given parenterally or PO. A low-phosphate milk (e.g., breast milk or Similac PM 60/40) should be used when oral feeding is started. Calcium can be added directly to the formula if necessary.

(2) Treatment of hypocalcemia is rarely necessary for more than 4–5 days unless other complications are present. During treatment, calcium levels should be monitored q12–24h and the dose gradually tapered as indicated. By 1 week of age, most infants of diabetic mothers remain normocalcemic on a regular formula or breast milk, and supplements are not needed.

e. The **risk of treatment** can be minimized by noting the following: Most hypocalcemia causes no symptoms and does not need rapid correction. **Aggressive, rapid therapy of asymptomatic hypocalcemia often causes more problems than it solves.**

(1) A rapid push of calcium can cause a sudden elevation of serum calcium, leading to bradycardia or other cardiac arrhythmias. This is especially true if the umbilical vein is being used. The injection rate should be no faster than 1 ml per minute. A cardiac monitor should be in place in infants receiving parenteral calcium as a bolus or as maintenance.

(2) Extravasation of calcium solutions into subcutaneous tissues can cause severe tissue necrosis. This occurs most often when an infusion pump is used. However, an infusion pump is best to provide a steady dose of calcium. The only way to minimize this problem is to use a reliable access (IV catheter) and closely observe the vein.

(3) Calcium cannot be mixed with $NaHCO_3$, because this may produce $CaCO_3$ precipitation.

(4) Calcium can cause necrosis of the liver if it is administered via an umbilical vein catheter that is in the portal system.

(5) Calcium pushed into the aorta may be a factor in necrotizing enterocolitis. Therefore, it should be given only by slow maintenance drip if an umbilical artery catheter is used for access.

f. Associated hypomagnesemia

(1) Symptomatic hypocalcemia that is unresponsive to calcium therapy may be due to hypomagnesemia and will not respond unless the hypomagnesemia is treated. Normal magnesium levels in newborns are 1.5–2.5 mEq per liter. Associated with neonatal hypomagnesemia are maternal magnesium deficiency, maternal hypoparathyroidism,

maternal diabetes, small-for-gestational-age infants, intestinal magnesium malabsorption, liver disease, exchange transfusions with citrated blood, and increased phosphate intake.

(2) Seizures caused by acute hypomagnesemia are treated with 0.1–0.2 ml/kg of 50% $MgSO_4$ IV (infuse slowly and monitor heart rate) or IM (may cause local tissue necrosis) repeated if necessary q6–12h. Maintenance magnesium therapy consists of oral administration of 50% $MgSO_4$, 100 mg or 0.2 mg/kg/day. If significant malabsorption is present, the dose can be increased two- to fivefold.

g. **Persistent hypocalcemia.** If the infant remains hypocalcemic despite adequate calcium supplementation and normal magnesium levels, a search for other causes of hypocalcemia must be started (see Chap. 11, p. 319).

h. For the long-term calcium needs of premature infants, see Chap. 5, p. 134.

VII. **Infection.** Infection accounts for 10–20 percent of infant deaths. For a more comprehensive discussion of infectious diseases, see G. Peter (Ed.), *Report of the Committee on Infectious Diseases* (22nd ed.). American Academy of Pediatrics, 1991.

A. **Congenital and natal infections**
1. **TORCH.** (Classically includes toxoplasmosis, rubella, CMV, and herpesvirus [HSV]. Syphilis, hepatitis B virus [HBV], and AIDS virus [human immunodeficiency virus, see 3] are often also included.)

a. **Evaluation and diagnosis**
(1) **Maternal history.** Most maternal infections with these agents are asymptomatic. *Screening* should be considered with the following maternal history:
(a) Known history of congenital infection
(b) Habitual abortion
(c) Infertility
(d) Contact with cats or mice
(e) Ingestion of raw meat
(f) Immunosuppressive therapy
(g) Rash
(h) Unexplained adenopathy
(i) Unexplained illness during pregnancy
(j) Oral or genital lesion
(k) Occupational exposure to congenital infection (e.g., neonatal nurses, dialysis workers)

(2) **Maternal diagnosis.** All mothers should be screened early in pregnancy for antibody to syphilis, rubella, and hepatitis B surface antigen. Serologic testing is available for HSV, CMV, HBV, and human immunodeficiency virus (HIV). Viral cultures are available for HSV, rubella, CMV, and enterovirus. Maternal vaginal cultures are used to diagnose maternal gonorrhea and group B streptococcal colonization.

(3) **Neonatal manifestations** include prematurity, intrauterine growth retardation, failure to thrive, and hepatomegaly with elevated direct bilirubin. **Disease-specific manifestations** include:
(a) **Syphilis.** Mucocutaneous lesions (snuffles), periostitis, osteochondritis, hepatomegaly, and rash
(b) **Toxoplasmosis.** Chorioretinitis, hydrocephalus, and intracranial calcifications
(c) **CMV.** Microcephaly with periventricular calcifications, thrombocytopenia, and hepatosplenomegaly
(d) **Rubella.** Retinopathy, cataracts, patent ductus arteriosis, pulmonary artery stenosis, deafness, and thrombocytopenia
(e) **HSV.** Skin vesicles, hepatitis, pneumonia, encephalitis, and DIC
(f) **HBV.** Hepatitis between 1 and 6 months of age
(g) **Enterovirus.** Encephalitis, sepsis-like syndrome, hepatitis, and DIC
(h) HIV (see 3ff for complete discussion)

(4) **Laboratory examination** (see also Chap. 14)

(a) Draw sera for a TORCH screen (5–10 ml blood) (before **transfusions**) or use cord blood (serum), and pair with a sample from the mother, drawn at the same time. This should include a search for immunoglobulin M (IgM)-specific immunofluorescent antibodies. Convalescent serum from the mother and baby must be sent in 2–8 weeks, depending on the clinical situation. Sera may be required at 3–6 months.

(b) Measure cord blood IgM (normal < 20 mg/ml).

(c) Viral cultures (HSV, rubella, CMV, enterovirus)

(d) Tzanck preparation smear of vesicles from the infant or mother

(e) Urine cytologic study after millipore filtration for CMV

(f) Histologic study of the placenta

(g) Hepatitis B surface antigen (HBsAg), antibody to surface antigen (anti-HBs), hepatitis B core antigen (HB_cAg), and antibody to hepatitis B core antigen (anti-HB_c)

(h) Liver enzymes, serum glutamic oxaloacetic transaminase (SGOT), and serum glutamic pyruvic transaminase (SGPT)

(i) Platelet count and clotting studies

b. Treatment (see also Chap. 14)

(1) No specific treatment is available for rubella.

(2) HSV has been successfully treated with both vidarabine and acyclovir (see Chap. 14, pp. 429 and 430). Topical idoxuridine eyedrops and large doses of gamma globulin (10–20 mg IM) have been used.

(3) Treatment is available for toxoplasmosis (see Chap. 15, p. 455).

(4) Experimental therapy for severe systemic CMV is under study at several centers in the United States.

(5) If varicella develops in the mother less than 5 days before delivery, there will be insufficient time for transfer of maternal antibody to the fetus. These infants should receive 125 U varicella-zoster immune globulin (VZIG) IM. Infants born to mothers in whom varicella develops within 2 days postpartum should also be treated with VZIG. In both cases the infant should be isolated from the mother until she is no longer infectious.

c. Prevention

(1) Congenital **rubella** is prevented by adequate immunization of child-bearing women.

(2) **Toxoplasmosis** (see Chap. 15, p. 455) may possibly be prevented by avoiding cats and the eating of raw meat during pregnancy.

(3) Because the majority of neonatal **HSV** infections is acquired at the time of vaginal delivery, the infants of mothers with active genital herpes should be delivered by cesarean section. If the membranes are ruptured, the baby should be delivered by cesarean section as soon as possible. Postnatal infection can be acquired from mothers with active lesions. If the mother has a primary HSV infection with positive cultures at the time of delivery, the infant should be isolated from other infants in the nursery and cultures should be obtained from the oropharynx/nasopharynx and conjunctivae at 24 hours of age. Infants with positive cultures or in whom symptoms of infection develop should have their culture repeated and antiviral treatment (acyclovir, 8–10 mg/kg IV q8h) started.

(4) Infants born to mothers in whom **hepatitis A** develops within 2 weeks of delivery should be given immune serum globulin (ISG), 0.15 ml/kg IM. Infants born to mothers who are HB_sAg positive should receive both hepatitis B immune globulin (HBIG), 0.5 ml, and hepatitis B vaccine, 0.5 ml, at birth. The hepatitis B vaccine is repeated at 1 and 6 months. Recommendations for routine immunization for HBV are covered in Chap. 2, pp. 24–25.

2. Syphilis (see also Chap. 14, p. 417)

a. Etiology. Transplacental transmission of *Treponema pallidum*

b. Evaluation and diagnosis
   (1) Perinatal clinical signs include stillbirth, fetal hydrops, and prematurity.
   (2) Postnatal manifestations include failure to thrive, persistent rhinitis, lymphadenopathy, rash, jaundice, anemia, hepatosplenomegaly, nephrosis, and meningitis.
c. Laboratory tests
   (1) Mother. Rapid plasma reagin (RPR) with titers and fluorescent-treponemal antibody absorption test (FTA–ABS) with titers. Test at first antenatal visit and in third trimester.
   (2) Infant
      (a) RPR with titer and FTA–ABS with titer
      (b) If available, IgM–FTA–ABS is most specific for fetal infection.
      (c) X-rays of long bones may provide evidence of metaphyseal demineralization of periosteal new bone formation.
      (d) Dark-field examination of any nasal discharge
      (e) Cerebrospinal fluid (CSF) examination
d. Treatment (see also Table 14-10)
   (1) Pregnant women with primary, secondary, or latent syphilis are treated as follows:
      (a) Benzathine penicillin G. The dose is 2.4 MU IM (1.2 MU in each buttock initially). Repeat 7 days later. The total dose is 4.8 MU. Alternatively, give **aqueous procaine penicillin G,** 600,000 U per day IM for 15 days. The dose of procaine penicillin is 1.2 MU per day for patients who are also HIV positive.
      (b) If penicillin allergy is present, skin testing and desensitization therapy should be considered, since penicillin is by far the most effective therapy.
      (c) Mothers with syphilis of more than 1 year's duration (latent syphilis of indeterminate or more than 1 year's duration, cardiovascular syphilis, late benign syphilis, neurosyphilis)
      (d) Penicillin
         (i) Benzathine penicillin G, 7.2 MU total, 2.4 MU IM per week for 3 successive weeks, *or*
         (ii) Aqueous procaine penicillin G, 9.0 MU total, 600,000 units IM daily for 15 days
      (e) The same considerations should be made for patients who are penicillin allergic.
   (2) Infant
      (a) If the infant's serologic test results are negative and he or she has no disease, *no* treatment is necessary.
      (b) If the serologic test results are positive, treat the **symptomatic** infant. Treat the **asymptomatic** infant when:
         (i) The titer is three to four times higher than the mother's.
         (ii) The FTA is 3–4+.
         (iii) The mother was inadequately treated or untreated.
         (iv) The mother is unreliable, and follow-up is doubtful.
         (v) The mother's infection was treated with a drug other than penicillin.
         (vi) The mother had a recent sexual exposure to an infected person.
         (vii) The mother was treated in the last month of pregnancy.
         (viii) The mother has HIV and was treated for syphilis with less than neurosyphilis regimen.
      (c) If the baby has a positive RPR or FTA, or both, and the history and clinical findings (including x-ray) make infection unlikely, it is safe to await the IgM report and repeat RPR and FTA titers. Any significant rise in titer or any clinical signs require treatment. If the antibodies are transferred maternal antibodies, the

baby should have a falling titer and be negative by 4 months. If the serology is not negative by 6 months of age, treat.

(d) For infants with no evidence of CNS infection, give procaine penicillin G in aqueous suspension, 50,000 U/kg IM in 1 daily dose for 10–14 days, or aqueous crystalline penicillin G, 100,000–150,000 U/kg/day q8–12h IM or IV for 10–14 days (see Table 14-12). Infants with CNS infection (CSF pleocytosis, elevated CSF protein, positive CSF serology) should be treated with aqueous procaine penicillin, 50,000 U/kg/day IM for 3 weeks, or aqueous crystalline penicillin, 150,000 U/kg/day q8–12h IM for 2–3 weeks. For infants at low risk for infection for whom follow-up is doubtful, treatment with benzathine penicillin G, 50,000 U/kg/day IM as a one-time dose, can be given.

3. **Acquired immunodeficiency syndrome** (see also Chap. 14, p. 435)
   a. **Etiology.** Maternal infection and transplacental passage of HIV.
   b. **Evaluation and diagnosis.** The diagnosis should be considered in infants when the mother or mother's partner is in a high-risk group:
      (1) Intravenous drug abuser
      (2) Prostitute
      (3) Sexual partner of HIV-positive man
      (4) Sexual partner of hemophiliac
      (5) Recipient of blood transfusion between 1979 and 1985
   c. **Laboratory tests**
      (1) **Informed consent** is required for testing of mother or baby.
      (2) **Maternal** HIV antibody status should be tested using an enzyme-linked immunosorbent assay (ELISA) with confirmation by Western blot analysis.
      (3) If the mother is positive, the **infant** may test positive for HIV antibody because of passive placental transfer of maternal antibody without transfer of HIV. Referral of such infants to a pediatric HIV program as soon as possible after birth is recommended. Some centers recommend T_4/T_8 cell studies to make judgments about *Pneumocystis* prophylaxis. A combination of clinical, virologic, and serologic parameters can be used for early detection of HIV infection including HIV culture and p24 antigen. At 18 months of age, it is believed that the results of HIV antibody testing represent the child's own, rather than maternal, antibodies.
   d. **Treatment.** There is currently no known treatment for AIDS other than supportive therapy.
   e. **Breast feeding.** Postnatal transmission of HIV from infected mothers to infants by means of breast milk is well documented. Although the risk for postnatal infection is small, it is currently recommended that HIV-positive mothers in developed countries not breast feed.
   f. **Universal precautions**
      (1) Gloves, gowns, and eye protection should be worn in the delivery room.
      (2) Direct oral endotracheal suctioning for meconium should be routinely avoided; DeLee suction trap or special suction device should be used.
      (3) Infants should be bathed carefully on admission.
      (4) Linens and disposables should be placed in separate marked containers.
      (5) Laboratory and PKU tests should be specially labeled and enclosed.

4. **Gonorrhea**
   a. **Etiology.** Intrapartum infection with *Neisseria gonorrhoeae*
   b. **Evaluation and diagnosis**
      (1) **Gonococcal ophthalmia** usually presents within 3 days of birth. If the eyes are infected before birth in association with premature rupture of the membranes, symptoms may be present at birth. Usually, a watery, then mucopurulent, then bloody conjunctival

discharge develops. There is prominent edema of the conjunctiva and lids, followed by corneal edema and ulceration. Perforation of the globe with panophthalmitis may be present. A presumptive diagnosis is made by demonstration of gram-negative diplococci on Gram stain of the exudate. Definitive diagnosis is by culture. Conjunctivitis from silver nitrate, HSV, staphylococci, pneumococci, *Escherichia coli,* and *Chlamydia* should be considered in the differential diagnosis. If there is doubt, treatment should begin, pending results of cultures.

    (2) Other gonococcal infections are rhinitis, anorectal infection, arthritis, sepsis, and meningitis.

  c. Treatment (see Table 14-11)

    (1) Asymptomatic infants. If a Gram stain or culture from a maternal or neonatal source is positive for *N. gonorrhoeae,* the infant should be treated with one dose of aqueous crystalline penicillin G (50,000 U for term and 20,000 U for preterm infants) IM or IV or ceftriaxone, 125 mg (50 mg/kg for preterm infants) IV or IM, in addition to ocular prophylaxis.

    (2) Symptomatic infants (ophthalmia, arthritis, sepsis) should be treated with 100,000 U/kg/day q12h of aqueous crystalline penicillin G for 7 days (see Table 14-11).

    (3) Frequent saline irrigations will help.

    (4) The possibility of penicillin-resistant gonococcus should be considered (see Table 14-11). Sensitivity testing should be done on all positive cultures. Cefotaxime, 100 mg/kg/day divided q8h (q12h for preterm infants) for 7 days, may be a more appropriate therapy until antibiotic sensitivities are obtained.

  d. Prevention

    (1) Pregnant women should have endocervical cultures for gonorrhea. Cultures should be repeated at delivery for high-risk women.

    (2) Application of erythromycin 0.5% ophthalmic ointment, tetracycline 1% ophthalmic ointment, or 1% silver nitrate to the infant's eyes at the time of birth will usually prevent gonococcal ophthalmia.

    (3) Infants born to mothers with positive cultures should be treated as in **c.(1).**

B. Acquired infections (see also Chap. 14). The incidence of sepsis in the newborn is 2 in 1,000. The meninges will be involved in 25 percent of the cases of neonatal sepsis.

  1. Sepsis

    a. Predisposing factors include:

      (1) Premature onset of labor

      (2) Prolonged rupture of membranes

      (3) Maternal fever or other signs of chorioamnionitis

      (4) Maternal colonization with group B streptococci

      (5) Indwelling catheters

      (6) Tracheal intubation

    b. Etiology. Organisms associated with neonatal infections are listed in Table 6-8.

    c. Evaluation. Sepsis should be suspected in the following situations:

      (1) Any sudden change for the worse

      (2) Temperature control problems, metabolic acidosis, and infant "not doing well"

      (3) Common symptoms include poor feeding, lethargy, apnea, vomiting, and diarrhea.

      (4) Signs include tachypnea, respiratory distress, abdominal distention, cyanosis, ileus, pustules, petechiae, purpura, omphalitis, and seizures.

      (5) Laboratory and radiographic evaluation

        (a) Leukopenia below 5,000 mm^3, a total neutrophil count under 1,000 mm^3, and a ratio of immature (band) to total neutrophils of

Table 6-8. Organisms associated with newborn infection

Early infection
  Group B streptococci
  Escherichia coli
  Klebsiella-Aerobacter
  Enterococcus
  Listeria monocytogenes
  Streptococcus (Diplococcus) pneumoniae
  Group A streptococci
  Haemophilus influenzae
  Neisseria gonorrhoeae
  Anaerobes: *Clostridium, Bacteroides*
Late nursery infection (>5 days of age)*

Staphylococcus aureus	*Pseudomonas*
E. coli	*Serratia*
Klebsiella-Aerobacter	*Staphylococcus epidermidis*
Candida albicans	

* The causative organisms vary with the flora of the nursery and with its personnel.

greater than 0.2 have all been correlated with an increased risk of bacterial infection.

  (b) **Cultures.** Blood cultures should be obtained from a peripheral site that has been thoroughly cleaned with an antiseptic agent. CSF cultures should be obtained in infants believed to be at high risk for bacterial infection. Urine cultures are generally not helpful in the immediate perinatal period.

  (c) **Chest x-ray** in infants with abnormal respiratory signs may be helpful.

  (d) **Antigen detection methods** such as latex agglutination assays may be helpful, especially in the setting of antenatal maternal antibiotic treatment or parenchymal lung disease with negative blood cultures. There is, however, a significant false-positive rate with urine specimens.

  d. **Treatment** of sepsis (see Chap. 14; see also Table 14-1 and 14-2)

  (1) When sepsis is suspected, treatment should begin **before** culture results are available.

  (2) IV antibiotics should be initiated (Table 6-9).

  (3) Newborns at high risk for sepsis, or in whom the diagnosis of sepsis is suspected, should be treated for the pathogens of greatest concern— group B streptococcus (GBS), *E. coli (ECK1)*, and *Listeria* (see Table 6-9). In this group, ampicillin and an aminoglycoside, gentamicin, generally are recommended for initial therapy. Ampicillin is used for initial therapy because of its effectiveness against streptococci, *Listeria monocytogenes,* enterococci, and some gram-negative bacteria. Third-generation cephalosporins may be useful in the treatment of gram-negative infections. They, however, have limited activity against *Listeria* and may place neonates with significant hyperbilirubinemia at increased risk for kernicterus because they displace bilirubin from albumin-binding sites.

  (4) Although ampicillin and gentamicin provide excellent broad coverage for perinatal pathogens, this combination may not be preferred for neonates at risk for nosocomial infections (usually more than 1 week in the nursery or NICU). These pathogens often include *E. coli, Klebsiella-Aerobacter, Pseudomonas, Serratia,* and *Staphylococcus epidermidis.* **The pattern of antibiotic susceptibility of the common agents causing nosocomial infections in the nursery should be**

Table 6-9. Recommended antibiotic regimens for neonatal sepsis and meningitis

Organism	Site of infection	Antibiotic therapy[a]	Duration of therapy
GBS	Blood	Penicillin, 200,000 U/kg/day	10–14 days
	CNS	Penicillin, 400,000 U/kg/day	Complete 14–21 days
ECK1	Blood	Cefotaxime, 50–100 mg/kg/day or other third-generation drug	Complete 14 days
	CNS	Cefotaxime, 100 mg/kg/day (? gentamicin,[b] 5 mg/kg/day for 5–10 days for synergy)	Complete 21 days
Listeria	Blood	Ampicillin, 100–200 mg/kg/day (? gentamicin,[b] 5 mg/kg/day for up to 1 week for synergy)	Complete 14 days
	CNS	Ampicillin, 300 mg/kg/day (? gentamicin,[b] 5 mg/kg/day for up to 1 week for synergy)	Complete 14–21 days

[a] In all cases, therapy with ampicillin (300 mg/kg/day) and gentamicin (5 mg/kg/day) is initiated until an organism has been identified and antibiotic sensitivities are determined. Doses are divided q12h for term newborn infants and should be adjusted for increased renal clearance beyond the first week of life.
[b] Gentamicin is always 2.5 mg/kg/dose, with the interval adjusted based on gestational age and serum levels. In general, the intervals are q24h for infants less than 1,000 gm, q18h for infants of less than 35 weeks' gestation, and q12h for infants more than 35 weeks.
Source: J. P. Cloherty and A. R. Stark [Eds.], *Manual of Neonatal Care* (3rd ed.). Boston: Little, Brown, 1991.

known. Considering the predominance of coagulase-negative staphylococci as the principal cause of nosocomial sepsis, vancomycin has become a principal agent for presumptive gram-positive bacterial coverage. Presumptive gram-negative coverage can continue to be provided with an aminoglycoside. Ampicillin and an aminoglycoside remain the antibiotics of choice when meningitis or a urinary tract infection is suspected.

(5) Careful attention should be paid to temperature, hydration, caloric intake, acid-base balance, and any coagulopathy.

(6) When cultures are positive, antibiotics should be "tailored" to the sensitivities of organism(s) recovered.

(7) Drug levels (peak and trough) should be obtained around the third to fifth dose for aminoglycosides and vancomycin.

(8) Infants who fail to respond to the preceding therapy may benefit from exchange transfusion, fresh-frozen plasma, or white cell transfusions.

2. Meningitis

a. Etiology. Group B streptococci and *E. coli* account for 70 percent of all cases of neonatal meningitis in North America. *L. monocytogenes*, miscellaneous gram-positive and gram-negative organisms, *Haemophilus influenzae*, and anaerobes account for the rest.

b. Evaluation and diagnosis

(1) Any infant suspected of having sepsis should have a lumbar puncture. Normal values are given in Table 6-10.

(2) Neonatal meningitis is rapidly fatal, and few, if any, clinical signs may be present up to and including its terminal stages.

(3) A full fontanel is a late sign of meningitis.

(4) Fever may or may not be present.

(5) **Laboratory studies** (see B.1.c.(5))

(6) The diagnosis is suspected when more than 20–25 WBC/mm³ are

Table 6-10. Cerebrospinal fluid findings in high-risk neonates without meningitis

Laboratory study	Full-term	Preterm
WBC count (cells/mm^3)		
No. of infants	87	30
Mean	8.2	9.0
Median	5	6
S.D.	7.1	8.2
Range	0–32	0–29
± 2 S.D.	0–22.4	0–25.4
Percentage neutrophils	61.3%	57.2%
Protein (mg/dl)		
No. of infants	35	17
Mean	90	115
Range	20–170	65–150
Glucose (mg/dl)		
No. of infants	51	23
Mean	52	50
Range	34–119	24–63
CSF and blood glucose (%)		
No. of infants	51	23
Mean	81	74
Range	44–248	55–105

Source: Modified from L. D. Sariff et al., *J. Pediatr.* 88(3):473, 1976.

present in CSF (see Table 6-10) and is confirmed by a positive CSF culture.

c. **Treatment** (see also Chap. 14, p. 407)

   (1) The initial empiric therapy for meningitis is ampicillin (300 mg/kg/ day) and gentamicin (5 mg/kg/day) (see Table 6-9).

   (2) The Gram stain of CSF or recovery of specific bacterial antigens may guide therapy until cultures are ready. Broad-spectrum coverage should not be dropped until an organism is identified.

   (3) Specific therapy is given when the organism and its antibiotic sensitivities are known.

   (4) For meningitis in low-birth-weight infants who have been in the nursery for several weeks and in those infants with long-term vascular lines, a penicillinase-resistant penicillin or vancomycin should be added to the regimen or substituted for ampicillin because of the risk of *staphylococcus aureus* or *epidermidis* infection.

   (5) The morbidity and mortality in gram-negative neonatal meningitis caused by penicillin-resistant organisms remain so high that early, aggressive therapy must be instituted. The poor penetration of systemically administered gentamicin into the cerebrospinal space may result in an inadequate bactericidal activity against gram-negative organisms. If the organism is ampicillin resistant, there will often be poor results. Intrathecal and intraventricular therapy with gentamicin have not been useful. This has led to therapy with third-generation cephalosporins.

   (6) To ensure rapid sterilization of the blood and CSF, repeat cultures of blood and CSF should be done in the patient who is receiving therapy.

   (7) General supportive care of the patient is essential. Attention must be paid to electrolyte balance (inappropriate antidiuretic hormone secretion), clotting factors (DIC), seizures, nutrition, and ventilation.

(8) Treatment of meningitis is IV, for 14–21 days. Gram-negative meningitis requires 21 days of treatment.

3. Group B streptococcal infection. The group B streptococcus is now the major cause of sepsis in most nurseries in the United States. The overall incidence of neonatal sepsis varies between 1 and 8 cases per 1,000 live births.

a. Etiology. Group B streptococci are recovered from the vaginal cultures of 25 percent of American mothers at the time of delivery. Of their infants, 25 percent have positive skin or nasopharyngeal cultures, or both. For every 100 colonized infants, 1 will become ill.

b. Evaluation

(1) The early-onset type may present as mild respiratory distress or "transient tachypnea of the newborn," progressing rapidly to shock and death in an infant with few or no risk factors for infection. If the disease presents within a few hours of birth, the mortality is high, irrespective of therapy.

(2) Late infections may present as meningitis at 2–4 weeks of age.

(3) Laboratory studies include CBC, chest x-ray, blood culture, urinalysis and culture, lumbar puncture, and gastric aspirate.

c. Diagnosis

(1) The **diagnosis** is confirmed by positive blood, urine, or CSF cultures.

(2) The chest x-ray may show pneumonia, "retained lung fluid," or a pattern not unlike that of HMD.

(3) The gastric aspirate may show gram-positive chains with neutrophils.

(4) The latex agglutination test may be helpful in cases in which the mother was treated with antibiotics before delivery so that neonatal cultures are unreliable. Because of the high false-positive rate associated with urine latex agglutination tests, a positive result must be interpreted in the context of the clinical picture.

d. Treatment

(1) Infants with documented group B streptococcal pneumonia or sepsis should be treated with aqueous penicillin, 200,000 units/kg/day in three to four doses per day (see Table 6-9).

(2) If sepsis or meningitis is proved, treatment should be carried out for 14–21 days at 400,000 units/kg/day.

(3) The use of exchange transfusion and immunoglobulin has been advocated for very sick infants.

e. Prevention

(1) Polyvalent **group B streptococcus vaccine** is being evaluated for use in nonimmune pregnant women.

(2) Administration of **ampicillin** to colonized pregnant women with fever, a history of previously GBS-infected newborns, preterm labor, or prolonged rupture of membranes (more than 12–18 hr), at any gestational age, has been shown effective in preventing neonatal group B streptococcal infection.

4. Pneumonia

a. Etiology

(1) Congenital pneumonia. Transplacental agents include TORCH agents, enteroviruses, *T. pallidum, L. monocytogenes, Mycobacterium tuberculosis,* and genital *Mycoplasma.*

(2) Perinatally acquired pneumonia is associated with inhalation of infected amniotic fluid (often caused by prolonged rupture of the membranes) or hematogenous miliary seeding of the lungs. These pneumonias are due to maternal vaginal flora and are caused by group B streptococci, *E. coli,* other gram-negative enteric bacteria, staphylococci, pneumococci, anaerobic organisms, *Chlamydia, Mycoplasma,* and HSV.

(3) Nosocomial pneumonia acquired after birth may come from nursery personnel, other infants in the nursery, or nursery equipment. Staphylococci, gram-negative enteric bacteria, enteroviruses, respiratory syncytial virus, adenovirus, parainfluenza virus, *Chlamydia*, and HSV are among the common agents.

b. Evaluation

(1) **A history** of maternal fever, premature delivery, prolonged rupture of membranes, excessive obstetric manipulation, or foul-smelling amniotic fluid should increase suspicion of neonatal pneumonia.

(2) **Physical examination.** Fever, lethargy, tachypnea, grunting, flaring of nasal alae, retractions, irregular breathing, rales, and cyanosis may be present.

(3) **Laboratory tests** should include a CBC, a chest x-ray for evidence of pulmonary infiltrate or pleural effusion, and a gastric aspirate for Gram stain and cultures. The presence of neutrophils is correlated with pneumonia more than is the finding of bacteria. Cultures, and Gram stain of the blood, urine, CSF, and tracheal aspirate (if intubated), should be obtained.

(4) If large amounts of pleural fluid are present, a **pleural tap** can be done. Direct lung aspiration or lung biopsy is rarely indicated in cases that are unresponsive to therapy.

c. Diagnosis. The diagnosis of pneumonia is usually made by the presence of physical signs (see **B.1.c**) and a chest x-ray showing a pulmonary infiltrate.

d. Treatment

(1) **General supportive measures** include:

(a) Fluid, electrolyte, and acid-base balance

(b) Maintenance of hematocrit, blood volume, and blood pressure

(c) Nutrition

(d) Temperature control

(2) **Respiratory support** includes:

(a) Respiratory physical therapy; oxygen as needed

(b) Intermittent positive pressure ventilation, if indicated

(c) Drainage of pleural fluid if the fluid is compromising respiration

(3) **Antibiotics** are used as in the treatment of sepsis, depending on the suspected cause.

5. Omphalitis. The devitalized umbilical cord is an excellent culture medium for many bacteria. In areas where there is poor maternal immunity to tetanus and inadequate aseptic technique, neonatal tetanus due to omphalitis is a major cause of death.

a. Etiology. The cord is colonized shortly after birth with the local flora. Infection with streptococci and staphylococci is common. **Phlebitis** may spread to the liver, causing liver abscess or thrombosis of the hepatic vein. **Arteritis** may interfere with postnatal obliteration of the umbilical vessels and cause bleeding.

b. Evaluation and diagnosis

(1) Infection can cause peritonitis and septic emboli to the lungs, pancreas, kidney, skin, and bone.

(2) If true omphalitis is present, the infant should have a full evaluation for sepsis, including, blood, urine, and CSF cultures.

c. Treatment

(1) As in sepsis, IV antibiotics are administered before culture results are available. Because *Staphylococcus* is a common agent, oxacillin and either gentamicin or kanamycin are preferred. Treatment should continue for 7–10 days.

(2) Any catheter in the umbilicus should be removed.

(3) Leaving the cord open to the air to dry may decrease the number of flora.

6. Tuberculosis in the newborn. In the United States, when maternal tuberculosis (TB) is present or suspected at the time of delivery, management of the newborn is a major clinical problem. For a brief discussion see Chap. 14, p. 425. For a complete discussion, see J. P. Cloherty and A. R. Stark [Eds.], *Manual of Neonatal Care* (3rd. ed.). Boston: Little, Brown, 1991.

7. **Urinary tract infection** may be secondary to sepsis or a primary source of infection. The diagnosis is by examination and culture of urine obtained by a bladder tap or sterile catheterization. Initial systemic treatment with ampicillin and an aminoglycoside is indicated. Medication can be changed after sensitivities are known. Parenteral treatment should be given for 14 days. Ultrasound and contrast studies of the urinary tract are indicated after treatment.

8. **Skin pustules** may be caused by staphylococci and will show gram-positive cocci on Gram stain, as opposed to erythema toxicum, which will show eosinophils on Wright stain. When only a few pustules are present, bathing with chlorhexidine solution and local application of bacitracin ointment may suffice. If there are multiple pustules or the infant appears sick, a sepsis evaluation and systemic treatment with oxacillin are indicated. Wounds from scalp monitors or abrasions related to delivery may cause both local and systemic infection. Organisms will include the maternal vaginal flora, especially group B streptococci, coliforms, and anaerobic organisms. Local treatment with warm saline soaks and application of Betadine may be adequate therapy. Systemic illness or local spread in spite of local therapy requires the use of systemic parenteral antibiotics and occasionally incision and drainage.

9. **Septic arthritis or osteomyelitis** may result from a bacteremia or local trauma (heel sticks). *Diagnosis* is by clinical examination, aspiration of fluid, and occasionally bone scan. **Treatment** involves systemic antibiotics for 3–4 weeks after local signs are gone. Open surgical drainage is recommended for diagnosis and relief of pressure in some joints (e.g., hip, shoulder), but needle aspiration may be sufficient for others (e.g., knee, wrist). Immobilization of joints is recommended until local signs have resolved and physical therapy can be initiated.

C. **Isolation guidelines.** Guidelines for obstetric-neonatal isolation procedures can be found in the American Academy of Pediatrics and the American College of Obstetricians and Gynecologists, *Guidelines for Perinatal Care,* 1992.

VIII. **Fluid and electrolyte management.** The goal of therapy is to provide fluid and electrolytes for maintenance and growth, and to replace losses due to pathologic states. The principles are the same as in older children (see Chap. 7). In the newborn, problems can occur because of differences in body composition (Table 6-11), the type and amounts of losses of fluid and electrolytes (Tables 6-12 and 6-13), and the limitations in the renal function of premature and newborn infants.

A. **Electrolytes**
1. **Sodium**
a. The usual maintenance requirement for sodium is 2–3 mEq/kg/day start-

Table 6-11. Body fluid in premature and newborn infants

Gestational age	TBW as percentage of body weight*	ECW as percentage of body weight*	ICW as percentage of body weight*
Premature at 32 weeks	80	52	28
Full-term infant	75	40	35

TBW = total body water; ECW = extracellular water; ICW = intracellular water.
* There is a 10% loss of body weight in the first 7–10 days of life. This is mostly a loss of ECW.
Source: Adapted from H. S. Dweck, *Perinatology* 2:183, 1975; and J. C. Sinclair et al., *Pediatr. Clin. North. Am.* 17:863, 1970.

Table 6-12. Fluid losses in infants at basal metabolic rate

Source of loss[a]	ml/kg/24h
Insensible water loss (IWL)[b]	26–35
Pulmonary	8–10
Skin	18–23
Urine (at 300 mOsm/liter)[c]	30–40
Stool	4
Total	60–70[d]

[a] The major variable in infants is the amount of insensible water loss.
[b] Will vary. See Table 6-13.
[c] Will vary with osmolar load plus renal function.
[d] Extra fluid will be required for growth.
Source: Adapted from H. S. Dweck, *Perinatology* 2:183, 1975; and J. C. Sinclair et al., *Pediatr. Clin. North Am.* 17:863, 1970.

ing on the second or third day. Preterm infants may require 4–8 mEq/kg/day. This amount will gradually decrease after the first few weeks.
   b. Some causes of **hyponatremia** in the newborn are:
      (1) Maternal. Hypotonic fluid overload, diuretics, and oxytocin use in labor, which causes an increase in antidiuretic hormone (ADH) in the mother and fetus
      (2) Neonatal. CNS disease, causing increased ADH; decreased renal resorption of sodium due to prematurity, adrenal insufficiency, or diuretics; water intoxication from nebulization or excess free water; and low salt intake in premature infants fed breast milk or low-sodium formula
   c. **Hypernatremia** is caused by sodium overload, diarrhea and vomiting, and failure to provide adequate free water in infants with increased insensible water loss (e.g., extremely immature infants).
   d. Treatment of hyponatremia and hypernatremia is similar to that used in older children (see Chap. 7, pp. 207 and 209).
2. **Potassium**
   a. The usual maintenance requirement for potassium is 2–3 mEq/kg/day. This is usually started on the second or third day.
   b. **Hyperkalemia** in the newborn may be caused by adrenal insufficiency, exchange transfusion with old blood, and excessive potassium administration. The ECG may show peaked T waves.
   c. **Hypokalemia** in the newborn is often seen in the failure to replace

Table 6-13. Insensible water loss (IWL) and body weight

IWL* (ml/kg/hr)	Body weight (gm)
2.7	< 1,000
2.3	1,000–1,250
1.5	1,250–1,500
1.0	1,500–1,750
0.8	1,750–2,000

* Factors that increase IWL are ambient-temperature-above-neutral thermal environment, fever, activity, radiant warmer, and phototherapy. Factors that decrease IWL are assisted ventilation with warm and humidified air, heat shield, and incubation with high humidity.
Source: Adapted from H. S. Dweck, *Perinatology* 2:183, 1975; and J. C. Sinclair et al., *Pediatr. Clin. North Am.* 17:863, 1970.

ongoing potassium losses, in association with vomiting as in pyloric stenosis or with use of diuretics. The ECG may show depressed T waves.
   d. For treatment of hypokalemia and hyperkalemia, see pp. 205 and 230.
   3. **Calcium.** See Chap. 7, p. 197.
B. **Renal factors in the newborn.** As compared with the kidneys of older children, the newborn kidney has a limited ability both to dilute and to concentrate urine; has a decreased glomerular filtration rate, blood flow, and tubular resorption of glucose, sodium, and bicarbonate; and has an inability to excrete an acid and a phosphate load. These limitations of function are more severe with decreasing gestational age.
C. **Fluid and electrolyte monitoring** in the newborn should include:
   1. **A physical examination**
   2. **Blood.** Sodium, potassium, chloride, total CO_2, glucose, BUN, and, occasionally, osmolarity
   3. **Urine.** Specific gravity or osmolarity, and sodium, potassium, and glucose when there is an electrolyte imbalance
   4. An **accurate record of intake and output.** A calibrated infusion pump is necessary for accurate hourly infusions. A pediatric urine collector should be used to measure output. In small male infants, the penis can be inserted in a test tube to facilitate accurate assessment of output. Weighing diapers or pads before and after voiding can be done to avoid the use of tape, with consequent breakdown of skin.
   5. Fluid and electrolyte therapy must be adjusted frequently, depending on the size of the infant and the results of the preceding determinations.
D. **Fluid and electrolyte requirements**
   1. **Term infants**
      a. **Fluid requirements:** 60–80 ml/kg for day 1, 80–100 ml/kg for day 2, 100–120 ml/kg for day 3, and 120–150 ml/kg for day 4 and thereafter. Requirements are **decreased in** renal failure, cardiac failure, decreased insensible water loss (IWL), and increased ADH states. Requirements are **increased in** excess IWL, low humidity, fever, activity, and increased renal loss.
      b. **Sodium.** 2–3 mEq/kg/24h starting on day 2
      c. **Potassium.** 2–3 mEq/kg/day starting on day 2
      d. **Calcium.** 30–45 mg/kg/day (only when hypocalcemia is noted)
   2. **Premature infants**
      a. **Fluid requirements** (ml/kg/day):

Body weight (gm)	Days 1–2	Day 3	Days 15–20
2,000–1,750	80	110	130
1,750–1,500	80	100	130
1,500–1,250	90	120	130
1,250–1,000	100	130	140
1,000–750	105	140	150

      b. Premature infants weighing under 1,000 gm may require up to 200 ml/kg/day because they are often on open beds and under radiant warmers and phototherapy (see Table 6-13). Failure to provide this amount of fluid will lead to significant hypernatremia. Pay close attention to infused sodium loads when providing such high fluid intake.
      c. Small premature infants may be unable to metabolize the glucose load in 10% D/W, and hyperglycemia and glucosuria will develop. Glucose intake can be measured as gm/kg/hr and gradually increased until the infant can tolerate the glucose load. Some useful numbers to help with this calculation are:

Infusion rate		Amount of glucose received	
ml/kg/hr 5% D/W	ml/kg/hr 10% D/W	gm/kg/hr	gm/kg/hr
4	2	0.2	4.8
6	3	0.3	7.2
8	4	0.4	9.6
10	5	0.5	12.0

For example, 2 ml/kg/hr of 10% D/W will provide 0.2 gm/kg/hr or 4.8 gm/kg/day glucose.

   d. **Electrolyte requirements**
   (1) Sodium. Premature infants require at least 2–3 mEq/kg/day starting on day 2 or 3. Many require up to 4–8 mEq/kg/day. Serum and urine sodium should be monitored.
   (2) Potassium. 2–3 mEq/kg/day should be started on day 2 or 3 if there is no renal problem.
   (3) Calcium. Acute requirements are often 30–45 mg/kg/day. Long-term calcium requirements are 100–150 mg/kg/day.
IX. Neurologic problems (see also Chap. 19)
   A. Neonatal seizures (see Chap. 19, p. 529)
   B. Intraventricular hemorrhage. Periventricular–intraventricular hemorrhage (PV–IVH) is the most common neonatal intracranial hemorrhage. It has an incidence of 30–40 percent in infants weighing under 1,500 gm and is associated with prematurity and hypoxia.
   1. Evaluation
      a. The catastrophic syndrome progresses rapidly in minutes to hours with shock, stupor, coma, bradycardia, respiratory irregularity, and apnea. Tonic seizures, decerebrate posturing, dilated pupils, flaccid quadriparesis, a full fontanel, a fall in hematocrit, temperature abnormalities, and metabolic acidosis may occur.
      b. The saltatory presentation may progress over hours to days. The signs are a change in level of consciousness, hypotonia, abnormal eye movements, changes in respiration pattern, and an unexplained fall in hematocrit.
      c. The condition should be suspected in premature infants who have any abnormal neurologic signs. A real-time **ultrasound sector scanner** should be used to confirm the diagnosis. Lumbar puncture often reveals xanthochromia, elevated protein, and late hypoglycorrhachia. Meningeal irritation from blood may cause a CSF pleocytosis and raise concerns about infection.
      d. Because most bleeds are clinically inapparent, we routinely scan all infants with a birth weight of less than 1,500 gm.
   2. Diagnosis. Intraventricular hemorrhage is usually classified as follows:
      a. Grade I. Subependymal bleeding
      b. Grade II. Intraventricular hemorrhage without ventricular dilation
      c. Grade III. Intraventricular hemorrhage with ventricular dilation
      d. Grade IV. Intraventricular hemorrhage with parenchymal hemorrhage
   3. Therapy
      a. General supportive measures to treat seizures, hypoxia, apnea, hypercapnia, acidosis, hypothermia, and hypoglycemia should be instituted.
      b. Cerebral perfusion should be maintained to prevent hypoxic–ischemic damage to the brain. The blood pressure should be maintained in the normal range and no wide swings permitted. This must be done carefully because excess cerebral perfusion may increase cerebral bleeding.
      c. Avoid arterial hypertension, hypercapnia, infusion of hyperosmolar solutions, or rapid expansion of intravascular space.

d. If the infant survives the acute insult, daily head circumference measurements and weekly ultrasound assessment of hemorrhage and ventricular size should be done.

e. Grade I and II hemorrhages have a good prognosis and usually need only supportive care.

f. If progressive ventriculomegaly with evidence of increased intracranial pressures develops, serial lumbar punctures can be tried to postpone definitive shunting. Furosemide (Lasix), 1 mg/kg/day, and acetazolamide (Diamox), 50–100 mg/kg/day, are used as ancillary treatments. In some cases this will arrest the hydrocephalus and allow resolution.

g. In acute hydrocephalus that is unresponsive to serial lumbar punctures, a temporary ventriculostomy may be necessary.

h. A ventriculoperitoneal shunt is used if a shunt is necessary after a ventriculostomy has been in place for 5–7 days or in slowly progressive hydrocephalus if lumbar punctures, furosemide, and acetazolamide are ineffective.

4. Prevention. Most PV–IVHs occur in the first 2–3 days of life in premature infants. Preventing major fluctuations in brain perfusion may prevent PV–IVH.

C. Periventricular leukomalacia (PVL). Watershed infarcts in the boundary zones between cerebral arteries may be seen in the preterm infant, particularly following severe hypotension. The white matter injury produced may result in spastic diplegia. Later ultrasound scans (at 4–6 weeks) are necessary to identify parenchymal resorption and cyst formation.

X. Necrotizing enterocolitis (NEC)

A. Etiology is not clearly defined. The primary event is believed to be damage to the intestinal mucosa that allows invasion of the bowel wall and circulation by intestinal flora with subsequent sepsis and perforation. Factors suggested to cause mucosal damage include ischemia, feeding of hypertonic formulas or medications, and bacterial or viral invasion.

B. Evaluation and diagnosis

1. Bloody diarrhea in a small premature infant with abdominal distention and bloody or bile-stained gastric aspirates suggest NEC. Other frequently associated systemic signs include temperature instability, ileus, apnea, and lethargy.

2. Clinical and laboratory abnormalities often associated with NEC include shock, DIC, neutropenia, thrombocytopenia, acidosis, hyponatremia, hyperkalemia, hypoglycemia, and reducing substances in stool.

3. Evaluation should include ABGs; CBC; differential; platelet count and smear; electrolytes; glucose; BUN; creatinine; prothrombin time and PTT; cultures of blood, stool, and CSF (if stable); KUB, and cross-table lateral abdominal x-ray.

4. The presence of pneumatosis intestinalis on abdominal x-ray confirms the diagnosis. Free peritoneal gas or gas in the portal venous system may be seen. Both are ominous signs.

C. Treatment

1. The infant should receive nothing by mouth.

2. A nasogastric tube should be placed for drainage.

3. After appropriate cultures have been obtained, the infant should be started on broad-spectrum systemic antibiotics, including ampicillin and gentamicin (unless the nursery has a high incidence of gentamicin-resistant pathogens or the surveillance stool cultures for the infant with NEC yield gentamicin-resistant organisms, in which case an alternative aminoglycoside should be selected based on the known sensitivity). Clindamycin may be necessary for coverage of anaerobic bacteria, especially if perforation has occurred.

4. Correction of shock, acidosis, hyponatremia, thrombocytopenia, or DIC should be instituted as detailed in the individual sections dealing with these problems.

5. Frequent vital signs and clinical examinations are essential. Follow serial abdominal x-rays, CBC with platelet count, electrolytes, and pH q6h until the individual variables are stable and the infant is improving.

6. Early surgical consultation is essential. The usual indications for surgery include perforation or the persistent clinical deterioration of the infant on optimal medical management.

7. Peripheral or central hyperalimentation should be instituted.

8. Treatment should be continued for 10–14 days.

9. Because intestinal strictures are a possible sequela of NEC, the infant should be observed closely for symptoms of obstruction when refeeding is initiated.

XI. Drug withdrawal in the newborn

A. Etiology. Withdrawal symptoms may be seen in infants born to mothers taking narcotics, methadone, diazepam, phenobarbital, alcohol, ethchlorvynol, pentazocine, chlordiazepoxide, or other drugs that may cause addiction.

B. Evaluation and diagnosis

1. **Maternal history.** Discrete, sensitive history taking is necessary to elicit a history of drug abuse. Such a history may also put the infant in a high-risk category for congenital viral infection (see sec. **VII.A**).

2. The **infant's symptoms** include disturbed patterns of sleeping and waking rhythms; nasal congestion, sneezing, and yawning; high-pitched cry; increased sucking, ravenous appetite; irritability, jitteriness; hypertonicity, hyperreflexia, and clonus; sweating and tachypnea; vomiting, diarrhea, and dehydration; fever; and seizures and tremors.

3. **Infants of methadone-treated mothers** may have severe, prolonged withdrawal. Some have "late" withdrawal that may be of the following two types:

   a. The first group shows symptoms shortly after birth, improves, then relapses at 2–4 weeks.

   b. The second group shows no symptoms at birth, but symptoms develop 2–3 weeks later. These infants may also have a history of a sudden, tremendous increase in appetite.

4. The effects of maternal cocaine addiction are not yet clearly delineated. There appears to be a significant risk of intrauterine growth retardation and of placental abruption following acute intoxication. Infants may be irritable and jittery.

5. Blood and urine samples from the mother and infant for toxicology screen within 24 hours after delivery may help, but drugs given to the mother during labor can sometimes confuse the results. Clinical suspicion and careful history usually lead to the diagnosis.

C. Treatment. The goal of treatment is an infant who is not irritable, is not vomiting, has no diarrhea, is growing, and can sleep between feedings, yet is not heavily sedated.

1. Swaddling, holding, and rocking may help infants who are not severely affected.

2. **Drugs.** Infants in whom the preceding therapy is inadequate will need medication.

   a. Phenobarbital, 5–8 mg/kg/day IM or PO in three divided doses, and tapered over 2 weeks, can be given. The side effects are sedation, poor sucking, and heightened sensitivity to pain.

   b. Chlorpromazine, 1.5–3.0 mg/kg/day in four divided doses, is given initially IM, then PO. This dose is maintained for 2–4 days, then tapered as tolerated every 2–4 days. The length of treatment is from 1–6 weeks. Methadone-dependent infants tend to need a longer course of treatment.

   c. Paregoric, 0.05 ml/kg or 2 drops/kg/dose, is given q4–6h. The dose is increased by 2 drops/kg (0.05 ml/kg) at the end of each 4-hour period until the desired response is achieved. Some babies will need medication more often than q4h. Once the adequate dose is determined, it can be tapered by 10 percent daily. The length of treatment is 1–6 weeks. Paregoric contains opium 0.4%, equivalent to morphine 0.04% (0.4 mg/ml). **Side effects** include sleepiness and constipation. **The effects of oral benzoic**

acid on bilirubin binding to albumin are not known. Camphor is a CNS stimulant.

 d. Neonatal opiate solution (formerly known as diluted tincture of opium [DTO], USP). For the above reasons, if a narcotic is to be used it may be best to use tincture of opium, USP, a 10% solution (equal to 1.0% morphine). **Dilute this 25-fold** to a concentration equal to that of paregoric (0.4 mg/ml morphine) and give in the same dose as paregoric.

 e. Diazepam. The dose is 0.1–0.3 mg/kg IM q8h until symptoms are controlled. The dose is then halved, then changed to q12h, then halved again. The length of treatment ranges from 2–7 days, and it seems to be effective in a shorter time than are other medications. The major side effect is respiratory depression. **Note that sodium benzoate included in parenteral diazepam interferes with bilirubin binding.**

 f. Methadone should not be routinely used until more data on toxicity are available. **Methadone is excreted in breast milk,** and thus methadone-treated mothers should not breast feed. When administration has been necessary, the doses used have been 0.5–1.0 mg q4–8h.

 3. The major problem for these children is proper disposition and follow-up. Most states require reporting of these infants to social service authorities, and these agencies should be involved in the decision for disposition (see Chap. 3, p. 74). Some risk factors to consider in sending infants home with their mothers are:

  a. Maternal age. The risk increases as age decreases.

  b. Length of drug use. The risk increases as length of usage increases.

  c. Availability of a drug program

  d. Drug use while on methadone suggests increased risk.

  e. Inability of the mother to make and keep commitments suggests a high risk to the child.

XII. Surgical emergencies

 A. Tracheoesophageal fistula (TEF) with or without esophageal atresia (EA)

  1. Etiology. Esophageal anomalies in the newborn are classified anatomically. Their frequency is given in Table 6-14.

  2. Evaluation. Depending on the presence and location of the fistula and the presence or absence of esophageal atresia, symptoms include excessive salivation, regurgitation of feedings, coughing from aspiration of feedings or gastric contents, abdominal distention, or a scaphoid, airless abdomen.

  3. Diagnosis

   a. EA is diagnosed by the inability to pass a catheter from the nose or mouth into the stomach. If EA is present, a plain chest film may show a dilated upper esophageal pouch. It will also demonstrate a catheter coiled in the upper pouch.

Table 6-14. Relative incidence of esophageal anomalies

Type	Relative incidence* (%)
EA with distal TEF	88
EA without TEF	8
TEF without EA	2
EA with proximal and distal TEF	0.6
EA with proximal TEF	0.8

EA = esophageal atresia; TEF = tracheoesophageal fistula.
* TEF/EA is often associated with other major malformation; 20% have congenital heart disease, and 10% have imperforate anus. TEF/EA is sometimes associated with Down syndrome or the VATER syndrome of: vertebral and vascular defects, imperforate anus, EA with TEF, radial dysplasia, and renal defects. Of infants with EA, 20% are premature, and another 20% are small for gestational age.

b. The absence of abdominal gas on x-ray suggests EA without a distal TEF. Diagnostic maneuvers are the same as in **a.**

c. TEF without EA may be suspected because of recurrent aspiration with feeding and excessive gas in the bowel. Diagnosis may be difficult. A barium swallow in the face-down position or simultaneous esophagoscopy and bronchoscopy with a dye placed in the trachea may be diagnostic. When clinical symptoms make the diagnosis very likely, surgical exploration of the neck should be considered.

4. Treatment. Once the diagnosis of EA with TEF is made, the pediatrician's role is to prevent aspiration and to provide nutrition and support until definitive surgical therapy is carried out. Measures should include:

a. Sump catheter drainage of the upper pouch

b. Provision of a reliable IV line for nutrition and fluids

c. Keeping the baby in a 30-degree head-up position

d. Close monitoring for signs of infection

e. Provision of adequate respiratory support

f. If the baby has complications that will delay primary repair, a **gastrostomy** is usually indicated to decompress the abdomen and prevent aspiration of gastric contents. This is urgent if mechanical ventilation becomes necessary. Definitive repair can be early, delayed, or staged.

B. Omphalocele and gastroschisis

1. Omphalocele

a. Etiology. An omphalocele is caused by failure of development of part of the abdominal wall. The defect, which is evident at birth, is covered with a translucent membrane holding the bowel and viscera. This membrane may rupture at delivery. Omphalocele may be associated with other anomalies, including cardiac, genitourinary, anorectal, and limb anomalies, or may be part of a syndrome such as Beckwith-Wiedemann and trisomies 13, 18, and 21.

b. Emergency medical treatment includes:

(1) Insertion of a nasogastric tube, which is placed to suction.

(2) Protecting the lesion by

(a) Covering the sac with petrolatum-impregnated gauze then wrapping it with Kling gauze to support the intestinal viscera in the abdominal wall

(b) If ruptured, placing a saline-soaked gauze over the exposed intestine and then wrapping the baby in a dry, sterile towel to prevent heat loss

(c) Starting IV fluids

(d) Starting antibiotics (ampicillin and gentamicin)

(e) Monitoring temperature and blood pressure

(f) Arranging immediate surgical treatment. The sac should not be pushed back into the abdomen, because this may impede venous return and respiration.

2. Gastroschisis is managed medically in the same manner as omphalocele until definitive surgical treatment is carried out. Antibiotics are **always used** because there is no membrane. Infants with gastroschisis should be evaluated for malformation of the colon and intestinal atresia.

C. Intestinal obstruction

1. Etiology. The causes are listed in Table 6-15.

2. Evaluation

a. The **symptoms** of intestinal obstruction vary with the site of the lesion. Lesions below the pylorus present with bile-stained vomiting. Lesions high in the gut such as malrotation with midgut volvulus will present with little abdominal distention, and lesions low in the bowel such as ileal atresia will show distention. There may be a history of polyhydramnios.

b. Laboratory tests include hematocrit, CBC, electrolytes, ABGs and pH, an x-ray of the abdomen taken with the infant in the left lateral decubitus

Table 6-15. Etiology of intestinal obstruction in newborn

Mechanical obstruction

Congenital

Intrinsic
Pyloric stenosis
Duodenal atresia
Jejunoileal atresia or stenosis
Imperforate anus
Intraluminal cysts
Meconium ileus with or without
cystic fibrosis

Acquired
Intussusception
Adhesions
Mesenteric artery thrombosis
Formation of intestinal concretions (lactobezoars)
Stenosis secondary to healed necrotizing enterocolitis

Extrinsic
Malrotation with or without midgut
volvulus
Volvulus without malrotation
Peritoneal bands
Incarcerated hernia (premature
infants)
Annular pancreas
Duplications
Aberrant vessels
Hydrometrocolpos

Functional obstruction

Prematurity
Defective innervation (Hirschsprung's
disease)
Drugs
Hypermagnesemia
Heroin
Hexamethonium bromide

Sepsis
Enteritis
CNS disease
Necrotizing enterocolitis
Endocrine disorders such as hypothy-
roidism and adrenal insufficiency

and flat positions, a barium swallow or enema, and a sweat test in cases
of meconium ileus.
3. The **diagnosis** of some common causes of intestinal obstruction in the
newborn are:
   a. **Pyloric stenosis.** This may present in the newborn period as nonbilious
   projectile vomiting. An enlarged pylorus can be palpated. A large gastric
   air shadow may be seen on x-ray. Abdominal ultrasound is diagnostic.
   b. **Duodenal atresia** may be associated with other anomalies, such as Down
   syndrome, cardiovascular malformations, and other GI malformations.
   The patient may have a history of polyhydramnios. Symptoms and signs
   are bilious vomiting and upper abdominal distention. A plain x-ray of the
   abdomen will show air in the stomach and upper part of the duodenum
   ("double bubble").
   c. **Jejunoileal atresia** presents with abdominal distention, bilious vomiting,
   and failure to pass stools. X-ray films show air-fluid levels and a barium
   enema shows a microcolon. There may be multiple atretic segments.
   d. **Volvulus with or without malrotation** of the bowel is an emergency. It
   may present as bile-stained vomiting without much abdominal distention
   in an infant who has previously been passing stools. There may be
   abdominal tenderness. X-rays may show duodenal obstruction with little
   air in the rest of the bowel. A barium enema may show the cecum in the
   upper right or central abdomen. Demonstration of absent or abnormal
   position of the ligament of Treitz confirms the diagnosis of malrotation.
   e. **Meconium ileus** is often associated with meconium peritonitis, a positive
   sweat test for cystic fibrosis, and an x-ray showing dilated small bowel

filled with a granular-appearing material or tiny bubbles. Treatment of this functional obstruction may require enemas. Meglumine diatrizoate (Gastrografin) enemas can be used after adequate and continuous intravenous hydration. Occasionally surgery is necessary.

f. **Functional obstruction** due to disorders such as prematurity, meconium plug syndrome, and hypermagnesemia will often respond to glycerin suppositories, gentle enemas (one-half strength saline in a dose of 5 ml/kg body weight) given with a soft rubber catheter, or rectal stimulation with a soft rubber catheter. Frequent small feedings and adequate hydration are also helpful. A barium enema, performed in an infant who has functional obstruction due to prematurity, may compound the problem. If contrast enemas are to be done, consideration should be given to using Gastrografin after adequate and ongoing intravenous hydration. Hirschsprung's disease should always be considered when a newborn has difficulty passing stools.

4. **Treatment** of most causes of mechanical intestinal obstruction includes:
   a. Nasogastric suction
   b. Fluid and electrolyte therapy; volume replacement (colloid) if indicated
   c. Antibiotics if there is a question of integrity of the bowel or the infant appears sick
   d. Surgical consultation

D. **Diaphragmatic hernia** occurs once in every 3,000 births. Most diaphragmatic hernias of Bochdalek are on the left side.
   1. **Evaluation.** Mortality in this disease is high due to the hypoplastic lungs and abnormal pulmonary vasculature. There are often severe complications due to the persistence of the fetal circulation pattern and myocardial dysfunction secondary to hypoxia and acidosis. Infants with large diaphragmatic hernias may present at birth with cyanosis, respiratory distress, a scaphoid abdomen, decreased or absent breath sounds on the side of the hernia, and heart sounds heard best on the side opposite the hernia. Small hernias, right-sided hernias, and substernal hernias of Morgagni may have a more subtle onset, manifested by feeding problems and mild respiratory distress.
   2. **Diagnosis.** The diagnosis is confirmed by chest x-ray.
   3. **Treatment.** When a diaphragmatic hernia is suspected, the following measures should be employed:
      a. A large tube should be placed into the stomach and put to suction to remove air and gastric contents, which, if allowed to accumulate, will increase mediastinal shift and lung compression.
      b. The infant should receive oxygen and respiratory support as needed. Any positive pressure should be administered through an endotracheal tube.
      c. A reliable IV line should be placed.
      d. Hypoxia and acidosis should be treated.
      e. Prompt surgical correction should be carried out.
      f. **Extracorporeal membrane oxygenation (ECMO)** is available at selected neonatal centers. Its use in cases of severe lung hypoplasia appears promising.

Fluid and Electrolytes

Norman Rosenblum

I. **General principles**
   A. **Renal function.** The glomerular filtration rate (GFR) is relatively depressed in infants and reaches a "normal" adult value (corrected for surface area) only at age 1–2 years. Other functions that are similarly depressed include renal plasma flow (RPF), free-water clearance, acid excretion, phosphate excretion, and maximal rate of tubular absorption (T_m) glucose (Table 7-1).
   B. **Fluid and volume physiology.** At birth the total body water (TBW) constitutes 75–80 percent of the infant's weight. The TBW falls to 60 percent in childhood (see **C.1.b**). A rapid diuresis ensues over the first few days of life, during which 7 percent of TBW is lost.
   1. **Body fluids**
      a. The TBW comprises the following two major compartments.
         (1) **Extracellular fluid (ECF)** constitutes 35–45 percent of body weight in infants and 20 percent in adults (15% interstitial and 5% intravascular).
         (2) **Intracellular fluid (ICF)** constitutes 40 percent of body weight in both infants and adults.
   2. **Regulatory mechanisms**
      a. The **kidney** regulates water balance, osmolality of fluids, and the distribution of body water.
      b. **Principles**
         (1) **Tonicity** (concentration, osmolality) is conserved in preference to volume.
         (2) The kidneys provide better protection against **dilution** of body fluids than against **dehydration.**
         (3) ECF volume is controlled by **sodium;** hence sodium control is the key to volume control.
      c. **Osmolality** refers to the number of osmotically active particles per 1,000 gm water in a solution (units = mOsm/kg), whereas **osmolarity** refers to the number of osmotically active particles per unit volume of solution (units = mOsm/liter). The serum osmolality is generally higher than the osmolarity due to the high specific volume of proteins. The terms *osmolality* and *osmolarity* frequently are confused. The term *osmolality* is theoretically more appropriate than *osmolarity* for the calculation of osmotic relationships.
         (1) ECF osmolality is somewhat higher than that of the ICF because of the contribution by plasma proteins.
         (2) Water flux follows ionic (osmolal) flux to equalize fluid concentrations.
         (3) Osmolality is determined by freezing point depression of the solution. Also, as a rule of thumb:

$$\text{Osmolality} = 2(\text{Na}^+) + \frac{\text{BUN}}{2.8} + \frac{\text{glucose}}{18}$$

Osmolal excretion depends on the concentrating ability of the kidney. To produce a minimal urinary volume requires a maximum osmo-

Table 7-1. Normal values of renal function*

Measurement	At birth	1–2 weeks	6 months– 1 year	1–3 years	Adult
GFR (ml/min/m²)	15 ± 11	31 ± 15	45 ± 12	55 ± 13	68 ± 10
RPF (ml/min/m²)	51 ± 12	89 ± 20	203 ± 42	310 ± 70	354 ± 53
T_m PAH (mg/min/m²)		8 ± 1	30 ± 12	38 ± 11	46 ± 7
T_m glucose (mg/min/m²)		10 ± 12			196 ± 29

m² = body surface area in square meters; T_m = maximum rate of tubular reabsorption; PAH = para-aminohippurate.
* Mean ± S.D.

lality: Maximal osmolality ranges from 1,200 mOsm/kg in the healthy child (600–700 mOsm/kg in the healthy infant), down to 300 mOsm/kg in the diseased kidney.

   d. Volume is a sine qua non for organ function. Regulatory factors include cardiac output, peripheral resistance, the renin-angiotensin-aldosterone axis, prostaglandins, and catecholamines. Because the body's sodium content determines ECF distribution, maintenance of total body sodium is essential to volume regulation. Angiotensin II causes peripheral vasoconstriction and enhanced sodium reclamation by the proximal tubule. Aldosterone enhances distal tubular sodium transport resulting in sodium conservation. Active transport of cation brings about passive water transfer, thereby restoring ECF volume. In addition, antidiuretic hormone (ADH) release, in response to hyperosmolarity, augments water retention and thereby aids volume repletion.

   e. "Third space" accumulations occur in many disease states, trapping fluids, electrolytes, and drugs outside their normal boundaries, thus robbing the body of effective volume.

C. Electrolyte physiology

   1. Sodium (Na⁺). 1 mEq = 23 mg; 1 gm = 43.5 mEq; plasma concentration = 135–140 mEq/liter. **Note:** 1 gm salt (NaCl) = 18 mEq Na⁺.

   a. Na⁺ is the principal volume regulator. Normally, Na⁺ accounts for 90 percent of extracellular cationic osmolality.

   b. Although Na⁺ is principally distributed in the ECF, the true Na⁺ space is the TBW (about 80% body weight in the term newborn, 75% body weight at age 3 months, 70% body weight at 6 months, and 60% body weight by age 1 year). The serum Na⁺ concentration is determined by the total body Na⁺ load and the TBW.

   c. Measurement of Na⁺ by flame photometer is artifactually depressed in hyperlipemic and hyperglycemic states. **Rule of thumb:** Na⁺ is depressed 5 mEq/liter for every 200 mg/dl glucose concentration above 100 mg/dl.

   d. Requirements for Na⁺ vary. A typical daily requirement is 40–60 mEq/M² or 1–3 mEq/dl water requirement.

   e. In the newborn, the Na⁺ and volume regulatory mechanisms are functionally limited. Excretory capacity is reduced by a relative concentrating defect (maximal urine osmolality approximately 600–700 mOsm/liter). Therefore, obligatory solute loads require extra free water for their elimination (see Table 5-3 for solute contents of various infant diets). Because infants cannot control their fluid intake, sufficient fluid must be provided to balance needs for solute excretion.

   2. Potassium (K⁺). 1 mEq = 39.1 mg; 1 gm = 25.6 mEq; plasma concentration 3.4–5.5 mEq/liter (may be higher in neonates).

   a. K⁺ is the principal cation of the ICF and contributes to the maintenance of intracellular tonicity and the cell membrane resting potential. The ICF contains 98 percent of the body K⁺ and thereby is the "hidden" storage pool of K⁺.

b. The proportion of K^+ in the ECF is controlled by multiple factors, including serum pH and body Na^+ and K^+ load. Thus, measurement of serum K^+ provides only an indirect assessment of total body K^+ stores and may therefore be misleading (e.g., diabetic ketoacidosis). **No practical estimate of K^+ space can be given for therapeutic replacement purposes.**

c. A typical daily K^+ requirement is 30–40 mEq/m²/24 hr or 1–3 mEq/dl fluid. There is an obligatory K^+ loss via the urine since the tubular resorption generally cannot lower U_{K^+} below 10 mEq/liter.

d. A maximal intravenous dose of K^+ is 1 mEq/kg/hr, preferably administered into a large vein via intravenous pump. IV administration of K^+ in concentrations > 40 mEq/liter often leads to phlebitis.

e. The danger of an **abnormal serum K^+** is exacerbated by abnormalities of calcium in the opposite direction.

f. Hypokalemia due to some renal tubular defects, starvation, chronic diarrhea or vomiting, diabetic ketoacidosis, hyperaldosteronism, chronic use of diuretics, or inadequate long-term IV replacement is usually accompanied by chloride depletion with metabolic alkalosis.

    (1) Symptoms include muscle weakness, cramps, paralytic ileus, decreased reflexes, lethargy, and confusion.

    (2) Acid urine in the presence of metabolic alkalosis (paradoxical aciduria) also indicates K^+ depletion. Hypokalemic metabolic alkalosis is usually accompanied by a K^+ deficit of at least 4–5 mEq/kg.

    (3) Cardiac effects indicated by electrocardiogram (ECG) are a low-voltage T wave, the presence of a U wave, and a prolonged Q-T interval.

    (4) Chronic exposure to low potassium damages the kidney's concentrating ability, thus producing a vasopressin-resistant diabetes insipidus.

g. Hyperkalemia occurs with renal failure, hemolysis, tissue necrosis, Addison's disease, congenital adrenal cortical hyperplasia, certain diuretics, and overdose of K^+ supplements.

    (1) Hypocalcemia, hyponatremia, and acidosis all exacerbate the dangerous effects of hyperkalemia.

    (2) The toxic effects are mainly cardiac. Rising K^+ interferes with normal nodal and bundle conduction. ECG changes include peaked T wave, increased P-R interval and widened QRS, depressed S-T segment, and atrioventricular or intraventricular heart block. As serum K^+ rises beyond 7.5 mEq/liter, there is grave danger of heart block, ventricular tachycardia, and ventricular fibrillation.

3. Chloride (Cl^-). 1 mEq = 35.5 mg; 1 gm = 28 mEq; 1 gm salt (NaCl) = 18 mEq Cl^-; plasma concentration = 99–105 mEq/liter.

a. Cl^- is the principal anion of both intravascular fluid and gastric fluid. Although Cl^- may undergo active renal tubular transport, it can be considered to behave passively and in parallel to Na^+.

b. Abnormal losses occur with vomiting, diuretic therapy, and cystic fibrosis, and tend to lead to metabolic alkalosis.

c. Paradoxical aciduria occurs in the face of Cl^- depletion with dehydration. In the absence of Cl^-, HCO_3^- is reabsorbed with Na^+. In addition, the accompanying secondary hyperaldosteronism causes the distal tubular secretion of H^+ (and K^+), resulting in an acid urine. This cycle of events can only be interrupted by the replacement of Cl^- as NaCl.

4. Calcium (Ca^{2+}). 1 mEq = 20 mg; 1 gm = 50 mEq; plasma concentration = 9.5–10.5 mg/dl or 4.7–5.2 mEq/liter except in the newborn and premature infant.

a. Free ionized Ca^{2+} constitutes about 47 percent of total serum calcium. Approximately 40 percent of total serum calcium is bound to serum proteins and 80–90 percent of this calcium is bound to albumin. The calcium space is approximately 25 percent of body weight.

b. A change in serum albumin of 1 gm/dl changes serum Ca^{2+} concentration, in the same direction, by 0.8 mg/dl.

    c. The ionized portion of Ca^{2+} carries out functions in enzyme regulation, stabilizing neuromuscular membranes, coagulation processes, and bone formation. Acidosis increases ionized Ca^{2+}, whereas alkalosis decreases it, even to the point of symptomatic tetany.

    d. Hypocalcemia is most commonly seen in rickets, renal insufficiency, and the hypoalbuminemic states of liver disease or nephrosis, and in the neonate who is fed cow's milk formulas. Other conditions that produce lowered calcium are discussed in Chap. 11.

    Drugs that cause hypocalcemia include furosemide, glucagon, calcitonin, mithramycin, bicarbonate, and corticosteroids. **Exchange transfusion with acid citrate–preserved blood can produce hypocalcemia** (see Chap. 16).

    (1) Symptoms of depressed ionized Ca^{2+} include Chvostek's and Trousseau's signs, carpopedal spasm, and, occasionally, mental confusion. Neonates commonly become jittery and may have seizures with tetany of the newborn (see Chap. 6, p. 173).

    (2) The ECG shows prolongation of the Q-T interval relative to the rate.

    (3) Treatment of hypocalcemia includes IV and PO administration of Ca^{2+}. An IV bolus of Ca^{2+} will only transiently (for about 1 hr) raise the serum Ca^{2+} level. Continuous IV administration is hazardous (cardiac arrhythmias, phlebitis, subcutaneous calcifications) and should be reserved for critical situations.

    e. Hypercalcemia is seen with hyperparathyroidism, vitamin D intoxication, sarcoidosis, cancer, immobilization, thyroid disease, Addison's disease, hypophosphatasia, and the milk-alkali syndrome in those taking antacids. **Symptoms** of excess Ca^{2+} include nausea, anorexia, vomiting, constipation, polyuria, dehydration, mental confusion, and eventually coma. Chronic elevation of Ca^{2+} can lead to nephrocalcinosis, extraskeletal calcification, and renal calculi.

D. Acid-base physiology

    1. General principles. Blood pH is maintained within a very narrow range by a regulatory system that includes **blood buffering,** changes in **ventilation,** and **renal** compensatory mechanisms. Children ingest 1–2 mEq/kg/day "fixed" acid in their diet as sulfate from amino acids, nitrate, and phosphate (from phosphoproteins) and produce organic acids from incomplete oxidation of fat and carbohydrate (e.g., lactic acid). Blood chemical buffers and increased elimination of carbon dioxide provide immediate defense against this tide of acid, but the kidney maintains long-term pH homeostasis. A shift of 0.1 pH units, at pH 7.40, represents a change of only 10 nanoequivalents (nEq)/liter in hydrogen ion concentration.

    a. Blood buffers include erythrocyte hemoglobin, organic and inorganic phosphates, carbonate (from bone), and both plasma and red cell bicarbonate. About half the buffering capacity derives from bicarbonate and roughly one third from hemoglobin.

    b. Alveolar ventilation normally eliminates thousands of milliequivalents of carbon dioxide per day and maintains arterial PCO_2 at approximately 40 mm Hg. This prevents the accumulation of the weak acid, H_2CO_3, formed when CO_2 remains dissolved in plasma. Alveolar ventilation is controlled by central chemoreceptors.

    c. The **kidneys** regulate the systemic levels of HCO_3 by means of recovery of filtered HCO_3 and generation of "new" HCO_3 by the process of net acid excretion. Generation of new HCO_3 replaces the HCO_3 that has been consumed by normal endogenous acid production. Net acid excretion occurs by excretion of titratable acids and excretion of NH_4^+.

    2. Determination of acid-base status requires measurement of blood pH and bicarbonate. Bicarbonate, total CO_2 content, and CO_2 combining power provide the same basic information. Total CO_2 (TCO_2) is 1–2 mEq/liter lower than combining power.

    3. Laboratory values. Ideally, arterial samples are obtained for the diagnosis of acid-base disturbances. Venous samples may prove inaccurate in patients with impaired peripheral circulation, local tissue damage, or blood stasis caused by a tourniquet. Normal values for arterial and venous blood are given in Table 7-2.

4. **Acid-base abnormalities.** By convention, acid-base disorders are divided into the following categories (Fig. 7-1): **respiratory** versus **metabolic, acute** versus **chronic, simple** versus **mixed,** and **pure** versus **compensated** and resulting in either **acidosis** or **alkalosis,** depending on pH. In pure imbalances of pH, the disequilibrium results from a deviation of either PCO_2 (respiratory) or HCO_3^- (metabolic) from the norm. As can be seen from the Henderson-Hasselbalch equation,

$$pH = pK + \log \frac{base}{acid} = 6.1 + \log \frac{HCO_3^-}{0.3 \times PCO_2},$$

where pK is $-\log$ of the dissociation constant for the bicarbonate buffer ($H_2CO_3 - HCO_3^-$). A rise in PCO_2 increases the denominator and pH falls; this constitutes **respiratory acidosis.** Conversely, a fall in PCO_2 diminishes the denominator and pH rises, leading to **respiratory alkalosis.** Similarly, retention of HCO_3^- causes **metabolic alkalosis,** and a drop in HCO_3^- results in **metabolic acidosis.**

These situations prevail only for brief periods. The change in the internal milieu brings compensatory mechanisms into play. Compensation is rarely sufficient to offset the primary disturbance completely, and the condition is usually only partially corrected, so that the patient has a compensated acid-base disorder (Table 7-3).

   a. **Respiratory acidosis** results from *retention of CO_2* and a consequent *increase in H_2CO_3.* Normally, a rise in PCO_2 stimulates a ventilatory effort to eliminate the hypercapnia. In the acute phase of respiratory acidosis, available buffering mechanisms and renal compensation are minimal, and pH falls rapidly as PCO_2 exceeds 50 mm Hg (for a discussion of acute respiratory failure, see Chap. 3). When hypercapnia is sustained, renal compensation leads to an increase in plasma bicarbonate. Net acid excretion is increased primarily through an increase in the excretion of NH_4^+. As well, tubular resorption of bicarbonate increases while that for chloride decreases. By acidifying the urine, the kidney can raise ECF bicarbonate to 40 mEq/liter or more to compensate for marked hypercapnia. Plasma bicarbonate increases by about 0.3 mEq/liter for each 1-mm increase in $PaCO_2$. *Usually, neonates are incapable of this adaptation and will remain severely acidotic with respiratory distress syndrome.*

   b. **Respiratory alkalosis** is not a common pediatric problem.
      (1) **Hyperventilation** occurs in patients without parenchymal disease who are managed with mechanical ventilators, in the early phase of salicylate intoxication, in anxious or hysterical states, and in hypermetabolic states.
      (2) **Rapid correction** of metabolic acidosis can result in respiratory alkalosis, since correction of the pH in the cerebrospinal fluid lags behind the ECF, and continuing central nervous system (CNS) acidosis stimulates the medullary ventilatory drive.

Table 7-2. Normal blood values*

Blood sample	pH	PCO_2	HCO_3^-	TCO_2
Arterial	7.38–7.45	35–45 mm Hg	23–27 mEq/liter	24–28 mEq/liter
Venous	7.35–7.40	45–50 mm Hg	24–29 mEq/liter	25–30 mEq/liter

* In children less than 1 year of age, the normal range for TCO_2 is 20–24, and pH is lower by approximately 0.05.

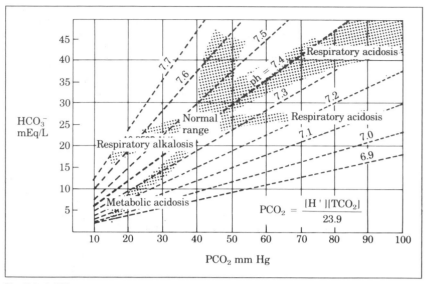

Fig. 7-1. Acid-base nomogram.

(3) **Acute respiratory alkalosis** can precipitate tetany (see **C.4.c**) and causes a feeling of lightheadedness. In psychogenic cases, symptoms of an acute anxiety state often dominate.

(4) **Laboratory diagnosis** rests on the triad of *decreased PCO_2, elevated pH,* and *normal bicarbonate.*

(5) **Hypocapnia** alkalinizes body fluids and elicits a prompt but modest reduction in plasma HCO_3 secondary to titration of HCO_3 buffer. This is followed by a net decrease in renal acid excretion, decreased tubular HCO_3 resorption, and enhanced tubular Cl reabsorption. Plasma bicarbonate decreases by about 0.4–0.5 mEq/liter for each 1-mm decrease in $PaCO_2$. Urinary loss of HCO_3 results in simultaneous loss of sodium and contraction of the ECF volume.

c. **Metabolic acidosis** results from an *increased acid burden,* which overcomes renal generation of HCO_3; *renal defects* in the secretion of H^+; and *loss of extracellular HCO_3.* In these situations bicarbonate and other blood buffers are consumed and TCO_2 falls.

(1) The **anion gap** is an estimation of anionic substances that are not measured by the usual laboratory techniques. The anion gap is the difference between the serum cations (Na^+) and anions (Cl^- and HCO_3^-). It normally is ~12 mEq/liter, but is somewhat higher in newborn infants. Increases in the anion gap occur when the fall in plasma bicarbonate is balanced by a rise in an anion that is not

Table 7-3. Compensation in acid-base disturbances

Acid-base disturbances	pH	HCO_3^-	PCO_2	Compensation
Metabolic acidosis	↓	↓		↓ PCO_2; acid urine
Respiratory acidosis	↓		↑	Acid urine
Metabolic alkalosis	↑	↑		↑ PCO_2; alkaline urine
Respiratory alkalosis	↑		↓	Alkaline urine

commonly measured (increased anion gap acidosis). When the fall in plasma bicarbonate is balanced by a rise in the plasma chloride, an anion that is usually measured, the acidosis is termed a *normal anion gap acidosis*. By contrast, in lactic acidosis (e.g., secondary to shock), the large anion gap reflects accumulation of the "unmeasured" anion.

(2) In response to the acidemic stress, both the kidney and lung undertake corrective measures. There is a prompt increase in minute ventilation, and PCO_2 falls. Urinary acidification maximizes over a few days within the limits of both reduced circulation and GFR.

(3) In children, chronic metabolic acidosis most commonly can be traced to a kidney abnormality, either parenchymal disease, obstruction, or a tubular disorder. Growth failure invariably accompanies chronic acidemia.

d. **Metabolic alkalosis** is a disorder characterized by *elevated plasma bicarbonate* and *decreased concentrations of proton and chloride* in the ECF. Metabolic alkalosis usually occurs as part of a generalized derangement in fluid and electrolytes. Although the list of possible etiologies is long, the cause of metabolic alkalosis in the majority of affected children is *loss of acid from the gastrointestinal tract* (e.g., vomiting secondary to pyloric stenosis).

(1) **Potassium plays a central role in both the development and correction of metabolic alkalosis.** In acute alkalosis, K^+ moves from the ECF to the ICF to help maintain electroneutrality in the face of H^+ ion depletion. *Although serum K^+ may then be low, total body K^+ remains normal.*

(2) **Paradoxical aciduria.** Conditions that produce K^+ depletion also stimulate aldosterone production. In volume-depleted states such as diarrhea, renal Na^+ reabsorption is increased. In the distal tubule Na^+ is exchanged predominately for H^+ since the total body stores of K^+ have been partially depleted. The outcome is aciduria, coexisting with systemic alkalosis.

e. **Mixed disorders** of acid-base homeostasis result from disturbances in both respiratory and renal function. Their diagnosis is simplified by reference to Fig. 7-1. Since the shaded areas in Fig. 7-1 represent the 95 percent confidence bands for each disturbance (including the normal compensatory response), any combination of values of PCO_2 and HCO_3^- that falls outside these areas represents a mixed disturbance.

f. As a rule, **compensatory mechanisms** modify the acid-base disturbances as shown in Table 7-3 to the following degree:

(1) **Metabolic acidosis:** PCO_2 ↓ 1.0–1.5 × fall of HCO_3^-
(2) **Metabolic alkalosis:** PCO_2 ↑ 0.5–1.0 × rise of HCO_3^-
(3) **Acute respiratory acidosis:** HCO_3^- ↑ to maximum 30 mEq/liter
(4) **Chronic respiratory acidosis:** HCO_3^- ↑ 4 mEq/liter/10 mm PCO_2
(5) **Acute respiratory alkalosis:** HCO_3^- ↓ 2.5 mEq/liter/10 mm ↓ PCO_2 (to minimum 18 mEq/liter)
(6) **Chronic respiratory alkalosis:** HCO_3^- falls to 15 mEq/liter.

II. **Maintenance of normal fluid and electrolyte balance**

A. **Estimation of fluid requirements**

1. **Rationale.** Fluid is continually lost from the body in the form of insensible and urinary losses. *Maintenance fluid requirement* is the amount of fluid required to keep total body fluid in balance. There are several methods of **estimating** the maintenance fluid requirements for an average patient under average conditions; the **actual** maintenance requirements may vary considerably from the usual estimations because of unusual circumstances (see 3 and Table 7-4).

2. **Components of maintenance fluid requirements**

a. **Insensible losses** account for about 50 percent of the total fluid lost per day. The usual sources of insensible losses and their respective contribution to total insensible losses are:

Table 7-4. Conditions affecting normal fluid requirements

Condition	Adjustment
Increased metabolic rate	
Fever	Increase H_2O by 12%/°C
Hypermetabolic state	Increase H_2O by 25–75%
Decreased metabolic rate	
Hypothermia	Decrease H_2O by 12%/°C
Hypometabolic state	Decrease H_2O by 10–25%
Unusual insensible losses	
High environmental humidity	Decrease IWL to 0–15 ml/100 calories
Hyperventilation	Increase IWL to 50–60 ml/100 calories
Excessive sweating	Increase H_2O by 10–25 ml/100 calories

IWL = insensible water loss.

    (1) Respiratory (humidification of exhaled air) = 15 percent.
    (2) Skin (evaporation, not sweat) = 30 percent.
    (3) Feces = 5 percent.
  b. Urine losses account for the other 50 percent of fluid loss. Actual urine volume depends mainly on the level of hydration, but a minimal obligatory urine volume is required to dissolve excreted metabolic waste products and electrolytes.
  c. Intrinsic fluid sources. The water of oxidation is water gained as a by-product of normal metabolism; it can replace about 15 percent of the usual fluid losses. This is normally considered when estimating maintenance fluid requirements (i.e., maintenance fluid requirement = insensible losses + urine losses − intrinsic fluid sources).
3. Methods of estimating maintenance fluids
  a. Surface area. Levels of renal function and body fluid requirements correlate best with body surface area (BSA). Hence, the unit of measurement used is the square meter (m^2), and water needs are expressed as ml/m^2/24 hr. This system works well for children **weighing more than 10 kg** and has the advantage that a single formula can be used for all ages. The normal water requirement is about 1,500 ml/m^2/24 hr (Table 7-5).
  b. Calories expended. This method computes water requirements from metabolic expenditure. Figure 7-2 depicts energy use as a function of

Table 7-5. Fluid balance in children

Losses	
Respiratory and skin	775 ml/m^2/24 hr[a]
Gastrointestinal	100 ml/m^2/24 hr
Urine	875 ml/m^2/24 hr[b]
Total	1,750
Sources	
Water of oxidation	250 ml/m^2/24 hr
Net maintenance requirement	
Water	1,500 ml/m^2/24 hr

[a] Varies with size of child; e.g., 1,200 ml/m^2 in a toddler versus 700 ml/m^2 at age 8–10 years.
[b] Based on excretion of isotonic urine, 300 mOsm/liter, and minimal solute intake, e.g., dextrose in water.

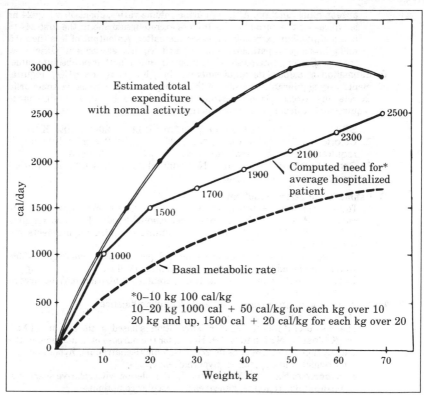

Fig. 7-2. Comparison of energy expenditure in basal and ideal state. (Reproduced with permission from W. E. Segar, Parenteral fluid therapy, *Curr. Probl. Pediatr.* 3(2):4, 1972. Copyright © 1972 by Year Book Medical Publishers, Inc., Chicago.)

weight. To calculate fluid requirement, one allows 100–150 ml/100 calories metabolized.

c. **Body weight**

(1) General rule is

100 ml/kg for the **first** 10 kg body weight
50 ml/kg for the **next** 10 kg body weight
20 ml/kg for the weights **above** 20 kg

Example: A 25-kg child would require:

100 ml/kg × 10 kg =	1,000 ml for first	10 kg
50 ml/kg × 10 kg =	500 ml for next	10 kg
20 ml/kg × 5 kg =	100 ml for last	5 kg
Total	1,600 ml	25 kg

(2) The main advantage of this method is that it is easy to remember and calculate.

d. **Allowances for unusual maintenance requirements.** Changes in normal maintenance requirements are affected by several conditions, shown in Table 7-4.

4. **The fluid needs of the newborn** (see Chap. 6)

5. **Urine output** accurately reflects both circulatory status and adequacy of hydration. Unless severe oliguria is present, **urine output cannot be used to**

assess renal function. Although urine volume varies, about 50 ml/kg/24 hr is typical for the normal child. Infants excrete less urine in the first 24–48 hours of life, but excretion increases thereafter. An output of less than 0.5 ml/kg/hr suggests pathologic oliguria and requires assessment. Otherwise, the reporting of relative rate of urine output (ml/kg/hr) has no absolute value.
B. **Estimation of electrolyte requirements.** Na^+, K^+, Cl^-, and HCO_3^- requirements vary significantly because of the kidney's ability to conserve them or to excrete any excess. General estimates of Na^+ and K^+ daily maintenance requirements calculated by three methods follow.

1. **BSA**	20–50 mEq Na^+/m^2 BSA	20–50 mEq K^+/m^2
2. **Caloric**	2–4 mEq $Na^+/100$	2–3 mEq $K^+/100$
requirement	calories	calories
3. **General method**	2–4 mEq $Na^+/100$ ml	2–4 mEq $K^+/100$ ml
(body weight)	fluid	fluid

C. **Estimation of caloric requirements**
  1. To reduce protein catabolism and avoid ketosis, 75–100 gm glucose/m^2/day is required. However, this will **not meet caloric needs.** To do so requires 1,200–1,500 calories/m^2/24 hr, not accounting for extra requirements imposed by illness.
  2. Dextrose solutions (5–10%) are tolerated peripherally, whereas 15–30% glucose can be administered through a central IV line.
  3. To provide high caloric content, total parenteral nutrition may be needed (see Chap. 10, p. 269).
III. **Assessment of abnormalities of fluid and electrolyte balance**
A. **General comments**
  1. The most useful way to consider dehydration is based on the amount of **Na^+** and **K^+ lost in relation to water.** Hence, for the purpose of management, the dehydration states are considered as isotonic (isonatremic), hypotonic (hyponatremic), and hypertonic (hypernatremic).
    a. **Hypotonic.** $Na^+ < 125$ mEq/liter; ECF depletion with relative sparing of intracellular ions; hence, early vascular compromise.
    b. **Isotonic.** $Na^+ = 130$–150 mEq/liter; balanced loss of water and ions
    c. **Hypertonic.** $Na^+ > 150$ mEq/liter; ICF depletion; allows more chronic dehydration; the vascular space is relatively protected.
  2. The best indicator of **short-term quantitative fluid loss** is change in body weight. Table 7-6 presents a rough clinical estimate of signs and degree of dehydration.
  3. **Role of solute load**
    a. In understanding dehydration states, it is important to consider the contribution of **intake** in producing a negative balance as well as the role played by **output** via diarrhea or vomiting.

Table 7-6. Estimation of dehydration

	Degree of dehydration		
Clinical signs	Mild	Moderate	Severe
Weight loss (%)	5	10	15
Behavior	Normal	Irritable	Hyperirritable to lethargic
Thirst	Slight	Moderate	Intense
Mucous membrane	May be normal	Dry	Parched
Tears	Present	±	Absent
Anterior fontanel	Flat	±	Sunken
Skin turgor	Normal	±	Increased

     b. Renal solute load hastens dehydration by causing obligatory urinary free-water loss in the infant who is struggling to excrete an ingested solute load. This means that *the solute stress of a given feeding is different from the formula's measured osmotic load.*

     c. Because infants cannot effectively concentrate urine much beyond 600 mOsm/kg, cow's milk causes free-water losses **three times greater** than those of human milk, while boiled skim milk imposes a fourfold free-water loss. Thus, to avoid hypertonic dehydration, **renal solute load should be minimized in infants with fluid losses.**

  4. Initial assessment of the dehydrated child should include the following:

     a. History. Urine output, weight change, infectious disease contacts, and estimate of stooling or vomiting frequency

     b. Clinical. Urine output, skin turgor, mucous membrane moisture, eye turgor, fullness of fontanel, and mental state

     c. Laboratory. Weight, complete blood count (CBC), serum and urine Na^+, K^+, Cl^-, pH, TCO_2, blood urea nitrogen (BUN), creatinine, osmolality, glucose, and calcium; **urinalysis** and appropriate cultures

  5. Urinalysis is particularly important. The **specific gravity** should be well above 1.015 unless intrinsic renal disease is contributing to the problem. **Ketonuria** often accompanies dehydration without diabetes. Trace or 1+ **protein** can be present, along with cellular debris and a few hyaline casts. However, a very active sediment signals underlying primary renal disease. **Alkaline urine** should raise the question of renal tubular acidosis.

  6. Water and electrolyte losses. Estimates of deficits in moderate to severe dehydration are given in Table 7-7.

B. Assessment of Na^+ and K^+ losses

  1. General. There is no practical means of assessing true K^+ loss; serum K^+ does not accurately reflect total body K^+ stores (see sec. **I.C.2.b**). Nonetheless, one can assume in most instances that K^+ losses are equivalent to Na^+ losses.

  2. Estimations of Na^+ and K^+ deficits in a child who appears severely dehydrated and in whom the serum Na^+ is known can be made using Table 7-7.

  3. Calculation of Na^+ deficit is based on the current (dehydrated) serum Na^+ concentration, the desired "normal" serum Na^+ concentration (usually 135 mEq/liter), and the volume of distribution of Na^+, the TBW (see sec. **I.C.1**). The assumption on which the calculations are based is that Na^+ is the **sole** cation used for rehydration. This is a prudent assumption, since rehydration preferentially should preserve the ECF (and thus the vascular space) over the ICF. In practice these calculations actually provide the deficits of total cations (Na^+ and K^+). This should be remembered when both Na^+ and K^+ are provided in the solutions used for rehydration. The total body Na^+ deficit ($TBNa_d^+$) is the difference between the normal total body Na^+ ($TBNa_n^+$) and the current (dehydrated) total body Na^+ ($TBNa_c^+$).

Table 7-7. Deficits in moderate to severe dehydration

Type of dehydration	Range of Na^+ (mEq/liter)	Water (ml/kg)	Na^+ (mEq/kg)	K^+ (mEq/kg)	$Cl^- + HCO_3^-$ (mEq/kg)
			Losses		
Isotonic	130–145	100–150	7–11	7–11	14–22
Hypotonic	< 125	40–80	10–14	10–14	20–28
Hypertonic	> 150	120–170	2–5	2–5	4–10

Source: Modified from R. W. Winters, *Principles of Pediatric Fluid Therapy.* North Chicago, IL: Abbott Laboratories, 1970. P. 56.

$$TBNa_d^+ = TBNa_n^+ - TBNa_c^+$$

Thus, $TBNa_d^+ = (TBW \times 135) - [(TBW - FL) \times NA_c^+]$

or $TBNa_d^+ = TBW(135 - Na_c^+) + FL\,(NA_c^+)$

where $TBW = 0.6 \times$ normal weight, FL = the fluid loss (or equivalent of weight change), and Na_c^+ = the current serum sodium concentration (mEq/liter).

C. **Ongoing losses**
   1. **General.** *Ongoing losses* are **abnormal** losses of fluids or electrolytes, or both, that occur while the patient is under observation. The losses may be continuous or sporadic, and while the changes in renal output can often accommodate small ongoing losses, appropriate management dictates that the losses be replaced in an orderly fashion.
   2. **Estimation of ongoing losses**
      a. **Fluid.** Abnormal losses (nasogastric suction, surgical drainage, vomitus) usually can be measured directly.
         (1) In the absence of direct measurement, **weight changes** can be used to determine fluid losses. Daily changes in weight can be assumed to reflect losses or gains of TBW.
         (2) Patients receiving maintenance fluids and calories should remain at a constant weight.
         (3) Patients receiving maintenance fluids, but insufficient calories, should lose about 0.5 percent of their weight per day. This weight loss accounts for the body fat stores metabolized to H_2O and other by-products.
         (4) Newborn infants should lose weight over the first 3–5 days of life and subsequently gain weight consistent with the usual growth curves (approximately 30 gm/day for full-term infants) if given sufficient nutrition.
      b. **Electrolytes**
         (1) The electrolyte content of abnormal body fluid losses frequently can be **measured directly.** This is particularly important for **abnormal** urine losses, since the composition can vary widely.
         (2) The usual composition of body fluids is shown in Table 7-8.
         (3) The gastric Na^+ content will vary directly with the pH of gastric fluid. Above pH 2.0 ($H^+ = 0.01$ molar or 10 mEq/liter), the Na^+ content of the gastric fluid may be 100 mEq/liter or higher. If gastric fluid losses are large, direct measurement of electrolyte concentrations is mandatory for accurate replacement.

Table 7-8. Composition of body fluids

Source	Na^+ (mEq/liter)	K^+ (mEq/liter)	Cl^- (mEq/liter)	HCO_3^- (mEq/liter)	pH	Osm (mOsm/liter)
Gastric	50	10–15	150	0	1	300
Pancreas	140	5	50–100	100	9	300
Bile	130	5	100	40	8	300
Ileostomy	130	15–20	120	25–30	8	300
Diarrhea	50	35	40	50	Alk	
Sweat	50	5	55	0		
Blood	140	4–5	100	25	7.4	285–295
Urine	0–100*	20–100*	70–100*	0	4.5–8.5	50–1,400

* Varies considerably with intake.

3. **Strategy for replacement of ongoing losses**
   a. Generally, ongoing losses of fluids and electrolytes are measured or calculated over fixed time periods and replaced evenly over an equivalent period of time.
   (1) If there are **large** ongoing losses, these periods should be **short** (e.g., every half hour or hour).
   (2) If losses are small, adjustment can be made daily.
   b. **Patients without deficits at the initiation of therapy**
   (1) The therapy is designed to provide **maintenance** fluid and electrolytes and to replace the **ongoing** losses.
   (2) If there are unusual urine losses or if the urine output is erratic, therapy is designed to provide **insensible** fluid losses plus urine and ongoing losses.
   c. **Patients who are dehydrated at the initiation of therapy** (e.g., vomiting or diarrhea)
   (1) The measured or extenuated *ongoing* losses are **added to** the calculated replacement of maintenance and deficit fluid and electrolytes. Adjustments should be made **frequently.** *Urine losses are ignored, since they are accounted for in the maintenance calculations.*
   (2) It is important **not** to recalculate the overall deficits in rehydrating a dehydrated patient with ongoing losses; this usually leads to an **underestimation** of true deficits. **Add** ongoing losses to previously estimated deficits.
   d. When providing replacement for large or unusual ongoing losses, periodically monitor and reassess the patient's condition (see sec. **V**).

IV. **Correction of abnormalities of fluid and electrolyte balance**
   A. **Acute fluid management and resuscitation: general concepts** (see also Chap. 3)
   1. Weigh the patient.
   2. If shock is present, or if no urine is produced in the first half hour, give 20–30 ml/kg Ringer's lactate or normal saline with 5% dextrose (D5NS) or 5% albumin IV until adequate circulation returns.
   3. After the first hour, give 10 ml/kg/hr Ringer's lactate or D5NS until shock is alleviated and actual fluid and electrolyte deficits can be accurately calculated.
   4. If the patient is asymptomatic and/or dehydration is hyponatremic or isotonic, one half the fluids calculated for 24 hours should be administered in the first 8 hours. The remaining half should be given in the remaining 16 hours.
   5. If hypertonic dehydration is present after correcting shock, correct the deficit **slowly and evenly** over 48 hours.
   6. Temperature will affect total maintenance needs; with **fever**, add 12 percent of the maintenance amount per degrees centigrade (see Table 7-4).
   7. In most situations, **do not add K⁺ to the IV solutions until after the patient has voided.** If the patient has hemolytic-uremic syndrome or acute tubular necrosis, IV K⁺ may lead to severe hyperkalemia.
   8. In **diabetic ketoacidosis**, however, **K⁺ can be added** to the initial solution, since rapid correction of dehydration, acidosis, and hyperglycemia may precipitate severe hypoglycemia and hypokalemia (see Chap. 13, p. 352).
   9. **Adequacy of therapy** is indicated by adequate urine output (see sec. **II.A.5**), normal circulation, and restoration of weight.
   B. **Hypotonic dehydration.** In this condition the fluid loss comes mainly from the *IVF* and *ECF* compartments rather than the intracellular reservoir. Circulatory compromise appears early, and there is marked loss of turgor. Patients arrive at this state when marked enteric losses are replaced with low-solute fluids (e.g., fruit juice, Coca-Cola).
   1. **Clinically,** infants present soon after the onset of illness because **symptoms** become apparent early. For a given weight loss, the clinical signs are more marked than in isotonic or hypertonic dehydration. Thus, estimates of weight loss should follow a 3, 6, 9 percent rule of thumb for mild, moderate,

and severe, respectively. Seizures occur infrequently, even with marked hyponatremia, but generalized lethargy is common, and **vascular collapse can occur early.**

2. **General principles of treatment**
   a. Because loss is mainly ECF, replacement therapy can advance rapidly, with volume and Na^+ restored by the end of 24–36 hours.
   b. Calculate or estimate the total deficits of fluid and electrolytes and add the maintenance requirement. Subtract the amount given during the initial resuscitation period. The result is the remaining deficit and maintenance to be provided in the first day.
   c. If the patient is asymptomatic and dehydration is hypotonic or isotonic, one half of the remaining deficit and maintenance fluids and electrolytes should be administered in the next 8 hours and the other half over the subsequent 16 hours.

C. **Symptomatic hyponatremia.** Regardless of the cause, whether Na^+ loss or water excess, therapy is directed at raising the Na^+ concentration **quickly,** to stop symptoms.

1. Use *hypertonic* saline (3% = 513 mEq Na^+/liter) to deliver approximately 5 mEq/kg/hr. Calculation of the approximate Na^+ deficit is given in sec. **III.B.3.**
2. Symptomatic hyponatremia may be seen with a serum Na^+ concentration of 130 mEq/liter *if* the change in concentration has been sudden. Thus, the patient's symptoms, if any, must be taken into account to determine the speed of correction of the serum Na^+ concentration.
3. The following is a **sample calculation** for a 10-kg child with no volume deficit but with serum Na^+ of 120 mEq who manifests irritability and diminished consciousness:
   a. 10 kg × 0.6 × (15 mEq deficit) = 90 mEq (total Na^+ deficit = 90 mEq)
   b. To raise Na^+ 5 mEq/liter acutely requires 5 mEq × 0.6 × 10 kg = 30 mEq:

$$\text{Dose of 3\% NaCl} = \frac{30 \text{ mEq Na}^+}{0.513 \text{ mEq Na}^+/\text{ml}} = 60 \text{ ml}$$

$$\text{Dose of 5\% NaCl} = \frac{30 \text{ mEq Na}^+}{0.856 \text{ mEq Na}^+/\text{ml}} = 35 \text{ ml}$$

Following acute correction, *the patient's acidosis may worsen.* Sodium bicarbonate (1 mEq/ml) can be mixed with the hypertonic saline to supply some of the Na^+ dose while also providing bicarbonate as the anion.

D. The therapy of **asymptomatic hyponatremia** requires *gradual* correction of the Na^+ deficit in increments of 10 mEq/liter.

1. The following is a **sample calculation** for a 10-kg child with 10 percent dehydration and a serum Na^+ of 125 mEq/liter:
   a. Volume deficit = 10% × 10 kg = 1.0 liter
   b. Volume maintenance = 100 ml/kg × 10 kg = 1.0 liter; total = 2.0 liters
   c. Deficit Na^+ can be calculated in two ways:
      (1) Based on calculations of the total body Na^+ (see sec. **III.B.3**),

$$
\begin{aligned}
\text{TBNa}_d^+ &= \text{TBNa}_n^+ - \text{TBNa}_c^+ \\
&= (\text{Na}_n^+ \times \text{TBW}) - [(\text{TBW} - \text{FL}) \times \text{Na}_c] \\
&= [135 \times (10 \times 0.6)] - (5 \times 125) \\
&= 184 \text{ mEq}
\end{aligned}
$$

      (2) Based on the analysis that the Na^+ deficit consists of two components, an isotonic loss and an extra Na^+ loss,

$$
\begin{aligned}
\text{Isotonic loss} &= (\text{TBW}_n - \text{TBW}_c) \times \text{Na}_c^+ \\
&= [(10 \text{ kg} \times 0.6) - 1 \text{ liter}] \times 125 \text{ mEq} \\
&= 125 \text{ mEq}
\end{aligned}
$$

$$\text{Extra Na}^+ \text{ loss} = \text{TBW}_n \times (\text{Na}_n{}^+ - \text{Na}_c{}^+)$$
$$= (10 \text{ kg} \times 0.6) \times (135 - 125)$$
$$= 60 \text{ mEq}$$

The total deficit Na^+ is, therefore, 185 mEq.

d. Maintenance $\text{Na}^+ = 3 \text{ mEq/kg} \times 10 \text{ kg} = 30 \text{ mEq Na}^+$

Thus, $\dfrac{\text{total Na needed} = 215 \text{ mEq}}{2.0 \text{ liters (total volume deficit)}} = \dfrac{108 \text{ mEq Na}^+}{1.0 \text{ liter}} = \text{¾ normal saline}$

2. Administer one half of the total fluid in the first 8 hours and the rest over the remaining 16 hours.

E. K^+ **deficit** and **acidosis** both require specific therapy for correction. Hemoconcentration and prerenal azotemia will resolve with restoration of fluids.

F. Isotonic dehydration. Children with enteric losses, taking an intermediate solute load (e.g., breast milk), arrive at a balanced dehydration. The deficit is lost only from the ECF since the net fluid loss is isotonic. For a given weight loss, symptoms will be less dramatic than for hypotonic dehydration—assume a weight loss of 5, 10, or 15 percent for clinical estimation of mild, moderate, and severe involvement, respectively.

Treatment is similar to that for hypotonic dehydration (see **B.2**). However, a slower tempo in completing deficit repair is acceptable. Aim to restore about two thirds of the total estimated volume deficit during the first day. During day 2, the emphasis should be on restoring both K^+ deficit and acid-base balance.

1. After acute therapy, supply **maintenance** plus deficit from estimated weight loss.

2. The solutions used are hypotonic, but since the normal kidney needs only ¼ N solution for true maintenance, these ½ N solutions provide sufficient solute even for correction of isotonic losses.

G. Hypertonic dehydration results when inappropriately high solute loads are given as replacement fluid, or when a renal concentrating defect produces a large free-water loss. Usually, hypernatremia represents the principal excess solute, but agents such as glucose, urea, and mannitol can produce the same disturbance.

1. The **clinical presentation** in these infants can be deceptive. Shock is a late manifestation. When it supervenes, one can be certain that fluid loss exceeds 10 percent of body weight.

  a. Skin turgor does not exhibit the usual tenting of advanced dehydration, but has a thick, doughy consistency.

  b. Other findings include a shrill cry or mewling sound, muscle weakness, tachypnea, and intense thirst in toddlers.

  c. In assessing these infants, be sure to check *serum glucose* and *calcium,* since **hyperglycemia** is present in half the patients, and **calcium deficiency** has been noted in 10 percent.

2. Treatment. The total fluid deficit must be replaced **slowly** over 48 hours or more, dropping serum Na^+ by 10 mEq/liter/day. **Rapid correction floods the intracellular space with fluid, leading to cerebral (and sometimes pulmonary) edema.** In general, *the more dilute the solution being used to correct the deficit, the slower it should be infused.*

  a. If shock is present, infuse 20 ml/kg of 0.9% saline over 20–30 minutes.

  b. First hour. The goal is to reestablish satisfactory circulation and urine flow. Give 10–20 ml/kg Ringer's lactate to reduce the Cl^- load in favor of lactate (alkali).

  c. Over the next 4 hours, the goal is to ensure urine output and reduce the serum Na^+. There is no **best** regimen.

   (1) The rate of IV infusion is determined by the tonicity of the solution; i.e., isotonic solutions can be infused more rapidly.

   (2) Infuse 10 ml/kg/hr of 5% D in Ringer's lactate, Ringer's lactate, or a mixture of 2% dextrose and $\frac{1}{2}$ N saline to which is added $\frac{1}{4}$ N bicarbonate (17 ml of 8% $NaHCO_3$/500 ml solution), depending on the degree of acidosis or hyperglycemia.

(3) This should establish a steady urine flow, which then permits addition of potassium to the infusion.

d. **The next 48 hours** are utilized to replenish the volume lost; infusion should proceed at a steady rate, based on calculated deficits. The serum Na^+ should decrease by about 0.5 mEq/hr.

Calculation of water deficit:

Water deficit (liters) = usual body water − current body water

$$\text{Usual body water} = \text{current body water} \times \frac{\text{current Osm}}{\text{normal Osm}}$$

Current body water = current weight × 0.6

Example: For a dehydrated child who currently weighs 10 kg and whose serum Osm = 340 (Na^+ = 160):

$$\text{Water deficit} = 10 \text{ kg} \times 0.6 \text{ liters/kg} \times \frac{340}{290} - (10 \text{ kg} \times 0.6 \text{ liters/kg})$$
$$= 7 \text{ liters} - 6 \text{ liters}$$
$$= 1 \text{ liter}$$

(1) Children with hypernatremic dehydration are usually **not** significantly deficient in Na^+. **Do not try to correct the water deficit rapidly with Na^+ (normal saline or greater) solutions,** because it may lead to severe Na^+ overload and possibly to an increased serum Na^+ concentration.

(2) **Do not allow the IV infusion to run rapidly,** because there is grave danger of CNS damage from acute osmotic shifts if fluid flow is unchecked.

(3) It is unwise to attempt rapid control of **hyperglycemia;** the presence of extra glucose acts as an "osmotic buffer" under whose cover the necessary ion shifts can occur as reequilibration proceeds. Slow sugar metabolism then provides a continuous source of free water delivered at a gentle rate.

(4) **Treatment of acute salt poisoning** requires dialysis or furosemide diuresis (1 mg/kg), replacing the urine output with a 10% dextrose in water (D/W) solution, monitoring Na^+ values q4h and repeating the administration of furosemide.

e. If the serum Na^+ concentration > 180 mEq/liter, **dialysis** may be required to correct the abnormalities. In this case, peritoneal dialysis may be preferable to hemodialysis, since the correction is relatively slow. The peritoneal dialysate can be prepared with a relatively high Na^+ concentration initially (e.g., 165 mEq/liter) and then reduced in a gradual stepwise fashion.

V. Monitoring fluid and electrolyte therapy

A. Since the rationale for provision of maintenance and replacement of deficits and ongoing losses of fluids and electrolytes rests on several estimations and calculations, assess the results of therapy periodically and adjust accordingly.

B. **The usual variables to monitor include:**

1. **Weight.** The patient's weight should be increasing and decreasing as predicted by the calculations of treatment. While it is frequently difficult to obtain accurate weights in sick patients, weight is the single most accurate variable to follow in planning treatment.

2. The **vital signs** indicate the stability of the vascular volume.

3. **Laboratory tests.** Serum electrolytes, osmolality, blood sugar, BUN, creatinine, and urine electrolytes and osmolality

4. Total **inputs** and **outputs** of both fluids and electrolytes

C. A well-conceived **flow sheet** is an efficient means of assessing the adequacy of therapy and making appropriate adjustments for patients with complications.
   1. Equally spaced time intervals are listed along the top of the flow sheet.
   2. The flow sheet should indicate both the interval and overall totals for both fluid and electrolytes.
D. Indicators that may indicate that the ECF (and vascular volume) is being expanded and stabilized include:
   1. Stabilization of vital signs: increased blood pressure and central venous pressure, decreased pulse and respirations
   2. Decreasing hematocrit (in the absence of blood loss)
   3. Improvement of acidosis with improved peripheral perfusion
   4. Decreased BUN and creatinine
   5. Decreased serum osmolarity and K^+
   6. Increased urine output with decreasing urine concentration (decreased urine-specific gravity and osmolarity)
   7. Increased urine Na^+ excretion

Renal Disorders

Lisa Guay-Woodford

I. Proteinuria

A. **Etiology.** Significant proteinuria can occur *with* or *without* intrinsic renal disease.

1. **Mild to moderate proteinuria** (200–500 mg/day) may be seen transiently with fever, dehydration, exercise, cold exposure, hypermetabolic states, heart failure, constrictive pericarditis, or urinary tract infection.

2. **Orthostatic proteinuria** is not associated with serious renal disease or the risk of progressive decline in renal function.

3. **Glomerular diseases** are usually associated with proteinuria. In glomerulonephritis, proteinuria **and** hematuria are typically evident. The degree of proteinuria varies from the mild to the nephrotic range.

   a. **Minimal** proteinuria **with** hematuria suggests a focal nephritis, vascular disease, or infection.

   b. **Massive** proteinuria **with** hematuria suggests significant glomerulopathy (with or without systemic disease), or malignant hypertension. **Without** hematuria, it suggests minimal lesion nephrotic syndrome or membranous nephropathy and is consistent with diabetic nephropathy.

4. **Tubulointerstitial processes** such as tubulointerstitial nephritis or drug toxicity can cause mild to moderate proteinuria.

B. **Evaluation and diagnosis.** In children, protein excretion varies with age and body surface area. Generally, for children less than 10 years old, significant proteinuria is defined as >100 mg/24 hr. Nephrotic range proteinuria is defined as >1 gm/24 hr and indicates significant glomerular disease. Alternatively, for patients with stable renal function, the **ratio** of protein to creatinine in a spot urine sample can be useful in identifying significant proteinuria. The normal urine protein/creatinine ratio is < 0.2. Nephrotic range proteinuria is indicated by a ratio >3.

1. Note how the sample was collected; look for fever, metabolic stress, etc., which might cause proteinuria. Check the urine on two more occasions to confirm the presence of proteinuria.

2. Look for orthostatic (postural) proteinuria: Check AM and PM urines with a dipstick; AM should be negative. Obtain 12-hour daytime (active) urine and 12-hour nighttime (recumbent) urine collections. The recumbent urine collection should have **completely normal** protein excretion.

3. **Urinalysis** and **culture** are necessary. If proteinuria is detected in the context of a urinary tract infection, recheck the urine 1–2 weeks after completion of an appropriate antibiotic course.

4. Persistent, constant proteinuria may require referral to a nephrologist for further evaluation and possible renal biopsy.

C. **Treatment.** No therapy is needed for orthostatic proteinuria. The treatment of proteinuria due to other causes depends on the diagnosis (Fig. 8-1).

II. Nephrotic syndrome.

The nephrotic syndrome is characterized by massive proteinuria, edema, hypoalbuminemia (albumin ≤ 2.5 mg/dl), and hyperlipidemia. The nephrotic syndrome occurs in 2–3 in 100,000 children (<16 years of age) per year. The peak incidence is between 2 and 4 years (75% of cases occur in children under 5 years of age). Boys are affected slightly more frequently than girls. In children

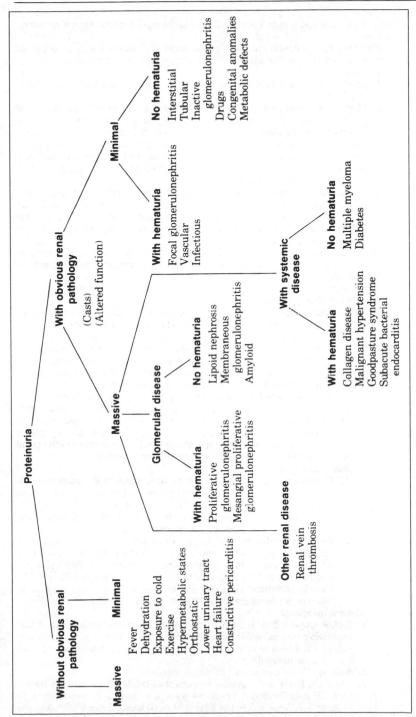

Fig. 8-1. Proteinuria with and without obvious renal pathology.

under 10 years of age, minimal change disease is the most common form of nephrotic syndrome.

A. Etiology. The nephrotic syndrome can occur as an isolated entity or as part of a progressive glomerulonephritis. The pathogenesis remains unclear.

B. Evaluation

1. **History.** A history of antecedent infection with concomitant nephritis is sought.

2. **Physical examination.** A careful assessment should include weight, blood pressure, sites and extent of edema, and respiratory and cardiac status.

3. **Laboratory evaluation** includes quantitative 24-hour urine protein excretion, selective protein index (ratio of immunoglobulin G–transferrin clearances), and 24-hour creatinine clearance. Serum studies should include blood urea nitrogen (BUN) and Cr, electrolytes, lipid profile, and serum protein electrophoresis with C3 and A/G ratio.

4. The presence of gross hematuria, elevated blood pressure, a low C3, non-selective proteinuria (selective protein index > 0.2), age at presentation below 1 year or over 10 years, or failure to respond to corticosteroids suggests diagnoses other than minimal change nephrotic syndrome and a renal biopsy should be performed.

C. Diagnosis. A combination of the defined clinical features with proteinuria in excess of 1 gm/m²/24 hr confirms the diagnosis. **However, all features need not be present,** especially early in relapse.

D. Treatment

1. **Minimal change nephrotic syndrome**

   a. **Corticosteroids** are the treatment of choice, usually 2 mg/kg/day prednisone PO in divided doses (not to exceed maximum dosage/day of 80 mg). This regimen is continued until the urine is protein free for 5–7 days. Following this, a further alternate-day regimen is generally given in a reduced dosage (1.0–1.5 mg/kg/day as one dose q48h) for a month; after that the steroids are tapered over 2–3 weeks and discontinued. Lack of response by 8 weeks suggests corticosteroid resistance.

   b. **Cytotoxic therapy.** Cytotoxic therapy with agents such as cyclophosphamide has been shown to be effective in prolonging remission in patients who are frequent "relapsers" and require multiple or prolonged courses of prednisone; it appears less effective in those who show no response to corticosteroids. **Cytotoxic therapy should only be undertaken after renal biopsy and consultation with a pediatric nephrologist.**

   c. **Diuretics and albumin**

      (1) **The use of a diuretic alone can be hazardous in the presence of a low serum albumin,** because this can aggravate existing contraction of the circulating blood volume. However, diuretics can be used alone in patients who have problems with recurrent edema. Consultation with a pediatric nephrologist is recommended.

      (2) When accumulation of edema fluid is severe, i.e., marked ascites or scrotal edema, or when the nephrotic patient has a concomitant infection, diuresis can be prompted by administration of 25% albumin in a dose of 0.5–1.0 gm/kg IV slowly q12h, followed by IV furosemide, 1 mg/kg. **Caution:** Too-rapid administration of albumin may cause pulmonary edema and congestive heart failure (CHF).

2. **General measures**

   a. **Diet.** A low-salt diet (1–2 gm/m²) is advised for edematous patients. Fluid restriction may be self-imposed if salt is restricted. For very edematous patients, fluid can be restricted to insensible losses plus urine output until remission is induced.

   b. **Activity.** No restriction of activity is required.

   c. **Infection.** Early and vigorous treatment of **bacterial** infection is important. Of note, bacterial infections were the leading cause of death in nephrotic patients before the advent of antibiotics. Since **viral** infections can lead to relapse, the urine should be monitored closely during such infections. *Nonimmune patients who are exposed to varicella while receiving high-dose steroids should receive prompt administration of zoster immune globulin.*

   d. Instruction of family. Parents and child should be well informed about nephrosis and should be taught to test urine for albumin with dipsticks. A written diary of urine protein should be kept.

 E. Prognosis

   1. In minimal change nephrotic syndrome, 80–90 percent of children show an initial response to corticosteroids. Of these, 80 percent will have further relapses.

   2. The rate of relapse in a group of children tends to decrease after the first 10 years. A child who remains relapse free for up to 3–4 years has a 95 percent chance of remaining in remission thereafter. However, after one relapse, the subsequent course cannot be predicted, and the number of relapses per se does not affect the ultimate outcome.

III. Hematuria. Normal children excrete 200,000–500,000 red blood cells every 24 hours through the urinary system. Based on average urinary volumes, hematuria is defined as the presence of more than five red blood cells per high-power microscopic field on at least two properly performed urinalyses. While it is sensitive, the urine dipstick test has a high false-positive rate. Thus, red urine or a positive urine dipstick test, or both, mandate microscopic examination of the urine.

 A. Etiology

   1. More than five red blood cells per high-power field may be caused by any lesion from the renal artery to the tip of the urethra. In addition, high fever and vigorous exercise can cause a transient, benign increase in red cell excretion rate.

   2. Positive dipstick in the absence of red cells on microscopic examination suggests free hemoglobinuria or myoglobinuria (Table 8-1). Both pigments, hemoglobin and myoglobin, may be associated with nephrotoxicity, and full evaluation, with attempts at forced diuresis and urine alkalinization, should proceed.

 B. Evaluation should include a complete history, physical examination, and baseline laboratory profile.

   1. History. Any possible precipitating event is noted.

   a. Particular attention is focused on possible antecedent streptococcal infection, symptoms of cystitis, or renal colic.

   b. The **past medical history** focuses on hemoglobinopathies or any previous hemorrhagic tendencies and details of any drug or travel history.

   c. Any **family history** of hematuria, renal disease, renal failure, collagen vascular diseases, or deafness is delineated.

   d. A **review of systems** includes recent rashes, arthralgias, arthritis, and abdominal pain, and notes fevers, malaise, anorexia, weight loss, exercise pattern, and trauma.

Table 8-1. Hemoglobinuria versus myoglobinuria

Observation	Myoglobinuria	Hemoglobinuria
Color of serum	Clear	Pink
Level of serum haptoglobin	Normal	Decreased
Mix urine with 80% $(NH_4)\ S_2O_4$ and filter	Pink	Clear
Muscle tenderness and elevated serum creatinine-phosphokinase	Present	Absent
Clinical setting	Crush injuries, trauma, infection, rhabdomyolysis	Transfusion, disseminated intravascular coagulation

2. A thorough **physical examination** is required, with careful attention to height, weight, blood pressure, rashes, and edema. Anomalous features on abdominal or perineal examination are noted.

3. **Baseline laboratory profile.** Basic laboratory tests include a urinalysis with complete microscopic examination, urine culture, complete blood count (CBC), erythrocyte sedimentation rate, platelet count, prothrombin time, partial thromboplastin time, and a purified protein derivative (PPD) skin test for tuberculosis.

C. **Differential diagnosis** (Fig. 8-2). The baseline investigations may provide the diagnosis **without further evaluation.** If not, the causes of hematuria can be separated into the following categories: **asymptomatic microscopic hematuria, symptomatic microscopic hematuria, and gross hematuria.** Table 8-2 shows ways of distinguishing renal from nonrenal hematuria. For discussion of hematuria associated with primary glomerular diseases or with serious underlying systemic disease, see sec. **IV.**

1. **Etiology can be suggested by baseline evaluation.**
   a. An abdominal mass with hematuria requires exclusion of **Wilms' tumor, cystic kidney disease,** or **hydronephrosis.**
   b. Perineal excoriation or meatal inflammation implicates **local factors.**
   c. Hematuria occurs in association with **sickle cell trait** and S-C **hemoglobin.**
   d. A family history of asymptomatic hematuria suggests **benign familial hematuria,** whereas a family history of hematuria, deafness, and renal insufficiency suggests **Alport's hereditary nephritis.**
   e. Hematuria with casts and proteinuria can occur in the critically ill child with **acute tubular necrosis (ATN), renal infarction, renal cortical necrosis,** or **renal vein thrombosis** (see sec. **X**).
   f. Multiple telangiectasias and characteristic mucous membrane lesions indicate **hereditary hemorrhagic telangiectasia** (Rendu-Osler-Weber disease).

2. **Asymptomatic hematuria**
   a. **Glomerulonephritis** should be the first consideration in asymptomatic hematuria (see sec. **IV**).
   b. In **subacute bacterial endocarditis** and **neurologic shunt infection,** hematuria is immunologically mediated and represents focal areas of glomerulonephritis.
   c. Family members should be screened with urinalyses to rule out **benign familial hematuria,** which is inherited as an autosomal dominant trait.
   d. **Extraglomerular hematuria** may be asymptomatic; anatomic lesions can be detected by an intravenous pyelogram (IVP) or renal ultrasound. **Hypercalciuria** may be associated with microhematuria. **Milk allergy** may be associated with hematuria.
   e. In a large group of patients, asymptomatic microscopic hematuria may persist without serologic or radiologic abnormalities. Follow-up of such children with **idiopathic hematuria** has shown no deterioration in renal function. Such patients should be followed closely, with periodic examinations and urinalyses. During the follow-up period, the appearance of proteinuria, active urinary sediment with casts, deterioration in renal function, or development of hypertension suggests the need for a renal biopsy.

3. **Symptomatic hematuria**
   a. A clinical picture of **cystitis** accompanied by hematuria, mild proteinuria (trace to 1+ unless hematuria is gross), and leukocyturia suggests bacterial, viral, or traumatic involvement of the bladder or lower urinary tract. A **Gram stain** of the unspun urine and culture should be done. When bacterial infection is documented, **a voiding cystourethrogram** and either a renal ultrasound or an IVP are performed 4–6 weeks following successful antimicrobial therapy (see Chap. 14, p. 413).
   b. Culture-negative cystitis may be secondary to **viral infection.** Adenovi-

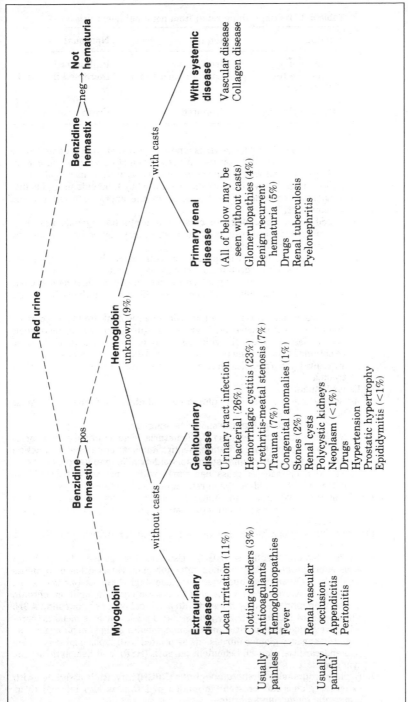

Red urine

Benzidine hemastix > pos

Benzidine hemastix > neg → **Not hematuria**

Myoglobin

Hemoglobin unknown (9%)

without casts

with casts

Extraurinary disease

Local irritation (11%)

Usually painless { Clotting disorders (3%)
Anticoagulants
Hemoglobinopathies
Fever

Usually painful { Renal vascular occlusion
Appendicitis
Peritonitis

Genitourinary disease

Urinary tract infection bacterial (26%)
Hemorrhagic cystitis (23%)
Urethritis-meatal stenosis (7%)
Trauma (7%)
Congenital anomalies (1%)
Stones (2%)
Renal cysts
Polycystic kidneys
Neoplasm (<1%)
Drugs
Hypertension
Prostatic hypertrophy
Epididymitis (<1%)

Primary renal disease

(All of below may be seen without casts)
Glomerulopathies (4%)
Benign recurrent hematuria (5%)
Drugs
Renal tuberculosis
Pyelonephritis

With systemic disease

Vascular disease
Collagen disease

Fig. 8-2. Differential diagnosis of red urine. The percentages indicate the frequency of the category in an unselected population of pediatric patients.

Table 8-2. Distinguishing renal from nonrenal hematuria

Finding	Renal	Nonrenal
Urine color	Brown, smoky	Pink or red
Three-tube test	Same in each tube	Increased in 1 or 3
RBC casts	±	−
Clots	−	±
RBC morphology	Crenated	Fresh

ruses 11 and 21, influenza virus, and a papovavirus-like organism have been implicated. Viral cystitis with resolution of hematuria and normal findings on urinalysis at follow-up requires no further investigation.

    c. Culture-negative cystitis may also be caused by **tuberculosis and schistosomiasis** and should be suspected in the appropriate clinical and endemic settings.

    d. In addition to **gonococcal** or **chlamydial urethritis,** vigorous masturbation and mechanical trauma to the urethra may also cause symptomatic hematuria with urethritis.

    e. In younger children with apparent cystitis, particularly girls aged 2–6, urethral or vaginal **foreign bodies** may be present.

    f. Hematuria accompanied by moderate to severe abdominal pain is characteristic of **nephrolithiasis.** True renal colic is rare in the pediatric age group.

    g. Microscopic hematuria following abdominal or flank **trauma** is common and often benign. However, if gross hematuria occurs or if microscopic hematuria is detected following seemingly minor trauma, an IVP should be obtained to determine the extent of renal damage as well as to identify structural abnormalities that might predispose to bleeding with minor trauma.

  4. Gross hematuria

    a. Both acute and recurrent **glomerulonephritis** can present with gross hematuria.

    b. Evidence for **coagulopathy** should be sought.

    c. Nonglomerular causes of gross hematuria include: **urinary tract infection, trauma, perineal irritation, nephrolithiases; ureteropelvic junction (UPJ) obstruction, meatal stenosis, epididymitis, and tumor.**

    d. Repeated episodes of gross hematuria with a normal IVP should be followed with a voiding cystourethrogram and cystoscopy.

IV. Glomerulonephritis. When asymptomatic hematuria occurs in the context of hypertension, active urinary sediment with casts, or proteinuria, glomerulonephritis should be suspected.

  A. Etiology. Glomerulopathies can be divided into acute, rapidly progressive, and chronic processes.

    1. Acute glomerulonephritis (AGN). Usually, the patient has had an **antecedent group A streptococcal infection** manifest as either pharyngitis or cellulitis. **Other infectious agents** include staphylococcus, pneumococcus, influenza A, Epstein-Barr virus, and Coxsackie virus. In addition, **chronic glomerulonephritides may present with a clinical picture suggesting AGN.** These entities include primary glomerular diseases such as membranoproliferative glomerulonephritis and immunoglobulin A (IgA) nephropathy, as well as secondary glomerular lesions associated with lupus nephritis, infective endocarditis, Henoch-Schönlein purpura (HSP), and hemolytic-uremic syndrome (HUS).

    2. Rapidly progressive glomerulonephritis (RPGN) is typically associated with extensive glomerular crescent formation and thus is also referred to as **crescentic glomerulonephritis.**

      a. RPGN can occur as an idiopathic process associated with deposition of antiglomerular basement membrane (anti-GBM) antibodies (Goodpasture's disease) or immune complexes. In RPGN with neither finding, circulating antineutrophil cytoplasmic antibody (ANCA) may be detectable.

   b. Diffuse crescent formation can be superimposed on other primary glomerular diseases such as membranoproliferative glomerulonephritis and IgA nephropathy.

   c. RPGN can be associated with glomerular lesions that are secondary either to infectious processes (poststreptococcal glomerulonephritis, infective endocarditis, hepatitis) or to systemic processes, such as lupus, HSP, and vasculitis.

   3. Chronic glomerulonephritis should be considered in patients with persistent microscopic hematuria, particularly in the context of hypertension, active urinary sediment with casts, or proteinuria.

B. Evaluation

   1. A thorough physical examination is required, with careful attention to height, weight, blood pressure, rashes, joint involvement, and edema. The patient's respiratory and cardiac status should also be carefully assessed.

   2. Laboratory evaluation should include BUN and serum creatinine, antistreptolysin O (ASLO) titer, anti-deoxyribonuclease (DNase) B titer or streptozyme profile, and serum protein electrophoresis with complement levels. An antinuclear antibody (ANA) test should be performed to delineate the subgroup with lupus nephritis. Renal biopsy is usually indicated to identify the histopathologic lesion and provide prognostic information.

C. Diagnosis

   1. Acute poststreptococcal glomerulonephritis (APSGN) is suggested by a history of the appropriate antecedent infection, elevations in ASLO titer and anti-DNase B titer, and depression of the C3 level for 4–8 weeks.

   2. Persistent hypocomplementemia suggests membranoproliferative glomerulonephritis, systemic lupus erythematosus (SLE) nephritis, nephritis associated with infective endocarditis, or shunt infection.

   3. Henoch-Schönlein purpura should be readily diagnosed by the typical rash (see Chap. 6). Renal biopsy is reserved for atypical cases.

   4. IgG-IgA mesangial nephropathy (Berger's disease) is characterized by baseline microscopic hematuria and proteinuria punctuated by recurrent episodes of macroscopic hematuria that are typically precipitated by intercurrent respiratory illnesses.

   5. Focal and segmental glomerulosclerosis is suggested by significant proteinuria often in the nephrotic range, a nonselective protein index (>0.2), and failure to respond to corticosteroid treatment.

D. Treatment

   1. For APSGN, the treatment is entirely symptomatic.

      a. Appropriate antibiotics are given to eradicate the streptococcal infection (see Table 14-2).

      b. A 1- to 2-gm salt diet is prescribed until the patient is asymptomatic. Then, a normal diet is resumed. There is no need for protein restriction in the usual case.

      c. Bed rest is maintained until there is clinical improvement. Normal activity is resumed within a few weeks in most instances.

      d. Hypertension (see sec. VI).

   2. Patients with RPGN, chronic glomerulonephritis, or nephritis associated with a systemic disease should be managed in consultation with a pediatric nephrologist.

E. Prognosis

   1. In APSGN, the usual course ends in complete recovery. Up to 5 percent of patients who appear clinically to have acute poststreptococcal glomerulonephritis may have a continuously downhill course and progress to renal insufficiency. Renal biopsy in such patients usually reveals evidence of an underlying chronic glomerular disease. The urine sediment may remain

abnormal for a prolonged period. Proteinuria often resolves before hematuria, which can persist for up to 2–3 years following the illness. However, even these patients make a complete recovery.

2. **Membranoproliferative glomerulonephritis, focal and segmental glomerulosclerosis, and IgA nephropathy** are chronic renal diseases. They are characterized by occasional clinical remissions, but generally progress to renal insufficiency.

V. **Hemolytic-uremic syndrome.** The triad of acute nephropathy, hemolytic anemia with fragmented red cells, and thrombocytopenia constitutes one of the most common syndromes of acute renal failure seen in childhood. It is endemic in Argentina, California, South Africa, and the Netherlands. It is often preceded by gastroenteritis or upper respiratory tract infection (URI).

A. **Etiology.** No discrete causes are known for the syndrome. Multiple reports note an association between infections with 0157:H7 *Escherichia coli* and epidemic HUS. The occurrence of familial clustering suggests that genetic factors are important.

B. **Evaluation.** Evaluate as for acute renal failure (see sec. **VII**).
   1. Do a CBC with a smear in any patient with acute renal failure.
   2. Suspect HUS if a viral gastroenteritis or URI precedes marked hematuria and/or renal failure.
   3. Separate into mild or severe categories, as follows:
      a. **Mild.** No single 24-hour period of anuria. The patient may have oliguria, hypertension, or convulsions but not all.
      b. **Severe.** Anuria or oliguria plus hypertension or convulsions is present.

C. **Diagnosis**
   1. The patient usually has a history of a prodromal illness.
   2. Microangiopathic hemolytic anemia is found, including low hematocrit, burr cells, helmet cells on smear, low platelets, and consumption coagulopathy.

D. **Treatment** is as for acute renal failure. In addition, note the following:
   1. Early dialysis may be lifesaving.
   2. **Transfuse with only washed, white cell–poor blood, because these patients may be renal transplant candidates in the future.**
   3. Control hypertension (see sec. **VI**).
   4. Do not use heparin or streptokinase; studies to date indicate no benefit from either.
   5. Antiplatelet agents are probably not indicated.

E. **Prognosis.** Mildly affected patients tend to do well, with little or no long-term proteinuria, hypertension, or azotemia. At least 20 percent of those with severe HUS will have long-term sequelae, such as hypertension, proteinuria, and/or progressive renal insufficiency.

VI. **Hypertension.** Hypertension is not a common pediatric problem. It is estimated to occur in 1 to 3 percent of children. Most of these children have essential or primary hypertension with mild elevations in their blood pressure. The younger the child and the more elevated the blood pressure, the more likely it is that there is a secondary cause of hypertension. Unless blood pressure is routinely recorded as part of the general physical examination, hypertension may be overlooked for considerable periods of time.

A. **Etiology**
   1. **Essential or primary hypertension** can begin in childhood, generally in children >10 years old. As in adults, the pathogenesis is unclear. However, genetic and racial factors appear to play a role.
   2. **Secondary hypertension** is associated with a variety of conditions.
      a. **Newborn infants:** Renal artery thrombosis, renal artery stenosis (particularly following umbilical artery lines), congenital renal malformations, coarctations of the aorta
      b. **Infancy–6 years:** Renal artery stenosis, renal parenchymal diseases, coarctation of the aorta
      c. **Children 6–10 years:** Renal artery stenosis, parenchymal diseases
      d. **Adolescence:** Renal parenchymal diseases

B. **Evaluation**
   1. **History.** Careful attention should be given to the neonatal and family history. Information about constitutional symptoms, abdominal pain, voiding abnormalities, muscle or joint complaints, edema, and rashes, as well as drug use, should be elicited.
   2. **Physical examination.** Measurement of blood pressure by auscultation requires an appropriate sized cuff that covers two thirds of the upper arm. The fourth Korotkoff's sound (K_4) is best to use in children, because K_5 often does not occur clearly. When possible, K_1 (onset), K_4 (muffling), and K_5 (disappearance) should be recorded. Height and weight should be plotted on appropriate growth charts. Coexisting features suggestive of renal disease, collagen vascular disease, endocrine disorders, genetic syndromes, or cardiac or vascular disease should be sought. In addition, careful neurologic evaluation should determine whether sequelae of chronic hypertension are present.
   3. **Laboratory evaluation** should include CBC, urinalysis, urine culture, serum electrolytes, BUN, and serum creatinine. If the child is obese or if the family history is suggestive, a serum lipid profile should be included.
   4. An **echocardiogram** provides information about the chronicity and the severity of the hypertension and serves as a useful marker to follow treatment efficacy.
C. **Diagnosis.** Hypertension is suggested by blood pressure values that are 2 S.D. above the mean or above the 95th percentile for age. Values for various age groups are depicted in Figs. 8-3 to 8-5.
D. **Treatment.** Any **diastolic blood pressure** above 95 mm Hg in a small child or above 110 mm Hg in a larger child requires immediate control. Acute control is also necessary if blood pressure elevation is associated with central nervous system (CNS) or cardiac symptoms.
   1. **Hypertensive crisis.** In acute, severe hypertension, the immediate short-term goal is blood pressure control. Simultaneously, there should be a program of medical or surgical investigation, or both, and treatment aimed at long-term control. The usual effective doses of antihypertensive medications are given in **a–h**; many patients require less, some more. **Intravenous diuretics**, given concomitantly, are often helpful.
      a. **Labetalol** (Normodyne, Trandate) is an adrenergic receptor blocking agent with selective alpha and nonselective beta effects.
         (1) **Dosage.** Initial dose is 0.25 mg/kg, with an additional 0.5 mg/kg at 15-minute intervals to a total cumulative dose of 1.25 mg/kg. It can also be given as a slow IV infusion of 1–3 mg/kg/hr. For the oral dose, see Table 8-3.
         (2) **Advantages.** One of the drugs of choice for hypertensive crisis. Not associated with reflex tachycardia as with other vasodilators. Dosing is independent of renal function. Labetalol is not cleared significantly either by peritoneal dialysis or hemodialysis. It has no significant effect on glucose metabolism, as do other beta-blocking agents. The onset of action is rapid (within 30 minutes), and its half-life is 5–8 hours. Once blood pressure control is achieved, labetalol treatment can be continued orally.
         (3) **Disadvantages.** Rare cases of hepatocellular injury are seen with both acute and chronic labetalol therapy. Injury is usually reversible, but hepatic necrosis has been reported. **LFTs need to be followed and at the first sign of hepatic injury, labetalol should be discontinued.**
      b. **Sodium nitroprusside (Nipride)** *must be used as an IV drip with constant intensive care unit monitoring.* It is universally effective, because it causes immediate vasodilation. The effects disappear when the IV drip is stopped.
         (1) The dose is 0.5–8.0 µg/kg/min. **Note:** The prepared solution is inactivated by light. **Do not use with other drugs in the same IV line.**
         (2) *Blood levels of thiocyanate must be checked daily,* because nitroprus-

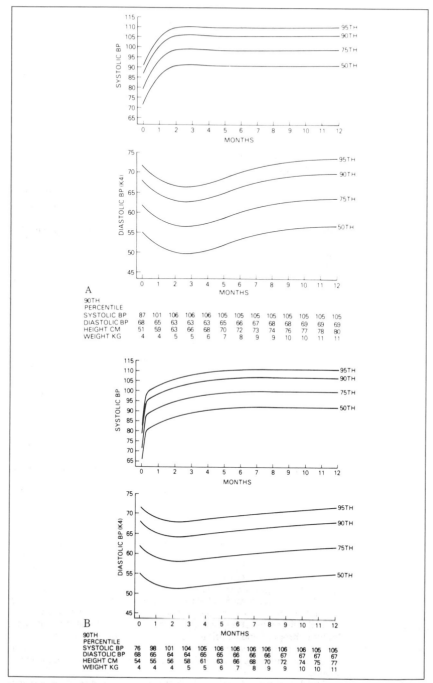

Fig. 8-3. Blood pressure in the first year of life in boys (A) and girls (B). (From Report of the Second Task Force on Blood Pressure Control in Children—1987. *Pediatrics* 79:1, 1987. Copyright 1987, American Academy of Pediatrics.)

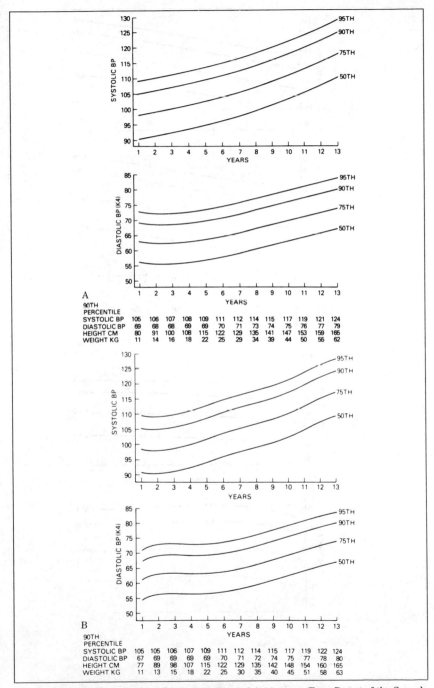

Fig. 8-4. Blood pressure in boys (A) and girls (B) aged 1–13 years. (From Report of the Second Task Force on Blood Pressure Control in Children—1987. *Pediatrics* 79:1, 1987. Copyright 1987, American Academy of Pediatrics.)

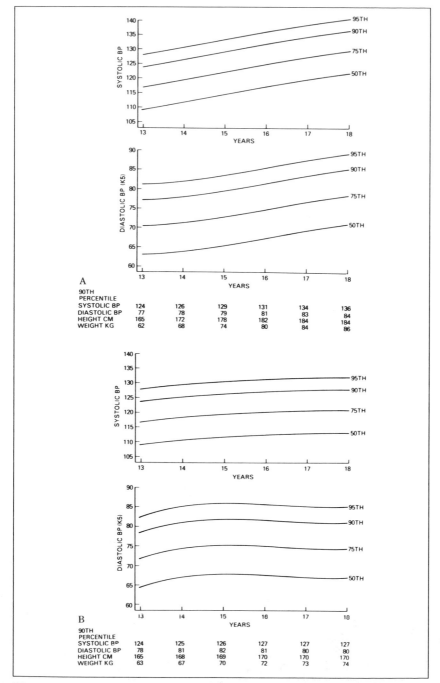

Fig. 8-5. Blood pressure in boys (A) and girls (B) aged 13–18 years. (From Report of the Second Task Force on Blood Pressure Control in Children—1987. *Pediatrics* 79:1, 1987. Copyright 1987, American Academy of Pediatrics.)

side is converted to thiocyanate by the hepatic enzyme, rhodanase. **Caution** is necessary in the presence of hepatic insufficiency.

(3) **Advantages.** The onset of action is instantaneous. Nitroprusside is effective when all other drugs have failed. The rate of infusion can be titrated against desired blood pressure.

(4) **Disadvantages.** Nitroprusside requires constant supervision in the intensive care unit. Discontinuance of the IV drip means instantaneous loss of the pharmacologic effect.

c. **Calcium-channel blockers** (nifedipine and others), given sublingually, have an onset of action within 15–30 minutes.

(1) **Dosage.** Use 0.25–0.50 mg/kg sublingually. Can give PO (see Table 8-3).

(2) **Advantage.** While calcium-channel blockers have not been studied extensively in children, these agents are very useful in adult hypertensive crises, given their rapid onset of action and sublingual administration.

(3) **Disadvantage.** Sublingual dose is difficult to administer precisely to small children.

d. **Diazoxide (Hyperstat)** is a useful second-line drug for acute blood pressure control. A benzothiazide with no diuretic effect, it acts directly on the vessels' smooth muscles, promptly and effectively reducing muscle tone. Diazoxide does not reduce renal blood flow.

(1) It is administered only IV (1 mg/kg/dose) **as fast as possible** to achieve maximal action on the smooth muscle and minimal binding to serum protein. The effects last 3–15 hours. If the initial dose proves ineffective, further doses can be repeated in 15- to 20-minute intervals. Maximum dose is 5 mg/kg.

(2) **Disadvantages.** The effect of diazoxide cannot be titrated. It produces hyperglycemia and can cause sodium and fluid retention. Transient tachycardia often follows administration.

e. **Enalaprilat (Vasotec IV)** is an angiotensin converting enzyme (ACE) inhibitor. This agent has not been studied extensively in children and the pediatric dose is not clearly established. However, oral ACE inhibitors (captopril and enalapril) are successfully used in managing pediatric hypertension. As with all ACE inhibitors, the dose should be adjusted in patients with renal impairment.

f. **Hydralazine (Apresoline)** is most effective when given in combination with diuretics or other IV antihypertensive agents, or both. Hydralazine is a direct vasodilator. When it is given intramuscularly, the onset of action is within 15–30 minutes. Onset after IV administration is immediate.

(1) **Dosage.** Hydralazine is given parenterally at an initial dose of 0.15 mg/kg. This dose can be progressively increased q6h according to the response up to 10 times the initial dose. When given with diazoxide, the dose needed may be smaller than when given alone. For the oral dose, see Table 8-3

(2) **Advantages.** Hydralazine does not reduce renal blood flow. It is effective fairly rapidly and it seldom produces hypotension. Hydralazine can be used with labetalol, diazoxide, calcium-channel blockers, or ACE inhibitors.

(3) **Disadvantages.** The most important side effects are tachycardia, nausea, vomiting, headache, diarrhea, and positive lupus erythematosus (LE) and rheumatoid factor (RF) reactions (very rare in children). The drug should be avoided in patients with arrhythmias and heart failure. It is not consistently effective.

g. **Beta blockers. Esmolol (Brevibloc)** is a selective β_1 blocker with a very short duration of action (approximately 9 min). It is administered as a continuous infusion of 50–200 µg/kg/min, though experience in children is very limited. **Propranolol** is a nonselective beta blocker and is most safely given PO. The usual pediatric IV dose is 0.5–1.0 mg under careful monitoring conditions. IV propranolol is reserved for life-threatening situations. (For discussion, see Chap. 9, p. 260).

h. **Methyldopa (Aldomet)** is an inhibitor of dopa decarboxylase and is metabolized to alpha-methyl norepinephrine, a weak pressor that displaces norepinephrine at nerve endings.

(1) **Dosage**

(a) **IV dosage** is from 10–50 mg/kg/day, administered in four divided doses q6h. Begin with 10 mg/kg/24 hr and double each subsequent dose until the desired effect is obtained. Methyldopa should be diluted in 5% dextrose in water (D/W) and given over 30–60 minutes. A paradoxical rise in blood pressure can be seen with too-rapid injection.

(b) **Oral dose** (see Table 8-3).

(2) **Advantages.** Gradual lowering of blood pressure is achieved. The renin level is also lowered.

(3) **Disadvantages.** Side effects include drug fever, hemolytic anemia with a positive Coombs test, positive LE cell reaction, positive RF, granulocytopenia, and thrombocytopenia and CNS depression. Methyldopa is not recommended for patients with pheochromocytoma. Both methyldopa and its metabolites produce false-positive blood and urine tests for pheochromocytoma.

2. **Mild and/or chronic hypertension.** It is important to identify children with primary or essential hypertension, so as to optimize their diet and their weight, control their hypertension, and educate them about the long-term implications of hypertension. For children with secondary causes of hypertension, it is important to identify the cause and to treat the hypertension. While epidemiologic data are inconclusive about the contribution of childhood hypertension to cardiovascular disease in adulthood, severe uncontrolled hypertension can cause significant end-organ damage in children. Several approaches to lowering blood pressure should be considered.

a. **Nonpharmacologic therapy.** Changes in diet, and dynamic exercise and relaxation techniques, may be effective, especially in essential hypertension. Weight reduction may help lower blood pressure.

b. **Diuretics** can be used if mild hypertension fails to respond to diet.

c. **Antihypertensive agents** should be added if techniques in **a** and **b** do not control blood pressure *or* if hypertension is moderately to severely elevated (see **D.1**). The dosages are shown in Table 8-3.

VII. **Renal tubular acidosis (RTA).** This syndrome is characterized by hyperchloremic metabolic acidosis secondary to defects in the renal tubular excretion of bicarbonate and acid. Generally, the glomerular filtration rate (GFR) is normal or mildly decreased.

A. **Proximal renal tubular acidosis (type II RTA)**

1. **Etiology.** Bicarbonate reclamation in the proximal tubule is impaired, resulting in a lowered renal threshold for bicarbonate reabsorption.

2. **Evaluation and diagnosis**

a. Patients often present with failure to thrive, vomiting, and severe bone disease.

b. Arterial blood gases (ABGs) and serum electrolytes reveal a hyperchloremic acidosis with low potassium.

c. Urine pH varies with the degree of acidemia. **All urine for pH should be collected under oil and measured while fresh.** Urine pH can be <5.5 with marked acidosis (serum $NaHCO_3$ < 16–18). Urine pH is inappropriately high in mild to moderate acidemia (serum $NaHCO_3$ 18–22).

d. A **bicarbonate titration test** can be done by infusing $NaHCO_3$ slowly (e.g., 1–2 mEq/kg over 1 hr) when the patient is acidotic and measuring serum HCO_3^- levels, urine pH, titratable acidity, and ammonium excretion. The renal threshold for HCO_3^- resorption in proximal RTA will be below the norms for children of comparable age.

Table 8-3. Oral antihypertensive agents

Agent	Form	Daily dose	Dose interval	Comments
Vasodilators				
Hydralazine	10, 25, 50 mg	0.1–3.0 mg/kg	q4–6h	
Minoxidil	2.5, 10 mg	0.2 mg/kg to max. 40 mg	qd–q12h	For severe hypertension; risk of hirsutism
Calcium-channel blocker				
Nifedipine	10, 20 mg	1.0–1.5 mg/kg	q6–8h	
Converting enzyme inhibitors				
Captopril	12.5, 25, 50, 100 mg	0.5–1.0 mg/kg to max. 6 mg/kg	q6–8h	Risk of renal failure, hyperkalemia
Enalapril	2.5, 5, 10, 20 mg	5 mg qd in adult; pediatric dose not established		
Beta blockers				
Propranolol	10, 20, 40, 60, 80 mg	0.5–1.0 mg/kg to max. 2 mg/kg	q6–12h	Contraindicated in asthma, congestive heart failure
Metoprolol	50, 100 mg	2.0 mg/kg	q12h	
Nadolol	40, 80, 120, 160 mg	40 mg/day in adults	qd	Long acting
Atenolol	50, 100 mg	50 mg/day in adults	qd	Long acting
Beta blocker/ vasodilator				
Labetalol	100, 200, 300 mg	200 mg in adults	q12h	
Alpha blocker				
Prazosin	1, 2, 5 mg	25–150 mcg/kg	q6h	
False transmitter				
Methyldopa	125, 250 mg tablets; 25 mg/5 ml suspension	10–40 mg/kg	q6–12h	Contraindicated in pheochromocytoma; active liver disease

    e. Children with proximal RTA who also have *glycosuria* and *aminoaciduria* should be evaluated for Fanconi's syndrome.

3. Treatment

    a. Large doses of bicarbonate (10–25 mEq/kg/day) are required to maintain the serum pH. Some patients require treatment with a combination of sodium and potassium bicarbonate. In primary proximal RTA the dosage is decreased after 6 months to determine if the threshold is still abnormal. If so, the acidosis will redevelop when the therapy is stopped.

  b. A repeat bicarbonate titration test should be performed. In some children, the disorder improves spontaneously after 2–3 years.
  c. Dietary salt restriction and thiazides can be useful adjuncts.
B. Distal renal tubular acidosis (type I RTA)
  1. Etiology. A defect in the distal tubule is present, resulting in an inability to establish a hydrogen ion gradient between blood and tubular fluid.
  2. Evaluation
    a. The presenting symptoms are usually growth failure, polyuria, and polydipsia.
    b. ABGs and serum electrolytes reveal a hyperchloremic acidosis, with hypokalemia seen in a number of patients.
    c. The urine pH is rarely below 6.5, even in the face of severe existing acidemia.
    d. Urinary concentrating ability is frequently impaired.
    e. Nephrocalcinosis is often present due to increased urinary calcium excretion and decreased urinary citrate.
    f. Ammonium chloride loading test. To distinguish proximal from distal RTA, an ammonium chloride loading test can be done (Table 8-4). Ammonium chloride ($75\ mEq/m^2$) is administered PO followed by serial measurement of the urine pH, titratable acidity, and ammonium excretion. Concomitant blood pH and CO_2 should be checked hourly for 5 hours. The serum HCO_3 concentration should fall to 17 mEq/liter or less. If it does not, a larger dose of ammonium chloride ($150\ mEq/m^2$) should be given cautiously on a second test day.
  3. Diagnosis is confirmed by an inability to acidify the urine below 6.5, with depressed excretion rates of titratable acid and ammonium in the context of marked acidemia.
  4. Treatment
    a. Bicarbonate or citrate in daily doses of 5–10 mEq/kg will correct the acidosis, minimize the risk of nephrocalcinosis, improve growth, and normalize the GFR.
    b. There is no indication at present that children will recover spontaneously from distal tubular acidosis, and treatment must be continued for life.
    c. The dosage of bicarbonate or citrate should be adjusted according to the blood pH. Daily urine calcium excretion should be kept below 2 mg/kg. Plasma potassium must be monitored. Some patients require all their bicarbonate as potassium bicarbonate.
C. Type IV RTA
  1. Etiology. In this disorder, the aldosterone-mediated mechanisms for distal tubule acidification are defective.
  2. Evaluation and diagnosis
    a. History includes significant urologic abnormalities or recurrent urinary tract infections.
    b. ABGs and serum electrolytes reveal a hyperchloremic acidosis, with **hyper**kalemia and hyponatremia.
    c. The urine pH is usually <5.5 with severe acidemia.
    d. Serum aldosterone levels are often elevated.

Table 8-4. Ammonium chloride loading test (normal values)

Age*	Urine pH	Titratable acid ($\mu Eq/min/1.73\ m^2$)	Ammonium excretion ($\mu Eq/min/1.73\ m^2$)
1–12 months	5.0	62 (43–111)	56 (42–79)
4–15 years	5.5	52 (33–71)	73 (46–100)

* Although current data are sparse, normal values for ages 1–4 years appear to approximate those of older children.
Source: Adapted from C. Edelmann et al., *Pediatr. Res.* 1:452, 1967; *J. Clin. Invest.* 46:1309, 1967.

e. In these patients, a careful urologic evaluation is indicated.

3. Treatment

a. Sodium chloride supplementation, potassium restriction, and/or furosemide (Lasix) treatment are efficacious.

b. For some patients, fludrocortisone is beneficial.

c. While surgery to correct urologic abnormalities and treatment of urinary infections should be pursued, the associated type IV RTA is usually not reversible.

VIII. Acute renal failure (ARF). Acute renal failure is defined as the acute cessation of glomerular filtration.

A. Prerenal failure. All patients with apparent ARF must be assessed for a prerenal cause.

1. Etiology. Dehydration, hypovolemia, or hemodynamic factors can compromise renal perfusion and intrarenal blood flow.

2. Evaluation

a. Review the history and physical findings for evidence of volume depletion, shock, decreased intravascular volume, and/or decreased cardiac output.

b. Measure the blood pressure and central venous pressure (CVP).

c. Insert an indwelling bladder catheter to ascertain the urine output (<0.5 ml/kg/hr indicates severe oliguria) and to obtain urine for urinalysis, sodium, potassium, creatinine (Cr), and osmolality. **Do not** leave the catheter indwelling after the initial evaluation.

3. The **diagnosis** of prerenal failure is suggested by:

a. Urinary sodium < 15 mEq/liter, fractional sodium excretion (FE_{Na}) < 1.0 (FE_{Na} = urine/P_{Na} divided by U/P_{Cr} × 100), renal failure index (RFI) $<$ 1 (RFI = U_{Na} divided by U/P_{Cr} × 100) (Table 8-5). **Note:** RFI can be <1.0 in acute glomerulonephritis (GN), interstitial nephritis, early acute obstruction, and polyuric ATN.

b. A ratio of U/P urea $> 10 : 1$, U/P creatinine $> 40 : 1$, urine osmolality $>$ 500

c. Urinary potassium ≥ 40 mEq/liter

d. Increased urine output in response to rehydration or increased intravascular volume, or both

e. Improved renal function with improved cardiac function

4. Treatment. Treatment is aimed at restoring renal blood flow and function.

a. Insert an IV line for infusion of fluids and solute. In some patients, CVP monitoring is useful.

b. Reestablish an effective circulating blood volume (see Chap. 3).

c. If, after restoration of extracellular fluid (ECF) volume, oliguria or anuria persists, mannitol, 0.5 gm/kg of a 20% solution, should be infused over 10–20 minutes. This should result in an increase in urine output of approximately 6–10 ml/kg over the next 1–3 hours. **If no increase in urine flow occurs, no further mannitol should be given.**

d. A trial dose of furosemide, 1 mg/kg IV, should be administered **after** the ECF volume is restored. **Note:** Diuretics cause changes in urine electro-

Table 8-5. Diagnostic indices in acute renal failure

Index	Prerenal oliguria	Oliguric renal failure
Urine sodium	<15 mEq/liter	>40 mEq/liter
Urine osmolality	>500 mOsm/liter	<350 mOsm/liter
Urine/plasma Cr	>40	<20
FE_{Na}	<1	>3
RFI	<1	>1

Key: Cr = creatinine; FE_{Na} = (U/P_{Na} divided by U/P_{Cr}) × 100; RFI = (urine Na divided by U/P_{Cr}) × 100.

lytes and osmolality, making distinction between prerenal and renal oliguria more difficult.

  e. If marked oligoanuria persists, assess the patient for intrinsic renal or postrenal failure (see **B** and **C**).

B. Intrinsic renal failure

 1. **Etiology.** Renal parenchymal injury can result from a variety of causes. A history of severe and/or prolonged decreased renal perfusion suggests ARF due to ATN. Acute renal failure may be associated with acute glomerulonephritis, hemolytic-uremic syndrome, accelerated hypertension, uric acid nephropathy, or vasculitis.

 2. **Evaluation and diagnosis.** First, assess the patient for prerenal or postrenal causes of ARF.

  a. Stabilize the patient's condition **before** any invasive diagnostic procedures are performed.

  b. Obtain estimates of renal function (see Table 8-5).

   (1) U/P creatinine ratio < 20

   (2) Urine osmolality < 350

   (3) Urinary sodium concentration > 40, FE_{Na} > 3, RFI > 1

   (4) A radionuclide renal scan can be useful in assessing renal perfusion and function as well as in distinguishing intrinsic renal failure from cortical necrosis. Abdominal ultrasound is helpful in ruling out obstruction and shows characteristic patterns in chronic renal damage.

 3. **Treatment**

  a. The use of an indwelling catheter **should be discontinued** as soon as possible in a severely oligoanuric patient in whom intrinsic renal failure is established.

  b. Weigh the patient bid (or use a metabolic bed with a scale).

  c. Measure intake and output.

  d. **Fluid management**

   (1) Fluid and electrolyte replacement should be calculated as insensible losses (see Chap. 7) plus urine output (if the patient is not edematous or does not have fluid overload).

   (2) Give as many calories as possible, orally if practical. A peripheral IV line can tolerate 10–15% glucose; a central line can tolerate up to 30% glucose.

   (3) When diuresis begins, increasing urine volume must be replaced with a solution containing approximately the same electrolytes as are being excreted. If the patient has been hyperkalemic, **do not replace potassium until the serum potassium has returned to normal.**

  e. **Hyperkalemia**

   (1) If the serum potassium is 5.5–7.0 mEq/liter, sodium polystyrene sulfonate (Kayexalate) in sorbitol at a dose of 1 gm/kg can be given PO or PR and repeated q4–6 hours until potassium is lowered. **Warning: 1 mEq sodium enters the body for each mEq potassium that is removed. Over time, hypernatremia may result.**

   (2) If the serum potassium is above 7 mEq/liter and/or if electrocardiogram changes are present, one or both of the following therapies are indicated immediately. Monitor the patient's ECG.

    (a) Give 10% calcium gluconate, 0.5–1.0 ml/kg IV over 5–10 minutes, with ECG monitoring.

    (b) Give sodium bicarbonate, 2 mEq/kg, as an IV push over 5–10 minutes.

   (3) If hyperkalemia persists, administer insulin, 0.1 U/kg IV with 25% glucose as 0.5 gm/kg (2 ml/kg) over 30 minutes. This dose can be repeated in 30–60 minutes if necessary. Monitor the blood sugar with Dextrostix. Prepare to dialyze the patient.

   (4) Acute dialysis is usually necessary if the potassium is above 7.5 mEq/liter, if the measures in (2) fail, or if (3) is needed.

  f. **Acidosis** can usually be alleviated by providing glucose for calories as well as 1–3 mEq/kg/day exogenous bicarbonate, citrate, or lactate. **Warning: A milliequivalent of bicarbonate contains 1 mEq sodium or potassium.** If the acidosis is severe and treatment is difficult due to fluid overload, dialysis is indicated.

   g. Nutrition. Optimal calories and protein nitrogen will help to decrease catabolism, lower BUN, ameliorate the uremic state, and improve healing and the immune response. With restricted fluids, little nitrogen and only 15–25 percent of calories can be given by a peripheral IV line.

   (1) If the patient can take POs, optimize the calories of dietary solids and increase the caloric density of fluids with glucose polymers (Polycose). The estimated caloric needs in ARF are 40–80 calories/kg/day, though some patients require more calories to suppress catabolism. Provide 3–5 percent of the total calories as protein.

   (2) If the patient will be NPO for over a week and renal failure is profound, consider total parenteral nutrition (see Chap. 10).

   h. Hypertension. If hypertension is acute and severe (2 S.D. above the age-appropriate norms), treat as outlined for hypertensive emergencies in sec. **VI.D.1. Note:** In acute renal failure:

   (1) Antihypertensive agents with rapid onset of action should be selected.

   (2) Hemodialysis or phlebotomy is indicated when hypertension is severe and unresponsive to medical management.

   i. Congestive heart failure (see also Chap. 9)

   (1) Congestive heart failure can usually be prevented by proper **fluid restriction.**

   (2) There is no place for diuretics in the anuric patient.

   (3) Digitalis will not produce a dramatic effect. If CHF is severe, dialysis is indicated.

   j. Drug therapy. Adjust the dosage of all drugs metabolized or excreted by the kidney.

   k. Indications for dialysis

   (1) Volume overload with severe hypertension or CHF

   (2) Hyperkalemia refractory to medical management

   (3) Severe acidosis associated with either fluid overload or hypernatremia

   (4) Symptomatic uremia (e.g., drowsiness, irritability) or rapidly rising BUN, Cr

   (5) Marked calcium/phosphorus imbalance (e.g., symptomatic hypocalcemia associated with severe hyperphosphatemia)

   (6) Support for parenteral nutrition

C. Postrenal failure

   1. Etiology. Obstruction is usually due to congenital anomalies, urethral valves or stricture, hematuria with clots, tumor compression, or retroperitoneal fibrosis.

   2. Evaluation and diagnosis. Obstruction is suggested by a history of genitourinary abnormalities, or lower abdominal trauma, or by the finding of flank masses or an enlarged bladder. Bilateral ureteral obstruction is suggested by absolute anuria.

   a. Do a renal ultrasonogram and a radionuclide scan. If facilities for these studies are unavailable and the serum creatinine < 5 mg/dl, an IVP can be attempted. The patient should be adequately hydrated and minimal amounts of a low-osmolality contrast agent should be used.

   b. Urologic consultation should be obtained.

   c. A cystoscopy and a unilateral retrograde pyelogram should be considered if anuria is present and obstruction is suspected.

   3. Treatment consists of surgical correction or bypass, as required.

IX. Uric acid nephropathy

   A. Etiology. Uric acid nephropathy may be associated with the following:

   1. Malignancies, especially leukemias and lymphomas **due to the large tumor burden and rapid cell turnover.** Uric acid nephropathy is a particular risk during induction chemotherapy.

      2. Regional enteritis, due to increased intestinal absorption of uric acid

  B. Evaluation

      1. Determine **uric acid levels** in all children with malignancies, especially before and during cytoreductive therapy. Measure uric acid levels in patients with regional enteritis.

      2. Measure **renal function** in all at-risk patients. If acute renal failure is developing, evaluate as in sec. **VIII.**

  C. Treatment. The prevention of renal failure is the most important aspect of therapy.

      1. Begin **allopurinol,** 10 mg/kg/day in three to four divided doses, in all children about to undergo massive cytoreductive therapy.

      2. Force fluids to two to three times maintenance.

      3. Alkalinize the urine, so that its pH is above 6.5, with IV sodium bicarbonate. Start with 1–2 mEq/kg/day and increase as needed. (Uric acid is more soluble in alkaline urine.)

      4. If oliguria or anuria develops, **hemodialysis** is indicated.

X. Chronic renal failure (CRF)

  A. Etiology

      1. Approximately half have congenital lesions: obstructive uropathy, renal dysplasia, juvenile nephronophthisis, or polycystic kidney disease.

      2. About a third of cases are due to glomerulopathy.

      3. Chronic pyelonephritis leading to CRF occurs primarily in the presence of an obstructive congenital lesion or marked vesicoureteral reflux.

      4. Other causes include hemolytic-uremic syndrome, malignant hypertension, interstitial nephritis, renal vein thrombosis, and nephrectomy for malignancy.

  B. General therapeutic measures

      1. Water and salt balance

        a. Fluid. The aim is to replace insensible losses and urine output (see Chap. 7). **For the patient with chronic renal failure, fluid restriction may be more detrimental than overhydration.**

        b. Sodium

          (1) To avoid arterial hypertension, sodium intake should be limited except in patients with significant renal sodium wasting. A "no-salt-added" diet is usually sufficient, as it provides 40–90 mEq sodium per day (2–4 gm sodium). If diet alone is not effective in controlling blood pressure, antihypertensive drugs, diuretics, or both can be added.

          (2) If salt wasting occurs, free salt intake may be necessary (see Chap. 7). Daily requirements are estimated by monitoring the patient's volume status (e.g., weight, blood pressure, and peripheral edema) and the urinary sodium excretion.

      2. Potassium

        a. Hyperkalemia. Conditions that usually lead to hyperkalemia include:

          (1) The onset of severe renal failure or sudden oliguria due to vomiting or diarrhea, or both, or to gastrointestinal bleeding

          (2) The indiscriminate administration of aldosterone antagonists (spironolactone) or inhibitors of distal tubular sodium-potassium exchange (triamterene); use of ACE inhibitors (captopril, enalapril)

          (3) Drugs that contain potassium, such as potassium penicillin

          (4) Massive hemolysis or tissue destruction

          (5) Treatment. Serum potassium levels below 5.8 mEq/liter are usually well handled by further restrictions in potassium intake, using the following guidelines:

            (a) Fruits high in potassium: Bananas, oranges (citrus), cantaloupe, watermelon, apricots, raisins, prunes, pineapples, and cherries

            (b) Vegetables high in potassium*: Green leafy vegetables, potatoes, avocado, artichoke, lentils, and beets

---

* Cooking leaches out potassium; cook these foods.

(c) **Meats and fish high in potassium:** All have potassium content (lowest are chicken liver, shrimp, and crab).

(d) **Breads and flours highest in potassium:** Pumpernickel, buckwheat, and soy

(e) **Miscellaneous foods high in potassium:** Chocolate, cocoa, brown (not white) sugar, molasses, nuts, and peanut butter.

The potassium content of commonly used beverages is given in Table 8-6. For serum levels that are chronically above 5.8 mEq/liter, treatment with an exchange resin is indicated to remove potassium from the body, and dialysis should be considered.

b. **Hypokalemia.** Hypokalemia is a common complication in patients with renal tubular dysfunction or polyuric renal disease complicated by an acute GI disorder. Unless renal failure supervenes, none of these patients will require any dietary potassium restrictions. Rather, they will need potassium supplementation, as follows:

(1) Potassium chloride, a 300-mg tablet with 4 mEq/tablet, or a 1 mM/ml solution. **Enteric-coated tablets should not be used** because of their intestinal insolubility. Of the available preparations, K-Lor (a pineapple-orange–flavored powder, 25 mEq/packet) is the most palatable. If chloride is chosen because of alkalosis, K-Lor can be mixed in fruit juice and given in three to four doses over the day.

(2) Potassium bicarbonate, 300-mg capsules with 3 mEq/capsule, or Shohl's solution, 140 gm citric acid + 100 gm sodium citrate or potassium citrate dissolved in water to 1 liter.

Note: The potassium requirement may range from 1–2 to 2–5 mEq/kg/day and even higher in long-standing renal tubular disease.

(3) Triamterene (smallest available tablet = 50 mg) can aid in the prevention of urinary potassium losses and works well for chronic conditions such as cystinosis or Bartter's syndrome. **Note:** In Bartter's syndrome, inhibitors of prostaglandin synthetase (aspirin, indomethacin) have produced striking improvements in potassium balance. Doses of 2–4 mg/kg per day or on alternate days can substantially reduce the need for potassium supplements when urinary loss is a major factor.

(4) **Prolonged hypokalemia** will lead to secondary metabolic alkalosis and possible paradoxical aciduria if the patient also has a sodium deficit. If the hypokalemia is severe (<2 mEq/liter serum), IV replacement should be given at 4–5 mEq/kg/day as potassium chloride, at least in the first 24 hours. Subsequent therapy is determined by the laboratory results and urinary output.

(5) **In RTA**, cystinosis, postobstructive diuresis, and ATN, serum potassium levels < 1 mEq/liter may be evident. The required replacement may exceed the maximal recommended peripheral IV fluid potassium concentration of 40–80 mEq/liter and require administration in a central vein.

3. **Nutrition.** Growth failure can be marked with decreased GFR, but may be improved by appropriate dietary management.

Table 8-6. Potassium content of beverages

High K	mEq/liter	Low K	mEq/liter
Milk	36	Ginger ale	0.1
Cola	13	Pepsi-Cola	0.8
Orange juice	49		
Grape juice	31		
Tomato juice	59		

a. **Calories.** In fasting conditions, an obligatory loss of 25–35 calories/kg/day occurs. Since 50 percent is normally contributed by carbohydrates, the minimal administration of glucose necessary to avoid increased tissue breakdown is 400 gm/m^2 daily, or 3–4 gm/kg in the small child.

b. **Protein**

  (1) Since the kidney is the obligatory route for the excretion of nitrogenous waste, progressive restriction of dietary protein is necessary with declining renal function. While the GFR remains above 25 percent of normal, any reasonable diet is usually tolerated.

  (2) The progression of renal disease decreases osmotic tolerance, and some protein restriction is necessary. (Each gram of protein contains 6 mOsm urea.) As the GFR decreases from 25 to 10 percent of normal, a decrease of urinary concentration ability from 900 to 300 mOsm/liter occurs, forcing a restricted protein diet of 1.5–2.0 gm/kg/day. At these levels, proteins of high biologic value (egg, meat, milk) should be used in order to satisfy essential amino acid requirements.

  (3) For infants, the appropriate caloric intake can be provided by supplementing proprietary formulas with carbohydrates and fats.

  (4) As renal function falls below 10 percent of normal and approximates zero, further restrictions are necessary until dialysis is started.

    (a) Once dialysis is instituted and adjusted to achieve sufficient urea clearance, liberalization of the protein intake is then possible to a daily intake of 2–3 gm protein/kg, 2 gm sodium, and 2 gm potassium.

    (b) A gradual increase in protein intake to 2 gm/kg or more daily can produce growth in a substantial number of children in renal failure.

4. **Mineral metabolism in renal disease.** Secondary hyperparathyroidism and metabolic bone disease occur in renal insufficiency (GFR < 25% of normal) unless vigorous measures are taken.

  a. **Hyperphosphatemia.** If the serum phosphate level is over 5 mEq/liter, or if alkaline phosphate is elevated, dietary phosphate must be restricted and oral phosphate binders administered. Once phosphate is normalized, vitamin D (as D$_3$ analogues or dihydrotachysterol) therapy should begin. Because of evidence that aluminum accumulation may cause osteomalacia and CNS problems in CRF patients, aluminum-containing preparations are not recommended as oral phosphate binders. Similarly, because of the risk of hypermagnesemia, magnesium-containing preparations are not recommended. **Only calcium-containing preparations should be used as oral phosphate binders** (Table 8-7). Preparations such as Os-Cal, Cal-Sup, or Titralac are palatable and also replace calcium (see below). Phosphate binders must be given with or just after all meals and snacks to bind the phosphate in the diet; otherwise, they are ineffective.

  b. **Calcium balance.** In general, good control of serum phosphorus levels should precede the administration of supplemental calcium, but seizures or other complications make immediate treatment with calcium unavoidable.

    (1) **Hypocalcemia** (see also Chap. 7)

      (a) **Acute replacement** is needed only if the patient is symptomatic, i.e., has hypocalcemic seizures or tetany. Then 10–15 mg elemental calcium/kg is given IV as 10% calcium gluconate. The correcting effects last only a few hours, and a new infusion or further PO administration is required.

      (b) **Oral preparations.** See Table 8-7 for the elemental calcium content of various oral calcium preparations. Therapy should be designed to provide the minimal allowance of 500–1,000 mg elemental calcium per day.

    (2) **Hypercalcemia.** Although hypercalcemia is not common in renal

Table 8-7. Phosphate binders

Trade name	Form	Elemental calcium	Active ingredients
OS-Cal*	500-mg tablet (chewable)	500 mg	Calcium carbonate
Phos-Ex	167-mg tablet	167 mg	Calcium acetate
	250-mg tablet	250 mg	
Phos-Lo	Tablet	169 mg	Calcium acetate
Titralac	Suspension	200 mg/5 ml	Calcium carbonate
Tums*	Regular tablet	200 mg	Calcium carbonate
	Extra-strength	300 mg	
	Suspension	400 mg/5 ml	

* Nonprescription.
Source: Courtesy of Nancy Spinozzi, R.D., Renal Nutritionist, The Children's Hospital, Boston, MA.

disease, it is a possible complication of indiscriminate use of vitamin D, severe secondary hyperparathyroidism, and inappropriate calcium concentration in the dialysate. If acute hypercalcemia occurs and immediate treatment is necessary, the following measures should be carried out:

(a) **Reduce calcium intake.** Discontinue the administration of vitamin D in any form (as in multivitamins). Special milk formulas are available with minimal calcium content (<100 mg/day).

(b) **Administer IV saline.** Use 1–2 liters/m^2 in acute severe hypercalcemia, if urine output is adequate.

(c) **Decrease the absorption of calcium.** Decrease gut absorption by administration of corticosteroids (prednisone, 1–2 mg/kg/day). This strategy requires days for optimal effect.

(d) Phosphate salts are best reserved for patients who are unresponsive to the preceding measures. Because IV infusion of sodium phosphate is itself dangerous, often producing metastic soft tissue calcification and an abrupt fall in calcium, the preferred route of administration is PR. Sodium phosphate (Phospho-Soda contains 3.3 gm/5 ml) can be given as an enema, or one can simply administer a Fleet enema.

(e) **Hemodialysis** can be used to control severe hypercalcemia.

c. **Vitamin D.** The use of vitamin D preparations is recommended to improve intestinal resorption and increase the parathyroid hormone end-organ responsiveness, thereby avoiding inappropriate hypertrophy of the parathyroid gland. Administration should start as soon as the GFR falls below 20–25 percent of normal and hyperphosphatemia is no longer present. If vitamin D toxicity develops and is recognized early, the loss in renal function is usually reversible. Patients should be cautioned to decrease their vitamin D intake when traveling or moving to areas that have higher sun exposure.

(1) 1,25-Dihydroxycholecalciferol (1,25-hydroxy vitamin D, calcitriol [Rocaltrol]) is recommended. The initial dose is 0.25 µg per day; the exact pediatric dose must be determined for each child. Follow-up should include periodic urinary calcium-creatinine ratios and serum calcium levels. The advantage of calcitriol is its short half-life, with pharmacologic activity lasting 3–5 days per dose.

(2) Dihydrotachysterol: Initial dose should be conservative (0.125 mg/m^2/day). The half-life is 2–3 weeks. One milligram of dihydrotachysterol is approximately equivalent to 3 mg (120,000 units) of vitamin D$_2$.

5. **Medications.** Daily administration of one to two standard multivitamin tablets or equivalent liquid preparations covers the basic requirements. Folic acid, 1–2 mg per day, should be added as more severe renal failure supervenes. Dosages of drugs excreted by kidneys must be adjusted.

6. **Hormone replacement therapy.** Anemia and growth retardation are significant problems for children with CRF. Recombinant human **erythropoietin (rHuEPO)** is now widely administered to adult CRF patients. Both rHuEPO and recombinant human growth hormone are under study in pediatric CRF patients.

7. **Anticonvulsant therapy** (see also Chap. 3, p. 67)

   a. The usual causes for seizures in the renal patient with preserved renal function are hypertensive encephalopathy, severe metabolic alkalosis with relative hypocalcemia, or hypomagnesemia.

   b. Since in CRF the appearance of seizures is most probably due to acute acid-base and electrolyte changes, these parameters must be assessed.

   c. Disequilibrium following dialysis may cause convulsions. This situation is best remedied by a change in dialysis procedures.

   d. Therapy depends on etiology.

8. **Dialysis therapy.** The indications for dialysis in renal failure are intractable CHF, increasing acidosis, intractable hyperkalemia, and continuing clinical deterioration. The decision to dialyze should not be made on the basis of one isolated laboratory value; rather, each case should be individualized.

   a. **Peritoneal dialysis**

      (1) Disposable catheter sets are available for pediatric peritoneal dialysis. However, even for short-term dialysis in acute renal failure, Tenckhoff catheters are preferable and should be surgically placed.

      (2) The usual amount of fluid exchanged is 20 ml/kg initially, with a gradual increase to 40–50 ml/kg per exchange. The initial loading fluid is not removed. The presence of such a reservoir will ensure that all the holes in the catheter are under water and will prevent air block. The fluid is usually warmed to body temperature, then permitted to run in as fast as is tolerated, allowed to equilibrate for 15–20 minutes, and then drained (usual time is 15–30 min).

      (3) **Factors affecting peritoneal dialysis**

         (a) **Clearance.** Urea is cleared at the rate of 14–30 ml per minute at 20°C. Creatinine is cleared at a slower rate of 10–15 ml per minute.

         (b) **Temperature.** Warming the solution to body temperature will decrease heat loss (especially important in small infants) and, more importantly, will increase urea clearance.

         (c) **Rate.** Increasing the flow of the dialysis fluid will shorten the time for dialysis, but will increase protein loss and aggravate hyperglycemia.

      (4) **Solutions**

         (a) Usually, 1.5% glucose and water with added electrolytes is used. Prepared solutions are strongly advised.

         (b) Prepared solutions contain no potassium; potassium should be added as required. In patients with hyperkalemia, except in those taking digitalis, no potassium needs to be added to the initial three to five exchanges. Subsequently, 2.5–3.5 mEq/liter can be added to the dialyzing fluid. The composition of a standard solution is given in Table 8-8.

         (c) The 1.5% glucose solution as used in dialysis is hyperosmolar (372 mOsm/liter) and thus can cause appreciable fluid loss (up to 200–300 ml/hr). For removal of excess fluid, glucose can be added to increase the osmolality of the solution as desired. However, the use of solutions of higher osmolality can rapidly dehydrate infants and children (4.25% glucose = 525 mOsm/liter; 6.5% glucose = 678 mOsm/liter).

Table 8-8. Composition of a standard peritoneal dialysate solution (Baxter)

Sodium	132 mEq/liter
Chloride	96 mEq/liter
Calcium	3.5 mEq/liter
Magnesium	0.5 mEq/liter
Lactate	45 mEq/liter
Potassium	Added as per patient requirement
Dextrose	1.5%, 2.5%, or 4.25%

    (d) Heparin (500 units/liter) should be added to each exchange for the first 1 to 2 days and continued if the fluid is not clear.

    (e) When dialyzing for certain toxins, various additives such as albumin are useful in increasing removal.

  (5) Complications in peritoneal dialysis

    (a) Infection is usually due to **staphylococcus and gram-negative organisms.** Antibiotics are not advised for routine use, but treatment should be initiated in a symptomatic patient even if culture results are not available (see Chap. 14, p. 368). If intraperitoneal antibiotics are used, they must be given with extreme care, because high blood levels can result from peritoneal absorption.

    (b) Hyperglycemia is a special problem in diabetic patients, but it can also occur in nondiabetic patients and result in nonketotic hyperosmolar coma. The blood sugar must be monitored routinely in patients dialyzed with a 4.25% solution.

    (c) Hypoproteinemia can occur; about 0.5 gm/liter protein is lost in dialysis.

 b. Hemodialysis for childhood acute or chronic renal failure is practical. Even small infants and neonates can be dialyzed without difficulty by experienced personnel. It is more efficient than peritoneal dialysis, permitting control of both clearance and ultrafiltration within narrow limits. Vascular access is necessary. A catheter placed in the femoral or subclavian vein is sufficient for a temporary access in older children. Permanent access consists of a surgically created connection between an artery and vein (fistula). Children have been maintained on hemodialysis for years. Appropriate consultation and referral should be made.

  (1) Clearance on hemodialysis. Blood flows are adjusted depending on the patient's weight, metabolic state, and dietary intake to achieve adequate urea clearance.

  (2) Complications of hemodialysis. Potential problems include hypotension from too-vigorous ultrafiltration and bleeding or infection at the vascular access site.

 c. Chronic ambulatory peritoneal dialysis (CAPD). This form of peritoneal dialysis, in which a patient with end-stage renal disease (ESRD) is dialyzed continually at a slow rate, is often used in children. Episodes of peritonitis are a major complication. A variation of CAPD, continuous cycling peritoneal dialysis (CCPD), is also available. In CCPD, overnight cycling of dialysis fluid is performed automatically and peritoneal infections tend to occur less frequently than in CAPD.

9. Transplantation is preferable to chronic dialysis for most children with CRF. Any child with CRF should be considered a transplant candidate. Though transplantation cannot be considered curative, long-term survival is the rule and transplantation offers the optimal chance for rehabilitation from CRF. Referral should be made to a transplantation center.

XI. Renal vein thrombosis (RVT). Thrombosis within the intrarenal veins may occur in one or both kidneys as an acute, potentially life-threatening event. The process rarely begins in a main renal vein. Most patients are less than 1 year of age (90%), and 75 percent are under 1 month of age.

A. Etiology. The slow dual capillary circulation of the kidney is particularly vulnerable to thrombosis. The risk of RVT is heightened in the presence of hypoperfusion, hemoconcentration, hypercoagulability, or hyperosmolality. In the neonate, associated conditions include perinatal hypoxia, sepsis, prematurity, maternal diabetes mellitus, and maternal thiazide usage.

B. Evaluation. In any sick infant with compromised circulation, the clinician must be vigilant for RVT. Newborns often present with the classic constellation of hematuria (gross or microscopic), flank mass(es), anemia, and thrombocytopenia. A CBC and coagulation studies are indicated. Renal ultrasound and radionuclide studies can support the diagnosis of RVT without using contrast agents.

C. Diagnosis is suggested by positive findings during the above evaluation. The differential diagnosis includes that for flank masses (e.g., hydronephrosis, cystic kidneys, renal or adrenal tumors), vascular lesions (e.g., ATN, cortical or medullary necrosis, arterial thrombosis, HUS, adrenal hemorrhage), and infection.

D. Treatment
1. Treat supportively for intravascular coagulopathy (see Chap. 16); the utility of heparin or other anticoagulants is unproven. Thrombectomy even with bilateral RVT or caval thrombosis is controversial.
2. Treat acute renal failure if present.
3. Treat associated hypertension.

E. Prognosis. In several series, 30–40 percent survival is reported. Long-term sequelae may vary from clinical health with residual evidence of renal parenchymal loss to frank renal failure. In affected infants, the nephrotic syndrome rarely occurs as a secondary event. Chronic hypertension may result.

XII. Wilms' tumor (nephroblastoma). Wilms' tumor accounts for a third of malignant intraabdominal tumors. The average age of presentation is 2 years. Most present with an abdominal mass. A fibroblastic cell or smooth muscle cell is the predominant tumor cell type. Some of the tumors are believed benign and are labeled **fetal renal hamartomas** or **congenital mesoblastic nephromas.**

A. The **etiology** is unknown, but its incidence is increased in congenital hemihypertrophy and in aniridia.

B. Evaluation. Most patients (80–90%) present with an abdominal mass. Other presentations include pain, fever, nausea, or anorexia. Hypertension may be present. Radiologic studies should include the following:
1. An abdominal ultrasound. This is usually useful in distinguishing the lesion from cystic lesions (multicystic kidney) and hydronephrosis. A computed tomographic (CT) scan with contrast aids in determining the degree of local extension and caval involvement.
2. A liver scan (to search for hepatic metastases), a bone survey, and a chest x-ray are indicated. Radionuclide bone scans are superior to skeletal surveys for detecting small lesions. Chest CT scan will detect pulmonary metastases more sensitively than chest x-ray.

C. Treatment
1. Presurgical treatment with x-ray and chemotherapy is indicated for a large or bilateral tumor.
2. Surgically remove and stage the tumor.
   a. **Stage I.** Limited to the kidney. Resect completely.
   b. **Stage II.** Local extension beyond the kidney or to local lymph nodes. Resect completely.
   c. **Stage III.** Residual gross or microscopic tumor in the abdomen after surgery or spill of tumor during surgery
   d. **Stage IV.** Hematogenic metastases are present (liver, lung, and/or bone).
   e. **Stage V.** Bilateral renal involvement
3. **Chemotherapy.** Wilms' tumor is a very chemosensitive tumor. Actinomycin D and vincristine are the most effective agents.

   4. Radiation therapy postoperatively for stages II–V
   5. A bilateral complete nephrectomy is performed if there is continued disease
   in stage V.
   D. Prognosis. The outlook has improved over the past decade. Nearly 90 percent
   of children under age 2 with stage I disease are free of tumor 2 years later.
   Long-term survivors may have problems with hypertension, proteinuria, and/or
   interstitial nephritis.
XIII. Congenital abnormalities of the kidney. Renal developmental abnormalities are
   diverse in their structural manifestations, physiologic consequences, and clinical
   findings. Some are characterized by renal maldevelopment, others by renal cyst
   formation, and others by both renal maldevelopment and cyst formation.
   A. Etiology. As shown in Table 8-9, some congenital renal anomalies result from
   spontaneous disruptions in urinary tract development; others are associated
   with more global developmental insults and others are caused by inherited
   genetic defects.
   B. Evaluation and diagnosis
   1. Assess the patient for associated systemic abnormalities.
   2. Assess renal function with BUN, creatinine.
   3. Anatomic studies are indicated to define the abnormality and to determine if
   it is unilateral or bilateral.
   a. Ultrasound and radionuclide scan
   b. Voiding cystourethrogram
   4. Consider early family counseling regarding genetics, ESRD.

Table 8-9. Common congenital renal abnormalities

Renal abnormality	Anatomic features	Radiologic features	Cause
Obstructive uropathy	Variably sized kidneys	Variably sized kidneys; typically dilated collecting system	1. Posterior urethral valves 2. UPJ obstruction 3. Neurogenic bladder 4. Severe VUR
Dysplasia	Small maldeveloped kidneys ± cysts	Small maldeveloped kidneys ± cysts	Renal maldevelopment
Cystic dysplasia		Variably sized kidneys with cysts	Associated with trisomies 13 and 18, and many genetic syndromes
Multicystic dysplastic kidney	Very large, grossly cystic kidney	Usually unilateral, very large kidney with diffuse, large cysts	Renal maldevelopment, most commonly renal abnormality
PKD	ADPKD cysts along the entire nephron	Large, echogenic kidneys ± cysts	Single gene defect
	ARPKD-CD cysts; liver bile ducts involved	Large, echogenic kidneys ± cysts	Single gene defect

UPJ = ureteropelvic junction; VUR = vesicoureteral reflux; PKD = polycystic kidney disease;
ADPKD = autosomal dominant PKD; ARPKD = autosomal recessive PKD; CD = collecting
duct.

C. **Treatment.** For anomalies not associated with obstruction, factors known to hasten the decline in renal function (e.g., hypertension, urinary tract infection) should be minimized. With urinary tract obstructions, correction by a pediatric urologist or pediatric surgeon is critical. In general, conservative management of renal function or tubular impairment, or both, will permit the patient the best growth and development. Vigilance against urosepsis is important.

D. **Prognosis.** Depends on the severity of the lesion, the prospect of surgical correction, and the reversibility of the associated renal damage

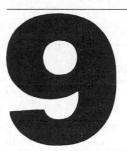

Cardiac Disorders

Edward P. Walsh

I. Congenital heart disease
A. General principles
1. The major clinical signs/symptoms of congenital heart disease include cyanosis, cardiac murmur, and/or congestive heart failure (CHF). The specific lesions are extremely varied, and will most often require consultation with a cardiologist for definitive diagnosis. However, a basic working knowledge of the common cardiac malformations is essential to the primary practitioner, in order to perform general screening and initiate proper referral.
2. The most common congenital heart defects are listed in Table 9-1, arranged in order of prevalence. The typical presentation is outlined for each lesion, along with the classic physical examination and laboratory findings.
3. Suspected congenital heart disease in the **neonate** requires prompt and aggressive evaluation. This topic is covered in detail in Chap. 6.
4. The basic diagnostic evaluation for structural heart disease begins with history and physical examination, and includes chest x-ray, electrocardiogram (ECG), and measurement of transcutaneous oxygen saturation. Detailed testing involves echocardiography and possible cardiac catheterization.
5. Definitive therapy for major cardiac malformations typically requires cardiac surgery. In recent years, a growing number of lesions are now being corrected with interventional catheterization procedures (e.g., patent ductus closure, atrial septal defect closure, relief of pulmonary/aortic/mitral stenosis).

II. Acquired heart disease
A. Myocarditis
1. **Etiology.** Infectious myocarditis is a common cause of acute congestive cardiomyopathy and may be caused by a variety of infectious agents, including viruses, rickettsiae, bacteria, mycobacteria, spirochetes, fungi, or parasites. Myocardial damage is effected by either invasion of the myocardium (e.g., echoviruses or Coxsackie viruses), production of a myocardial toxin (e.g., diphtheria), or autoimmune mechanisms (e.g., rheumatic fever). In North America, the most common etiologic agents are viruses. Myocarditis may be either acute or chronic.
2. **Presentation and evaluation.** The clinical presentation of infectious myocarditis ranges from the asymptomatic state to fulminant CHF, depending on the severity of myocardial involvement.
   a. **Symptoms** on presentation include fatigue, dyspnea, palpitations, and chest pain (usually secondary to associated pericarditis). **Signs** include tachycardia, protodiastolic gallop, and clinical evidence of CHF in severe cases.
   b. The **ECG** often shows ST and T-wave changes, arrhythmias, conduction defects, and occasionally a pattern of abnormal ventricular voltages.
   c. On **chest x-ray,** heart size ranges from normal to markedly enlarged.
   d. **Echocardiography** reveals dilated and/or hypocontractile ventricles. Pericardial effusion may be present.

Table 9-1. Classic findings for the 10 most common congenital heart lesions

Lesion	Presentation	Physical examination	ECG	X-ray
Ventricular septal defect	Murmur, CHF	Pansystolic murmur	LVH, RVH	+CE, ↑PBF
Pulmonic stenosis	Murmur, ±cyanosis	Click, SEM	RVH	±CE, NL or ↓PBF
Tetralogy of Fallot	Murmur, cyanosis	SEM	RVH	±CE, ↓PBF
Aortic stenosis	Murmur, ±CHF	Click, SEM	LVH	±CE, NL PBF
Atrial septal defect	Murmur	Fixed split S_2	Mild RVH	±CE, ↑PBF
Patent ductus	Murmur, ±CHF	Continuous murmur	LVH, ±RVH	±CE, ↑PBF
Coarctation of aorta	Hypertension	↓Femoral pulses	LVH	±CE, NL PBF
Transposition	Cyanosis	Marked cyanosis	RVH	±CE, NL or ↑PBF
AV canal defect	Murmur, ±CHF	Pansystolic murmur	"Superior" axis	±CE, ↑PBF
Single ventricle	(Variable)	(Variable)	(Variable)	(Variable)

CE = cardiac enlargement; CHF = congestive heart failure; LVH = left ventricular hypertrophy; NL = normal; PBF = pulmonary blood flow; RVH = right ventricular hypertrophy; SEM = systolic ejection murmur.

     e. Endomyocardial biopsy may be indicated in select cases to confirm diagnosis.

   3. The **diagnosis** depends in part on the features of the associated systemic illness. Viral etiology should be evaluated by obtaining viral cultures of throat washings, blood, feces, and pericardial fluid, as well as by acute and convalescent sera for virus neutralizing antibody, complement fixation, or hemagglutination inhibition titers.

   4. Treatment

     a. Treatment of infectious myocarditis should be supportive, with maintenance of adequate oxygenation.

     b. Monitoring and treatment, preferably in an intensive care unit, should be provided for arrhythmias, conduction abnormalities, and CHF.

     c. Since patients with myocarditis may be sensitive to digitalis glycosides, digoxin should be administered cautiously.

     d. Patients should remain at bed rest for 10–14 days.

     e. Corticosteroids are contraindicated in the acute phase of viral myocarditis.

     f. Immunosuppressive therapy has been used investigationally at some centers to reduce myocardial inflammation following the acute phase. Efficacy is unknown at this point.

 B. Pericarditis

   1. Causes

     a. Bacterial. Bacterial pericarditis may occur by hematogenous or contiguous spread. The most common causative organisms are staphylococci, pneumococci, *Haemophilus influenzae,* meningococci, streptococci, and *Mycobacterium tuberculosis.*

     b. Viral. Viral pericarditis is often preceded by a history of upper respiratory tract infection and occurs as part of the spectrum of viral myopericarditis.

The most common causative agents are Coxsackie virus, echovirus, adenovirus, influenza virus, mumps virus, varicella-zoster virus, vaccinia, or Epstein-Barr virus (i.e., infectious mononucleosis).

   c. **Noninfectious causes include** collagen diseases, uremic fibrinous pericarditis, radiation-induced pericarditis, and malignant pericardial effusion.

2. **Diagnosis**
   a. **Presenting clinical signs and symptoms** depend in part on the etiology, age of the patient, associated infection or systemic disease, and presence of tamponade.
   b. The **ECG** is characterized by diffuse ST and T-wave abnormalities. *Echocardiography* establishes the presence of fluid in the pericardial space and is the most useful test to confirm the diagnosis and follow the response to therapy.
   c. The chest x-ray often shows an increase in the size of the cardiac silhouette with normal pulmonary vascular markings; associated infection of the lung or pleural space may be evident.
   d. Pericardiocentesis for culture and examination of pericardial fluid should be performed in all patients who appear toxic, have evidence of tamponade, or in whom the cause of the pericarditis is uncertain.
   e. Additional studies should be done as appropriate to the cause (e.g., blood cultures; viral cultures of blood, urine, throat, and feces; tuberculin skin test; test for connective tissue disorders; blood urea nitrogen [BUN] and creatinine; complete blood count [CBC] and differential; cold agglutinins; heterophils; fungal serology; thyroid studies; rheumatic fever assessment).

3. **Treatment**
   a. **General measures** include bed rest, analgesia, and observation for and treatment of tamponade or cardiac decompensation.
   b. **Specific therapy** should be directed toward the etiology (e.g., antimicrobial agents, chemotherapy, dialysis). In acute purulent pericarditis, antibiotic therapy appropriate to the sensitivities of the causative organism should be combined with effective pericardial drainage (e.g., subxiphoid pericardial window, anterior pericardiectomy with tube drainage).

C. **Subacute bacterial endocarditis** (see Chap. 14, p. 421)

D. **Rheumatic fever** is covered in Chap. 14, p. 423.

E. **Kawasaki disease** is covered in Chap. 18, p. 517.

III. **Recognition of the innocent murmur.** The innocent murmur is one that occurs in the absence of either anatomic or physiologic abnormalities of the heart and lacks association with future cardiovascular disease. Innocent murmurs are audible in the majority of children.

A. **Clinical characteristics of innocent murmurs**
   1. **General**
      a. Systolic in time and of short duration
      b. Loudest along the left sternal border, transmission is usually not widespread; loudness may change with position but not respiration and is usually grade III or less and increases with exercise.
      c. Other heart sounds are normal (importantly, there is a normal split of the second sound). Thrills are absent.
      d. The ECG and chest x-ray are normal.
   2. **Specific**
      a. **Still's murmur** is usually grade I–III. It is a vibratory, buzzing, or musical systolic ejection murmur, loudest in the second to fifth left intercostal spaces and maximal in the supine position. It may intensify with exercise, excitement, and fever. It is not associated with a thrill.
      b. **Pulmonic systolic murmur.** A grade I–III, high-pitched, crescendo-decrescendo murmur, usually peaking in the first half of systole. It is maximal in the second left intercostal spaces, radiating upward and to the left. It is not associated with a thrill. It is best heard in the supine position

and more apt to be heard in persons with narrow anteroposterior diameter. It originates in the pulmonary trunk.

c. **Cardiorespiratory murmurs** are of extracardiac origin; they are usually located at the heart-lung margin. They are not well transmitted and seem to originate close to the ear. Their variable loudness and timing are associated with cardiac and respiratory cycles, and they often disappear in expiration. Their incidence is associated with intraabdominal masses or ascites, thoracic cage deformities, and pleural or pericardial adhesions.

d. **Cervical venous hum.** This is a grade I–VI continuous murmur with diastolic accentuation and is maximal in the supraclavicular fossa lateral to the sternocleidomastoid muscle. It may radiate below the clavicle, where it may be confused with the murmur of patent ductus arteriosus. It is elicited by turning the patient's head away from the side of the murmur and elevating the chin while in a sitting position. It is abolished by recumbency, turning the head to the ipsilateral side of the murmur, or digital compression of the ipsilateral internal jugular vein.

e. **Supraclavicular arterial bruit.** This is a crescendo-decrescendo early systolic ejection murmur. It is maximal over the supraclavicular fossa and prominent in the suprasternal notch. It may generate a carotid thrill. Radiation is more effective to the neck than to below the clavicles. The murmur is accentuated by exercise and abolished or diminished by hyperextension of the shoulders.

B. **Specific diagnosis.** The innocent murmur should be distinguished from the following lesions.

1. **Mitral valve prolapse**

   a. **Clinical evaluation.** Most commonly, mitral valve prolapse is characterized by an isolated variable mid- to late systolic click or a midsystolic click followed by a late systolic murmur. However, it may also present as an early systolic click, isolated late systolic murmur, pansystolic murmur, or precordial honk or whoop. Since the click in mitral valve prolapse is not always evident, auscultation should be carried out in four positions: supine, left decubitus, sitting, and standing. The click and murmur occur earlier with maneuvers that decrease left ventricular volume and/or increase left ventricular contractility (e.g., inspiration, standing, a Valsalva maneuver, isoproterenol, amyl nitrite inhalation). Opposite maneuvers (e.g., squatting, propranolol, phenylephrine) delay the onset of the click and murmur. Regurgitant murmurs become louder with maneuvers that raise arterial pressure and diminish with those that decrease it.

   b. **Laboratory data.** In approximately one third of patients with mitral valve prolapse seen by cardiologists, the **ECG** shows T-wave inversion with or without minimal S-T segment depression, characteristically noted in leads II, III, and Vf, with frequent additional involvement of the left precordial leads. A **chest x-ray** reveals a normal heart size in the absence of mitral insufficiency. The **echocardiogram** is abnormal in approximately 80 percent of subjects with the auscultatory findings of mitral valve prolapse.

   c. **Complications.** Although the prognosis in patients with mitral valve prolapse is generally excellent, rare complications include progression of mitral insufficiency, bacterial endocarditis, cardiac arrhythmias, cerebral ischemic events, and sudden death. Antibiotic prophylaxis against infective endocarditis should be used in patients with late or pansystolic murmurs (see Table 14-7). Their prophylactic use in patients with an isolated click is controversial.

   d. **Treatment.** Generally, no treatment is indicated unless mitral regurgitation advances or symptomatic arrhythmias are present. Beta blockers seem to be effective for the rare patient with ventricular arrhythmias associated with mitral valve prolapse.

2. **Idiopathic hypertrophic subaortic stenosis.** Auscultation is characterized by a harsh midsystolic ejection murmur that is maximal between the apex

and left sternal border and results from left ventricular outflow tract obstruction. Frequently, there is a separate pansystolic regurgitant murmur maximal at the apex, caused by mitral regurgitation. The systolic ejection murmur is augmented by maneuvers that increase contractility, decrease preload, or decrease afterload, i.e., Valsalva maneuvers, standing, postextrasystole, exercise, digitalis, amyl nitrite, or isoproterenol. Conversely, the murmur diminishes with squatting, isometric hand grip, alpha-adrenergic stimulation, or beta-adrenergic blockade.

IV. **Congestive heart failure.** Congestive heart failure is a clinical syndrome in which the heart is unable to supply an output sufficient to meet the metabolic requirements of the tissues.

A. **Etiology**

1. Congenital diseases of the heart, usually with large left-to-right shunts or obstructive lesions of the left or right ventricle
2. Acquired diseases of the heart, including myocarditis, acute or chronic rheumatic heart disease, and infectious endocarditis
3. Arrhythmias, including paroxysmal atrial tachycardia, atrial fibrillation or flutter, or complete heart block
4. Iatrogenic causes, including damage to the heart at surgery (ventriculotomy), fluid overload, or doxorubicin (Adriamycin) therapy
5. Noncardiac causes, such as thyrotoxicosis, systemic arteriovenous fistula, acute or chronic lung disease, glycogen storage disease, or connective tissue or neuromuscular disorders

B. **Clinical manifestations.** The signs and symptoms of CHF fall into the following three categories:

1. **Signs of impaired myocardial performance.** These include growth failure, sweating, cardiac enlargement, gallop rhythm, and alterations in peripheral pulses, including pulsus paradoxus and pulsus alternans.
2. **Signs of pulmonary congestion** include tachypnea, dyspnea with effort, cough, rales, wheezing, and cyanosis.
3. **Signs of systemic venous congestion** include hepatomegaly, neck vein distention, and peripheral edema.

C. **Treatment.** Whenever possible, the precipitating causes (e.g., arrhythmia) and underlying causes (e.g., structural abnormalities) of CHF should be removed. Control of CHF may be achieved by (1) *increasing cardiac contractile performance,* (2) *reducing cardiac workload,* and (3) *reducing the volume overload* responsible for congestive symptoms.

1. **Increasing cardiac contractile performance**

a. **Digitalis** therapy increases cardiac output by directly enhancing the myocardial contractile state. The inotropic effect of digoxin increases linearly with increasing dose until toxicity is reached. The optimal dose should be dictated by the patient's response and must be individualized. Guidelines for digoxin use are detailed in sec. **VII.B.**

b. **Other cardiotonic agents.** When CHF is associated with hypotension or is refractory to other modes of therapy, additional inotropic support may be achieved with the following:

(1) **Dopamine.** The usual therapeutic dose is 5–20 µg/kg/min by continuous IV infusion. Therapy is begun at a low dose (2 µg/kg/min) and gradually increased until the desired effect is achieved. At low doses (<5 µg/kg/min), dopamine causes renal vasodilation. At higher doses (>10 µg/kg/min), dopamine may have the undesirable effects of increasing total peripheral resistance and heart rate.

(2) **Dobutamine.** The usual therapeutic dose is 5–20 µg/kg/min, but should be titrated by the patient's response.

(3) **Amrinone** improves cardiac performance by combined effects on contractility and afterload. The usual loading dose is 1–3 mg/kg followed by an infusion of 5–20 µg/kg/min.

2. **Reducing cardiac workload**

a. **General measures**

(1) **Restriction of physical activity** and periods of **bed rest** reduce metabolic requirements in older children and adolescents. Activity restriction is usually counterproductive in young children.

(2) **Cool, humidified oxygen** by tent, mask, or nasal prongs may be useful in hypoxic patients.

b. **Afterload reduction.** Vasodilator therapy, which decreases peripheral resistance and ventricular filling pressures, is used in patients with CHF that is refractory to digoxin and diuretics. Vasodilator agents are most effective in patients with extremely decreased cardiac index, high systemic vascular resistance, and pulmonary congestion. Agents that alter arteriolar resistance have the greatest effect on cardiac index, while agents that increase venous capacitance reduce congestive symptoms caused by elevated ventricular filling pressures.

(1) **Acute therapy.** Sodium nitroprusside affects both arteriolar resistance and venous capacitance, thus treating both low output and congestive symptoms (see also Chap. 8, p. 224). Continuous IV infusion is usually begun at 0.5 μg/kg/min and increased until the desired effect is achieved or until arterial pressure falls by 10 percent. The average dose is 3 μg/kg/min. **Sodium nitroprusside should be administered in an intensive care unit setting with monitoring by an arterial line and a thermodilution Swan-Ganz catheter, with supervision by a physician experienced in its use.** *Thiocyanate levels should be measured when the drug is used for an extended period.*

(2) **Long-term maintenance**

(a) **Hydralazine** preferentially dilates the peripheral arteriolar bed, thus augmenting cardiac output. The initial dosage is 1 mg/kg/day PO given in three to four divided doses, with a gradual increase until the desired effect is achieved or adverse effects occur.

(b) **Captopril and enalapril** are angiotensin-converting enzyme inhibitors that block production of angiotensin II. They are "balanced" vasodilators with actions on both the arteriolar and venous beds. Dosages for captopril range from 0.5–3.0 mg/kg/day, in three divided doses. Enalapril is generally used only in older children at a dose of 2–10 mg bid.

3. **Reducing volume overload**

a. **Sodium restriction.** No-added-salt diets are used in children. Infants should receive a high-calorie, low-sodium formula.

b. **Fluid restriction** is necessary **only** when dilutional hyponatremia complicates far-advanced CHF. Formula intake should **not** be restricted in infants.

c. **Diuretics** (see also Chap. 8, p. 214). The effectiveness of a diuretic is dependent on renal perfusion and electrolytes and acid-base balance. Diuretic agents may cause profound changes in electrolyte composition, and therefore frequent electrolyte evaluations should be made. In the presence of shock or acute renal failure, diuretics will have little effect. **Potassium depletion, especially in the digitalized patient, is dangerous and may be lethal.** The characteristics of commonly used diuretics are given in Table 9-2.

(1) **Thiazides** are sulfonamide derivatives that share moderate potency and low toxicity. Those most commonly used in pediatrics are chlorothiazide (Diuril) and hydrochlorothiazide (HydroDIURIL).

(a) **Mechanism.** The thiazide diuretics inhibit resorption of sodium and chloride at the cortical diluting site of the ascending loop of Henle and the early distal convoluted tubule.

(b) **Route of administration, absorption, and metabolism.** The thiazides are rapidly absorbed from the gastrointestinal tract and begin to have a diuretic effect within 1 hour. The duration of action of chlorothiazide is about 6–12 hours, while that of hydro-

Table 9-2. Dosages and characteristics of various diuretics

Drug	Dosage	Action Onset	Action Peak	Action Duration	Contraindications	Adverse reactions	Mechanism of action
Furosemide (Lasix)	IV: 1.0 mg/kg/dose (over 1–2 min)	5 min	30 min	2 hr	Anuria	Hypovolemia	Blocks resorption of Cl^- in ascending loop of Henle
Ethacrynic acid (Edecrin)	PO: 2–3 mg/kg/day IV: 1 mg/kg/dose PO: 2–3 mg/kg/day	1 hr 5 min 30 min	1–2 hr 45 min 2 hr	4–6 hr 3 hr 6–8hr	Hypersensitivity Women with child-bearing potential	Hypokalemia Hyperuricemia Ototoxicity	
Chlorothiazide (Diuril)	PO: 20–30 mg/kg/day in 2 doses	2 hr	4 hr	6–12 hr	Anuria, progressive renal insufficiency	Hypokalemia	Blocks resorption of Na^+ in ascending loop of Henle
Hydrochlorothiazide (Hydro-DIURIL)	PO: 2–3 mg/kg/day in 2 doses	2 hr	4 hr	6–12 hr	Hypersensitivity to this or other sulfonamide-derived drugs	Hyperuricemia Hypersensitivity Dermatitis Photosensitivity	
Spironolactone (Aldactone)*	PO: 1–3 mg/kg/day in 2 doses		Several days		Renal insufficiency	Headaches Gynecomastia Nausea and vomiting Rashes	Blocks aldosterone exchange of K^+ for Na^+
Acetazolamide (Diamox)	PO: 5 mg/kg/day	1 hr	2 hr	24 hr	Hypokalemia Anuria Renal insufficiency Hyperchloremia Acidosis	Drowsiness Paresthesias Hypersensitivity	Carbonic anhydrase inhibitor

* Spironolactone is rarely given alone, but its potassium-sparing effect makes it useful in combination with other agents.

chlorothiazide is 12 hours or more. Excretion is via the kidney, with some subsequent resorption.

(c) **Dosage.** Give chlorothiazide, 20–30 mg/kg/day PO in two divided doses, or give hydrochlorothiazide, 2–3 mg/kg/day PO in two divided doses.

(d) **Toxicity**

   (i) **Potassium depletion** may occur with long-term use. Alternate-day therapy, intake of foods high in potassium, administration of liquid potassium, or the addition of a potassium-sparing diuretic such as spironolactone or triamterene may protect against potassium depletion. However, periodic measurements of serum potassium are necessary, especially early in therapy.

   (ii) **Allergic reactions,** such as thrombocytopenia, leukopenia, or vasculitis, are rarely seen. **Hyperglycemia** and **aggravation of preexisting diabetes or hyperuricemia** may occur.

(2) **Furosemide (Lasix) and ethacrynic acid (Edecrin).** These potent diuretics are different structurally from each other but have similar diuretic effects. Because of the massive diuresis that may be produced, they should rarely be used in previously untreated children unless careful observation of electrolytes, especially serum potassium, and blood volume is possible.

(a) **Mechanism.** Both furosemide and ethacrynic acid inhibit active chloride transport in the ascending limb of the loop of Henle, where 25 percent of sodium resorption occurs.

(b) **Route of administration, absorption, and metabolism**

   (i) Both drugs are well absorbed PO or can be given IV.

   (ii) When they are given PO, effects can be expected within 30–60 minutes. The onset of action after parenteral administration is within 5 minutes for furosemide and within 15 minutes for ethacrynic acid.

   (iii) The duration of action for the parenteral dose is 2–3 hours and 6–8 hours for the PO dose.

   (iv) Both drugs are bound to plasma protein, with approximately two thirds excreted by the kidney.

(c) **Dosage**

   (i) Ethacrynic acid is given in a 1-mg/kg dose over 1–2 minutes IV and 2–3 mg/kg/day PO. *Or*

   (ii) Furosemide can be given as a 1-mg/kg dose over 1–2 minutes IV or 2–3 mg/kg/day PO.

(d) **Toxicity.** Both drugs are potent, and clinical toxicity is usually manifested by **hypovolemia** or **hypokalemia.** Both drugs competitively inhibit urate secretion in the proximal tubule and may cause **hyperuricemia** and, in susceptible persons, gout. Transient or even permanent deafness has been reported, especially with ethacrynic acid (possibly due to electrolyte changes in the endolymph). **GI disturbances, bone marrow suppression, skin rashes,** and **paresthesias** have been reported occasionally.

(3) **Spironolactone (Aldactone)** is a weak diuretic by itself, but may be useful as an addition to diuretics previously discussed, both because of its different site of action and because of its potassium-sparing effects.

(a) **Mechanism.** The diuretic properties of spironolactone result from its structural similarity to aldosterone. It is a competitive inhibitor of the mineralocorticoids that normally stimulate sodium resorption and potassium excretion in the distal tubules.

(b) **Route of administration, absorption, and metabolism.** Spironolactone is absorbed orally, but the diuretic effects may not be manifested for 2–3 days. Its effects may persist for 2–3 days after cessation of therapy.

(c) The **dosage** is 1–3 mg/kg/day PO.

(d) **Toxicity.** The major complication is **hyperkalemia,** resulting from inhibition of potassium secretion with normal or increased potassium intake. Careful monitoring of serum potassium will avoid this problem. Spironolactone has been shown to be **oncogenic** in chronic toxicity studies in rats. Gynecomastia may be seen in adolescents.

V. Hypoxic or cyanotic spells. Paroxysmal dyspnea with marked cyanosis often occurs in infants and young children with tetralogy of Fallot. Rarely, it may occur in other types of cyanotic congenital heart disease. It is characterized by increasing rate and depth of respirations with increased cyanosis, progressing to limpness, loss of consciousness, and, in the more severe cases, convulsions, cerebrovascular accidents, or even death.

A. Etiology

1. Cyanotic spells are due to an acute reduction of pulmonary blood flow, increased right-to-left shunting, and systemic hypoxemia.

2. "Spasm" of the infundibulum of the right ventricular outflow tract has been suggested. Other explanations include inadequate systemic venous return, decreased systemic vascular resistance, and a vicious cycle of arterial hypoxemia due to hyperpnea.

3. Anemia, either absolute or relative to the child's oxygen saturation, may predispose to cyanotic spells.

B. Diagnosis

1. **Signs and symptoms** include:

    a. Reduction in intensity or disappearance of the pulmonary ejection murmur

    b. Hyperpnea

    c. Increased cyanosis

    d. Irritability, often leading to unconsciousness and occasionally to convulsions due to cerebral anoxia

2. **Laboratory findings** include:

    a. Hypoxemia and acidosis

    b. Diminished pulmonary blood flow on x-ray

    c. Increased voltage of the P wave on the ECG

C. Treatment

1. Place the child in a knee-chest position.

2. Give **oxygen** by hood or mask at 5–8 liters per minute.

3. Give **morphine sulfate,** 0.1–0.2 mg/kg IM or SQ.

4. If the spell is severe, give **sodium bicarbonate,** 1 mg/kg IV.

5. Volume expansion with crystalloid or blood should be given if cyanosis persists.

6. **Propranolol,** 0.1 mg/kg IV, may be effective in a protracted spell that does not respond to the preceding measures.

7. **Surgery** (corrective or palliative) may be necessary to increase pulmonary blood flow, or to prevent recurrence of spells, or both.

VI. Arrhythmias

A. Etiology

1. **Arrhythmias** result from disorders of impulse formation, impulse conduction, or both.

    a. Premature beats and **tachyarrhythmias** are due to abnormal impulse formation caused either by enhanced automaticity, reentry, or triggered activity.

    b. Bradyarrhythmias are due to either depressed automaticity or block of an impulse.

2. Arrhythmias may be a manifestation of cardiac, metabolic, or acquired systemic disorder.

    a. Congenital heart disease (pre- and postrepair)

    b. Acquired heart disease (e.g., rheumatic fever or myocarditis)

    c. Electrolyte disturbances, including potassium, calcium, and magnesium

   d. Drug toxicity or poisoning
   e. Disorders of endocrine, neurologic, or pulmonary systems
   f. In association with inherited disorders of metabolism, collagen diseases, or infection
B. Evaluation
   1. Careful physical examination with attention to blood pressure, perfusion, and respiratory status
   2. Full **12-lead** ECG with long rhythm strip
   3. Additional information can be obtained by manipulating sympathetic tone:
      a. Depress tone with vagal maneuvers such as Valsalva or carotid massage, or use bag to face.
      b. Enhance tone with controlled exercise (treadmill testing).
   4. Sporadic or infrequent arrhythmias can be studied with 24-hour ambulatory monitoring (Holter) or transtelephonic ECG transmission.
   5. If P waves are poorly seen on ECG, passage of an esophageal electrode can clarify atrial activity.
   6. Complicated, drug-refractory, or potentially serious arrhythmias may require electrophysiology study (EPS) with intracardiac catheters, which record electrical activity directly from the atrium, ventricle, and His-Purkinje system.
C. Diagnosis and treatment. Arrhythmias in an asymptomatic patient with a normal heart are generally benign. An arrhythmia should be diagnosed slowly and carefully, and should be judged to be an acute or potential danger to a patient before **any** drug therapy is undertaken. The toxicity and side effect profiles of antiarrhythmic agents are generally high (see sec. **VII**).
   1. Classification of arrhythmias
      a. Premature beats (atrial or ventricular)
      b. Tachycardias
         (1) Narrow QRS complex (supraventricular tachycardia)
         (2) Wide QRS complex (ventricular or complex supraventricular tachycardia)
      c. Bradycardias
         (1) Depressed pacemaker activity
         (2) Conduction block
   2. Premature beats
      a. Atrial premature beats (APBs) may be an incidental finding in normal infants or children. If frequent, or if the patient is symptomatic, consider myopathy, hyperthyroidism, or the presence of an abnormal conduction pathway.
         (1) Diagnosis. Early beats with QRS similar to sinus beats, preceded by an abnormal P wave, followed by a noncompensatory pause
         (2) Treatment. Not necessary in absence of underlying pathology
      b. Junctional premature beats (JPBs) are quite rare and usually benign. Considerations are the same as for APBs.
         (1) Diagnosis. Early beat with QRS similar to sinus beat, without preceding P wave
         (2) Treatment. Generally not indicated
      c. Ventricular premature beats (VPBs) are not uncommon in healthy normal patients, but could be a manifestation of serious cardiac pathology. Evaluation by a cardiologist is recommended for all children with VPBs.
         (1) Evaluation includes history and physical examination, ECG, chest x-ray, and, most often, Holter monitoring and echocardiogram.
         (2) Diagnosis. Wide bizarre QRS without a preceding P wave, usually followed by a full compensatory pause. Must be differentiated from APBs, which conduct to the ventricle with aberration
         (3) Grading of VPBs. Benign VPBs tend to be infrequent, of one morphology, and suppressed with exercise. If the VPBs are frequent,

multiform, or occur as couplets or runs of ventricular tachycardia, serious pathology is more likely to be present.

(4) Treatment. The goal in treating VPBs is not to suppress every ectopic beat, but to prevent degeneration to ventricular tachycardia or fibrillation.

(a) Acute suppression. Give IV lidocaine bolus (1.0 mg/kg); follow by infusion (10–50 μg/kg/min).

(b) Chronic suppression therapy should be chosen after consultation with a cardiologist, using agents such as beta blockers, quinidine, procainamide, and phenytoin (Dilantin).

3. Narrow complex tachycardia

a. General considerations

(1) Narrow complex tachycardias have a QRS morphology similar or identical to normal sinus rhythm.

(2) Narrow complex tachycardias include most, but not all, supraventricular tachycardias (SVTs) (some SVTs have a wide QRS complex).

(3) Narrow complex tachycardias are relatively well tolerated (at least acutely).

b. Sinus tachycardia (ST) is a normal response to fever, stress, dehydration, and anemia, but can be exaggerated at times and confused with a primary arrhythmia.

(1) Diagnosis. Normal P wave preceding each QRS; some variability in rate

(2) Treatment. Correct underlying cause.

c. Automatic ectopic atrial tachycardia (EAT) is an uncommon, but potentially serious, arrhythmia in children, caused by enhanced automaticity of a portion of atrial tissue

(1) Evaluation. Includes ECG and x-ray. A cardiac consult is suggested to evaluate for myopathy and congestive failure.

(2) Diagnosis. Rapid atrial rate of 160–240 per minute, with unusual (ectopic) P wave; variable rate depending on activity; occasionally with blocked conduction of some beats to the ventricle

(3) Treatment

(a) Often difficult! Cardioversion is **not effective.**

(b) Digoxin and beta blockers will slow the ventricular rate and occasionally stop the atrial tachycardia.

(c) Other drugs (e.g., amiodarone) may be needed if congestive failure is present.

(d) Ablation of the abnormal focus with surgery or catheter techniques can be employed in refractory cases.

d. Atrial fibrillation rarely occurs in a normal heart; if suspected, a cardiac consult is recommended.

(1) Evaluation. Consider myocarditis, valvular heart disease, hypertrophic myopathy, hyperthyroidism, and Wolff-Parkinson-White (WPW) syndrome.

(2) Diagnosis. The ECG shows irregular, rapid, low-amplitude atrial activity with a variable and irregular ventricular response. The QRS is normal, although occasional aberrant beats can occur (Ashman's phenomenon).

(3) Treatment

(a) If atrial fibrillation presents for more than a few days, anticoagulation is needed before converting rhythm, to minimize the risk of embolization of atrial clots.

(b) Digoxin will increase atrioventricular (AV) block and slow rate. Occasionally, digoxin will convert fibrillation.

(c) Quinidine or procainamide is often effective in converting atrial fibrillation, and they are good long-term maintenance drugs.

(d) Synchronized cardioversion will convert most cases.

e. Atrial flutter, like atrial fibrillation, is uncommon in a normal heart, and pathology should be expected.

  (1) Diagnosis. ECG reveals regular atrial "sawtooth" waves at rates of 250–350 per minute, best seen in leads 2, 3 avF. Conduction to the ventricle can vary (1 : 1, 2 : 1, etc.). The diagnosis is often hard during the 2 : 1 flutter, because every other flutter wave may be hidden in the QRS.

  (2) Treatment

   (a) Digoxin is effective in titrating the degree of AV block and in controlling the ventricular response rate. Rarely, digoxin will convert atrial flutter.

   (b) Quinidine and procainamide will frequently convert atrial flutter. If use of these drugs is contemplated, the patient should be **fully digitalized first,** because both drugs can acutely increase the ventricular response rate to flutter.

   (c) Synchronized cardioversion is almost always successful in converting atrial flutter.

   (d) Overdrive pacing with an esophageal or intracardiac pacing wire is frequently successful in terminating atrial flutter.

   (e) Maintenance therapy against recurrence can be accomplished with digoxin, beta blockers, or a quinidine/digoxin combination.

f. AV node reentry is a common narrow complex SVT mechanism, accounting for about one quarter of cases in children. Because a normal AV node frequently has dual pathways, an appropriately timed APB can cause reentry within the node.

  (1) Evaluation. AV node reentry usually occurs in otherwise normal hearts. It is well tolerated acutely, although hypotension and failure can occur if AV node reentry persists for many hours.

  (2) Diagnosis. The tachycardia rate is **strictly regular,** with normal QRS morphology. The P wave occurs quickly after the QRS (is sometimes buried in the QRS) and is inverted (retrograde P wave) in leads 2, 3 avF.

  (3) Treatment. The SVT due to AV node reentry is generally easy to convert. Enhancement of vagal tone will slow conduction within the AV node and frequently break the tachycardia. Carotid sinus massage, Valsalva maneuver, induced gag, or the application of ice to the face is effective. Ocular compression should be avoided because of reported retinal detachment.

   (a) If vagal maneuvers are not successful, intravenous **adenosine,** given by rapid push at a dose of 0.1 mg/kg, is highly effective for this disorder. The drug can be repeated at 0.2 mg/kg if the first dose fails.

   (b) Alternate drug therapy with digoxin (any age) or verapamil (over age 1 year) can be used.

   (c) Esophageal or intracardiac overdrive pacing is very effective in converting AV node reentry.

   (d) Immediate synchronized cardioversion is indicated in any patient with acute decompensation from this tachyarrhythmia.

g. Wolff-Parkinson-White syndrome refers to the presence of an accessory AV conduction pathway outside the AV node. The accessory connection can be located anywhere along the right or left AV groove. Patients with WPW may be asymptomatic, but often present with tachyarrhythmias. Congenital heart disease (particularly Ebstein's disease) is fairly common.

  (1) Mechanisms of arrhythmia in WPW include narrow QRS complex reentry SVT ("orthodromic"), atrial flutter, atrial fibrillation, and wide QRS complex reentry SVT ("antidromic").

  (2) Diagnosis. The sinus rhythm ECG of a patient with WPW reveals a short P-R interval and a slurred upstroke on the QRS (delta wave).

The ECG in tachycardia is variable, depending on the SVT mechanism. In children, orthodromic reentry (antegrade conduction over normal AV node, and retrograde conduction over the "Kent bundle") is most common, and presents a picture similar to that of AV node reentry.

(3) **Treatment** of tachyarrhythmias in WPW depends on the SVT mechanism and **must be approached with some caution.**

  (a) **Digitalis** and **verapamil** can speed up conduction over the Kent bundle in some patients, and, if atrial flutter or atrial fibrillation is present, serious acceleration in ventricular rate and ventricular arrhythmias can occur. Because atrial fibrillation is quite uncommon in infants with WPW, digoxin is sometimes used safely in the first year of life.

  (b) If the presenting arrhythmia is a **narrow QRS** tachycardia ("orthodromic reentry"), intravenous **adenosine** is the preferred initial agent if vagal maneuvers fail.

  (c) If the presenting arrhythmia has a **wide QRS** complex, one must be alert to the possibility that atrial flutter or fibrillation is present. In this setting, intravenous **procainamide or electrical cardioversion** is the preferred treatment.

  (d) For chronic therapy in WPW syndrome, oral agents, such as **beta blockers, quinidine, flecainide,** and **amiodarone,** can be used after consultation with a cardiologist.

  (e) If arrhythmia control is poor in a WPW patient, intracardiac electrophysiologic studies are indicated. The bypass tract can be localized, and acute drug testing can be tried to find an efficacious regimen.

  (f) Recently, effective therapy for difficult cases of WPW syndrome has become possible with **transcatheter ablation** of the abnormal pathway with radiofrequency energy, in both adults and children.

4. **Wide complex tachycardia**
  a. **General considerations**
    (1) **Patients presenting in wide QRS (>0.12 sec) tachycardia should be treated as an emergency.**
    (2) Differential diagnosis includes some complex SVT (from WPW syndrome or due to aberration), but ventricular tachycardia (VT) is a most important consideration.
    (3) Whenever one is unsure of the mechanism, the diagnosis is **VT until proved otherwise!**
  b. **Ventricular tachycardia** is generally associated with severe congenital or acquired heart disease.
    (1) **Diagnosis.** The ECG reveals rapid wide bizarre QRS complexes at regular rapid rates. Often the atrial rhythm is independent of the VT, and P waves can be seen to "march" through.
    (2) **Acute treatment.** Any hypotensive or unresponsive patient should be treated **immediately** with synchronized electrical cardioversion. Thereafter, sinus rhythm can be maintained with IV lidocaine, procainamide, and/or bretylium.
    (3) **Long-term management.** Response to drugs can be evaluated with serial Holter monitoring or electrophysiologic studies with intracardiac catheters. Drugs commonly used for long-term therapy include procainamide, quinidine, disopyramide, Dilantin, and beta blockers. Second-line agents include mexiletine, tocainide, amiodarone, and flecainide.

5. **Bradycardia due to depressed pacemaker activity**
  a. **Sinus bradycardia** is rarely a primary cardiac disorder and more often is associated with increased vagal tone, hypoxia, central nervous system (CNS) disorder, hypothyroidism, hypothermia, or drug intoxication. It is a normal finding in healthy athletic teenagers.

(1) **Diagnosis.** The ECG reveals a normal P wave with normal AV conduction at rates less than 100 beats per minute in neonates or less than 60 beats per minute in older children. Escape rhythms of atrial or junctional origin may be seen.

(2) **Treatment.** No intervention is necessary if cardiac output is maintained. If needed, atropine, 0.01 mg/kg IV, will increase rate by reducing vagal tone.

b. **Sick sinus syndrome** refers to profound sinus node dysfunction, often with bursts of SVT (tachy-brady syndrome), seen most often several years following open heart surgery.

(1) **Diagnosis.** The ECG reveals slow atrial or junctional rhythm with often abrupt pauses. Episodic SVT (e.g., atrial fibrillation or flutter) can occur.

(2) **Treatment.** No acute treatment is required unless the patient is symptomatic. Bradycardia can be handled acutely with atropine, but long-term management necessitates a pacemaker implant. If SVT episodes occur, a pacemaker is necessary before beginning antiarrhythmic medications.

6. **Bradycardia due to conduction block**

a. **First-degree heart block** is associated with increased vagal tone, digitalis and beta blocker administration, inflammatory disease involving the conduction system, and congenital heart disease (especially atrial septal defects, endocardial cushion defects, corrected transposition).

(1) **Diagnosis.** The ECG reveals a P-R interval that is prolonged for age: approximately 0.15 second in an infant, 0.18 second in a child, and >0.20 second in an adult.

(2) **Treatment.** None necessary

b. **Second-degree heart block** refers to episodic interruption of AV conduction of one beat's duration.

(1) **Diagnosis**

(a) **Mobitz type 1 (Wenckebach) block** consists of a regular P wave with progressive prolongation of P-R interval and ultimately a dropped QRS. The R-R interval shortens progressively during a Wenckebach sequence, causing "grouped beating" of the QRS.

(b) **Mobitz type II block** has regular P waves, a typically normal or constant P-R interval, and an abrupt and unpredictable dropped QRS.

(2) **Treatment** for either form of second-degree heart block is generally unnecessary in the absence of symptoms. Progression to third-degree heart block can occur, and close monitoring is needed in select patients.

c. **Third-degree (complete) heart block** may be congenital or acquired in children and associated with inflammatory processes or structural heart disease (corrected transposition or endocardial cushion defects). Acquired heart block occurs occasionally following cardiac surgery.

(1) **Evaluation**

(a) Complete heart block in a **fetus** or **newborn** suggests congenital heart disease or possible inflammation secondary to maternal connective tissue disease (particularly systemic lupus erythematosus [SLE]). All such infants should be evaluated with an echocardiogram, and maternal serum testing for antinuclear antibody (ANA) should be performed.

(b) **Older children** likewise should be screened for structural cardiac defects and inflammatory disease including endocarditis and vasculitis.

(2) **Diagnosis.** The ECG reveals a normal P-wave rate that is independent of the slower escape mechanism. The escape rhythm may be a narrow QRS complex junctional rhythm (suggesting a block in an AV node or the proximal His-Purkinje system) or a wide QRS complex ventricular rhythm (suggesting a distal His-Purkinje block).

(3) **Treatment** for complete heart block involves pacemaker implantation, and the decision to pace is based on the cause of the conduction defect, the presence or absence of symptoms, and the rate and stability of the escape rhythm.

    (a) **Congenital complete heart block** in the absence of structural heart disease is usually well tolerated in children. Pacing is reserved for symptomatic patients, those with wide QRS complex escape rhythms, and any patient with associated ventricular arrhythmias.

    (b) **Postoperative acquired complete heart block** is generally an indication for pacing.

    (c) **Acquired heart block** can be managed acutely with IV atropine, isoproterenol infusion, or temporary transvenous pacing.

    (d) Permanent pacemakers are inserted transvenously in older children. Epicardial wires are placed via a thoracotomy in infants or in any patient with right-to-left intracardiac shunts.

    (e) Current technology allows a variety of pacing modalities. The ventricle alone can be paced (ventricular demand) or the pacemaker can be connected to both atrium and ventricle, thus allowing pacing and sensing in both chambers (AV sequential pacing).

VII. Antiarrhythmic therapy

  A. Classification of antiarrhythmic drugs is based on the mechanism of drug action at the cellular level. Only those agents in common use for the pediatric population are discussed here.

    1. Type I agents are local anesthetics and act on the fast sodium current. They are subdivided based on their cardiac cell action potential effects as follows:

      a. Type IA: quinidine, procainamide, disopyramide

      b. Type IB: lidocaine, Dilantin, tocainide, mexiletine

      c. Type IC: flecainide

    2. Type II agents are beta-adrenergic blockers; propranolol is the prototype.

    3. Type III agents are unique drugs that prolong action potential repolarization; amiodarone is the prototype.

    4. Type IV agents are calcium-channel blockers, which act primarily on cells with slow calcium-channel characteristics such as the AV node; verapamil is the prototype.

    5. Digoxin and adenosine are classified separately.

  B. Digoxin

    1. General considerations

      a. Although many digitalis glycosides are available, digoxin (isolated from *Digitalis lanata*) is the formulation of choice for infants and children.

      b. A relatively narrow gap exists between optimal therapeutic doses and toxicity. **Care must be taken when digoxin dosage is ordered;** avoidable disasters have occurred because of a misplaced decimal point!

    2. Indications

      a. Control of ventricular rate in atrial fibrillation or atrial flutter

      b. SVT (non-WPW)

      c. Indirectly, for arrhythmias secondary to CHF

    3. Electrophysiology and ECG effects

      a. Digoxin acts directly on cardiac cells and indirectly through the CNS.

      b. Digoxin slows sinus node automaticity and prolongs the AV node refractory period to account for the prominent ECG effects of sinus slowing and increased P-R interval.

      c. Ventricular tissue refractory periods are decreased; the ECG may show a shortened Q-T interval and some abnormality of the S-T segment.

    4. Digoxin pharmacology

      a. Digoxin can be given PO, IM, or IV.

      b. Orally, approximately 75 percent is absorbed, with onset of action within 15–30 minutes and peak effect at 1–5 hours.

c. "Total digitalizing doses" (TDD) are generally based on estimate of oral digoxin dosages. If digoxin is given IV (100% absorbed), the TDD should be reduced 25 percent.

d. Digoxin is excreted primarily by the kidney.

5. Digoxin dosage

a. Before administration, a baseline ECG, serum electrolyte determination (particularly potassium), and some estimation of renal function are required.

b. Digoxin is administered in two stages. Initial digitalization establishes the body stores, given over 24 hours in three divided doses: ½ TDD at time 0 hours, ¼ TDD at 12 hours, and ¼ TDD at 24 hours. Maintenance therapy is then administered, which is generally calculated as ⅛ TDD q12h (thus, ¼ TDD per day).

c. Approximate total digitalizing doses (reduced 25% if IV)

(1) Premature: 0.020 mg/kg PO

(2) Full-term newborn: 0.030 mg/kg PO

(3) Under 2 years: 0.040 mg/kg PO

(4) Over 2 years: 0.030–0.040 mg/kg PO

(5) Adult: maximum of 1.0 mg total PO

d. Digoxin is not removed with dialysis or cardiopulmonary bypass. Patients with renal failure must be monitored closely if digoxin is administered.

e. Drug interaction occurs with quinidine, verapamil, and amiodarone, requiring a dosage reduction of approximately 50 percent.

6. Toxicity (see also Chap. 4)

a. Manifestations of digoxin toxicity

(1) Arrhythmias. In children, sinus bradycardia and first- or second-degree AV block are the most common arrhythmias with mild to moderate intoxication. Severe acute overdose can precipitate SVT, complete heart block, and serious ventricular arrhythmias.

(2) GI. Nausea and vomiting are common. Abdominal cramping and diarrhea can occur.

(3) CNS. Hazy or blurred vision and perceptual color disturbances (yellow and green) may occur in patients with subacute or chronic intoxication. Lethargy and fatigue may be present.

b. Treatment of intoxication

(1) Stop the drug! Oral doses of digoxin, particularly the elixir, are rapidly absorbed. Cholestyramine resins or activated charcoal can bind some digoxin in the GI tract and reduce absorption.

(2) Check electrolytes and serum digoxin level. If serum potassium is significantly low, it should be replaced slowly and carefully because sensitivity to digoxin is much increased in hypokalemic states.

(3) Lidocaine and phenytoin are often effective in treating ventricular arrhythmias induced by digoxin toxicity.

(4) Temporary transvenous pacing is indicated for a digoxin-induced, high-grade AV block.

(5) Cardioversion is risky in digoxin-toxic patients; it can precipitate ventricular fibrillation, which may be impossible to correct. It should be reserved as a last resort.

(6) A rapid and effective treatment for serious digoxin-induced rhythm disorders is digoxin-specific "Fab" antibody fragments (Digibind, Burroughs-Wellcome). IV infusion generally corrects life-threatening arrhythmias within 30 minutes.

c. Digoxin elixir is a very **pleasant-tasting** preparation, quite appealing to toddlers, and **families should be warned about the necessity for secure storage out of reach of children.**

C. Quinidine (type IA)

1. General considerations

a. Quinidine and quinine are both isolated from *Cinchona* bark. Both are antipyretic, antimalarial, and vagolytic, but only quinidine has antiarrhythmic activity. **Quinidine is a potent but potentially dangerous agent. It should be used only with careful monitoring.**

2. **Indications**
   a. In conjunction with digoxin for atrial fibrillation or flutter
   b. SVT in patients with WPW that is unresponsive to beta blockers
   c. **High-grade** ventricular ectopy or VT

3. **Electrophysiology and ECG effects**
   a. Increased effective refractory period of atrial and ventricular tissue
   b. Vagolytic effects may enhance AV conduction.
   c. In normal doses, the major ECG change is a moderate increase in Q-T interval. In sensitive or toxic patients, the QRS duration may increase, and the Q-T interval can be markedly increased (30% from baseline).

4. **Pharmacology**
   a. Quinidine is available as the sulfate (half-life 6 hr) or gluconate (half-life 8 hr).
   b. Administer by oral route only. The IV formulation can cause profound hypotension and is contraindicated.
   c. The liver and kidneys are involved in its metabolism and excretion.

5. **Dosage**
   a. An initial test dose should be given with careful ECG monitoring. If idiopathic QRS widening or profound QT prolongation occurs, the drug should be withheld.
   b. Dose for children: 15–60 mg/kg/day, divided q6h for sulfate, or q8h for gluconate

6. **Precautions and side effects**
   a. GI symptoms of nausea and diarrhea are common and may necessitate discontinuation.
   b. A small percentage of patients may experience a worsening of ventricular arrhythmias, TV (*torsades de pointes*), or both, even at therapeutic serum levels of quinidine.
   c. Hemolytic anemia and thrombocytopenia have been reported.

7. **Drug interactions**
   a. Reduces renal digoxin excretion by half
   b. Reduces hydroxycoumarin requirements
   c. Can shorten phenytoin half-life

D. **Procainamide (type IA)**
   1. **General considerations**
      a. **Procainamide** is the esterified form of procaine (synthetic local anesthetic).
      b. Like quinidine, it is a potent agent with a potentially high number of side effects. Close monitoring is required.
      c. Procainamide, unlike quinidine, can be administered IV, although some hypotension can still occur (usually reversed easily with volume expansion).
   2. **Indications**
      a. Used in conjunction with digoxin for atrial flutter or fibrillation
      b. Acute management of SVT, including WPW patients
      c. High-grade ventricular ectopy and VT
   3. **Electrophysiology and ECG effects** are similar to those of quinidine.
   4. **Pharmacology**
      a. The liver and kidneys are involved in its excretion and metabolism.
      b. Procainamide has a short half-life (3–5 hr) and requires frequent dosing. A slow-release form contained in a wax matrix is available for q6h dosing.
      c. Infants may need very large oral doses to obtain therapeutic serum levels, probably because of poor absorption.
   5. **Dosage**
      a. **IV dosage**
         (1) Infants: 7 mg/kg over 1 hour
         (2) Children: 7–15 mg/kg over 1 hour

    b. Oral dosage: 15–50 mg/kg/day, divided q4–6h

    c. Serum levels can be followed.

  6. Precautions and side effects

    a. Like quinidine, procainamide can be "proarrhythmic" and worsen ventricular arrhythmia or cause *torsades de pointes.*

    b. Drug-induced lupus syndrome is a well-recognized complication. Up to 70 percent of adult patients will develop positive serology (+ ANA), but only 30 percent develop symptoms that force discontinuation of the drug.

E. Disopyramide (type IA)

  1. General considerations

    a. Disopyramide, as a type IA agent, is similar to quinidine and procainamide. With the exception perhaps of treatment of arrhythmias in hypertrophic myopathy, it has little advantage over these other IA drugs, but it is a useful substitute if patients develop intolerable side effects to them.

    b. Depression of myocardial contractility may be slightly greater with disopyramide than with other IA agents; it should be used with caution in patients with poor ventricular function.

  2. Indications

    a. Similar to those of quinidine and procainamide

    b. Arrhythmias in patients with hypertrophic myopathy

  3. Electrophysiology and ECG effects are similar to those of quinidine and procainamide.

  4. Pharmacology and dosage

    a. For oral use only

    b. Infants: 10–20 mg/kg/day, divided q6h

    c. Children: 5–15 mg/kg/day, divided q6h

  5. Precautions and side effects

    a. Not for use in patients with depressed ventricular function

    b. As with quinidine, disopyramide may be "proarrhythmic," and careful monitoring is indicated.

    c. Anticholinergic side effects, such as dry mouth, blurred vision, and urinary retention, may occur.

F. Lidocaine (type IB)

  1. General considerations

    a. An effective IV agent, quite well tolerated even in the face of myocardial dysfunction, with few side effects at standard doses

    b. Local anesthetic

  2. Indications

    a. Acute suppression of ventricular arrhythmias

    b. Precardioversion prophylaxis against ventricular arrhythmias for patients receiving digoxin

    c. Possible predictor of response to oral IB agents (tocainide, mexiletine, Dilantin)

  3. Electrophysiology and ECG effects

    a. Lidocaine has its major effect on abnormal Purkinje and ventricular cells, where spontaneous automaticity is suppressed.

    b. ECG is unaffected.

  4. Pharmacology

    a. Lidocaine is metabolized quickly on its first pass through the liver. An IV bolus will produce an acute effect within 5 minutes, but peak levels decay after only 30 minutes. Additional boluses or constant infusion is necessary to maintain levels.

    b. Patients with hepatic dysfunction may require lower infusion rates.

  5. Dosage

    a. IV bolus, 1.0 mg/kg, can be repeated q10min for three doses.

    b. Constant infusion, 10–50 μg/kg/min.

    c. Monitor serum levels if prolonged infusion is required.

6. **Precautions and side effects**
   a. In patients with marked sick sinus syndrome or complete heart block, in which a ventricular rhythm serves as the "escape" rhythm, lidocaine is **not** indicated!
   b. At therapeutic serum levels, side effects are virtually nonexistent (although some patients may complain of mild nausea).
   c. Toxic levels can produce GI distress with nausea and vomiting, and CNS difficulties such as ataxia and seizures. Hypotension may occur at very elevated serum levels.
   d. Treatment for toxicity is to withhold the drug. Elimination is generally rapid.

G. **Phenytoin (Dilantin) (type IB)** (see also Chap. 19)
   1. **General considerations**
      a. In addition to having well-known anticonvulsant properties, phenytoin is an effective antiarrhythmic agent in select patients.
      b. Although phenytoin is classified in the same category as lidocaine based on cellular electrophysiologic effects, its clinical effects are not equivalent.
   2. **Indications**
      a. Very effective for arrhythmias due to digoxin toxicity
      b. Useful drug for late ventricular arrhythmias following repair of congenital cardiac defects (e.g., tetralogy of Fallot)
   3. **Electrophysiology and ECG effects**
      a. The antiarrhythmic effects of phenytoin in digoxin toxicity may be, at least in part, mediated through CNS effects.
      b. Cellular action is similar to that of lidocaine. As with lidocaine, minimal ECG effects occur.
      c. Phenytoin may be particularly useful in reducing ventricular arrhythmias due to "delayed after depolarizations."
   4. **Pharmacology.** Phenytoin is metabolized by the liver and excreted into the gut. There is minimal renal involvement.
   5. **Dosage** (dosage and therapeutic levels similar to anticonvulsant dosage)
      a. **IV use**
         (1) IV loading: 2.5 mg/kg over 10 minutes
         (2) Repeat q15min to total of 10 mg/kg
      b. **Oral**
         (1) Oral loading: 15 mg/kg over 24 hours, divided q6h
         (2) Maintenance: 5 mg/kg/day PO, divided q12h
      c. The GI absorption may be extremely poor in neonates and infants.
   6. **Precautions and side effects**
      a. **IV phenytoin can cause hypotension, bradycardia, and shock. IV administration is contraindicated in patients with very poor ventricular function.**
      b. Signs of toxicity include ataxia, nystagmus, vertigo, drowsiness, and respiratory depression.
      c. Hypersensitivity to the drug may be manifested by serum sickness, Stevens-Johnson syndrome, leukopenia, thrombocytopenia, and lymphoid hyperplasia.
      d. Gingival hyperplasia, megaloblastic anemia, and GI upset can occasionally occur even at therapeutic levels.

H. **Tocainide and mexiletine (type IB)**
   1. These agents have electrophysiologic properties similar to those of lidocaine, but can be given orally on a long-term basis.
   2. **Experience with these drugs in pediatrics is limited, and their use should be restricted to patients under the supervision of a cardiologist.**
   3. Nausea and CNS side effects (tremor, headache) are common.
   4. Little suppression of cardiac function. Well-tolerated drugs from hemodynamic point of view

I. **Flecainide (type IC)**

1. This agent is a potent blocker at all levels of the conductive system
2. Its use in children is still largely limited to investigational protocols.
3. Useful in suppression of ventricular arrhythmias and in prevention of SVT that is difficult to control (including WPW syndrome)
4. Moderate suppression of myocardial performance. Can worsen CHF
5. Can be "proarrhythmic." Careful monitoring is required.

J. Beta blockers (type II)
1. **General considerations.** Several beta blocker formulations are now available for routine use.
   a. **Propranolol** is still the most widely used agent, but must be taken q6–8h.
   b. Longer-acting agents (**atenolol** and **nadolol**) are useful in older children, with doses given once or twice a day.
   c. Short-acting agents (**esmolol**) can be used for acute arrhythmia management.
2. **Indications**
   a. Effective for SVT (including WPW); acts by blocking reentry circuits through AV node
   b. Useful in acute and chronic treatment of ventricular arrhythmias, including arrhythmias associated with a long Q-T interval
3. **Electrophysiology and ECG effects**
   a. At normal levels, beta blockers do not directly change cellular electrical activity. Their major action appears to be secondary to beta blockade.
   b. On the ECG, the slowing of sinus rate and a slight increase in P-R interval are noted.
   c. The heart rate response to exercise is blunted in patients receiving long-term beta blockade.
4. **Pharmacology and dosage**
   a. IV esmolol dosage: 0.5 mg/kg rapid push
   b. Oral propranolol dosage: 1–3 mg/kg/day, divided q6h
   c. IV propranolol dosage (for emergency use only): 0.025 mg/kg q15min to maximum of four doses
   d. Oral atenolol dosage: 1.0 mg/kg once a day
5. **Precautions and side effects**
   a. IV administration can cause hypotension and bradycardia. Whenever possible, oral administration is preferred.
   b. **Beta blockers are generally contraindicated in patients with asthma.**
   c. Noncardiac beta blockade side effects, such as aggravation of bronchospasm in asthmatic patients, may be reduced **somewhat** with "cardioselective" beta blockers. However, the "selectivity" is **never** absolute with any preparation.
   d. Severe hypoglycemia at times of stress can be caused by long-term beta blocker therapy.
   e. Beta blockers in combination with **verapamil** (IV or oral) are **contraindicated** because of profound additive myocardial suppression.
   f. Fatigue, depression, and decreased exercise tolerance can occur in patients taking beta blockers. However, occasional CNS side effects of fatigue and depression may be reduced **somewhat** by beta blockers with low CNS penetration.

K. Amiodarone (type III)
1. Amiodarone is a potent antiarrhythmic agent that has proved quite useful in difficult arrhythmias when all conventional medications have been unsuccessful. The side effect profile is unfortunately quite high, and the drug should be reserved for refractory life-threatening rhythm disturbances such as recurrent VT or WPW with dangerously rapid SVT.
2. Use of amiodarone in children is still largely limited to investigational protocols.
3. The pharmacology of amiodarone is not completely understood. The half-life is exceedingly long (several weeks). Giving oral loading doses for 10 days,

followed by a once-a-day maintenance dose, is the usual method of administration. In the hospital, monitoring during the loading period is generally required.

4. The ECG effects of amiodarone reflect its diffuse suppression of all elements of the conduction system. Sinus slowing, increased P-R interval, increased QRS duration, and prolongation of QT are all observed.

5. Side effects include allergic pneumonitis (can be fatal), hyperthyroidism or hypothyroidism, photosensitive skin rash, peripheral neuropathy, corneal microdeposits, hepatitis, and blue skin coloration.

L. **Verapamil (type IV)**
1. **General considerations**
   a. Calcium-channel blocking agents act primarily on the cells of the sinoatrial (SA) node and AV node. Verapamil is quite effective, therefore, in interrupting and preventing SVT, which involves the AV node in its circuit.
   b. Verapamil can speed up conduction over accessory bypass tracts in patients with WPW syndrome and should be used with caution.
   c. **Verapamil is contraindicated in children less than age 1 year.** Profound hypotension and circulatory collapse have been observed following its administration in infants.
   d. **Verapamil should never be administered to patients who are receiving quinidine or beta blockers** because of the additive myocardial suppression of the drugs.
2. **Indications**
   a. SVT, particularly AV node reentry
   b. To slow ventricular response acutely to atrial fibrillation or flutter
   c. Certain ventricular arrhythmias, which may be due to enhanced automaticity
3. **Electrophysiology and ECG effects**
   a. Decreases automaticity of sinus node and slows conduction over AV node
   b. ECG reveals sinus slowing and increased P-R interval
4. **Pharmacology and dosage**
   a. Metabolized by the liver
   b. IV administration of verapamil is usually effective within minutes in interrupting usual AV node reentry SVT. The dose is 0.05–0.10 mg/kg (maximum 5.0 mg) IV push. This dose can be repeated q15min three times.
   c. Oral dose is 4–15 mg/kg/day, divided q8h.
5. **Precautions and side effects**
   a. IV verapamil may cause significant hypotension, bradycardia, and AV block even in older children with good myocardial function. This problem can often be corrected acutely with the administration of IV calcium or isoproterenol, or both.
   b. Oral verapamil can worsen CHF in patients with poor ventricular function.
   c. Generally a well-tolerated drug from the noncardiac point of view. Nausea is a rare side effect.

M. **Adenosine** is a new and promising agent that is extremely effective in the acute management of SVT. It has largely replaced verapamil, digoxin, and beta blockers for this purpose.
1. **General considerations**
   a. Adenosine is an endogenous nucleoside that can produce profound but transient block of the sinus node and AV node when administered as a large rapid bolus.
   b. Because of rapid metabolism (<10 seconds) this drug must be given as close to the central circulation as possible (e.g., antecubital vein rather than a hand vein), and pushed quite rapidly, followed by a saline flush.
2. **Indications**

> **a.** Reentry SVT involving the AV node as part of the circuit (e.g., AV node reentry, orthodromic reentry in WPW syndrome)
> **b.** As a diagnostic tool (e.g., to uncover atrial flutter waves by transiently slowing AV conduction)
> **3. Dosage** is 0.1 mg/kg by rapid IV push. The dose can be doubled and repeated as a second IV push after 5 minutes. Maximum dose is 12 mg.
> **4. Side effects are few.**
> > **a.** Transient sinus bradycardia and AV block are seen, but last less than 15 seconds.
> > **b.** Patients may complain of short-lived chest pain, facial flushing, shortness of breath, or dizziness.

N. Cardioversion is the use of a synchronized, direct-current shock applied to the heart to convert certain arrhythmias to normal sinus rhythm.

> **1. Indications**
> > **a. Atrial fibrillation.** Immediate cardioversion is indicated if atrial fibrillation is of short duration, if a rapid ventricular rate cannot be controlled, or if hemodynamic compromise exists. When cardioversion is elective, patients should receive anticoagulant therapy with a coumarin derivative before cardioversion. Cardioversion may be unsuccessful in restoring normal sinus rhythm in patients with an enlarged left atrium (e.g., mitral stenosis).
> > **b. Atrial flutter** converts often at low energy levels (0.5 watt-sec/kg). For this condition, cardioversion should be performed as an emergency procedure only in hemodynamically compromised patients; otherwise, cardioversion can be performed electively.
> > **c. Supraventricular tachycardia vagotonic** maneuvers and medical therapy should be used initially unless hypotension or CHF is present. Energy settings of 0.25–0.5 watt-sec/kg should be sufficient. Prophylactic lidocaine is often given for patients receiving digoxin.
> > **d. Ventricular tachycardia.** Cardioversion is the treatment of choice for sustained VT. During preparation for cardioversion, a bolus of IV lidocaine (1–2 mg/kg) can be given. Cardioversion is usually accomplished with 1–2 watt-sec/kg.
> > **e. Ventricular fibrillation.** Immediate cardioversion with an **unsynchronized** discharge at an energy level of 2–6 watt-sec/kg is required for ventricular fibrillation in children (see Chap. 3).
> **2. Contraindications** include sinus tachycardia, digitalis-induced arrhythmias, multifocal or automatic atrial tachycardia, complete AV block, and the supraventricular arrhythmias associated with hyperthyroidism. Patients with sick sinus syndrome should have a temporary pacing wire placed before cardioversion.
> **3. Techniques.** One must be prepared for complications, and **the procedure should only be done in an intensive care unit.** Cardioversion should be performed at the lowest possible energy level to minimize complications.
> > **a.** Analgesia should be obtained with IV administration of a short-acting barbiturate such as methohexital (Brevital, 0.5–1.0 mg/kg as a bolus in a 1% solution) or diazepam (0.25 mg/kg IV). Use of these drugs for elective cardioversion should only be done in an intensive care unit with an anesthesiologist in attendance. The child should be preoxygenated before the procedure. When the patient's lid reflex is lost, cardioversion can be attempted.
> > **b.** The cardioverter should be synchronized on the R wave to avoid the ventricular vulnerable period. **For treating ventricular fibrillation, the synchronizing switch must be turned off.**
> > **c.** The electrode paddles should be liberally covered with conductive paste and placed in the second right intercostal space and the fifth left interspace in the anterior axillary line in older children and adults, or in the third space in the parasternal area and below the left scapula in younger children.

d. Postconversion arrhythmias are not uncommon and include APBs, VPBs, and delayed recovery of the SA node, manifested by slow junctional rhythm or sinus bradycardia. Occasionally, these must be treated. Lidocaine (IV), atropine (IV), and isoproterenol (IV) should be drawn up in advance, accessible for rapid delivery if necessary.

10

Gastroenterology
John D. Snyder

I. **General principles**
A. **Nutrition**
   1. **Assessment**
      a. **Height and weight** (specifically the following indices):
         (1) Weight/age
         (2) Height/age
         (3) Weight/height (see Chap. 2, p. 13)
      b. **Anthropometrics**
         (1) Triceps skin fold
         (2) Arm circumference
         (3) Head circumference
      c. **Blood tests**
         (1) Complete blood count (CBC) with lymphocyte count
         (2) Purified protein derivative (PPD) and *Candida* (skin tests)
         (3) Total protein, albumin, transferrin, and globulins
         (4) Liver function tests and alkaline phosphatase
         (5) Iron and total iron-binding capacity
         (6) Minerals
      d. **Urine tests**
         (1) Creatinine and creatinine/height index (*Pediatrics* 46:696, 1970)
         (2) Nitrogen
         (3) Minerals
   2. **Diets** prescribed for the management of a specific nutritional deficiency can be obtained by writing to the Nutrition Department at The Children's Hospital Medical Center, Boston, MA 02115. For patients in whom the oral route is not appropriate, nasogastric (NG) or nasojejunal feedings are indicated, utilizing elemental formulas (Table 10-1). Indications for the selection of enteral formulas are found in Table 10-2.
   3. **Therapy**
      a. **General approach.** Remember that patience is an important principle in the management of malnourished patients. The following measures are suggested:
         (1) Correct fluid and electrolyte disorders (hyponatremia, hyposmolality, acidosis, hypomagnesemia, hypokalemia, hypophosphatemia). Watch for the development of hypophosphatemia.
         (2) Therapy for infections
         (3) **Protein load.** Start with 1 gm/kg/day and increase as tolerated.
         (4) **Caloric load**
            (a) For *severely malnourished children,* start with 50 kcal/kg/day, and increase by 25 kcal/kg/day every 2–3 days as tolerated.
            (b) For **mild to moderate malnutrition,** start with 80–100 calories/kg/day.
         (5) Formulas without lactose or sucrose to prevent diarrhea secondary to disaccharidase insufficiency may be needed.

Table 10-1. Enteral hyperalimentation chart

	General				Milk-base	
	Formula 2	Compleat	Vitaneed	Meritene	Instant breakfast	Nutri 1000
Calories/ml	1	1.07	1	1	1.05	1
Carbohydrate source	Lactose, sucrose	Hydrolyzed cereal solids, fruit, vegetables, maltodextrin, lactose	Corn syrup solids, maltodextrin	Lactose, corn syrup, sucrose	Sucrose, corn syrup, lactose	Sucrose, lactose, corn syrup solids
Protein source	Wheat, beef, egg, milk	Beef, skim milk	Beef caseinate	Skim milk, sodium caseinate	Nonfat milk, sodium caseinate, soy protein	Skim milk
Fat source	Egg yolk, corn oil, beef fat	Corn oil, beef fat	Soy oil, soy lecithin	Corn oil	Whole milk	Corn oil
Protein (gm/liter)	38	43	35	58	57	40
Fat (gm/liter)	40	43	40	32	31	55
Carbohydrate (gm/liter)	123	128	130	110	134	101
mOsm/kg	435/510	405	400	505	500	500
Na/K (mEq/liter)	26/45	56/36	24/32	38/41	42/71	23/39
Residue	High	High	High	Medium	Medium	Medium
Vitamin content	Yes	Yes	Yes	Yes	Yes	Yes
Producer	Cutter	Sandoz	Organon	Doyle	Carnation	Cutter
Flavors	Orange	Natural flavor	Natural flavor	Varied	Varied	Chocolate, vanilla
Form	Ready to use	Ready to use	Ready to use	Ready to use	Powder	Ready to use
Uses/features	Blenderized tube feeding, requires digestion and absorption	Blenderized tube feeding, requires digestion and absorption	Blenderized tube feeding, requires digestion and absorption, low Na, lactose free	High protein, supplemental, tube feeding, requires digestion and absorption	Supplemental, easily available, requires digestion and absorption	Supplemental, tube feeding, requires digestion and absorption

Table 10-1. (continued)

	Sustacal	Pediasure	Lactose free					
			Isocal	Osmolite	Ensure	Ensure Plus	Enrich
Calories/ml	1	1	1.06	1.06	1.06	1.5	1.1
Carbohydrate source	Sucrose, corn syrup	Sucrose, hydrolyzed corn starch	Maltodextrins	Hydrolyzed corn starch	Corn syrup, sucrose	Corn syrup, sucrose	Hydrolyzed corn starch, sucrose, soy polysaccharide
Protein source	Calcium and sodium caseinate, soy protein isolates	Sodium caseinate, low-lactose whey	Calcium and sodium caseinate, soy protein isolates	Calcium and sodium caseinate, soy protein isolates	Sodium and calcium caseinate, soy protein isolates	Sodium and calcium caseinate, soy protein isolates	Sodium and calcium caseinate, soy isolate
Fat source	Partially hydrogenated soy oil	Partially hydrogenated soybean oil	Soy oil, MCT oil	MCT oil, corn oil, soy oil	Corn oil	Corn oil	Corn oil
Protein (gm/liter)	61	30	34	37	37	55	40
Fat (gm/liter)	23	49	44	38	37	53	37
Carbohydrate (gm/liter)	140	110	133	145	145	200	162
mOsm/kg	625	325	300	300	450	600	480
Na/K (mEq/liter)	41/53	16/33	23/34	24/26	37/40	49/54	37/40
Residue	Low	Low	Low	Low	Low	Low	High
Vitamin content	Yes	Yes	Yes	Yes	Yes	Yes	Yes
Producer	Mead Johnson	Ross	Mead Johnson	Ross	Ross	Ross	Ross
Flavors	Varied	Varied	Unflavored	Unflavored	Varied	Varied	Vanilla, chocolate
Form	Ready to use	Ready to use	Ready to use	Ready to use	Ready to use	Ready to use	Ready to use
Uses/features	High protein, supplemental, tube feeding, requires digestion and absorption	Supplemental, lactose, gluten and cholesterol free, lactose free	Tube feeding, requires digestion and absorption, low sodium, lactose free	Supplemental, tube feeding, lactose free, low sodium, requires absorption	Supplemental, tube feeding, lactose free, requires digestion and absorption	Supplemental, tube feeding, lactose free, requires digestion and absorption	Tube or oral feeding with fiber, lactose free, requires digestion and absorption

Chemically defined formulas

	Reabilan HN	Vital HN	Vivonex TEN	Nutramigen	Portagen	Pregestimil	Alimentum
Calories/ml	1.33	1	1	0.67	0.67	0.67	0.67
Carbohydrate source	Maltodextrin, tapioca, starch	Hydrolyzed corn starch, sucrose	Maltodextrin	Corn syrup solids	Corn syrup solids	Corn syrup	Sucrose modified tapioca
Protein source	Casein and whey peptides	Whey, soy, and meat protein; hydrolysate; free essential amino acids	Free amino acids	Hydrolyzed casein	Sodium caseinate	Hydrolyzed casein	Casein hydrolysate
Fat source	Soybean oil	Sunflower oil, MCT oil	Safflower oil	Corn oil	MCT oil 85%, corn oil 12%, soy lecithin 12%	Corn oil 20%, MCT oil 60%, safflower oil 20%, soy oil	MCT oil, safflower oil
Protein (gm/liter)	58	42	38	19	24	19	24
Fat (gm/liter)	52	11	2.8	26	32	37	37
Carbohydrate (gm/liter)	158	185	206	90	80	70	70
mOsm/kg	490	460	630	320	220	320	370
Na/K (mEq/liter)	43/42	20/34	20/20	14/19	16/22	14/19	13/20
Residue	Low	Low	Low	Low	Low	Low	Low
Vitamin content	Yes	Yes	Yes	Yes	Yes	Yes	Yes
Producer	O'Brien	Ross	Norwich Eaton	Mead Johnson	Mead Johnson	Mead Johnson	Ross
Flavors	Unflavored	Varied	Varied				
Form	Liquid	Powder	Powder	Powder	Powder	Powder	Powder
Uses/features	Supplemental, tube feeding, lactose free	Supplemental, tube feeding, absorbed in upper gut, low sodium	Supplemental, tube feeding, lactose free, no pancreatic stimulus, absorbed in upper gut	Supplemental, tube feeding, lactose free, isotonic, absorbed in upper gut	Supplemental, tube feeding, lactose free, hypotonic, absorbed in upper gut, fat malabsorption	Supplemental, tube feeding, lactose free, isotonic, absorbed in upper gut	Supplemental, tube feeding, lactose free, isotonic, absorbed in upper gut

Table 10-1. (continued)

	Special formulation				Caloric additives				
	TraumaCal	Pulmocare	Microlipid	Citrotein	Polycose (powder)	Polycose (liquid)	Sumacal	Corn oil	MCT oil
Calories/ml	1.5	1.5	4.5	0.66	3.8/kg/gm	2	3.8	8.4	7.7
Carbohydrate source	Corn syrup, sucrose	Sucrose, corn starch		Sucrose, maltodextrin	Hydrolysis of corn starch	Hydrolysis of corn starch	Maltodextrins		
Protein source	Sodium and calcium caseinate	Sodium and calcium caseinate		Egg albumin					
Fat source	Soy oil, MCT oil	Corn oil	Safflower oil, soy lecithin	Soy oil				Corn oil	Fractionated coconut oil
Protein (gm/liter)	83	60		41					
Fat (gm/liter)	68	92	50	2					
Carbohydrate (gm/liter)	143	106		122					
mOsm/kg	490	520	32	405	570	680		930	930
Na/K (mEq/liter)	51/36	57/49		31					
Residue	Low	Low	Low	Low	Low	Low	Low	Low	Low
Vitamin content	No	Yes	No	Yes	No	No	No	No	No
Producers	Mead Johnson	Ross	Sherwood	Sandoz	Ross	Ross	Sherwood	Organon	Mead Johnson
Flavors	Varied	Vanilla	Unflavored	Punch	Unflavored	Unflavored	Cherry, lemon, lime		
Forms	Ready to use	Ready to use	Ready to use	Powder	Powder	Liquid	Ready to use	Oil	Oil
Uses/features	Supplemental, tube feeding, high protein needs	Lower carbohydrate content to reduce CO_2 production, high caloric density, vitamins and minerals	Supplemental, pure fat emulsion, low osmolarity, low electrolytes, lactose free	Supplemental, lactose free	Supplemental, lactose free	Supplemental, lactose free	Supplemental, lactose free	Excellent source of linoleic acid, readily available	Lipase and bile salts not necessary for digestion and absorption

Table 10-2. Indications for selecting enteral formulas

Conditions	Formula description	Suggested formulas Infants	Suggested formulas Older children
Supplemental caloric needs (normal functioning intestine)	Nutritionally complete		Carnation Instant Breakfast Meritene
Lactose intolerance	Lactose free	Isomil Nursoy Prosobee	Citrotein Enrich Ensure Isocal Osmolite
Abnormal nutrient digestion and absorption with starch, lactose, or sucrose malabsorption	Hydrolized protein, MCT oil, and glucose	Pregestimil	Vivonex TEN
Severe steatorrhea (e.g., bile acid deficiency)	Contains MCT oil	Alimentum Portagen Pregestimil	Fesocal Isotein HN Osmolite Peptamen Reabilan HN Tracemocal Travasorb (HN) Vital HN Vivonex TEN
Pulmonary compromise	High-fat formulation		Pulmocare
Increased protein needs	High-protein formulation		TraumaCal
Complete formula with fiber			Enrich Jevity
Caloric additives		Corn oil (fat) MCT oil (fat) Polycose (glucose) Sumacal (glucose)	Same as for infants

(6) If the infant is anorectic, nasogastric feeding should be considered.

(7) Vitamin and mineral supplementation

b. Total parenteral nutrition (TPN). *Intravenous alimentation* is delivery of a mixture of hypertonic dextrose and crystalline amino acid solutions utilizing a central high-flow vein. This method should be used if the enteral route is not possible. IV alimentation should be used in all patients who will be allowed nothing PO for 2 weeks or more. Periods of poor intake from 2–3 days to 2 weeks should be managed with peripheral IV alimentation.

(1) Nitrogen sources are generally provided as either protein hydrolysate or a mixture of pure crystalline amino acids. The usual daily requirement of each is 2–4 gm/kg in infants and children. The bulk of the caloric content of hyperalimentation fluid is derived from glucose. The amount required in most infants is 25–30 gm/kg/day. The rest of the metabolic needs (i.e., water, electrolytes, minerals, and vitamins) are provided in the customary amounts.

(2) **Intralipid** (soybean oil), a fat emulsion that provides 1.1 calories/ml (10% solution) or 2.0 calories/ml (20% solution) is necessary to prevent essential fatty acid deficiency and should be given as 5–10 percent of the total calories. The following are the recommended rates:
   (a) 5–10 ml/kg for the first 10 kg
   (b) 2.5–5.0 ml/kg for second 10 kg
   (c) 1.25–2.5 ml/kg for all weights above 20 kg. The maximum infusion is 4 gm/kg/day. It is inadvisable to begin administering Intralipid at the same time as other parenteral nutrition solutions.
(3) **Caloric densities utilized:**
   (a) Amino acids, 3.33 calories/ml
   (b) 10% dextrose, 0.34 calories/ml
   (c) 20% dextrose, 0.68 calories/ml
   (d) 30% dextrose, 1.02 calories/ml
   (e) PN 10, 0.39 calories/ml
   (f) PN 20, 0.73 calories/ml
(4) **Peripheral hyperalimentation** is usually administered as a 10% glucose solution with 2% protein that contains water, electrolytes, minerals, and vitamins. If given at a rate of 150 ml/kg/day, 50 calories/kg/day are supplied, which is sufficient to prevent a negative nitrogen balance.
(5) **Indications for TPN.** Any patient who is unable to maintain nutrition adequate for metabolic needs is a candidate for TPN. Some specific disease states in which TPN is employed include chronic diarrheal states, inflammatory bowel disease with growth failure or fistulas, postoperative status, chronic pancreatitis and pseudocyst, short-bowel syndrome, and esophageal injury.
(6) **Management of hyperalimentation program**
   (a) A central venous catheter is placed and its position checked radiographically.
   (b) A 10% glucose solution is given IV as maintenance fluid (see Chap. 7, p. 201). Adequate electrolytes should be provided. Continue the infusion for 12–24 hours.
   (c) A 20% glucose–amino acid solution is then given as maintenance fluid for 12 hours.
   (d) The infusion rate is increased approximately 10 percent q12h until fluid intake is 135 ml/kg/day, *irrespective of age.* An infusate with 20% glucose and 3 gm per day of protein provides the equivalent of 110 calories/kg/day. Generally, no more than 200 ml/kg/day is used in infants. It may be necessary to decrease the protein content of the infusate at such rates.
   (e) **Intralipid infusion**
      (i) Intralipid is commonly administered by use of connector tubing (Y) proximal to the millipore filter so that Intralipid will join to the glucose–amino acid–electrolyte solution just before the infusion site.
      (ii) The initial rate of a 10% Intralipid infusion via a peripheral vein should provide 15 ml/kg/day given over 6–12 hours. If the patient's serum is not lipemic, the infusion is increased by 5 ml/kg/day until 30–40 ml/kg/day is attained.
   (f) Only multiple-lumen catheters are used to safely permit administration of parenteral nutrition *and* IV medication.
   (g) If possible, the administration of parenteral nutrition is cycled to permit infusion at night, with capping of the central venous line during the day to permit freedom of movement.
(7) **Monitoring the patient receiving TPN**
   (a) Daily weights should be measured.

(b) Intake and output and qualitative sugar and acetone are measured on all urine specimens.

(c) Sodium, potassium, chloride, blood urea nitrogen (BUN), and glucose are determined daily while increasing fluid and then weekly when fluid requirements have been reached.

(d) CBC, magnesium, calcium, phosphorus, total protein, aspartate aminotransferase (AST; SGOT), alanine aminotransferase (ALT; SGPT), lactic dehydrogenase (LDH), alkaline phosphatase, bilirubin, and creatinine are measured initially and then weekly.

(e) Copper, zinc, and iron levels are measured at the beginning of therapy and then monthly.

(f) Lipemia checks daily

(g) 24-hour urine for creatinine, Ca^{2+}, PO_4^{2+}, and Mg^{2+} is obtained every 2 weeks.

(8) Complications of TPN

(a) Infection is the most serious complication of TPN. Fungi (usually *Candida albicans*) and bacteria are the infecting agents.

    (i) Care of the central venous line must be scrupulous.

    (ii) Unexplained glycosuria may be the first clue. Several blood cultures should be obtained from the patient and from the line.

    (iii) *When sepsis is documented, the central venous line should be withdrawn if possible.*

(b) Hepatic complications.

    (i) Abnormalities in liver function test results are common during the course of TPN. Hepatomegaly with elevations of serum transferases (often to high levels), with prolongation of prothrombin time (PT) and partial thromboplastin time (PTT), may be seen, and liver biopsy reveals a fatty liver.

    (ii) Cholestatic liver disease frequently develops in premature infants.

(c) Metabolic complications

    (i) Hyperglycemia is common in septic patients, premature infants, and patients with renal disease.

    (ii) Hypoglycemia is a common and severe complication **if TPN is stopped abruptly.**

    (iii) Acidosis occurs in patients with renal compromise or prematurity when large (4 gm/kg/day) protein loads are administered.

    (iv) Hypomagnesemia may occur in patients with low endogenous magnesium stores (e.g., those with chronic diarrhea).

    (v) Hyperlipemia occurs with excess Intralipid administration.

    (vi) Hyperammonemia

    (vii) Hypocalcemia

    (viii) Carnitine and selenium deficiencies have been described.

(d) Trace metal deficiency

    (i) Copper deficiency is not uncommon and is manifested by anemia, neutropenia, and rash.

    (ii) Zinc deficiency is common and is manifested by an erythematous, maculopapular rash (acrodermatitis enteropathica) involving the face, trunk, metacarpophalangeal joints, and perineum. *Low* serum alkaline phosphatase is common.

(e) Mechanical complications

    (i) Arrhythmias may occur with an improperly placed catheter.

    (ii) Venous thrombosis is rare.

    (iii) Air embolus occurs only after accidental coupling of the IV line.

    (iv) Skin sloughs may occur from infiltration of peripheral venous infusions.

(f) Complications of Intralipid administration
(i) Bilirubin. Intralipid displaces bilirubin from albumin and is contraindicated in jaundiced infants.
(ii) Eosinophilia may be present.
(g) Contraindications to the use of Intralipid include *hyperlipemic states* and *severe liver disease*.

B. **Evaluation of gastrointestinal disease**
1. **Examination of the stool**
   a. Examine the stool for consistency, odor, blood, and mucus. The presence of gross blood and mucus indicates colitis. Use saline and Lugol's solution to look for parasites.
   b. **Clinitest to detect the presence of reducing substances**
      (1) Mix one part **fresh** stool in two parts water. (To detect sucrose intolerance, hydrolyze with 1 N HCl, boiling for 30 sec.)
      (2) Centrifuge and add 15 drops of supernatant to one Clinitest tablet.
      (3) The test is positive if 0.5 percent or more of reducing substance is present. The presence of reducing substance is *always* abnormal and indicates sucrose or disaccharide intolerance, or both.
   c. **pH**
      (1) Normal stool pH is 7–8.
      (2) A decreased pH suggests the presence of organic acids, as seen in disaccharide intolerance.
      (3) An increased pH suggests secretory diarrhea.
   d. **Hemoccult** or **guaiac test** for blood
   e. **Sudan stain for fat.** Place a representative sample on two slides. On the first slide, put two drops of 95% ethyl alcohol and several drops of Sudan black III. Place a cover slip and examine for neutral fats. On the second slide, put two to four drops of 35% acetic acid and several drops of Sudan black III. Place a cover slip, heat the slide to boil, and examine for split fats (*N. Engl. J. Med.* 264:85–87, 1961). The presence of fat (red) globules in the slide indicates a positive test. The amount of fat globules correlates with the 72-hour fecal fat assay.
   f. **Fecal leukocytes**
      (1) Stain with Loeffler's methylene blue, or Wright or Gram stains.
      (2) Infections or inflammatory processes with leukocytes include *campylobacter, salmonella,* Shigella, *typhoid fever, invasive* Escherichia coli, Clostridium difficile, *ulcerative colitis,* and *Crohn's disease.* A predominance of band forms suggests shigellosis.
   g. **Cultures for ova and parasites.** Commercially available preservative kits increase the rate of identification of parasites.
2. **Fecal fat excretion.** Although often distasteful to patient and clinician, this is the best method for detecting steatorrhea.
   a. All stools are collected for 72 hours.
   b. Because fecal fat excretion is expressed as a percentage of intake, the patient must keep a diary of food intake during this period, so that the amount of fat in the diet can be estimated. *The diet should contain at least 35 percent fat.*
   Coefficient of absorption (CA):

   $$\frac{\text{Dietary fat} - \text{fecal fat}}{\text{Dietary fat}} \times 100$$

   c. **Normal values.** (Values for breast-fed infants are lower but are not precisely known.)
   Normal CA:
      Prematures: 60–75%
      Newborns: 80–85%
      10 mo–3 yr: 85–95%
      Older than 3 yr: 95%
3. **D-Xylose excretion.** This test reflects enteric mucosal absorption. Its reliabil-

ity for detecting mucosal disease is controversial, but it remains a useful screening test.

   a. Give 14.5 gm/m^2 after an overnight fast.

   b. Measure serum xylose at 1 hour; above 25 mg/dl is normal.

   c. Delayed gastric emptying may cause falsely low levels.

4. The **breath hydrogen test** is useful for detection of lactose and sucrose malabsorption.

   a. After an overnight fast, the patient is given a loading dose of the disaccharide to be studied.

   b. A breathing mask is placed over the nose and mouth, and 3–5 ml expired air is collected in a syringe at 30-minute intervals for 3 hours.

   c. H$_2$ excretion is measured; excretion of >11 ppm H$_2$ indicates disaccharide malabsorption.

   d. False positives and false negatives may be seen due to natural or antibiotic-induced changes in bacterial flora. *No antibiotics should be administered within 1 week before the test.*

5. Jejunal biopsy is an invaluable tool for the diagnosis of intestinal mucosal disease, including gluten-sensitive enteropathy, Whipple's disease, abeta-lipoproteinemia, and agammaglobulinemia.

   a. All patients must have a platelet count, PT, and PTT before the procedure.

   b. After an overnight fast, patients over 6 months of age and under 6–7 years are premedicated with chlorpromazine (Thorazine), 1 mg/kg intramuscularly, and pentobarbital, 4 mg/kg IM. Older patients require no premedication; instead, an anesthetic spray (e.g., tetracaine [Pontocaine or Cetacaine]) is used to anesthetize the pharynx.

   c. The biopsy specimen is sent for histologic examination, assay of small intestine disaccharides, and touch prep for *Giardia.*

6. Duodenal fluid should be obtained by a nasogastric tube or at the time of biopsy. The fluid is examined for parasites, especially *Giardia lamblia,* and sent for bacterial culture (aerobic and anaerobic).

7. Sweat test. Pilocarpine iontophoresis for sweat electrolytes diagnoses cystic fibrosis in 99 percent of cases (see sec. **II.D.1.c**).

8. The Schilling test measures the ability to absorb ingested vitamin B$_{12}$. It is used to evaluate patients with pernicious anemia, ileal dysfunction syndromes, malabsorption, pancreatic insufficiency, bacterial overgrowth, and Crohn's disease.

9. Esophageal manometry is designed to evaluate the motility characteristics of the esophagus and the upper and lower esophageal sphincter pressures. It provides information in diseases such as scleroderma, achalasia, diffuse esophageal spasm, and abnormal gastroesophageal reflux.

10. Rectal manometry is designed to evaluate the relaxation and pressure of the rectal sphincters. It is very useful in the diagnosis of Hirschsprung's disease.

11. Radiologic evaluation

   a. An **upper GI series** and small bowel follow-through

   b. Barium enema

   c. Oral cholecystogram

   d. Percutaneous transhepatic **cholangiogram**

12. Nuclear medicine and ultrasound

   a. Abdominal ultrasound to evaluate liver parenchyma, biliary tree, and pancreas

   b. Technetium-99 scans for evaluation of pathologic gastroesophageal reflux, aspiration pneumonia, or gastric emptying.

   c. Hepatobiliary iminodiacetic acid (Hida) scan (or other iminodiacetic acid derivatives) for evaluation of bilirubin excretion.

   d. A liver and spleen scan to evaluate the liver and spleen size as well as filling defects

13. Endoscopy

   a. Esophagogastroduodenoscopy

      b. Proctosigmoidoscopy
      c. Colonoscopy
      d. Endoscopic retrograde cholangiopancreatography
    14. A *computed tomographic (CT)* scan and magnetic resonance imaging
II. Specific entities
   A. Malabsorption. Because fat absorption depends on all the phases of digestion, the presence of *steatorrhea* (fat malabsorption) is the best indicator of a malabsorptive defect. Further tests will permit the localization of specific sites of abnormality.

   B. Diarrheal disease. Diarrhea is among the most common symptoms in pediatrics, and in underdeveloped countries *it is the most common cause of morbidity and mortality in childhood.*

   Evaluation of chronic diarrhea includes a history, with particular attention to blood or mucus in the stools, weight loss, failure to thrive, associated symptoms (fever, recurrent infection), drugs taken (particularly antibiotics), GI surgical procedures, family history, travel, age, and race.

   A **physical examination** should attend to nutritional status, hydration, edema, protuberant abdomen, abdominal masses, muscular habitus, rectal prolapse, and affect, particularly irritability. The cardiopulmonary system and neurologic status should be carefully evaluated.

   Laboratory studies include a CBC, erythrocyte sedimentation rate (ESR), urinalysis, serum protein analysis (SPA), stool examination, and sweat test. If the results of malabsorption screening are positive, the steps listed in this subsection should be followed.

    1. Acute gastroenteritis
      a. Etiology. This common condition has many causes. These are listed in Table 10-3.
      b. Evaluation. This condition is often manifested by a sudden onset of vomiting, followed by diarrhea. It is most often self-limited. Fever may or may not be present, but with a reduction of fluid intake and abnormal losses, dehydration may occur, especially in children under 3 years of age.
        (1) History. Record the following: weight loss, duration, presence of blood or mucus, type and frequency of stools, type and amount of feedings, frequency of urination, presence or absence of tears, associated symptoms (e.g., fever, rash, vomiting, localized abdominal pain) and current family illnesses, source of water supply, attendance at a day care center, contact with animals, and travel history.
        (2) Physical examination should include measurement of vital signs, assessment of postural changes, and description of the skin turgor, mucous membranes, fontanels, eyes (presence or absence of tears), activity state, irritability, and associated rashes.
        (3) Laboratory tests can be minimized in the milder clinical states, but a stool Wright stain for neutrophils may be helpful, and urinary specific

---

Table 10-3. Common causes of acute diarrhea in childhood

Viral enteritis (e.g., rotavirus in children <2 yr)
Bacterial enteritis
   Enterotoxin associated (*Escherichia coli, cholera, Clostridium perfringens, Staphylococcus*)
   Nonenterotoxin associated* (*Salmonella, Shigella, E. coli, Yersinia*)
Parasitic enteritis (amebiasis,* giardiasis, cryptosporidiosis)
Extraintestinal infection (e.g., otitis media, urinary tract infection, sepsis)
Antibiotic induced* (*Clostridium difficile*)
Hemolytic-uremic syndrome*
Inflammatory bowel disease* (ulcerative colitis, Crohn's disease)

---

* May be associated with blood in the stool.

gravity can detect early dehydration. The yield from stool cultures is much higher when the Wright stain is positive.

c. **Therapy**

(1) Children with acute diarrheal disease and minimal to moderate dehydration are treated most effectively with **oral rehydration therapy** (ORT) (Table 10-4). In the initial vomiting stage, small volumes (5–15 ml) of ORT should be given frequently; large-volume feedings should be avoided.

(2) **Boiled skim milk has a very high osmolar load and can cause hypernatremia.** High osmolar fluids (e.g., cola, ginger ale, apple juice, chicken broth) should be avoided.

(3) Once rehydration is accomplished (usually in 8–12 hours), easily absorbed foods from the regular diet should be started, for example, rice, rice cereal, bananas, dry cereal, crackers, and toast. Lactose- and sucrose-containing fluids can be diluted 1 : 1 with water if secondary disaccharidase deficiency is present.

(4) The value of drugs such as kaolin and belladonna-containing compounds remains unproved, and their use should be discouraged. An antispasmodic such as diphenoxylate (Lomotil) or camphorated opium tincture, or loperamide (Immodium) are not recommended for use in children (*MMWR* 41:1, 1992). Even when spasm is reduced, **fluid losses continue to occur into the lumen of the gut, but are not measurable and give a false sense of security.** In toxogenic diarrhea the elimination of the toxin is also **delayed** by these agents.

(5) Antiemetics such as promethazine (Phenergan) or dimenhydrinate (Dramamine) are not recommended for vomiting associated with acute diarrhea for use in children (*MMWR* 41:1, 1992). The side effects of these drugs preclude their long-term use. If vomiting persists, more vigorous evaluation and management are indicated.

(6) Close follow-up, including daily weights, is imperative, particularly in smaller infants, who may rapidly become dehydrated.

(7) **Specific therapy for acute diarrhea**

(a) **Enterotoxigenic *E. Coli.*** Bismuth subsalicylate (Pepto-Bismol)

(b) ***Shigella* species.** Trimethoprim-sulfamethoxazole (Bactrum)

(c) **Campylobacter fetus.** Erythromycin

(d) ***Clostridium difficile.*** Vancomycin, cholestyramine

(e) ***Giardia.*** Quinacrine, metronidazole (Flagyl), bacitracin

(f) ***Entamoeba histolytica.*** Metronidazole (Flagyl)

2. **Chronic gastroenteritis.** Diarrheal symptoms lasting more than 2 weeks are chronic. The causes of chronic diarrhea are listed in Table 10-5.

a. **Nonspecific diarrhea** is the most common cause of chronic diarrhea in childhood.

(1) The **etiology** is unknown. Psychosocial and family stress is often implicated.

(2) **Evaluation and diagnosis.** The classic history is of watery diarrhea with multiple formula and dietary changes in the age group 1–5 years. The physical findings and growth are normal. The findings of

Table 10-4. Approximate electrolyte content for oral rehydration solutions

Solution	Composition of oral rehydration fluids (mmole/liter)				
	Glucose	Na	K	Citrate	Osmolality
Pedialyte (Ross)	140	45	20	10	270
Ricelyte (Mead Johnson)	70	50	25	10	200
Rehydralyte (Ross)	140	75	20	10	305
WHO solution (ORS)	111	90	20	10	310

Table 10-5. Causes of chronic diarrhea

Chronic nonspecific diarrhea (irritable bowel syndrome)
Chronic infections: *Yersinia, E. coli, Giardia, Clostridium difficile, Cryptosporidium,* small bowel overgrowth
Cystic fibrosis
Gluten-sensitive enteropathy (celiac disease)
Disaccharide deficiency (particularly lactose intolerance)
Food allergy
Inflammatory bowel disease
Immunodeficiency states (including transient hypogammaglobulinemia)
Anatomic causes
    Short-bowel syndrome
    Malrotation
    Hirschsprung's disease
Endocrine
    Hyperthyroidism
    Addison's disease
    Congenital adrenal hyperplasia
Others
    Urinary tract infections
    Acrodermatitis enteropathica
    Neuroblastoma and ganglioneuroma

routine urinalysis and stool cultures are negative. The diagnosis is based on exclusion of other causes of diarrhea.

(3) Therapy. The goal of therapy is to stop diarrhea (and to ensure that normal growth continues).

(a) The family should be reassured that the illness is not too serious.

(b) Often, past dietary manipulations may have contributed to the production of symptoms, and correction of the diet may result in relief of the diarrhea. A decrease in the intake of fructose and sucrose-containing drinks, or changing the diet, may function as a placebo.

(c) Should reassurance and dietary adjustment fail, hospitalization may be necessary. The disappearance of diarrhea during hospitalization may help convince the family of the absence of significant disease and permit the examination of psychosocial factors.

(d) Antidiarrheal medication is not indicated.

(e) X-ray contrast studies should be done when it is necessary to rule out anatomic abnormalities.

C. Peptic ulcer disease. Peptic disease is no longer a rare diagnosis in infants and children.

1. Evaluation. Vomiting is frequently seen, especially in small children, and the pain is often atypical when compared to peptic disease in adults.

a. History should focus on vomiting, abdominal distention, hematemesis, melena, poor eating, abdominal pain, relation of pain to meals, pain affecting sleep, medications, associated underlying illness, and family history.

b. A **physical examination** should include a rectal examination looking for occult blood.

c. **Laboratory studies** include a CBC, reticulocyte count, and stool examinations for occult blood. Fasting and 60-minute postprandial gastrin levels should be obtained if the Zollinger-Ellison syndrome is being considered.

d. Diagnostic procedures

(1) An upper GI series will demonstrate an ulcer in approximately 50–67 percent of cases.

(2) Fiberoptic endoscopy is the most accurate tool for diagnosing peptic ulcers.

(3) *Helicobacter pylori* should be sought on gastric antral biopsies.

2. **Treatment**

a. **Antacids.** The recommended dose is 0.5–1.0 ml/kg 1 and 3 hours after each meal and at bedtime for 4–6 weeks. Alternating aluminum- and magnesium-containing antacids may reduce the incidence of diarrhea and constipation.

b. **H₂ blockers.** Cimetidine is given in a dosage of 20–40 mg/kg over 24 hours in four divided doses with meals and at bedtime for 4–6 weeks. Ranitidine is given in a dosage of 150 mg/1.73 m² bid, but has not yet been approved for use in small children. Children with symptoms that persist longer than 6 weeks can be given a single dose of an H₂ blocker at bedtime for 3–12 months. There is no evidence that using antacids and H₂ blockers together has any advantage over using either agent alone.

c. **Surface protective agent. Sucralfate** is a nonabsorbed sulfated disaccharide, which acts locally to form a barrier for irritated mucosa. The recommended dose is 1 gm/1.73 m², given ½ hour before meals and at bedtime for 4–6 weeks.

d. **Hydrogen pump antagonist.** Omeprazole inhibits hydrogen ion production. The recommended dose is 20 mg/1.73 m² once a day.

e. **Diet.** No form of diet (including bland) has been shown to be helpful in healing ulcers or in preventing their recurrence.

D. **Cystic fibrosis and Shwachman-Diamond syndrome**

1. **Cystic fibrosis (CF)** is the most common lethal hereditary disease among whites, with an incidence of approximately 1 in 2,000 births. CF is inherited as an autosomal recessive trait, apparently due to a mutation in a single gene on chromosome 7. The gene frequency within the North American white population is 1 : 20.

a. **Etiology.** The exact defect and cause of the disease are still unknown.

b. **Clinical manifestations.** CF is clinically characterized by exocrine gland dysfunction involving the sweat, pancreatic, bronchiolar, and biliary glands. These disturbances in exocrine function result in secondary effects such as abnormal sweat electrolytes and the production of viscous secretions, leading to pancreatic insufficiency, airway obstruction, and repeated infection associated with chronic bronchiectasis and progressive pulmonary destruction, as well as liver cirrhosis. Mean life expectancy is now between 20 and 30 years. An optimistic outlook needs to be maintained and issues of adult life addressed.

(1) Gastrointestinal. There are many GI manifestations of CF, and the disease should always be considered in patients with these features.

(a) Pancreatic insufficiency occurs in 85 percent of patients with CF. These individuals usually have a history of chronic diarrhea, with foul-smelling stools and failure to thrive.

(b) Meconium ileus presents with intestinal obstruction, often associated with ileal atresia, in the immediate neonatal period in 15 percent of patients.

(c) Rectal prolapse is a common presenting feature.

(d) Meconium ileus equivalent, distal intestinal obstruction in the older child or adult, presents with abdominal pain and may be associated with intussusception.

(e) Growth failure is quite common despite current therapy.

(f) Cirrhosis of the liver develops in 15–20 percent of patients. An elevated alkaline phosphatase is often the first sign of liver

involvement. Subsequent development of portal hypertension is common.
- **(g) Diabetes mellitus.** Overt diabetes occurs in 1 percent of patients. Abnormal results on glucose tolerance tests are routinely found. Ketoacidosis is rare.
- **(h) Gastroesophageal reflux.** The incidence is increased in patients with CF.
- **(i) Pancreatitis.** Recurrent acute pancreatitis may develop in patients with residual pancreatic function.
- **(j) Gallstones** occur in nearly one third of all CF patients, although acute cholecystitis develops in only a few.

(2) Pulmonary. Pulmonary complications cause the majority of morbidity and 98 percent of nonneonatal mortality. Manifestations include the following:
- **(a) Infancy.** Cough, slight increase in the anteroposterior diameter, tachypnea, and retractions. CF often presents with the picture of bronchiolitis.
- **(b) Childhood and adolescence.** Widespread bronchial plugging and large areas of segmental lobar atelectasis are characteristic.
- **(c) Pulmonary function tests.** The findings range from normal to the pattern of obstructive lung disease.
  - **(i)** An increase in residual volume (RV) because of air trapping
  - **(ii)** A slight increase in total lung capacity (TLC) until late in the disease, when TLC is decreased by extensive pulmonary fibrosis, leading to a greatly increased RV/TLC ratio
  - **(iii)** A decrease in vital capacity
  - **(iv)** Decreased flow rates, seen first at low lung volumes
  - **(v)** Reduction in PO_2 is an early pulmonary functional change.
- **(d) Chronic pulmonary infection** is marked by thick viscous sputum that is frequently rich in *Pseudomonas aeruginosa* and *Staphylococcus aureus*. Colonization by these organisms can occur early in childhood.
- **(e) Pneumothorax** (see Chap. 3, p. 62)
- **(f) Cor pulmonale**
- **(g) Hemoptysis.** With increasing lung disease bronchial vessels enlarge, become tortuous, and are at increased risk of endobronchial hemorrhage. Massive hemorrhage (300 ml/24 hr) can be treated with bronchial artery embolization (Gelfoam).
- **(h) Reactive airway disease**
- **(i) Allergic bronchopulmonary aspergillosis (ABPA)**
- **(j) Nasal polyps**
- **(k) Chronic sinusitis**

c. Diagnosis is made by pilocarpine iontophoresis for sweat electrolytes. Sweat weight should be greater than 100 mg. A chloride level above 60 mEq/liter or a sodium level above 60 mEq/liter is abnormal. The diagnosis can now be made by testing blood for the genetic marker for CF (ΔF-508).

d. Therapy
- **(1) Treatment of GI disorder**
  - **(a) Pancreatic preparations.** All patients with cystic fibrosis who have steatorrhea (85%) require supplemental pancreatic enzymes. Although fat absorption improves with these agents, it does not return to normal. Various pancreatic preparations are available. Dose is titrated on stool frequency, degree of steatorrhea, and growth. **Excessive dosage may result in the "meconium ileus equivalent," i.e., recurrent abdominal pain, palpable fecal masses, and obstruction.** Approximate dosage schedules for pancrelipase **(Pancrease)** are the following:

Infancy	¼–½ capsule per bottle. Enzyme is mixed with some vehicle, such as applesauce, immediately before feeding.
1–3 years	1–2 capsules/meal
School age	2–5 capsules/meal, 1–3/snack
Adolescents/adults	4–7 capsules/meal, 2–4/snack

(b) Diet. Should contain 130–150 percent of normal calorie needs based on weight, age, and activity level. Fat content should not be restricted and should approximate 30 percent of total calories. If weight gain and growth are inadequate, or if significant weight is lost due to exacerbation of disease, supplemental feeding should be considered via nasogastric or gastric tube as nighttime feedings. Titrate the dose of pancreatic enzyme replacement to the usual intake of food, infant formula, or supplemental feedings to minimize steatorrhea. If GI involvement is significant in infants, a semielemental formula such as Pregestimil should be used.

(c) Vitamins

(i) Multivitamins: twice the usual dosage

(ii) Vitamin E: 200 IU per day

(iii) Vitamin K: 2.5 mg biweekly until age 1 year, then supplement only if liver disease is present or when PT is prolonged

(iv) Vitamin D: 800 IU per day if serum levels of 25-hydroxy vitamin D are inadequate

(v) Calcium: Dietary or supplemental consumption should be 1,000–1,500 mg per day of elemental calcium.

(2) Treatment of pulmonary disorder

(a) Pulmonary toilet

(i) Adequate hydration, mobilization, and loosening of secretions are essential.

(ii) Chest physiotherapy should be administered by a properly trained provider.

(iii) Bronchodilators (see also Chap. 3, p. 62). Many patients with CF have significant bronchospasm. Beta agonists may also improve mucociliary clearance. Theophylline may improve diaphragmatic contractility.

(iv) Mist tents are no longer recommended.

(v) Endoscopy and bronchopulmonary lavage are not indicated on a routine basis.

(vi) Mucolytics. Clinical studies of their efficacy are inconclusive. Currently, they are not routinely used.

(vii) Antitussives are generally **not** recommended. Bronchodilators may help in cases in which cough is in part secondary to hyperactive airways.

(b) Antimicrobial therapy

(i) Long-term suppressive antibiotic therapy. The aim is to reduce pulmonary bacterial burden, retard pulmonary damage, and decrease the frequency of acute pulmonary exacerbations requiring hospitalization. Therapy is directed primarily against *Staph. aureus* and *Haemophilus influenzae* (Table 10-6).

(ii) Acute pulmonary exacerbation. Treatment is directed against the predominant pathogens isolated from sputum, usually *P. aeruginosa*, although *Staph. aureus*, and *Enterobacteriaceae* can also be found. Standard therapy employs the combination of an aminoglycoside and an antipseudomonal beta-lactam antibiotic selected on the basis of antibiotic

---

Table 10-6. Antibiotic therapy in cystic fibrosis

Chronic suppression
Trimethoprim, 10–20 mg/kg/day, and sulfamethoxazole, 50–100 mg/kg/day PO in
2–3 divided doses *and* cephalexin, 25–50 mg/kg/day PO in 3–4 divided doses
or dicloxacillin, 25–50 mg/kg/day PO in 3–4 divided doses

Acute pulmonary exacerbation
Tobramycin, 240 mg/m^2/day IV in 4 divided doses, *with* mezlocillin, 500 mg/kg/day
IV in 6 divided doses
or azlocillin, 450 mg/kg/day IV in 6 divided doses
or ticarcillin, 500 mg/kg/day IV in 6 divided doses
or ceftazidime, 150 mg/kg/day IV in 3 divided doses
or cefoperazone, 150 mg/kg/day IV in 3 divided doses
or timentin, 500 mg/kg/day IV in 6 divided doses if *Staph. aureus* and *P. aeruginosa* are isolated. Otherwise add oxacillin, 250 mg/kg/day IV in 6 divided doses,
in addition to the above

---

susceptibility testing. The pharmacokinetics of aminoglycosides and most beta-lactam antibiotics are altered in patients
with CF; higher dosages are required to achieve therapeutic
serum levels.

    (iii) A yearly **influenza vaccine** is recommended.

  2. Shwachman-Diamond syndrome (congenital hypoplasia of the pancreas) is
a rare disease characterized by exocrine pancreatic insufficiency, growth
retardation, metaphyseal dyschondroplasia, bone marrow hypoplasia, neutropenia, anemia, or thrombocytopenia. After CF, it is the most common
cause of pancreatic insufficiency in childhood.

    a. Etiology. This condition is probably hereditary.

    b. Evaluation. The **history** includes failure to thrive, chronic diarrhea, and
recurrent infection. **Physical examination** reveals a small, malnourished
child. **Laboratory investigation** includes a sweat test, stool examination,
CBC, platelets, 72-hour stool-fat test, pancreatic function test, bone
x-rays, bone marrow examination, and liver function tests.

    c. Diagnosis

      (1) The sweat test is normal.

      (2) A blood count reveals cyclic or constant *neutropenia*. Some patients
have *anemia* and *thrombocytopenia* as well.

      (3) A stool examination reveals positive Sudan stain.

      (4) A 72-hour stool-fat test reveals *steatorrhea*.

      (5) The bone marrow shows *maturation arrest* of the neutrophils.

      (6) A bone x-ray reveals *metaphyseal dysostosis* in 10–15 percent of
patients.

    d. Treatment

      (1) Replace pancreatic enzymes [see **1.d.(1)(a)**].

      (2) Give antibiotic therapy for recurrent infections.

 E. Gluten-sensitive enteropathy (GSE; celiac disease) is manifested clinically by
malabsorption and morphologically by a flat intestinal lesion. Both improve on
a gluten-free diet and are reexacerbated by the reintroduction of gluten into the
diet. It is a lifelong disease that presents most frequently between 9 and 18
months of age (earlier in formula-fed infants), but can be seen at any age.

  1. Etiology. The mechanism of gluten sensitivity is unknown. Genetic factors
play an important role. It is more common in Ireland (1 : 200) than in the rest
of the world (United States estimate is 1 : 3,000). Theories as to its cause
include immune mediation of gluten toxicity and an enzymatic defect.

  2. Evaluation

    a. The **history** may include a family history of GSE, failure to thrive,
irritability, anorexia, and chronic diarrhea.

    b. The **physical examination** classically reveals an irritable, malnourished child with a pot belly and proximal muscle wasting, characteristically including the buttocks. However, some patients present atypically with features only of a selective malabsorption, i.e., only growth failure, anemia, and rickets.

    c. **Laboratory investigations** should include a blood count, serum albumin, immunoglobulin (Ig), folate, iron, iron-binding capacity, stool examination, and sweat test. **Jejunal biopsy is mandatory for the diagnosis of GSE.** Recently, antigliadin and anticndomysial antibodies have been shown to be elevated in active celiac disease.

3. Diagnosis

    a. The findings of **stool examination,** including cultures for ova and parasites, are negative. Clinitest findings are variable. Sudan stain and a 72-hour stool-fat test usually reveal steatorrhea.

    b. The results of a D-xylose absorption test and lactose H_2 breath tests are usually abnormal.

    c. A series of three jejunal biopsies associated with gluten elimination and reintroduction are required to establish the diagnosis.

        (1) The *initial* biopsy reveals a flat, villous lesion; this is not a pathognomonic finding.

        (2) Clinical improvement, including a return to normal growth, is demonstrated on a gluten-free diet for 6 months. A *second* jejunal biopsy demonstrates a return to normal morphology.

        (3) A *gluten challenge* is done for up to 6 weeks. Gluten powder, where available, is sprinkled into food in a dose of 10 gm per day. In the absence of gluten powder, gluten-rich flour can be substituted. Gluten-containing foods can also be reintroduced, but children who taste previously restricted foods may resist a return to gluten restriction. A positive gluten challenge is the only available confirmatory test for GSE.

        (4) After 6 weeks of gluten challenge (or earlier if symptoms recur), a *third* jejunal biopsy is done. It is unusual for overt diarrheal symptoms to occur during the challenge period. Biopsy evidence of active enteritis confirms the diagnosis. A normal biopsy essentially rules out celiac disease, but a subsequent biopsy may be needed after 1 year on the normal diet if symptoms recur.

4. Treatment

    a. A gluten-free diet is begun immediately. Rye, oats, and barley should also be excluded.

    b. Lactose should be omitted for the first 6 weeks to ameliorate the secondary disaccharide intolerance that is usually associated with GSE. Pregestimil or a soy-based formula will accomplish this purpose in infants.

    c. Irritability is the first symptom to respond to therapy; diarrheal symptoms may linger for up to 6 weeks. If diarrhea persists, it may be necessary to alter the sugar base of the formula prescribed.

    d. Vitamins and minerals should be replaced according to specific losses. A multivitamin preparation and iron are usually administered for 2–3 months, after which resolution of malabsorption permits normal dietary replacement. Common specific deficiencies are vitamin D, folic acid, vitamin K, and iron.

    e. **A gluten-free diet is maintained for life.** For this reason, confirmation of the diagnosis must be as clear as possible.

5. Prognosis

    a. On adequate gluten restriction, patients achieve normal life expectancy and fertility.

    b. Spontaneous remission does not occur.

    c. Recent reports indicate that patients with GSE may have an increased incidence in the subsequent development of GI malignancy.

F. Disaccharidase deficiency may be primary (genetic) or secondary to intestinal mucosal damage. The most commonly seen disaccharidase deficiencies are of lactase and sucrase.

1. **Lactose intolerance (primary).** Primary lactase deficiency is extremely common in older children.
   a. **Etiology.** The condition is hereditary.
   b. **Evaluation**
      (1) Lactase deficiency usually presents in blacks *over* 3 years of age and whites *over* 5 years of age. Detection of lactose intolerance *before* these ages indicates a secondary lactose intolerance, except for the very rare congenital lactase deficiency.
      (2) The **history** includes recurrent abdominal pain and flatulence or diarrhea, or both. Family history is usually positive.
      (3) The **physical examination** is usually normal.
      (4) **Laboratory tests** include a stool examination, including pH and reducing substances. Jejunal biopsy is usually not indicated. The **lactose breath test** is an easy, reliable, noninvasive test for the diagnosis of lactase deficiency.
   c. **Diagnosis**
      (1) The stool may be positive for reducing substances.
      (2) The results of the lactose tolerance test are usually, but not always, positive.
      (3) Jejunal biopsy, if done, shows a normal morphologic picture and normal disaccharide levels except for lactase.
      (4) The lactose breath test is positive.
      (5) There is usually a dramatic response to milk withdrawal in both primary and secondary lactase deficiency. It does not distinguish one from the other.
   d. **Therapy**
      (1) A lactose-free diet is begun immediately.
      (2) A calcium supplement may be needed for long-term therapy (see Food and Drug Administration requirements). This can be supplied in patients over 5–6 years of age by commercially available calcium-containing antacid tablets (e.g., Tums, Rolaids).
      (3) Primary lactase deficiency persists for life. However, patients may reintroduce lactose in small amounts until symptoms supervene. LactAid, a commercially available lactase, appears to be of value in some patients who wish to try a limited amount of lactose.

2. **Sucrase-isomaltase deficiency**
   a. **Etiology.** This is a rare autosomal recessive disorder.
   b. **Evaluation**
      (1) **History.** These patients present with chronic diarrhea that starts with the introduction of sucrose-containing foods.
      (2) The **physical findings** are usually normal. Failure to thrive is *not* a feature of this disease.
      (3) **Laboratory tests** include stool examination, sucrose tolerance and breath tests, and jejunal biopsy.
   c. **Diagnosis**
      (1) The stools may be positive for reducing substances.
      (2) Sucrose tolerance test findings are usually positive.
      (3) The sucrose breath test is positive.
      (4) Jejunal biopsy shows a normal histologic picture and, except for low to absent sucrase-isomaltase, normal disaccharide levels.
   d. **Treatment**
      (1) A sucrose-free diet is instituted immediately, usually with a dramatic response.
      (2) Sucrase-isomaltase restriction is lifelong.
      (3) Dietary supplements are not indicated.

G. **Food sensitivity.** The most common food sensitivities associated with GI disease are cow's milk and soy protein.

1. **Cow's milk protein sensitivity.** The incidence of cow's milk protein sensitivity is estimated at 0.5–1.0 percent of infants under 6 months of age. GI involvement is usually limited to the upper GI tract or to the colon.
   a. **Etiology.** Systemic sensitivity (e.g., anaphylaxis, wheezing) to cow's milk appears to be mediated by immediate hypersensitivity, whereas GI disease may be mediated by other immune mechanisms.
   b. **Evaluation.** Sensitivity to cow's milk usually presents in infants.
      (1) The **history** may include pallor, edema, irritability, vomiting, diarrhea, colic, failure to thrive, and hematochezia.
      (2) The **physical examination** may reveal a pale, edematous child. Some infants may present with a colitis-like picture with profuse, bloody diarrhea.
      (3) **Laboratory tests** include a CBC, serum albumin and immunoglobulins, serum iron, iron-binding capacity, IgE, radioallergosorbent test (RAST) to milk sensitivity, gastric and intestinal biopsy, sigmoidoscopy, rectal biopsy (if the patient has grossly bloody diarrhea), and stool guaiac.
   c. **Diagnosis**
      (1) The CBC may show iron deficiency anemia and eosinophilia.
      (2) SPA may reveal low serum albumin and immunoglobulins.
      (3) IgE levels are usually normal and the RAST is negative in GI disease alone, but usually not in systemic allergic disease.
      (4) Gastric biopsy may reveal a gastritis with eosinophilic infiltration.
      (5) Biopsy of the small intestine reveals a patchy, flat, villous lesion.
      (6) In patients with colonic involvement, sigmoidoscopy reveals colitis.
      (7) **Occult blood** is always present in the stool.
      (8) Withdrawal of milk protein (not lactose) produces a dramatic clinical and morphologic response. Reintroduction of milk protein after remission exacerbates clinical and morphologic abnormalities. Unlike GSE, this disease is transient, and milk protein can be tolerated after the age of 1–2 years. **A milk challenge should not be attempted in patients with a history of milk anaphylaxis.** In other patients, the milk challenge should be performed in the presence of medical staff with resuscitation equipment available.
   d. **Therapy**
      (1) A milk-free diet is instituted immediately.
      (2) In view of associated secondary disaccharidase deficiency, a disaccharide-free formula or diet is introduced.
      (3) An iron supplement should be provided.
2. **Soy protein sensitivity.** The incidence of isolated soy sensitivity is unknown. It is estimated that 20–30 percent of patients with milk sensitivity have associated soy sensitivity.
   a. **Etiology.** The cause is unknown.
   b. **Evaluation.** The history, physical examination, and laboratory investigations are similar to those carried out in patients with cow's milk sensitivity. The syndrome is usually seen in infants for whom soy formulas have been prescribed.
   c. **Diagnosis**
      (1) The CBC may show iron deficiency anemia and eosinophilia.
      (2) The SPA may reveal low levels of serum albumin and immunoglobulins.
      (3) IgE levels are usually normal. The RAST reaction is usually negative in GI disease alone, but positive in systemic allergic disease.
      (4) Gastric biopsy may reveal a gastritis with eosinophilic infiltration.
      (5) Biopsy of the small intestine reveals a patchy, flat, villous lesion.
      (6) Sigmoidoscopy reveals colitis.
      (7) Withdrawal of soy protein produces a dramatic clinical response.
      (8) Rechallenge after remission will reproduce abnormalities in a manner similar to that occurring with milk challenge.

   d. Therapy
   (1) A soy protein–free diet is instituted.
   (2) An iron supplement is indicated.
   (3) Whether this lesion is transient or permanent is unknown.
3. **Eosinophilic gastroenteritis**
   a. Etiology. The cause is unknown.
   b. Evaluation
   (1) The history often reveals the onset of systemic allergy (usually asthma) and abdominal pain.
   (2) Growth failure is a prominent part of the syndrome. The physical findings may also include pallor and edema.
   (3) Laboratory investigations include a stool guaiac test, CBC, SPA, IgE, serum iron, and skin and RAST test reactions to various foods (see Chap. 17, p. 489).
   c. Diagnosis
   (1) The CBC may reveal peripheral eosinophilia and iron deficiency anemia.
   (2) SPA may reveal hypoalbuminemia and hypogammaglobulinemia.
   (3) Serum IgE may be elevated.
   (4) RAST and skin test reactions to many foods are often positive.
   (5) Gastric antral biopsy reveals gastritis with eosinophilic infiltration.
   (6) Jejunal biopsy reveals an abnormal antrum and abnormal gastric mucosa.
   d. Treatment
   (1) Dietary manipulations may alleviate acute symptoms (anaphylaxis) but may not affect the long-term course of disease.
   (2) Prednisone in a dose of 1–2 mg/kg/day may be used if dietary management fails. Then alternate-day corticosteroids may be used.
   (3) Vitamins and iron supplements are indicated.
   (4) Unlike cow's milk sensitivity, eosinophilic gastritis (like GSE) can be a lifelong condition in some patients.
H. Inflammatory bowel disease
1. **Ulcerative colitis**
   a. Etiology. Ulcerative colitis is a chronic inflammatory mucosal disease of unknown origin. Genetic, environmental, psychological, infectious, and immunologic mechanisms have been implicated.
   b. Evaluation
   (1) The **history** usually includes bloody diarrhea and recurrent abdominal pain.
   (2) Systemic manifestations, including arthritis, erythema nodosum, uveitis, episcleritis, and liver disease, may precede or accompany the GI symptoms.
   (3) The findings on **examination of the abdomen** are usually benign, unless local complications of toxic megacolon or perforation have occurred. Growth failure may be present.
   (4) **Laboratory tests** include CBC, stool examination, cultures, ova and parasites, SPA, sigmoidoscopy, rectal biopsy, barium enema, and upper GI series.
   c. Diagnosis
   (1) Stool examination reveals blood and fecal leukocytes.
   (2) Sigmoidoscopy reveals colitis, confirmed by rectal biopsy.
   (3) Stool cultures are negative, and ova and parasites are not present.
   (4) The CBC may reveal anemia, leukocytosis with left shift, thrombocytosis, and elevated ESR.
   (5) Serum albumin levels may be low or normal.
   (6) A barium enema reveals colitis (the findings may be normal in the early stages of the disease). An upper GI series is normal.
   (7) A tuberculin skin test is negative.
   d. Treatment depends on the severity of the symptoms and signs.

(1) **Sulfasalazine (Azulfidine)** is usually the drug of choice in mild to moderate cases. Therapy is begun at 500 mg per day and increased over 4–5 days to 2–3 gm per day in three divided doses. Side effects include leukopenia, agranulocytosis, hemolytic anemia, arthralgia, headache, rash, and, rarely, lower GI bleeding.

(2) **Corticosteroids** are the mainstay of therapy in inflammatory bowel disease. In the moderate case in which sulfasalazine alone is inadequate, prednisone, 1 2 mg/kg/day in a daily dose, is given. In patients who require IV therapy, methylprednisolone sodium succinate (Solu-Medrol), 1–2 mg/kg/day in two to four divided doses, is indicated. In limited rectal disease, methylprednisolone (Medrol) enemas are preferred to systemic therapy.

(3) **Immunosuppressive agents,** including azathioprine and 6-mercaptopurine, are sometimes tried in patients who respond poorly to or cannot be weaned from corticosteroids. Cyclosporin has also been tried in severe cases.

(4) **Parenteral alimentation** should be used in all patients who require IV therapy.

(5) **Enteral alimentation.** Elemental diets, which usually must be administered by NG tube, can be an effective treatment for Crohn's disease.

(6) **Psychiatric consultation** may be required to assist the patient or the parents, or both, to cope with chronic ulcers.

(7) **Surgery.** Colectomy is curative. The indications are:
   (a) Perforation
   (b) Toxic megacolon
   (c) Massive bleeding
   (d) Severe corticosteroid side effects that preclude further use
   (e) Poor growth
   (f) Chronically disabling disease
   (g) **Malignancy.** Patients with long-standing ulcerative colitis have a definite risk of developing colon cancer. Appropriate screening, such as colonoscopy and rectal biopsy, should be performed annually for more than 10 years on patients with the disease. Any sign of dysplasia on biopsy is an absolute indication for colectomy.

2. **Crohn's disease.** This is a chronic transmural and predominantly submucosal inflammatory disease that can affect any part of the GI tract from mouth to anus; it most often affects the distal ileum and colon while sparing the rectum.
   a. **Etiology.** The cause is unknown.
   b. **Evaluation**
      (1) The **history** commonly includes growth failure, recurrent fever, and abdominal pain. Diarrhea is less common than in ulcerative colitis. Systemic symptoms include arthritis, erythema nodosum, uveitis, aphthous ulcers, and perianal disease.
      (2) **Physical examination** may reveal evidence of malnutrition, localized abdominal signs or perianal disease on rectal examination, and blood and mucus.
      (3) **Laboratory tests** include a CBC, ESR, SPA, electrolytes, iron, iron-binding capacity, folate, sigmoidoscopy, barium enema, and upper GI series.
   c. **Diagnosis**
      (1) **Stools.** Cultures are negative for bacteria, ova, and parasites. Leukocytes are present. The guaiac test findings are positive if colitis is present.
      (2) A CBC reveals anemia, leukocytosis with left shift, and thrombocytosis. The ESR is often elevated.
      (3) A tuberculin skin test is negative.
      (4) Serum iron and folate levels are low, and iron-binding capacity is increased.

(5) SPA reveals a serum albumin level that may be low.

(6) Sigmoidoscopy may show colitis (if the colon is involved).

(7) A barium enema, or upper GI series, or both, may show involvement.

(8) **Growth failure.** Severe growth failure occurs in 30 percent of patients with Crohn's disease. Fewer than 5 percent of patients have malabsorption. The causes of growth failure are believed to be lack of caloric intake and disease activity.

(9) Periodic flare-ups are very common in the clinical course.

(10) The results of a Schilling test might be abnormal.

d. Treatment

(1) **Colonic Crohn's disease.** Sulfasalazine (Azulfidine) and corticosteroids are given as in ulcerative colitis.

(2) **Ileal Crohn's disease.** Corticosteroids are the drug of choice. Sulfasalazine is not useful for this specific disease. Azathioprine (Imuran) and 6-mercaptopurine have sometimes been successful in patients with dependence or undesirable side reactions to corticosteroids.

(3) **Perianal fistula.** Metronidazole (Flagyl), 250 mg PO tid, has been used with benefit.

(4) Antispasmodics have no place in the management of acute disease. However, in chronic disease, with diarrhea and tenesmus, their use is recommended (deodorized tincture of opium, diphenoxylate, and loperamide hydrochloride).

(5) The use of elemental formula supplementation has proved to be beneficial for patients with Crohn's disease and growth failure.

(6) TPN has been used with good success in prepubertal patients to promote growth and initiate puberty in those who fail to respond to corticosteroids.

(7) Psychiatric consultation is useful for the patients and their families in managing this chronic, often debilitating, disease.

(8) The indications for surgery are less clear-cut than for ulcerative colitis because of the chronic nature of this disease. They include:

  (a) Perforation

  (b) Obstruction

  (c) Extensive perianal or rectal disease unresponsive to other therapeutic modalities

  (d) Severe growth failure, in which a localized segment can be removed. (See Table 10-7 for a comparison of the features of ulcerative colitis and Crohn's disease.)

I. Hirschsprung's disease (congenital, aganglionic megacolon). Congenital absence of the intrinsic ganglionic plexus of Auerbach and Meissner, which involves varying lengths of the rectum and colon. The incidence is estimated at 1 in 5,000. A family incidence exists in 10 percent of cases.

1. Etiology. The cause is unknown.

2. Evaluation

  a. The **neonatal history** includes failure to pass meconium in the first 24 hours of life or bile-stained vomiting in the first week of life. In late infancy and childhood, the history reports increasing constipation.

  b. **Rectal examination** classically reveals a tight anal sphincter and an empty rectum followed by an explosive gush of stool and gas. In the *neonatal period* abdominal distention is a prominent feature, whereas in the older child, fecal masses are palpable.

  c. **Laboratory investigations** include a kidneys-ureters-bladder (KUB) study, barium enema, rectal manometry, and rectal biopsy.

3. Diagnosis

  a. X-rays of the abdomen reveal dilated loops of bowel on an anteroposterior film. Rectal air is absent.

  b. The **barium enema** may reveal a narrow aganglionic segment with a dilated colon above. (In the immediate neonatal period, this typical pattern may be absent.) An important clue will be a 24-hour film showing

Table 10-7. Clinical, pathologic, and radiographic features of ulcerative colitis and Crohn's disease

Feature	Ulcerative colitis	Crohn's disease
Diarrhea	Severe	Moderate or absent
Rectal bleeding	Common	Rare
Abdominal pain	Frequent	Common
Weight loss	Moderate	Severe
Growth retardation	Mild	Severe
Extraintestinal manifestations	Common	Common
Percentage with bowel involvement		
Anus	15	85
Rectum	95	50
Colon	100	50
Ileum	0 (except for backwash ileitis)	80
Distribution of lesions	Continuous	Skip areas
Pathologic features	Diffuse mucosal disease	Granulomas; focal disease
Radiographic features	Loss of haustra Superficial ulcers No skip areas	Thumbprinting Skip areas String sign
Cancer risk	High	Less than with ulcerative colitis but still increased

that the barium is still present. Rarely, in "low segment" Hirschsprung's disease, the barium enema findings may be normal or nondiagnostic. The patient should not receive a preprocedure enema.

   c. **Rectal manometry** may reveal absence of the normal relaxation reflex of the internal sphincter.

   d. **Rectal biopsy** is definitive. If a suction biopsy does not reveal ganglion cells, a full-thickness surgical biopsy is necessary. Rarely, if symptoms persist when laboratory findings are normal, a second or even a third biopsy may be needed.

4. Treatment

   a. The neonate is often extremely ill, with enterocolitis, shock, and sepsis.

     (1) A nasogastric tube is passed for decompression.

     (2) Urgent rehydration is begun.

     (3) Antibiotics are indicated.

     (4) An emergency colostomy is performed in an area of the colon where ganglion cells are seen.

     (5) Resection of the aganglionic segment is delayed for 6 months to 2 years.

   b. In infants and children who are relatively well, the definitive surgery can be performed with a diverting colostomy.

   c. **Surgical management.** Three types of operations have been in vogue.

     (1) **Swenson.** The aganglionic colon is resected, and the ganglion-containing bowel is anastomosed to the rectal stump.

     (2) **Duhamel.** A longer piece of rectum, usually 5–7 cm, is left and closed proximally. Ganglionic bowel is pulled down retrorectally to 1 cm from the mucocutaneous junction, leaving part of the internal sphincter intact. Colorectal anastomosis is achieved by clamping the posterior wall of the rectum to the anterior wall of the colon.

     (3) **Soave.** This operation leaves 10–20 cm of rectal stump. The mucosa is stripped and the ganglionic bowel pulled through.

d. Surgical complications

(1) Following colostomy

(a) Circulatory collapse resulting in severe enterocolitis may occur following colostomy for decompression. Treatment is supportive, i.e., fluid and electrolyte replacement and antibiotics.

(b) Persistent diarrhea, which is often due to disaccharide deficiency, may occur. A Clinitest is positive, and a change in the type of sugar in the formula will alleviate symptoms.

(2) After definitive surgery. Segmental obstruction with overflow incontinence is often a problem, especially in the first few months after surgery.

J. Hepatic failure

1. Etiology. Acute hepatic failure is a clinical syndrome resulting from severe hepatic dysfunction or massive hepatic necrosis. The causes are listed in Table 10-8.

2. Evaluation

a. The **history** may reveal evidence of a previous viral infection; exposure to blood products, drugs, or chemicals; circulatory collapse; preexisting liver disease; or a family history of liver disease.

b. The **physical examination** reveals progressive jaundice (except in Reye syndrome), asterixis ("liver flap"), fetor hepaticus, mental confusion, or coma.

Table 10-8. Causes of hepatic failure in childhood

Infections
Viral hepatitis, particularly hepatitis B, non-A,
  non-B hepatitis (rare in Type A)
Leptospirosis
Adenovirus
Coxsackie virus
Cytomegalovirus
Infectious mononucleosis
Q fever
Disseminated herpes simplex virus
Clostridium perfringens

Metabolic abnormalities
Reye syndrome
Wilson's disease

Drugs, chemicals, poisons
Acetaminophen
Salicylates
Tetracycline
Carbon tetrachloride
Ethanol
Phosphorus
Anesthetic agents
  Halothane (Fluothane)
  Methoxyflurane (Penthrane)
Mushrooms (*Amanita phalloides*)

Ischemia and hypoxia
Acute circulatory failure
Acute Budd-Chiari syndrome
Acute pulmonary failure
Ligation of hepatic artery
Heat stroke

    c. Laboratory investigations include urinalysis; CBC; platelet count; reticulocyte count; Monospot test; PT; PTT; BUN; electrolytes; glucose; creatinine; ammonia, AST (SGOT), ALT (SGPT), alkaline phosphatase; bilirubin; blood gases; serum albumin; serologic tests for hepatitis A, B, C, D, and E; slit-lamp examination for Kayser-Fleischer rings; serum copper; ceruloplasmin; 24-hour urine copper; alpha-1-antitrypsin level; and toxic screen.

3. Diagnosis

    a. The blood count may reveal leukocytosis or hemolytic anemia, or both. (*Always rule out Wilson's disease when liver disease and hemolytic anemia occur.*)

    b. PT and PTT are prolonged. Serum albumin may be low.

    c. SGOT and SGPT are increased.

    d. Alkaline phosphatase may be normal or increased.

    e. Except in Reye syndrome serum bilirubin is usually increased, both in direct and indirect fractions.

    f. Blood glucose may be low.

    g. BUN and electrolytes may reflect hypokalemia and hyponatremia.

    h. Blood gases may reveal a metabolic alkalosis or, less commonly, acidosis.

    i. Serologic tests for hepatitis A, B, C, D, or E may be positive.

    j. If serum copper and ceruloplasmin are low, and 24-hour urinary copper excretion is increased, further diagnostic tests for Wilson's disease are needed (see **L.3**).

    k. The findings of a toxic screen may be positive if ingestion has occurred.

4. Treatment. The purpose of therapy is to alleviate the systemic effects of liver failure and promote liver cell regeneration.

    a. Prepare a flow sheet to record laboratory data and daily intake and output.

    b. Give a 10–15% glucose solution IV at a rate dependent on renal function. Monitor blood glucose.

    c. Give vitamin K, 5–10 mg per day IV, for 3 days or while PT remains prolonged. If therapy is needed for more than 3 days, reduce this vitamin K dose to 1–2 mg daily. Fresh-frozen plasma may be required to control bleeding.

    d. To decrease ammonia production:

        (1) Initially, give 10 gm protein per day if the patient is able to take food orally.

        (2) Give lactulose, 1 ml/kg q6h, or neomycin, 50 mg/kg/day q6h, or both, to reduce the activity of endogenous flora.

    e. Pass a nasogastric tube to identify GI bleeding and as a route for medication.

    f. A central venous pressure line is needed to maintain fluid balance.

    g. Avoid all sedatives, especially those metabolized by the liver (e.g., barbiturates).

    h. Always culture urine, blood, and ascitic fluid.

    i. Treat GI bleeding vigorously. If gastritis or peptic ulcer disease is present, start cimetidine, 300 mg IV q6h (children under twelve years, 5–10 mg/kg q6h). Monitor gastric pH >5. If bleeding is due to varices, use a Sengstaken-Blakemore tube, or a vasopressin infusion may be necessary. In certain circumstances, emergency surgery can be undertaken.

    j. Monitor serum and urinary electrolytes daily. Characteristically, low urinary sodium and high urinary potassium with urine osmolarity greater than plasma osmolarity are found.

    k. If intravascular volume and serum albumin are low, give albumin, 1.75 gm/kg. This dose will increase serum albumin 1 gm/dl.

K. Pathologic gastroesophageal reflux is defined as the abnormal clearance of acid from the distal esophagus. It differs from *chalasia of infancy*, which is defined as the regurgitation of gastric contents into the esophagus *without* pathologic complications.

1. **Etiology.** The cause is unknown.
2. **Clinical manifestations** include (see also *Gastroenterology* 81:376, 1981):
   a. Recurrent emesis
   b. Recurrent pneumonia
   c. Asthma
   d. Sudden infant death syndrome, apnea
   e. Failure to thrive
   f. Sandifer syndrome
   g. Heartburn (pyrosis)
   h. Dysphagia
   i. Nocturnal cough and wheeze
   j. Hematemesis
   k. Rumination
   l. Iron deficiency anemia
3. **Evaluation and diagnosis**
   a. **Upper GI series** to assess anatomy, the presence of strictures, and the gastric outlet
   b. The **continuous intraesophageal pH probe** study is the best test to evaluate acid clearance. It is positive when a sustained pH <4 lasts for more than 4 minutes. It should be obtained over an 18- to 24-hour period.
   c. **A technetium-99m (^{99m}Tc) scan** (milk scan) to assess regurgitation of gastric contents into the lungs, and gastric emptying
   d. **Endoscopy** and **biopsy** to evaluate the presence of esophagitis (basal zone hyperplasia, infiltration of neutrophils, and the presence of intraepithelial eosinophils)
   e. **Esophageal manometry** to assess esophageal motility and lower esophageal sphincter pressure
4. **Therapy**
   a. **Treatment for children with chalasia of infancy.** Children are fed small, thickened feedings and are kept prone, with the head of the bed elevated after meals.
   b. For children with **abnormal acid clearance,** the following therapy is recommended:
      (1) **Antacid therapy** (alternating ALternaGEL and Mylanta). The dose is 0.5–1.0 ml/kg 1 and 3 hours after meals and at bedtime.
      (2) **Therapy to block acid secretion.** Cimetidine (H_2 blocker) is used. The recommended dosage is 5–10 mg/kg/dose q6–8h. A bedtime dose is indicated when the medication is tapered down.
      (3) **Therapy to increase sphincter pressure.** Bethanechol chloride (Urecholine), 2.9 mg/m^2/dose PO q8h. The maximum single dose is 50 mg.
      (4) **Therapy to lower sphincter pressure and enhance gastric emptying.** Metoclopramide (Reglan), 0.1–0.2 mg/kg/dose q6–8h.
   c. If intensive medical therapy fails, **surgical intervention** is indicated (Nissen fundoplication).
L. **Wilson's disease** is an autosomal recessive metabolic disorder, associated with consanguinity, and characterized by cirrhosis of the liver, bilateral softening of the basal ganglia of the brain, and greenish-brown pigmented rings in the periphery of the cornea (Kayser-Fleischer rings).
   1. The **etiology** is unknown.
   2. **Clinical manifestations** include:
      a. **Onset**
         (1) The majority of patients become symptomatic between 6 and 20 years of age.
         (2) The presenting features are variable and include the liver, kidney, and central nervous system (CNS).
      b. **Modes of presentation** include:
         (1) Acute hepatitis
         (2) Chronic active liver disease
         (3) Cirrhosis

(4) Fulminant hepatic failure
(5) Hemolytic anemia
(6) Neurologic disease
    (a) "Clumsiness," poor handwriting, tremors
    (b) Slurring of speech, dysarthria, behavioral disturbances
    (c) Dystonia, fixed facial expression, rigidity, athetoid movements
(7) **Renal disease**
    (a) Renal tubular acidosis
    (b) Reduced glomerular filtration rate
    (c) Increased urate clearance, decreased serum uric acid levels
    (d) Aminoaciduria (threonine, cystine), glycosuria, proteinuria
    (e) Hyperphosphaturia
(8) **Bones and joints**
    (a) Osteoporosis
    (b) Osteoarthritis

3. Evaluation and diagnosis
  a. **Clinical history** and **family history,** especially regarding psychiatric or neurologic disease and childhood deaths
  b. **Neurologic and general physical examination**
  c. **Slit-lamp** examination for Kaiser-Fleischer rings. *Gross inspection is inadequate.*
  d. **Laboratory**
    (1) **Blood.** Hemoglobin, reticulocytes, smear, iron, haptoglobin, ceruloplasmin, copper, other proteins, and PT
    (2) **Liver.** Liver function tests, ^{99m}Tc scan, and copper content
    (3) **Urine.** Aminoaciduria, protein, sugar, uric acid, and 24-hour copper level

4. Treatment
  a. **Penicillamine** (see also Chap. 4) (β_1 β-dimethylcysteine) is the treatment of choice. The dosage is 250 mg D-penicillamine hydrochloride PO qid before meals. If there is no improvement, the dosage can be increased to 2 gm per day. The side effects of penicillamine include skin rashes, leukopenia, nephrotic syndrome, a lupus-like syndrome, and hemolytic anemia.
  b. **Diet**
    (1) **Avoid** organ meats, shellfish, dried beans and peas, whole wheat, and chocolate.
    (2) Try to limit copper intake to 1 mg/day.
    (3) Measure tap water for copper.

M. **Acute pancreatitis** is a systemic disease characterized by acute inflammation of the pancreas. On a pathologic basis it is divided into two distinct entities: edematous (interstitial) and hemorrhagic (necrotic) pancreatitis.
  1. Etiology
    a. **Trauma:** blunt, penetrating, or surgical
    b. **Infectious.** Mumps, Coxsackie virus B, rubella, measles, *Mycoplasma,* and septic shock
    c. **Systemic disease.** Diabetes mellitus, systemic lupus erythematosus, periarteritis nodosa, uremia, hypercalcemia, *Henoch-Schönlein purpura, Reye syndrome, inflammatory bowel disease, and CF*
    d. **Drugs and toxins.** Azathioprine, thiazides, sulfonamides, furosemide tetracycline, corticosteroids, L-asparaginase, ethanol
    e. **Obstruction to flow**
      (1) **Congenital.** Absense of pancreatic duct, absence of common bile duct, stenosis of ampulla of Vater, pancreas divisum, and choledochal cyst duplications
      (2) **Acquired.** Trauma, gallstones, tumors, pseudocyst, infection in the ducts, *Ascaris*
    f. **Hereditary.** Hyperlipoproteinemia (types I and V), hyperparathyroidism
    g. **Miscellaneous.** Postoperative, graft-versus-host disease, idiopathic, penetrating peptic ulcer

2. **Clinical manifestations** include abdominal pain, nausea and vomiting, fever, ileus, and shock. It can also present as chronic upper abdominal pain and epigastric tenderness or ascites of unknown cause, or following abdominal trauma.

3. **Evaluation and diagnosis**
   a. Elevated serum or urine **amylase** or **lipase** only supports rather than proves the diagnosis of pancreatitis.
   b. Liver function tests (SGOT, SGPT, alkaline phosphatase)
   c. CBC, BUN, creatinine, and electrolytes
   d. Glucose and calcium levels should be monitored.
   e. Abdominal ultrasound
   f. A CT scan (abdomen)
   g. A chest x-ray to detect pleural effusion and pulmonary edema

4. **Treatment**
   a. Treat fluid and electrolyte imbalance, specifically hypovolemia, hypocalcemia, and hyperglycemia.
   b. Stop enteral feeding until the amylase level has fallen and there is no evidence of abdominal pain.
   c. Relieve pain using meperidine q3–4h by the IV route (see Chap. 1, p. 7).
   d. Aspiration by nasogastric tube (to reduce pancreatic stimulation and prevent paralytic ileus)
   e. Use of TPN (peripheral or central) (see sec. I.A.4.b).
   f. Anticholinergics, antacids, and H_2 blockers are very controversial, but can be used.
   g. Monitor for respiratory insufficiency and renal failure.
   h. Remember to be aware of further complications such as pancreatic pseudocyst and pancreatic fistula.

N. **Hepatomegaly and splenomegaly. Differential diagnoses** for childhood hepatomegaly and splenomegaly are listed in Tables 10-9 and 10-10.

O. **Protein-energy malnutrition.** Sustained deficits in the daily intake of protein or energy in relationship to specific requirements for nitrogen–amino acids and calories will result in the clinical syndrome of **protein-energy malnutrition.** This broad spectrum of protein-energy deficiency is conditioned by several factors: the severity of the deficiency, the duration, the age of the host, the cause of the deficiency, and the relative severity of protein versus energy deficiency (*Am. J. Clin. Nutr.* 23:67, 1970). Adequate nutrition is the most important aspect of therapy in acute and chronic illness.

1. **Classification**
   a. A child with **marasmus** has a caloric deficiency and an expected weight for age of less than 60 percent of normal. The clinical characteristics include the following:
      (1) The age of maximal incidence is 6–18 months.
      (2) No clinical evidence of edema with normal serum albumin ("skin and bones")
      (3) Poor nitrogen retention
      (4) No fatty infiltration of the liver
      (5) A slow response to dietary therapy during the first 4 weeks
   b. **Kwashiorkor** is predominantly a protein deficiency; usually, the child has a minimum weight not less than 60 percent of expected weight for age. Kwashiorkor has the following characteristics:
      (1) The age of maximal incidence is 12–48 months.
      (2) Clinical evidence of edema with low albumin
      (3) Fatty infiltration of the liver
      (4) Initial weight loss with delivery of edema
   c. Intermediate protein-energy malnutrition occurs in children who weigh less than 60 percent of the expected weight, but without the salient features of either marasmus or kwashiorkor (see *Br. Med. J.* 3:566, 1972).

2. **Diagnosis.** See sec. I.A.1 for assessment of malnutrition.

3. **Therapy.** See sec. I.A.4.a.

Table 10-9. Hepatomegaly

Mechanism	Entity
Inflammation	TORCH infections Hepatitis B, A, non-A non-B Hepatic abscess (pyogenic, amebic) Visceral larva migrans, schistosomiasis, liver flukes Toxin and drug injury Intra- and extrahepatic Biliary tract obstruction
Congestion	Hepatic cirrhosis/Wilson's disease Stenosis or thrombosis of portal or splenic vein Myeloid metaplasia Vinyl chloride Biliary atresia Congestive heart failure
Storage	Glycogen storage disease Mucopolysaccharidoses Gaucher's disease Niemann-Pick disease Gangliosidosis M_1 Alpha-1-antitrypsin deficiency Amyloidosis Porphyrias Wilson's disease
Infiltrative lesions	Erythroblastosis fetalis Metastatic tumor Histiocytosis Leukemia Lymphoma Hepatomas Hemochromatosis Amyloid Extramedullary hematopoiesis
Intrinsic	Cirrhosis, primary biliary cirrhosis Congenital hepatic fibrosis Multicystic liver and kidney disease Hereditary hemorrhagic telangiectasia
Kupffer cell hyperplasia	Sepsis Granulomatous hepatitis Hypervitaminosis A

Source: Modified from W. A. Walker et al. *Pediatr. Clin. North Am.* 22:929, 1975.

Table 10-10. Splenomegaly

Mechanism	Entity
Inflammation or immunologic	Subacute bacterial endocarditis
	Brucellosis
	Tuberculosis
	Mononucleosis
	TORCH infections
	Malaria
	Schistosomiasis
	Rheumatoid arthritis, systemic lupus erythematosus, Felty syndrome
	Sarcoidosis
	Typhoid fever
	Sepsis
Congestion	Congestive heart failure
	Budd-Chiari syndrome
	Congestive pericarditis
	Cavernous transformation
Sequestration	Sickle cell disease
	Thalassemia
	RBC enzyme deficiencies
	Rh and ABO incompatibility
	Autoimmune hemolytic anemia
	Galactosemia
	Wolman's disease
	Reye syndrome
	Tetracycline toxicity
Infiltrative lesions	Leukemia
	Lymphoma
	Histiocytosis
	Metastatic neuroblastoma
	Polycythemia
	Myelofibrosis
Other	Splenic trauma
	Splenic hemangiomas or cysts

Source: Modified from M. K. Younoszai et al. *Clin. Pediatr.* 14:378, 1975.

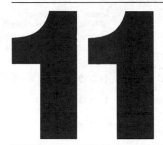

Disorders of the Endocrine System

Joseph I. Wolfsdorf and
Samir Najjar

I. **General approach to endocrine disorders.** Deviations from the normal rate or pattern of growth and secondary sexual development are frequent reasons that endocrine disorders are suspected in pediatric patients. Morphologic aberrations and behavioral changes are common in endocrine abnormalities.
   A. **The endocrine history**
      1. **A more directed history** is frequently necessary, expanding the review of systems to include such items as a detailed summary of the child's diet and eating habits, sleep patterns, bowel and bladder habits, activity level, and school performance.
      2. **The family history** provides essential information concerning the child's genetic growth potential and any unusual familial patterns of pubertal development. Actual height measurements of family members should be obtained whenever possible.
   B. **The physical examination** assesses somatic growth, sexual development, and the rate and sequence of bodily changes documented by serial measurements. Measurements are compared to normative data (Tables 11-1 and 11-2; see Figs. 2-1 to 2-4). Interpretation of the significance of the child's pattern and rate of growth is related to knowledge of the growth history of other family members.
   C. **Screening laboratory tests.** Few screening tests can be recommended as a routine. Rather, specific laboratory studies are suggested by the differential diagnosis. Bone age (obtained by an x-ray film of the left hand and wrist), an index of skeletal maturity, is compared to height age and to chronological age, and may suggest a specific category of growth disorder.
   D. **Therapy**
      1. Because most endocrine disorders are chronic diseases, **parent and patient education (and reeducation)** are essential if the family's lifestyle is to be as normal as possible. The social effects of an often highly visible condition must be approached with concern and support. The importance of relating the child to his or her chronological age, despite size or sexual development, should be emphasized.
      2. Hormonal therapy attempts to replace a deficiency of a specific hormone and rarely, if ever, mimics the normal pattern of hormone secretion. Success of therapy depends not only on prescribing the optimal dose, but also on the patient's ability and willingness to adhere to an often complex treatment plan.
      3. Personality and behavior may be affected directly by hormonal excess or deficiency. It may be difficult to determine the relative contributions of organic factors and psychological problems incurred because of a chronic disease.
      4. **Medic Alert bracelets** or **necklaces** should be worn by patients whose disease is associated with potentially life-threatening complications if therapy is omitted. Examples include diabetes mellitus, diabetes insipidus, congenital adrenal hyperplasia, and adrenal insufficiency.
II. **Disorders of growth**
   A. **Short stature**
      1. **Etiology** (Table 11-3)

Table 11-1. Tanner stages of sexual development

Stage	Characteristics	Mean age at onset (97th–3rd percentiles)*
Testis		
1	Prepubertal (<4 ml or long axis <2.5 cm)	
2	Testes enlarge (4 ml or long axis ≥2.5 cm)	11.5 (9.5–13.5)
3	Testes 12 ml (long axis 3.6 cm)	14.0 (11.5–16.5)
Pubic hair		
1	Prepubertal; no coarse, pigmented hair	
2	Minimal coarse, pigmented hair at base of penis	12.0 (9.9–14.0)
3	Coarse, dark curly hair spread over the pubis	13.1 (11.2–15.0)
4	Hair of adult quality but not spread to junction of medial thigh with perineum	13.9 (12.0–15.8)
Penis stage		
1	Prepubertal	
2	Earliest increased length and width	11.5 (9.2–9.7)
3	Increased length and width	12.4 (10.1–14.6)
4	Continued growth in length and width	13.2 (11.2–15.3)
Peak height velocity		13.5 (11.7–15.3)
Boys who mature at an average time		9.5 (7.1–11.9) cm/yr
Boys who mature early (+2 SD)		10.3 (7.9–12.5) cm/yr
Boys who mature late (+2 SD)		8.5 (6.3–10.7) cm/yr
Breast stage		
1	Prepubertal	
2	Breast buds palpable; areolae enlarge	10.9 (8.9–12.9)
3	Elevation of breast contour; areolae enlarge	11.9 (9.9–13.9)
4	Areolae and papillae form a secondary mound on the breast	12.9 (10.5–15.3)
Pubic hair		
1	Prepubertal; no coarse, pigmented hair	
2	Minimal coarse, pigmented hair mainly on labia	11.2 (9.0–13.4)
3	Dark, coarse, curly hair spreads over mons	11.9 (9.6–14.1)
4	Hair of adult quality but not spread to junction of medial thigh with perineum	12.6 (10.4–14.8)
Menarche		12.7 (10.8–14.5)
Peak height velocity		11.5 (9.7–13.3)
Girls who mature at an average time		8.3 (6.1–10.4) cm/yr
Girls who mature early (+2 SD)		9.0 (7.0–11.0) cm/yr
Girls who mature late (+2 SD)		7.5 (5.4–9.6) cm/yr

* 97th percentile refers to the earliest age and the 3rd percentile refers to the latest age at which the physical characteristic appears.

Source: Adapted from J. W. Tanner and P.W.S. Davies, *J. Pediatr.* 107:317, 1985.

Table 11-2. Penis and testis size

Age (yr)	Penis length (cm)*	Testis length (cm)*
0–2	2.7 ± 0.5	1.6 ± 0.4
2–4	3.3 ± 0.4	1.2 ± 0.4
4–6	3.9 ± 0.9	1.5 ± 0.6
6–8	4.2 ± 0.8	1.8 ± 0.3
8–10	4.9 ± 1.0	2.0 ± 0.5
10–12	5.2 ± 1.3	2.7 ± 0.7
12–14	6.2 ± 2.0	3.4 ± 0.8
14–16	8.6 ± 2.4	4.1 ± 1.0
16–18	9.9 ± 1.7	5.0 ± 0.5
18–20	11.0 ± 1.1	5.0 ± 0.3
Adult	12.4 ± 1.6	5.2 ± 0.6

* Mean ± SD.
Source: Data from J.S.D. Winter and C. Faiman, *Pediatr. Res.* 6:126, 1972.

2. **Evaluation**
   a. **History.** Gestational history, birth weight, perinatal events, rate of growth, nutritional history, symptoms suggestive of intracranial or hypothalamic dysfunction, psychosocial adjustment, review of systems, family history (stature and pattern of growth and pubertal development in the extended family)
   b. **Physical examination.** Accurate measurements of height, weight, upper and lower segments of the body, and arm span. Staging of pubertal development, neurologic examination including visual fields, and funduscopic examination
   c. **Laboratory tests** (Table 11-4)
   d. **Specialized tests.** Pharmacologic stimuli for growth hormone (GH) release, overnight frequent sampling to detect growth hormone pulses, thyrotropin releasing hormone (TRH) stimulation test, gonadotropin-

Table 11-3. Causes of short stature

Normal
Familial (genetic)
Constitutional growth delay
Pathologic

Disproportionate	**Proportionate**
Long bones	*Prenatal*
Rickets	Intrauterine growth retardation
Achondroplasia	Placental dysfunction
Hypochondroplasia	Intrauterine infections
Spine	Teratogens (ethanol, drugs, etc.)
Vertebral anomalies	Chromosomal anomalies (e.g.,
	Down syndrome)
	Postnatal
	Malnutrition
	Chronic disease
	Psychosocial deprivation
	Drugs
	Endocrine disorders (hypothyroidism, growth
	hormone deficiency, glucocorticoid excess,
	gonadal dysgenesis, pseudohypoparathyroidism,
	late effects of precocious puberty)

Table 11-4. Screening evaluation of children with growth failure

Detailed history and physical examination
Analysis of growth pattern from all available data
Urinalysis including pH and specific gravity
Tests of renal function: blood urea nitrogen (BUN), creatinine, electrolytes, venous pH, and TCO_2
Tests for rickets: calcium, phosphorus, alkaline phosphatase
Assessment of nutritional status: serum albumin, carotene, complete blood count; antiendomysial antibodies to rule out gluten enteropathy
Thyroid function: serum thyroxine, thyroid-stimulating hormone
Erythrocyte sedimentation rate to rule out inflammatory disease
IGF-I (somatomedin-C) and postexercise measurement of growth hormone for deficiency of GH
Radiograph of hand and wrist to assess skeletal maturity **(bone age)**
Cranial magnetic resonance imaging (MRI) to identify abnormalities in the area of the hypothalamus and pituitary
Karyotype to rule out abnormalities of the X chromosome in girls

---

releasing hormone (GnRH) stimulation test, magnetic resonance imaging (MRI) of the head, particularly the hypothalamus and pituitary

3. **Diagnosis**
   a. **Familial short stature (FSS) and constitutional delay (CD)**
      (1) History and physical examination are normal. Growth velocity is normal (0 to 12 months, 18–25 cm/yr; 1 to 2 years, 10–13 cm/yr; 3 to 5 years, 6.0–7.5 cm/yr; 5 years to puberty, 5–6 cm/yr).
      (2) Family history is frequently positive.
      (3) Bone age is commensurate with chronological age in FSS but is delayed and commensurate with height age in CD.
      (4) The onset of puberty is normal in FSS whereas it is delayed in CD.
   b. **Hormonal disorders** that result in short stature (see under specific hormones). The patient is usually overweight for height; the bone age is delayed, and growth velocity is subnormal.
4. **Treatment**
   a. Catch-up growth followed by normal growth velocity can be achieved if the underlying cause is treatable and is treated effectively.
   b. No treatment is currently available that increases the mature height of children with FSS or CD. Studies on the use of growth hormone in pharmacologic doses in these two conditions are ongoing.
   c. Anabolic hormones (e.g., oxandrolone) and small doses of long-acting testosterone (e.g., testosterone enanthate, 50 mg intramuscularly q1mo) can be used judiciously, the former to enhance growth, the latter to induce puberty and growth in boys with CD who have severe psychological problems and social maladjustment. Final adult height is not changed by such therapy.

B. **Tall stature**
   1. **Etiology**
      a. **Constitutional** (familial, genetic) tall stature is the most common cause.
      b. **Organic** causes include GH-producing tumors, cerebral gigantism, Beckwith syndrome, Marfan syndrome, homocystinuria, Klinefelter syndrome, syndromes with an extra Y chromosome, syndromes of insulin resistance (e.g., lipodystrophy), and thyrotoxicosis. Patients with excess androgens or estrogen have an accelerated growth velocity early before fusion of the epiphyses.
   2. **Evaluation and diagnosis**
      a. The probable diagnosis should be evident from the history and physical examination.
      b. Bone age is used to predict mature adult height.

c. **Laboratory tests** are used to confirm a suspected diagnosis and might include: MRI of the head; karyotype; urine amino acids; suppression of GH by glucose (oral glucose tolerance test); blood levels of androgens, estrogens, and gonadotropins; thyroid function tests; insulin-like growth factor-1 (IGF-I)/somatomedin-C; and insulin levels.

3. **Treatment**

a. When a prepubertal or early pubertal girl with constitutional tall stature is predicted to achieve a mature height exceeding 70–72 in., **estrogen therapy** to attempt to arrest growth may be warranted.

b. Treatment of organic causes of tall stature depends on the underlying cause.

C. **Obesity**

1. **Etiology**

a. **Idiopathic (exogenous) obesity** results from energy intake that exceeds the individual's energy expenditure. The factors that predispose to the development of obesity are still incompletely understood. A family pattern of obesity is common, suggesting genetic and environmental influences in the genesis of exogenous obesity. Psychosocial stress often leads to overeating.

b. **Organic conditions** associated with obesity include hyperinsulinism; hypothyroidism; pseudohypoparathyroidism; and Cushing, Turner, Prader-Willi, and Laurence-Moon-Biedl syndromes.

2. **Evaluation**

a. A person whose weight is more than 120 percent of the ideal weight for height is considered obese.

b. Most children with *idiopathic* obesity are of normal or tall stature. Patients whose obesity has an organic cause are usually short or have a deceleration in height velocity.

c. The **history** should elicit the age of onset of obesity, a complete dietary history (preferably of a 3-day food record with a calorie count), unusual eating or drinking patterns, food preferences, exercise habits, history of past central nervous system (CNS) injury or disease, intellectual ability, and symptoms suggestive of hypothyroidism, tetany, or the Cushing syndrome.

d. The severity of obesity should be assessed by expressing current weight as a percentage of ideal weight for height.

e. Particular attention should be directed to the distribution of body fat, facial abnormalities, funduscopic changes, presence of a goiter, abnormal secondary sexual development, signs of tetany, skin texture, short fourth metacarpals, and polydactyly. Striae and a buffalo hump may be present in patients with exogenous obesity and are not pathognomonic of Cushing syndrome.

f. **Growth data** should be obtained in all cases.

g. The following **screening tests** may help to rule out an organic cause of obesity: bone age, thyroid function, 8 AM and 8 PM serum cortisol levels or 8 AM serum cortisol after overnight dexamethasone suppression, serum calcium, and phosphorus.

3. **Diagnosis** of organic conditions should be made primarily by clinical evaluation and confirmed by laboratory tests and x-ray studies, as necessary.

4. **Treatment** of hypothyroidism or Cushing syndrome results in weight loss and accelerated linear growth. The only therapy for other forms of obesity is caloric restriction and increased activity to enhance calorie utilization.

a. For moderate obesity, the balanced calorie-deficit diet attempts to reduce the individual's usual caloric intake by at least one third. Weight loss is slow because expenditure of 3,500 calories of stored energy results in the loss of only 1 lb fat. In severely obese individuals, a protein-sparing modified fast is utilized, providing 1.5 gm protein per kilogram of ideal weight per day and 1.0 gm carbohydrate per kilogram of ideal body weight per day while allowing salads, low-calorie dressings, and fluids.

This diet is supplemented with calcium, potassium, and multivitamins.
   b. Counseling. Involvement of the other family members in the treatment
      will increase the likelihood of sustained weight loss in the obese child or
      adolescent.
   c. Medications are often ineffective and potentially dangerous.
   d. Surgical therapy with intestinal bypass and oral occlusion have been
      attempted successfully in some patients. Serious long-term side effects
      have occasionally developed.
III. Disorders of sexual development
   A. Ambiguous genitalia (intersex). The birth of a baby with ambiguous genitalia
      is a psychosocial emergency. It is essential to avoid announcing the sex
      assignment based on a first impression of the external genitalia before a
      complete evaluation has been performed by the pediatrician in consultation
      with a pediatric endocrinologist, pediatric urologist, radiologist, and geneticist.
      Inappropriate sex assignment can have catastrophic future consequences. The
      investigation must be performed expeditiously. Meanwhile, the parents should
      be told that an immediate decision cannot be made because the baby's sexual
      development is immature or incomplete; however, with appropriate treatment,
      genital appearance and sexual function will ultimately be normal.
      1. Etiology (Table 11-5)
      2. Evaluation and diagnosis
         a. The **history** should include an inquiry about maternal virilization and the
            possibility of maternal hormone ingestion. In taking the family history,
            one should ask about infants with ambiguous genitalia, unexplained
            infant deaths, and relatives with disorders of puberty, amenorrhea, or
            infertility.
         b. The baby's blood pressure, heart rate, and hydration must be monitored
            carefully. The **physical examination** should attempt to ascertain the
            presence of gonads in the labioscrotal folds. The phallus is carefully
            examined and measured; the position of the urethra and the degree of
            pigmentation, rugation, and fusion of the labioscrotal folds are noted. A
            rectal examination is done to determine the presence of a uterine cervix.
            Somatic stigmata suggesting a chromosomal abnormality are noted.
         c. Obtain a **karyotype,** measure serum **electrolytes,** and send a blood sample
            for measurement of all **steroid metabolites likely to be needed:** cortisol,
            17-hydroxyprogesterone, 17-hydroxypregnenolone, 11-deoxycortisol, de-
            hydroepiandrosterone (DHEA) and its sulfate (DHEA-S), androstenedi-
            one, and testosterone.
            (1) Measurement of plasma adrenocorticotropic hormone (ACTH) and
               plasma renin activity is valuable in cases of suspected *congenital
               adrenal hyperplasia.* Salt-wasting is not evident for 3 to 7 days or
               more after birth. In selected cases, measurements of plasma preg-
               nenolone, progesterone, deoxycorticosterone (DOC), corticosterone,
               18-hydroxylated corticosterone, and aldosterone levels are required
               for diagnosis.
            (2) A disorder of testosterone biosynthesis may be diagnosed from steroid
               hormone measurements in the basal state, but **stimulation with 3,000
               U/m^2 human chorionic gonadotropin (HCG) IM** and sampling after 48
               hours will often be valuable in determining the site of the block in
               testosterone biosynthesis. The diagnosis of androgen unresponsive-
               ness can be made in two ways:
               (a) Administer testosterone, 25 mg IM each month for 3 months, and
                  observe the change in the stretched length and width of the penis.
               (b) Androgen receptors can be determined in fibroblasts from skin
                  biopsy (only done in specialized research laboratories).
            (3) Pelvic ultrasonography is used to identify the presence of a uterus
               and ovaries. A **urogenital sinogram, laparoscopy** (to identify internal
               ducts and gonads), **surgical exploration, and histologic examina-
               tion of the gonads** (and excision of discordant gonadal and ductal

Table 11-5. Causes of ambiguous genital development (intersex)

Disorder	Phenotype		Karyotype
	External genitalia	Gonads	
Disorders of gonadal differentiation			
True hermaphroditism	Ambiguous	Ovarian and testicular tissue	46,XX; 46,XY; 46,XX/46,XY chimerism or mosaic
"Pure" gonadal dysgenesis	Female	Streak gonads or hypoplastic ovaries	46,XX
	Female or ambiguous	Dysgenetic testes or dysgenetic testes and streak gonads	46,XY
Mixed gonadal dysgenesis	Ambiguous	Streak gonad and dysgenetic testis	45,X/46,XY; 46,XYp⁻
Female pseudohermaphroditism (masculinization of the genetic female)			
Congenital adrenal hyperplasia			
21α-hydroxylase deficiency	Ambiguous	Ovaries	46,XX
11β-hydroxylase deficiency	Ambiguous	Ovaries	46,XX
3β-OH steroid dehydrogenase deficiency	Ambiguous	Ovaries	46,XX
Transplacental synthetic progestogens	Ambiguous	Ovaries	46,XX
Maternal androgen excess	Ambiguous	Ovaries	46,XX
Male pseudohermaphroditism (incomplete masculinization of the genetic male)			
Testicular unresponsiveness to HCG and LH (Leydig cell hypoplasia or agenesis)	Ambiguous	Testes	46,XY
Disorders of testosterone synthesis			
Side chain cleavage enzyme deficiency	Ambiguous	Testes	46,XY
17α-hydroxylase deficiency			
3β-OH steroid dehydrogenase deficiency			
17-lyase deficiency			
17-ketosteroid reductase deficiency			
End-organ resistance to testosterone			
Complete testicular feminization	Female	Testes	46,XY
Incomplete testicular feminization	Ambiguous	Testes	46,XY
Disorder of testosterone metabolism			
5α-reductase deficiency	Ambiguous	Testes	46,XY
Vanishing testes syndrome	Variable	Absent gonads	46,XY
Lack of müllerian inhibiting substance	Male	Testes, uterus, fallopian tubes	46,XY

Key: HCG = human chorionic gonadotropin; LH = luteinizing hormone.

tissue) may be necessary, depending on the features of the individual case.

3. **Treatment**

    a. Assignment of the sex of rearing is based on the diagnosis, but most importantly on the potential to achieve cosmetically and functionally normal external genitalia by surgical and hormonal therapy, and the potential for fertility. In rare cases (e.g., true hermaphrodite), when either a male *or* female sex assignment is possible, the decision is influenced by the preference of the parents. The decision to recommend a male sex of rearing is based on the size of the phallus and its potential for growth during childhood and puberty. In a phenotypic male with a microphallus (penile length < 2.5 cm), a trial of testosterone, 25–50 mg IM monthly for 3 months, can be performed to assess the potential for growth of the phallus. Failure of the penis to lengthen significantly suggests that the penis lacks the capacity for growth in later childhood and at puberty.

    b. A baby with **congenital adrenal hyperplasia** (see sec. **VI.B**) will usually be raised concordant with the chromosomal sex, with glucocorticoid and mineralocorticoid therapy to stop further virilization (if present), or testosterone to promote virilization (if undervirilization is the problem). Surgical therapy will be required to correct the external appearance. Reconstructive surgery on the genitalia of girls with congenital adrenal hyperplasia is performed early in the first year to reduce the size of an enlarged clitoris; definitive vaginoplasty is usually deferred until adolescence.

    c. Infants with **androgen resistance** are raised as girls. Ambiguity of the external genitalia occurs with **incomplete androgen resistance** and surgical reconstruction is necessary.

    d. In some instances, a **true hermaphrodite** can be raised either as a boy or girl, and the decision may be influenced by the presence of some normally functioning testicular or ovarian tissue. If surgical reconstruction resulting in either normal male or female genitalia is possible, the parents' preference may help to make the decision. In general, surgically creating a vagina is less difficult than constructing an adequate penis and penile urethra. Therefore, the size of the phallus is a crucial factor in making the decision about sex assignment.

    e. A child who would be expected to be unable to function as a male because of a small, probably androgen-unresponsive penis should *not* be raised as a boy because of the high likelihood of tragic psychological problems in the future.

    f. Reconstruction of the penis and correction of severe forms of hypospadias may have to be done in stages. To preserve valuable tissue for reconstruction, **circumcision is contraindicated.**

    g. If a genetic (46,XY) boy is to be raised as a girl, intraabdominal or inguinal testes are removed because of the high risk of future malignant degeneration, and the possibility of virilization during puberty.

    h. **Growth and sexual development** should be monitored closely and **hormone therapy** instituted as indicated (see below).

    i. The diagnosis and prognosis for sexual and reproductive function should be discussed frankly with the parents and later, at the appropriate time, with the patient. Psychological support, guidance, and repeated explanations, especially when the patient has reached adolescence, are of critical importance.

B. Delayed puberty

    1. Etiology

        a. Constitutional delay of pubertal development occurs more frequently in boys than in girls. These children characteristically grow below, but parallel to, the third percentile and their pubertal growth acceleration is delayed for several years.

b. **CNS abnormalities,** such as pituitary and hypothalamic tumors, congenital vascular anomalies, severe head trauma, birth asphyxia, psychosocial deprivation, and Kallmann and Laurence-Moon-Biedl syndromes, result in pubertal delay.

c. **Systemic conditions,** such as anorexia nervosa; severe cardiac, pulmonary, renal, or gastrointestinal disease; malabsorption syndromes; weight loss or weight gain; sickle cell anemia; thalassemia; chronic infection; hypothyroidism; or Addison's disease, are associated with an increased incidence of delayed or incomplete sexual development.

d. **Primary gonadal** insufficiency may be caused by the following: Turner, Noonan, Klinefelter, Reifenstein, and Sertoli-cell-only syndromes; testicular feminization; pure or mixed gonadal dysgenesis; cryptorchidism and anorchism; trauma; infection; pelvic radiation; and surgical castration.

2. **Evaluation.** Although there are normal variations in the normal time of onset of puberty, differential diagnosis of delayed puberty should be considered when a girl over 14 or a boy over 15 lacks any secondary sexual characteristics, or when an adolescent has not completed maturation over a period of 5 years.

a. The **history** should concentrate on the details and chronology of any sexual development, previous growth pattern, CNS symptoms, including anosmia, and nutrition. Any **family history** of abnormal puberty, amenorrhea, infertility, or ambiguous genitalia should be elicited.

b. The **physical examination** should include all growth measurements (height, weight, span, upper-lower ratio), sexual staging, careful observation of the genitalia for ambiguity, palpation for inguinal masses, a pelvic examination (or at least a rectal), and a search for stigmata suggesting a syndrome. Signs of virilization in the female or incomplete masculinization in the male strongly imply an underlying pathologic cause that must be pursued.

c. **Review of past growth data** is mandatory; a subtle increase in growth rate may be the first indication of impending sexual development. Conversely, deceleration may be a sign of active disease.

d. The initial **laboratory evaluation** usually includes a complete blood count, urinalysis, luteinizing hormone (LH), follicle-stimulating hormone (FSH), estrogen, testosterone, DHEA-S, bone age, and cranial computed tomographic (CT) or MRI scan. A karyotype is sometimes indicated.

3. **Diagnosis**

a. The diagnosis of constitutional or hereditary delay in an otherwise normal patient is always tentative because it can be confirmed only after normal sexual development has occurred.

b. Patients with hypothalamic or pituitary deficiencies have low (usually prepubertal) levels of LH or FSH, or both. A GnRH test may differentiate hypothalamic from pituitary lesions.

c. In primary gonadal failure, gonadotropins are usually elevated by age 12–13 years.

4. **Treatment.** Before therapy is begun the patient's height, growth potential, and emotional needs, and the risks of treatment, must be considered.

a. **Constitutional and genetic delay.** The patient and family should be reassured that no abnormalities are apparent, and normal development is anticipated, but that continued surveillance is important. Progression of development should be monitored and emotional support offered. For certain patients, temporary hormone therapy may be warranted for psychological reasons.

b. **CNS abnormalities.** Patients with hypogonadotropic hypogonadism (decreased production of LH and FSH) require hormonal therapy to induce sexual development. With the availability of GnRH analogues, therapy for these patients has been revolutionized. If the pituitary is intact, treatment with GnRH analogues makes it possible to mature completely and, ultimately, to reproduce.

    (1) In females, the replacement regimen includes an oral conjugated estrogen, e.g., Premarin, 0.3 mg per day, with the dosage gradually increased to 0.65–1.25 mg per day over 9–12 months; medroxyprogesterone acetate (Provera), 10 mg per day on days 12–25 of each month, is then added to induce cyclic bleeding.

    (2) In males, ideal therapy consists of HCG, 1,000–2,500 IU IM q5 days. Serum testosterone is helpful in monitoring dosage needs.

  c. Systemic conditions. Improvement of the underlying medical condition may be followed by normal puberty. In certain conditions, replacement therapy as outlined below may be necessary.

  d. Primary gonadal insufficiency

    (1) In girls, treatment consists of administering estrogens and progesterone [see **b.(2)**].

    (2) In boys, a therapeutic trial of HCG should be attempted if there is a possibility of testicular function. If no response is demonstrated, testosterone enanthate, 100–200 mg IM every 2–4 weeks, will induce virilization, normal libido, and sexual potency. The prognosis for fertility should be evaluated and discussed frankly.

C. Sexual precocity

  1. Etiology (Table 11-6)

  2. Evaluation should focus on the points emphasized in **B.2.**

    a. Skin should be examined for multiple small café au lait spots of neurofibromatosis or larger irregular brown macules of McCune-Albright syndrome. Dimensions of breast areolae and glandular tissue in girls, and testes and phallus in boys, should be recorded. Presence of pubic or axillary hair and apocrine odor should be noted. Asymmetry or nodules in the testes suggest the presence of a tumor. In girls a pale-pink vaginal introitus with developed labia minora suggests active estrogenization. Estrogenization can be quantitated using a vaginal smear fixed for

Table 11-6. Causes of sexual precocity

True central precocious puberty (pituitary gonadotropin secretion)
Idiopathic
Russell-Silver syndrome
Neurogenic (central nervous system disorder)
  Hypothalamic hamartoma
  Space-occupying lesions: astrocytoma, optic glioma with neurofibromatosis, tumors associated with tuberous sclerosis, teratoma
  Cerebral damage resulting from CNS anomalies, irradiation therapy, surgery, trauma, prior inflammation (encephalitis, meningitis), hydrocephalus
Pseudoprecocious puberty (source of sex steroids independent of pituitary)
Androgen- or estrogen-secreting tumors
  Ovarian (granulosa cell, theca cell, luteomas, follicular cysts)
  Testicular (Leydig cell, adrenal rest)
Congenital adrenal hyperplasia
Adrenal adenoma or carcinoma
Exogenous sex steroids (oral contraceptives, estrogen-containing creams, consumption of estrogen-fed poultry or cattle)
Exogenous human chorionic gonadotropin (HCG) in boys
McCune-Albright (polyostotic fibrous dysplasia)
Gonadotropin or HCG-producing tumors: chorioepithelioma, teratoma, hepatoblastoma (boys)
Familial male gonadotropin-independent precocity
Severe hypothyroidism (associated with ovarian cysts)
Incomplete sexual precocity
Premature thelarche
Premature adrenarche

cytologic examination to determine the maturation index. A rectoabdominal examination may reveal an adnexal mass if an ovarian tumor or cyst is present.

b. **The source of hormone secretion (adrenal or gonadal) must be determined.** One must establish whether sex steroid production is independent (usually a cyst or tumor) or the result of premature activation of the hypothalamic-pituitary-gonadal axis (central precocity).

c. For laboratory evaluation, see Table 11-7.

3. **Diagnosis**

a. **Isosexual precocity** refers to an abnormally early onset (girls <8 years of age, boys <9 years of age) of sexual characteristics appropriate to the child's sex, with eventual attainment of full sexual maturation and premature closure of epiphyses. Precocious puberty is much more common in girls than in boys and is usually idiopathic. Precocity in boys is more often caused by CNS lesions, hormone-secreting tumors, congenital adrenal hyperplasia, or familial male gonadotropin independent precocity. Masculinization of a female or feminization of a male is always pathologic and requires investigation.

b. **Precocious adrenarche (pubarche)** refers to the early appearance of pubic hair, axillary hair, and/or apocrine odor, which are effects of adrenal androgens. Increase in growth and skeletal maturation is minimal. Some of these children have mild adrenal enzyme defects (congenital adrenal hyperplasia; see sec. **VI.B**).

c. **Precocious thelarche** refers to the premature development of one or both breasts in 1- to 4-year-old girls without acceleration of growth or

---

Table 11-7. Laboratory evaluation of precocious puberty

Isosexual
Hormonal
Serum LH, FSH (may require GnRH stimulation test to document presence or absence of pubertal response)
Estradiol (girls)
Testosterone (boys)
Dehydroepiandrosterone sulfate (DHEA-S)
Beta HCG subunit (boys)
Radiographic
Bone age (left hand and wrist)
Pelvic ultrasound
Cranial MRI scan
Premature thelarche
Hormonal
Serum LH, FSH
Estradiol
Cytologic examination of vaginal smear for maturation index (bioassay of estrogen effect)
Radiographic
Bone age
Pelvic ultrasound
Premature adrenarche
Hormonal
DHEA-S
17-OH progesterone (8 AM)
Dehydroepiandrosterone (consider ACTH stimulation test for congenital adrenal hyperplasia)
Radiologic
Bone age

advancement of skeletal maturation. Estrogenization of the genitalia **is minimal or absent.**

4. **Treatment** of central precocious puberty with daily injections or depot formulations of potent analogues of GnRH can suppress LH, FSH, and gonadal steroids to prepubertal levels, resulting in cessation of menses and penile erections, slowing of accelerated growth, and partial regression of secondary sexual development. Therapy must be monitored closely in order to maximize gains in final height. Many 6- to 8-year-old girls with precocity may attain normal adult height without intervention and do not need therapy.

D. **Gynecomastia**

1. **Etiology**

   a. **Idiopathic gynecomastia** occurs in approximately 40 percent of all normal boys carefully examined during puberty.

   b. **Iatrogenic causes** may be estrogens, androgens, HCG, isoniazid, digitalis, reserpine, spironolactone, phenothiazines, cimetidine, tricyclic antidepressants, meprobamate, amphetamines, ketoconazole, or marijuana.

   c. **Organic conditions** include true hermaphroditism, male pseudohermaphroditism, disorders characterized by primary testicular failure (e.g., Klinefelter syndrome), estrogen-producing tumors of the adrenal gland or testis, hyperthyroidism, and hepatic disease.

2. **Evaluation**

   a. The **history** should focus on sexual development and function, symptoms of pain, tenderness, galactorrhea, hair loss, drug exposure, and systemic illness.

   b. The size and configuration of ductular tissue, color of the areolae, presence of galactorrhea (best elicited with the patient in the sitting position), size and consistency of the testes, and stage of sexual development should be noted.

3. **Diagnosis.** Idiopathic gynecomastia usually begins during Tanner stages II–III of puberty, resolves within 2 years, and is not associated with galactorrhea. It may be unilateral or bilateral and is often asymmetric. Plasma estrogen and testosterone concentrations are normal but the estradiol/testosterone ratio may be elevated. If the history and physical examination are otherwise normal, no special diagnostic tests are necessary.

4. **Treatment.** Spontaneous regression occurs after 1–3 years. Removal of the hormonal or pharmacologic agent usually results in disappearance of ductular tissue. Severe gynecomastia with more than 5 cm breast tissue and pronounced areolar changes will seldom resolve spontaneously or, if it does, will take several years. Because pronounced gynecomastia is difficult to conceal and can cause significant psychological problems, a reduction mammoplasty is recommended.

IV. **Disorders of the pituitary**

A. **Hypopituitarism.** Pituitary function depends on the integrity of the entire hypothalamic-pituitary axis.

1. **Etiology**

   a. **Tumors** of the pituitary and suprasellar tumors (especially craniopharyngioma) may disrupt pituitary function.

   b. **Tissue damage** involving the hypothalamus resulting from perinatal insult, trauma, hemorrhage, vascular anomaly, infectious/inflammatory disease, histiocytosis, previous irradiation, and infarction may cause isolated or multiple hormonal deficiencies.

   c. **Congenital anomalies,** such as septooptic dysplasia, midline malformations, and syndromes of abnormal forebrain development, may be associated with hypopituitarism.

   d. **Psychosocial deprivation** alters hypothalamopituitary function.

   e. **States of end-organ resistance** (Laron syndrome)

   f. **Isolated GH deficiency** is usually idiopathic but occasionally may be hereditary.

   g. Isolated gonadotropin deficiency occurs in association with Kallmann syndrome (anosmia and color blindness) and Laurence-Moon-Biedl syndrome (mental retardation, polydactyly, obesity, retinitis pigmentosa, nerve deafness, short stature, and diabetes insipidus [DI]).

   h. Isolated deficiencies of thyroid-stimulating hormone (TSH) and ACTH are rare.

  2. Evaluation. Systematic investigation of all anterior and posterior pituitary hormones is necessary to determine the status of current function and to establish a baseline for long-term follow-up.

   a. The **history** should review past growth, CNS symptoms (anosmia, visual changes, symptoms of increased intracranial pressure), and previous head or neck illnesses or therapy, specifically radiation therapy.

   b. The **physical examination** should include precise growth measurements, staging of sexual development, a neurologic evaluation including visual fields and funduscopy, and a search for the signs of hypothyroidism and hypoadrenalism.

   c. Further evaluation should include a carefully plotted height and weight curve and bone age. If pituitary insufficiency is suggested, an evaluation of both anterior and posterior pituitary hormonal status includes circulating basal and stimulated levels of GH, LH, FSH, thyroxine, ACTH, and cortisol. Serum and urine values of sodium and potassium and osmolality should be obtained.

   d. An MRI of the brain is useful to evaluate structural lesions.

  3. Diagnosis

   a. Patients with **isolated GH deficiency** have a normal weight and length; growth velocity begins to decrease at 6–18 months of age. Incidence is higher in neonates who had an adverse perinatal event (e.g., hypoxia, low Apgar score) or had a breech presentation. Neonatal cholestatic jaundice, hypoglycemia, and micropenis in boys are suggestive of the diagnosis.

    (1) Patients with GH deficiency have a subnormal rate of growth (<4.0 cm/year after the age of 4–5 years; see sec. II.A.3).

    (2) The weight age is usually greater than the height age, and the facies and body proportions are immature. These patients tend to have truncal obesity. They may have craniofacial disproportion with small midface and crowded teeth. Some have a high-pitched voice. The bone age is delayed and is usually commensurate with height age.

    (3) GH does not increase in response to pharmacologic stimuli, such as insulin-induced hypoglycemia and the administration of arginine, glucagon, clonidine, L-dopa, or propranolol.

    (4) Nocturnal and diurnal pulsations of GH are greatly diminished, both in frequency and amplitude.

   b. Deficiencies of LH and FSH may not become apparent until puberty. A micropenis suggests hypogonadotropic hypogonadism.

   c. Deficiency of TSH may be responsible for mild to severe clinical hypothyroidism. Serum TSH levels are low in pituitary hypothyroidism and normal or slightly elevated in hypothalamic hypothyroidism. TSH does not respond to TRH administration in pituitary hypothyroidism, but hyperresponds in hypothalamic hypothyroidism.

   d. Patients with **ACTH deficiency** often have a relatively mild form of adrenal insufficiency that may go undetected until they are under stress or later in adolescence. These patients are differentiated from patients with Addison's disease by their lack of hyperpigmentation or salt-craving. Serum cortisol may be low or, occasionally, within the normal range, but the cortisol response to ACTH or insulin-induced hypoglycemia is inadequate. Serum ACTH is low.

  4. Treatment

   a. Tumors are treated surgically, by irradiation, or by a combination of the two, depending on the characteristics, location, and size of the individual tumor.

    b. Growth hormone. GH-deficient patients are treated with biosynthetic growth hormone, 0.025 mg/kg/day SC administered in the evening.

    c. TSH deficiency is treated with L-thyroxine (as discussed in sec. **V**).

    d. ACTH deficiency usually requires no treatment except during the stress of surgery, trauma, or illness. In these circumstances, treatment with cortisone acetate, 50 mg/m^2/day IM, or in divided doses PO, is recommended. An additional 100 mg/m^2 hydrocortisone sodium succinate (Solu-Cortef) solution is administered intravenously during surgery. In the presence of hypoglycemia or symptoms of adrenal insufficiency, cortisol should be replaced, as discussed in sec. **VI.A.5.** When symptomatic (usually in adolescence), hydrocortisone should be replaced, 12 mg/m^2/day in divided doses.

B. Hyperpituitarism

  1. Etiology. Excessive levels of GH, TSH, ACTH, or prolactin result from autonomous hormone production by a primary pituitary tumor or from altered regulation at a hypothalamic level.

  2. Evaluation

    a. Clinical states reflecting hypersecretion may be a result of elevated serum levels of the hormone or of uninterrupted hormone secretion, with circulating hormone levels apparently within the normal range.

    b. Evaluation consists of documenting the onset of observed changes (serial photographs are very helpful), determining pituitary function, ascertaining any local effects of a space-occupying lesion in the region of the sella, and measuring the ability of pharmacologic stimuli to suppress pituitary secretion.

  3. Diagnosis

    a. GH excess results in an accelerated growth rate in the child before fusion of the epiphyses and acromegaly after fusion has occurred.

      (1) Physical findings and symptoms include weakness, thickened skin, hypertrichosis, headaches, excessive perspiration, and joint pains. Not infrequently, acral changes are found in children.

      (2) Laboratory diagnosis is established by elevated circulating levels of GH and IGF-I (somatomedin-C), and the inability of a glucose load to suppress the elevated levels of GH. Impaired glucose tolerance may be seen, along with elevations in circulating levels of immunoreactive insulin.

    b. Excess TSH results in a clinical picture of hyperthyroidism, with elevated thyroid hormone, TSH, and alpha subunit.

    c. Cushing's disease results from hypercortisolism secondary to excessive or inappropriate secretion of ACTH. The clinical picture is that of the Cushing syndrome with a pituitary adenoma (see sec. **VI.C**).

    d. Patients with **hyperprolactin states** usually have galactorrhea and oligomenorrhea, or amenorrhea.

  4. Treatment

    a. Complete eradication of the tumor can be difficult and often requires a combined approach that involves surgery (transphenoidal or frontal approach) and radiation (x-ray, proton beam, isotope implantation).

    b. Bromocriptine is useful in treating prolactinomas. A dose of 2.5 mg per day is used to begin therapy; this is increased in 2.5-mg increments (maximum is usually 7.5 mg/day) by increasing the frequency of dosage schedule from qd to bid or tid. When large tumors are present, surgery and radiation therapy may be necessary.

    c. Long-acting somatostatin (Octreotide) has been used successfully for the treatment of GH- and TSH-producing tumors.

C. Diabetes insipidus

  1. Etiology

    a. Central DI is caused by either primary deficiency of antidiuretic hormone (ADH) as a result of defective ADH synthesis or release, or is secondary to interruption of the neurohypophyseal transport of ADH by tumors, histiocytosis, granulomatous disease, and inflammatory, vascular, or traumatic lesions. The familial form is usually inherited in an autosomal dominant fashion. It may be associated with congenital intracranial defects or result from autoimmune destruction of the supraoptic and paraventricular nuclei. A rare form is associated with diabetes mellitus, optic atrophy, and nerve deafness (Wolfram syndrome).

   b. Nephrogenic DI is caused by renal unresponsiveness to ADH (both endogenous and exogenous) and is inherited in an X-linked fashion. Female heterozygotes have a partial concentrating defect.

2. **Evaluation.** The diagnosis should be suspected in any child with persistent *polydipsia* and *polyuria*.

   a. Excess water intake and urine output must first be documented. Urine volume usually exceeds 3 liters/m^2/day, and serum osmolality exceeds urine osmolality.

   b. Evidence should be sought for CNS or pituitary disease, and the workup should include a cranial MRI study.

   c. Screening for DI is done by measuring the osmolality of a fasting second voided morning urine sample. The duration of the fast should be determined from the patient's history of unusual fast duration to avoid excessive dehydration during the study. A urine osmolality >650 mOsm/kg makes the diagnosis of DI highly unlikely. Hyponatremia in a random blood sample is more indicative of primary polydipsia than DI.

   d. Primary renal disease (chronic failure) and tubular unresponsiveness to ADH secondary to hypercalcemia, hypokalemia, pyelonephritis, and sickle cell disease should be ruled out.

   e. Primary polydipsia (excessive water intake) should be considered, especially if psychiatric illness or psychosocial problems are present.

3. **Diagnosis. The water deprivation test** is used to confirm the diagnosis. Body weight, osmolality, and sodium concentration of serum and urine, and plasma ADH are measured before, during, and at the end of the period of water deprivation. The deprivation of water should be continued either until urine osmolality does not change significantly (<30 mOsm/kg) in three consecutive hourly determinations or until body weight has decreased by 5 percent or more. The test is positive when serum hypertonicity develops (osmolality ≥295 mOsm/kg) and plasma ADH does not rise appropriately in the face of persistent polyuria and hyposthenuria (urine osmolality <300 mOsm/kg). An injection of ADH at the end of the test should increase urine osmolality by more than 50 percent in patients with central DI. In nephrogenic DI, the urine osmolality does not increase significantly.

4. **Treatment**

   a. Acute DI may occur after surgery or trauma to the hypothalamopituitary region.

   (1) Initial treatment consists of matching input and output up to a maximum of 3 liters/m^2/day, with the first 1 liter/m^2 being one-fourth normal saline in 5% dextrose in water (D$_5$ ¼NS) and the remainder 5% dextrose in water (5% D/W). This will produce a baseline sodium of 150–155 mEq/liter.

   (2) Alternatively, an ADH (Pitressin) drip can be initiated at 1.5 mU/kg/hr, with restriction of fluids to 1 liter/m^2/day.

   (3) Frequent weighing and measurements of serum osmolality and electrolytes are used to guide therapy.

   b. Chronic therapy

   (1) Desmopressin acetate (DDAVP), a long-acting vasopressin analogue, is the treatment of choice, and is administered as a nasal spray. The dose varies with the patient's weight. Initially, a bedtime dose sufficient to eliminate nocturia should be established. If a second dose is required, it is given in the morning and should be slightly less than the evening dose to allow a period each day during which any fluid overload can be excreted. DDAVP can also be injected SC, IM, or IV.

Therapy is usually started with a dose of 2.5–5.0 μg and increased gradually in increments of 2.5 μg until satisfactory antidiuresis is attained.

(2) Therapy is monitored by measuring 24-hour urine volume and urine and plasma osmolalities. The patient's random serum sodium should be at least ≥140 mEq/liter to reduce the risk of water intoxication.

(3) Therapy in infants is more complicated because their nutrition is provided largely in liquid form, making the risk of fluid overload with DDAVP greater than in older children. Consequently, it may be preferable to avoid exogenous ADH and simply provide daily fluids at 3 liters/m²/day, divided on a 3- to 4-hour feeding schedule, to allow adequate caloric intake and reduce the risk of water intoxication.

(4) For older infants, addition of a single dose of short-acting intranasal lysine vasopressin at bedtime reduces fluid needs and allows a brief period of uninterrupted sleep.

c. **Hormone amplifiers.** Chlorpropamide, 4 mg/kg/day, can be effective in patients with residual ADH secretion. Hypoglycemia is a potential side effect. Because of its thirst-stimulating activity, chlorpropamide is the preferred treatment for patients with partial DI and for those with adipsia or hypodipsia (essential hypernatremia).

d. **Nephrogenic DI.** Treatment is more difficult than for central DI. Because no treatment is able to eliminate the polyuria, **polydipsia is essential for survival.** Proprietary formulas are diluted 25–50 percent with water to reduce the solute load, and chlorothiazide, 1 gm/m²/day or 30 mg/kg/day, is given in two or three divided doses to reduce glomerular filtration rate (GFR) and enhance proximal water reabsorption. These maneuvers reduce the urine volume by 50 percent but may not supply adequate calories for growth; therefore, the formula should be supplemented with corn syrup or other glucose polymers.

D. **Inappropriate ADH secretion**

1. **Etiology.** This usually occurs after head trauma or intracranial surgery. Other causes include intracranial tumors, CNS infections, intrathoracic diseases, drugs that stimulate ADH secretion, and lesions of the hypothalamus that cause a state of chronic ADH excess. Ectopic ADH production is rare in childhood. The majority of patients are also receiving parenteral fluids, which they are unable to excrete because of the inappropriate persistence of ADH secretion.

2. **Evaluation and diagnosis**

a. Urine output is decreased, there is progressive weight gain, and the patient has an altered state of consciousness if hyponatremia is severe (e.g., serum sodium < 120 mEq/liter).

b. **The laboratory findings** include a decreased serum sodium, urine osmolality inappropriately high (>100 mOsm/kg) for the concurrent serum hypoosmolality, and increased urine sodium. Serum levels of urea and uric acid are usually decreased. Renal and adrenal function are normal.

3. **Treatment** is with fluid restriction to about 800 ml/m²/24 hr. Loss of body weight and a steady rise in serum sodium and osmolality are evidence of therapeutic success. More aggressive therapy is indicated if hyponatremia is acute, with serum sodium concentrations below 120–125 mEq/liter in association with severe CNS symptoms. Slow IV infusion of 3% saline, calculated to correct serum sodium to 125 mEq/liter, is combined with furosemide to minimize further expansion of intravascular volume. Raising the serum sodium too rapidly to levels >125 mEq/liter may result in CNS damage such as central pontine myelinolysis. Treatment should aim to raise the serum sodium concentration by 1–2 mEq/liter/hr to 125 mEq/liter and then gradually to 135 mEq/liter over the next 24 hours.

4. **Prevention.** The effects of inappropriate ADH secretion can be prevented by carefully monitoring the patient's serum electrolytes and weight, and by restricting fluid intake to match insensible water loss plus urine output.

V. Disorders of the thyroid
  A. Hypothyroidism
  1. **Etiology**
    a. **Congenital** causes include ectopic thyroid gland, 40–60 percent; aplasia of the thyroid, 20–30 percent; and dyshormonogenesis, 10–25 percent. Rarely secondary to thyroid resistance
    b. **Transient** causes include iodine excess or deficiency, transplacental passage of drugs (iodine, radioactive iodine [^{131}I] antithyroid medications), and maternal antibodies (anti-TSH receptor-inhibiting antibodies [TBII, or TBA]).
    c. **Acquired** causes include autoimmune (Hashimoto disease), irradiation, and surgery.
  2. **Congenital hypothyroidism** is the most common preventable cause of mental retardation. The prevalence is 1 : 4,000 (blacks, 1 : 30,000; Hispanics and Orientals, 1 : 2,000). Prevalence is increased in children with Down syndrome. The only means to prevent mental retardation is early (in the first 4 weeks) and adequate therapy.
    a. **Evaluation and diagnosis**
      (1) **Clinical manifestations.** Babies appear normal at birth, birth weight is slightly above the average, length is normal, and head circumference is slightly above average. Early manifestations are nonspecific and include: feeding difficulties, respiratory difficulties, prolonged jaundice (unconjugated hyperbilirubinemia), hypotonia, constipation, excess sleep, little cry, large posterior fontanel, macroglossia, umbilical hernia, dry and mottled skin, and slow relaxation of deep tendon reflexes. The full-blown picture may take months to manifest, making early diagnosis very difficult. Only 10 percent of infants with congenital hypothyroidism have suggestive signs when examined at 4 to 6 weeks of age.
      (2) **Neonatal screening** is the only means of early diagnosis and is performed on dried blood samples. Thyroxine (T$_4$) is measured initially. If T$_4$ < 6.5 µg/dl, TSH is measured. If TSH is 20 µU/ml or more, patients are referred for evaluation. Screening is most effective using samples obtained 3 to 5 days after birth; blood samples obtained earlier may increase the incidence of false-positive tests as a result of the TSH surge soon after birth. If the screening test is positive, the patient should be referred for evaluation.
        (a) Premature babies may have relatively low serum T$_4$, but the TSH concentration is normal.
        (b) Infants with congenital hypothyroidism may be missed by neonatal screening programs either because of human errors (failure to collect a blood sample; errors in processing, analysis, and reporting), or because of biologic variants (delayed rise in serum TSH).
      (3) **Laboratory**
        (a) Repeat thyroid studies determining T$_4$, triiodothyronine (T$_3$), T$_3$ resin uptake (or thyroid binding globulin index), and TSH on whole blood.
        (b) Obtain a thyroid scan and radioactive iodine (^{123}I) uptake to define the anatomy of the thyroid gland and assess its function.
        (c) If the TSH is low, a TRH stimulation test is recommended to determine whether hypothyroidism is secondary to pituitary or hypothalamic dysfunction.
        (d) Bone age determination is useful in diagnosis and for evaluating the results of therapy.
    b. **Treatment** should be begun immediately if the clinical or laboratory evidence suggests the diagnosis.
      (1) L-Thyroxine (10–15 µg/kg/day) is recommended. This dose should maintain the total serum thyroxine in the upper half of the normal range for the method (10–16 µg/dl in the first 2 years of life). This dose

will normalize serum thyroxine in less than 3 weeks. Smaller doses (7–9 μg/kg/day) take an average of 74 days to raise T_4 levels to >10 μg/dl. On 10–15 μg/kg, TSH levels will drop to <10 μU/ml in the majority of cases. Occasionally, the serum TSH may remain above 20 μU/ml for 2–3 months or more. This is thought to be secondary to the resetting, in utero, of the feedback threshold for T_4 suppression of TSH.

(2) Therapy should be monitored by measuring serum T_4, T_3 resin uptake or thyroid binding globulin index and TSH 2 weeks after the initiation of therapy, and at intervals of 2 months during the first 18–24 months, and every 3–4 months thereafter, as well as 4–6 weeks after each change in the dose of thyroxine.

(3) Because neonatal hypothyroidism is occasionally transient, therapy can be withheld at 4–5 years of age for a trial period of 4–6 weeks to determine if the hypothyroidism is indeed permanent. This step will be obviated if at any time the serum TSH becomes elevated, whether as a result of inadequate replacement with thyroxine or poor compliance.

3. Acquired hypothyroidism
  a. Etiology
    (1) Chronic lymphocytic thyroiditis (Hashimoto disease) is the most common cause.
    (2) TSH deficiency secondary to hypopituitarism
    (3) Exogenous causes include thyroidectomy, radioactive iodine therapy, iodine excess or deficiency, fluorine, lithium, cobalt, perchlorate, thiocyanate, para-aminosalicylic acid, propylthiouracil, and anticonvulsant therapy.
  b. Evaluation and diagnosis
    (1) Symptoms may be insidious. Linear growth is particularly vulnerable. Weight gain continues despite a poor appetite. Constipation, dry skin, fatigue, anorexia, and cold intolerance may be present. Puberty is delayed.
    (2) Signs. Short and overweight for height but rarely obese. Immature facies, bradycardia, and small pulse pressure are rare. Pallor, dry skin, mottled skin, cold extremities, distended abdomen, delayed relaxation phase of deep tendon reflexes (ankle jerk). The thyroid gland may be enlarged. In Hashimoto thyroiditis the gland is usually but not necessarily firm in consistency with a "cobblestone surface." Enlargement of the prelaryngeal (Delphian) lymph node felt just above the isthmus, 2–3 mm in size, is very suggestive of the diagnosis.
    (3) Laboratory evaluation. Serum T_4 is low. TSH is elevated in primary hypothyroidism, low in pituitary hypothyroidism, and low to normal and occasionally slightly elevated in hypothalamic (tertiary) hypothyroidism. Serum T_3 is usually low, but, not infrequently, is normal. Antithyroglobulin or antimicrosomal antibodies, or both, are found in high titers in Hashimoto thyroiditis.
  c. Treatment
    (1) Treatment with L-thyroxine is begun with 0.025 mg per day, and the dosage is gradually increased by 0.025 mg every 1–2 weeks until the appropriate dosage is attained. Most children require 75–100 μg/m²/day.
    (2) Thyroid function tests are used to monitor the appropriateness of the dosage, compliance, or both. The serum level of TSH is the most sensitive guide to the adequacy of therapy.
    (3) Striking alterations in personality and behavior should be anticipated when the euthyroid state is restored in a child who has been chronically hypothyroid.
B. Hyperthyroidism
  1. Neonatal hyperthyroidism

a. **Etiology.** One to ten percent of women with **Grave's disease** have offspring with hyperthyroidism, presumably secondary to transplacental passage of TSH receptor-stimulating immunoglobulins (TSI or TRAb).

b. **Evaluation and diagnosis**

   (1) **Clinical manifestations:** irritability, failure to gain weight, diarrhea, vomiting, diaphoresis, exophthalmos, enlarged thyroid gland. The most serious threats to life are severe tachycardia with congestive heart failure, tracheal obstruction, and associated infections. The manifestations may last 8 weeks to 6 months.

   (2) **Laboratory tests.** Elevated serum T_4 and T_3, undetectable serum TSH using ultrasensitive assays, and the presence of high titers of thyrotropin-stimulating immunoglobulins (TSI) or thyrotropin-binding inhibiting immunoglobulins (TBII), or both.

c. **Treatment** should be initiated promptly with propylthiouracil, 5–10 mg/kg/day given q6h, and iodine (saturated solution of potassium iodide [SSKI]) or Lugol's solution, one drop q8h.

   (1) The infant must be carefully monitored for signs of **heart failure** and treated with digoxin if necessary.

   (2) **Respiratory distress** from a greatly enlarged goiter is encountered infrequently and is treated with elevation and extension of the neck. Rarely, however, it may be necessary to resect the thyroid isthmus or intubate to relieve respiratory distress from tracheal compression.

2. **Acquired hyperthyroidism**

a. **Etiology.** Almost exclusively secondary to Grave's disease (autoimmune thyrotoxicosis) where anti-TSH receptor autoantibodies bind to the TSH receptors and mimic TSH function. It is rarely caused by a functional adenoma, subacute thyroiditis, TSH-producing tumor of the pituitary, or pituitary resistance to thyroxine. Girls are affected six times more frequently than boys.

b. **Evaluation and diagnosis**

   (1) Patients present with increased activity, increased appetite, weight loss, irritability, restless sleep, heat intolerance, poor coordination, increased number of bowel movements (not necessarily diarrhea), excessive sweating, palpitations, and irregular menses.

   (2) **Physical examination** reveals a tachycardia, systolic hypertension with a wide pulse pressure, warm and wet skin, diffusely enlarged thyroid gland that is soft to firm in consistency with a bruit, fine tremors of the outstretched fingers, and hyperreflexia. The eye signs are usually mild and consist of exophthalmos, lid lag, inability to converge, and, rarely, injection of the conjunctivae, excess lacrimation, and paresis or paralysis of the extraocular muscles.

c. **Laboratory evaluation.** Serum T_4 and T_3 are elevated (on rare occasions only T_3 is elevated, T_3 toxicosis). Serum TSH measured by ultrasensitive assays is undetectable, except if secondary to a pituitary tumor or partial (pituitary) resistance to T_4. Thyrotropin-stimulating antibodies (TSI or TSAb) or TBII, or both, are present. TRH stimulation test shows failure to release TSH, but is rarely needed with the advent of ultrasensitive TSH assays.

d. **Treatment**

   (1) **Thyrotoxicosis**

   (a) **Propylthiouracil (PTU),** 50–300 mg or 5–7 mg/kg/day, depending on the age and size of the patient, is given in three equally divided doses at eight hourly intervals. The dose is increased until the desired effect is achieved. When euthyroidism has been restored, the dose is reduced to the minimum necessary to maintain normal thyroid hormone levels. Recent recommendations include adding a replacement dose of thyroid while maintaining a full blocking dose of PTU.

   (b) **Methimazole (Tapazole)** can be used instead of PTU. The dose is one-tenth that of PTU and is given in two or three equally divided doses.

(c) **Toxic side effects** of the thionamides, PTU and methimazole, may occur at any time during the course of therapy and include: erythematous rashes, urticaria, agranulocytosis, arthritis, lymphadenopathy, a lupus-like syndrome, and hepatitis. A complete blood count must be performed whenever the patient has a sore throat, and therapy should be stopped immediately if leukopenia or granulocytopenia is present. If the side effect is not severe, a trial of the other thionamide can be attempted, with extremely careful monitoring for recurrence of side effects.

(d) For patients who are allergic to thionamides, noncompliant with therapy, or nonresponsive to maximal doses, or who require several years of treatment because of frequent relapses, alternative therapy such as **subtotal thyroidectomy** or thyroid ablation with **radioactive iodine** should be considered.

(2) **Thyroid storm** is a rare medical emergency that requires immediate treatment.

(a) Thyroid hormone synthesis and release, and the peripheral conversion of T_4 to T_3, are inhibited with large doses of **propylthiouracil (PTU)**, 200–400 mg q6h.

(b) **SSKI** is given orally or sodium iodide is given IV in a dose of 1–2 gm to block thyroid hormone secretion.

(c) **Dexamethasone**, 1–2 mg q6h, is effective in reducing the serum level of T_3.

(d) **Propranolol** should be used judiciously because tachycardia is a compensatory mechanism for the high output failure. The dose is 2 mg/kg/day and can be increased to 4–6 mg/kg/day.

(e) A cooling blanket is used to **control hyperthermia** and **fluids** are given intravenously to correct dehydration.

VI. Disorders of the adrenals

A. Adrenocortical hypofunction

1. **Etiology.** The causes of **primary adrenocortical insufficiency** include the following:

    a. Congenital adrenal hyperplasia

    b. Adrenal hemorrhage

    c. Hypoplasia or aplasia of the adrenals

    d. Congenital unresponsiveness to ACTH

    e. Fulminating infections, especially meningococcemia

    f. Addison's disease (autoimmune adrenalitis), isolated or associated with polyglandular autoimmune disease

    g. Adrenal leukodystrophy

    h. Granulomatous infiltration (e.g., tuberculosis)

    i. Acquired immunodeficiency syndrome (AIDS)

2. **Secondary adrenal insufficiency** is caused by:

    a. Congenital hypopituitarism (e.g., pituitary aplasia, septooptic dysplasia)

    b. Acquired hypopituitarism

    (1) Iatrogenic adrenal suppression as a result of long-term glucocorticoid therapy

    (2) Tumor

    (3) Irradiation

    (4) Surgery

    (5) Trauma

3. **Evaluation**

    a. The onset is usually insidious with vague and nonspecific complaints. The major **clinical features** are: weakness, personality changes, increased pigmentation (primary insufficiency only), salt-craving, hypotension, hypoglycemia, anorexia, nausea, vomiting, diarrhea, weight loss, and menstrual abnormalities. GI symptoms may mimic influenza or simulate an acute abdominal condition.

  b. Adrenal crisis, usually precipitated by stress, is characterized by vomiting, dehydration, fever, hypoglycemia, and hypotension, culminating in shock and coma.

  c. A short ACTH test should be performed whenever adrenocortical insufficiency is suspected.

4. Diagnosis

  a. Decreased serum sodium, increased serum potassium, hypochloremic acidosis, hypoglycemia, increased urinary sodium (>20 mmole/liter), and decreased urinary potassium. Note that electrolyte changes are not always present, especially in secondary insufficiency.

  b. Eosinophilia and relative neutropenia may be present depending on the severity of the illness.

  c. Serum cortisol and aldosterone may be low or within normal range, but ACTH levels are significantly elevated (>200 pg/ml) in primary adrenal insufficiency (especially if they are obtained at the time of maximal stress), and low (<50 pg/ml) in secondary adrenal insufficiency.

  d. The short ACTH test will diagnose primary adrenal insufficiency and most cases of secondary insufficiency, but does not distinguish between the two. The insulin tolerance test is the definitive test to confirm secondary adrenal insufficiency.

  e. Adrenal autoantibodies are found with autoimmune adrenalitis.

  f. Adrenal imaging (CT and/or ultrasound) and cranial imaging with CT or MRI are indicated in certain circumstances.

5. Therapy

  a. Addisonian crisis

   (1) Shock must be treated by rapid volume expansion (20 ml/kg normal saline IV stat); then estimate the degree of dehydration and replace the deficit over the next 24 hours together with maintenance fluids.

   (2) Hypoglycemia is treated with an IV infusion of 0.5 gm/kg dextrose over 5–10 minutes, followed by 0.5 gm/kg/hr.

   (3) Hydrocortisone sodium succinate (Solu-Cortef), 50–100 mg, should be given IV stat; then hydrocortisone, 100 mg/m^2/day is given as a continuous infusion, gradually reducing the dose to maintenance over 5 days and changing to oral therapy when appropriate.

   (4) Pressor agents usually are not necessary if adequate fluid is administered.

  b. Maintenance therapy consists of hydrocortisone, 10–20 mg/m^2/day in divided doses tid, with a larger dose in the morning; fludrocortisone (Florinef), 0.05–0.3 mg per day; and table salt ad lib, especially in the summer.

  c. During periods of stress the hydrocortisone dosage should be doubled or trebled and the frequency of administration increased to q6h. Patients or parents, or both, should know how to use cortisone acetate, 25–50 mg IM, in emergencies. Patients should wear a Medic Alert identification tag.

  d. For **surgery** or **severe stress,** see sec. **IV.A.4.D.**

B. Congenital adrenal hyperplasia (CAH)

 1. Etiology

  a. Congenital adrenal hyperplasia refers to a group of autosomal recessive enzyme defects of cortisol synthesis. The most common enzyme deficiencies and their clinical and biochemical features are shown in Table 11-8.

  b. Two enzyme deficiencies, 18-hydroxylase and 18-dehydrogenase, result only in deficiencies of aldosterone synthesis.

 2. Evaluation and diagnosis (see also Table 11-8)

  a. Presentation

   (1) Hypertension may be present in patients with 11β-hydroxylase and 17α-hydroxylase deficiencies.

Table 11-8. Clinical and laboratory features of congenital adrenal hyperplasia

Enzyme deficiency	Clinical features					Laboratory findings							
	Newborn with ambiguous genitalia		Postnatal virilization	Salt-wasting	Hyper-tension	Urinary excretion			Circulating hormones				
	M	F				17KS	P'Triol	ALDO	17OHP	Δ4	DHEA	Testo	Renin
21-Hydroxylase													
Simple virilizing	A	P	P	A	A	+	+	N/+	+	+	N/+	+	N/+
Salt-wasting	A	P	P	P	A	+	+	-	+	+	N/+	+	+
"Late onset"[a]	A	A	P	A	A	+/N	+/N	N	+/N	+/N	N/+	N/+	N
11β-Hydroxylase	A	P	P	A	P	+	+	-	+/N	+/N	+	N/+	-[e]
3β-HSD	P	P[d]	P	P	A	+	N/-	-	N/+	N/+	+	F+/M-	+
17α-Hydroxylase	P	A	A	A	P	-	-	-	-	-	-	-	-
Side chain cleavage enzyme	P	A	A	P	A	-	-	-	-	-	-	-	+
18-Hydroxylase	A	A	A	P	A	N	N	-	N	N	N	N	+
18-Dehydrogenase	A	A	A	P	A	N	N	-	N	N	N	N	+
17,20-Lyase	P	A	A	A	A	N/+	N/+	N	N/+	-	N/-	-	N

17KS = 17-ketosteroids; P'Triol - pregnanetriol; ALDO = aldosterone; 17OHP = 17-hydroxyprogesterone; Δ4 = androstenedione; DHEA = dehydroepiandrosterone; Testo = testosterone; Renin = plasma renin activity; M = male; F = female; N = normal; A = absent; P = present; + = increased; - = decreased; HSD = hydroxysteroid dehydrogenase
[a] Also referred to as "nonclassic."
[b] Increased DOC and 11-deoxycortisol.
[c] Increased DOC and cortisone.
[d] Clitoral enlargement.
Source: Adapted from M.I. New and L.S. Levine, *Congenital Adrenal Hyperplasia.* Berlin: Springer-Verlag, 1984.

(2) The patient often has a family history of spontaneous abortion or early infant death.

b. Laboratory examination

(1) Patients with 21-hydroxylase deficiency typically have high serum levels of 17-hydroxyprogesterone. The level may be normal, however, in "late-onset" or "nonclassic" CAH. Urinary 17-ketosteroids (derived from degradation of adrenal androgens) are increased in the virilizing varieties of CAH. Serum cortisol and aldosterone may be normal or low.

(2) A karyotype is done to determine the gender of infants with ambiguous genitalia (see sec. **III.A**).

3. Treatment

a. Salt-losing crisis

(1) Salt loss is treated with infusion of normal saline.

(2) Hypotension is treated with a fluid bolus of 20 ml/kg followed by 1.5 times maintenance fluid requirement until the patient's condition is stable.

(3) Glucocorticoids are administered as described above (**A.4a**). Frequently, diurnal weight changes are dramatic.

(4) Fludrocortisone (Florinef), 0.05–0.3 mg per day, is used for mineralocorticoid replacement. This is begun when the patient's condition has stabilized and (s)he is ready for oral intake. A dosage of up to 0.3 mg per day may be necessary in some infants. Salt supplementation of 2–4 gm per day is used to replace urinary losses. This can be added to the formula or solids until the child is capable of ad lib salt supplementation.

b. The glucocorticoid-deficient varieties of CAH (21-hydroxylase, 11β-hydroxylase, 3β-hydroxysteroid dehydrogenase, 17α-hydroxylase, and side chain cleavage enzyme or cholesterol desmolase) require cortisol replacement.

(1) Initial treatment of the symptomatic neonate with CAH may require three to four times the usual maintenance dose of glucocorticoids to suppress ACTH levels. Newborns are treated with 5 mg hydrocortisone q8h for the first 3 days; thereafter, the dose is reduced to 2.5 mg q8h.

(2) Hydrocortisone, 10–25 mg/m^2/day in three divided doses, suppresses ACTH secretion and reduces adrenal androgen synthesis.

c. The mineralocorticoid-deficient varieties (salt-wasting 21-hydroxylase, 3β-hydroxysteroid dehydrogenase, side chain cleavage enzyme or cholesterol desmolase, 18-hydroxylase, and 18-dehydrogenase deficiency) are treated with a salt-retaining hormone such as fludrocortisone (Florinef), 0.05–0.3 mg per day, and 2–4 gm additional salt each day. Patients with simple virilizing 21-hydroxylase deficiency with high plasma renin levels also benefit from treatment with mineralocorticoids.

d. Therapy is monitored clinically by measuring blood pressure, growth, pubertal development, and skeletal maturity (bone age).

(1) Plasma androstenedione, 17-hydroxyprogesterone at 8 AM, plasma renin activity, and testosterone (in females and prepubertal boys) are used to monitor the adequacy of replacement therapy.

(2) Although useful because they provide a measure of integrated adrenal steroid production, 24-hour urinary excretion of 17-ketosteroids and pregnanetriol is less frequently used to monitor therapy because of the difficulty of obtaining complete 24-hour urine collections in children.

e. Girls with the **virilizing** forms of CAH (21-hydroxylase, 11β-hydroxylase, and 3β-hydroxysteroid dehydrogenase) usually have clitoromegaly and varying degrees of labial fusion requiring surgery in infancy. If necessary, vaginoplasty is deferred until adolescence.

f. Incomplete virilization occurs in boys with cholesterol desmolase (side chain cleavage enzyme) deficiency, 3β-hydroxysteroid dehydrogenase deficiency, and 17α-hydroxylase deficiency. In certain cases, it is preferable to raise the child as a girl; surgery is performed to remove the testes and correct the genital abnormality to conform to the assigned sex. **Sex hormone therapy** is instituted at the time of puberty to induce and maintain secondary sex characteristics.

C. Cushing syndrome

1. **Etiology.** Glucocorticoid excess may be caused by adrenal tumors, (adenoma and carcinoma), adrenal hyperplasia (bilateral micronodular dysplasia), an ACTH-producing tumor of the pituitary (Cushing's disease), an ectopic ACTH-producing tumor, or prolonged treatment with glucocorticoids.

2. **Evaluation and diagnosis**

   a. **Clinical manifestations**

      (1) Evidence of glucocorticoid excess includes increased appetite, weight gain, slowing or arrest of linear growth, weakness, fatigue, and personality changes.

      (2) Fat deposition occurs in the facial, nuchal, shoulder, and abdominal areas, producing the characteristic "moon" facies and "buffalo hump." The extremities often appear thin as a result of muscle wasting.

      (3) Hypertension, plethora, purple striae, ecchymoses, and weakness may be present.

      (4) Hirsutism as a result of excess adrenal androgens is consistent with ACTH excess, but virilization (enlarged clitoris or phallus) suggests an adrenal carcinoma.

   b. **Laboratory examination**

      (1) There is an increase in 24-hour urinary free cortisol. Serum cortisol may be normal. Serum androgens and urinary 17-ketosteroids may be increased in Cushing's disease, ectopic ACTH, and especially adrenal carcinoma, but tend not to be increased in adrenal adenoma. **The most specific diagnostic feature is absence of the normal diurnal variation in serum cortisol levels.** Serum ACTH should be low in primary adrenal tumors and markedly elevated (typically >200 pg/ml) with ectopic ACTH-producing tumors (very rare in children). Serum ACTH may be normal or elevated in Cushing's disease.

      (2) A single-dose overnight **dexamethasone suppression test** (10–20 μg/kg dexamethasone given at 11 PM, with plasma cortisol measured at 8 AM) is a useful screening test. Normally, plasma cortisol < 5 μg/dl; >10 μg/dl is consistent with Cushing syndrome. If the results are equivocal, a low-dose dexamethasone suppression test (5 μg/kg q6h for 2 days) should be performed.

      (3) Glucocorticoid excess may be accompanied by a hypokalemic alkalosis, polycythemia, eosinopenia, lymphopenia, and abnormal glucose tolerance with hyperglycemia. Bone age is delayed and osteoporosis may be present.

      (4) **Evaluation of hypothalamopituitary-adrenal function** (high-dose dexamethasone suppression, 20 μg/kg q6h for 2 days; metyrapone, corticotropin releasing factor (CRF) stimulation tests), MRI studies of the hypothalamopituitary region, and CT scan and ultrasonography of the adrenal glands are done to determine the cause of the Cushing syndrome. Inferior petrosal venous sampling is performed in specialized centers.

3. **Treatment** depends on the etiology.

   a. If the disorder is caused by an adrenal tumor, surgical resection is the treatment of choice. If an autonomously functioning adrenal adenoma is removed, the remaining adrenal gland and contralateral adrenal gland will be atrophic; therefore, the patient must be given supplemental glucocorticoid therapy before, during, and after surgery until normal adrenal function recovers. **Bilateral diseases** (tumors, adrenal hyperplasia, micronodular disease) require total adrenalectomy and lifelong adrenal steroid replacement.

b. Treatment of a **nonresectable adrenal carcinoma** is unsatisfactory. Excessive glucocorticoid secretion may be diminished using the adrenolytic agent o,p'-DDD (mitotane) or agents that inhibit cortisol synthesis such as metyrapone, an 11β-hydroxylase inhibitor, or aminoglutethimide, which blocks conversion of cholesterol to pregnenolone.

c. **Cushing's disease (bilateral adrenal hyperplasia)** caused by excessive pituitary ACTH secretion is treated by surgical removal of the pituitary adenoma. Postoperative ACTH deficiency, which is usually temporary, requires glucocorticoid replacement until pituitary-adrenal function recovers. Radiotherapy, either conventional external irradiation or radioactive implants, is used if surgery is not feasible or has been unsuccessful.

D. Pheochromocytoma

1. Etiology. The adrenal medulla is derived from the ectoderm of the neural crest and secretes the catecholamines epinephrine, norepinephrine, and sometimes dopamine. Overproduction of catecholamines may be caused by tumors of the adrenal medulla or of accessory chromaffin tissue. In children, >90 percent are intraabdominal, and as many as 20–30 percent of pheochromocytomas are extramedullary in location; in 25 percent of patients, more than one tumor may be found.

2. Evaluation

a. The **clinical manifestations** most commonly noted are hypertension, headache, tachycardia, weight loss, growth failure, visual changes, palpitations, nervousness, abdominal or chest pain, hyperhydrosis, anxiety, fatigue, facial pallor, polydipsia, polyuria, and tremors.

b. A **family history** of multiple endocrine neoplasia and neuroectodermal dysplasias, or pheochromocytoma, should be explored. The presence of a coexisting medullary carcinoma of the thyroid and parathyroid tumors must be carefully ruled out.

3. Diagnosis. Typically, symptoms and signs are intermittent. The diagnosis is made by demonstrating increased urinary excretion of free catecholamines and total metanephrines in a 24-hour urine specimen. CT scanning is useful for localizing the tumor(s). A ^{131}I-metaiodobenzylguanidine (MIBG) scan is useful for identifying very small or extraadrenal tumors, and for localizing metastases.

4. Treatment. Surgical excision of the tumor is the treatment of choice. Preoperative, intraoperative, and postoperative management of the patient with a pheochromocytoma is complex and should only be carried out in a center with the resources and expertise to manage such cases.

VII. Disorders of calcium homeostasis

A. Hypoparathyroidism

1. Etiology

a. Idiopathic

(1) Early onset of hypoparathyroidism (first year)

(a) X-linked recessive (mild)

(b) Congenital absence of parathyroids (DiGeorge's syndrome)

(2) Later onset. Boys and girls are equally affected.

(a) Associated with Addison's disease and mucocutaneous candidiasis (the **type 1 autoimmune polyglandular deficiency syndrome**); other components of the syndrome may include: hypothyroidism, chronic active hepatitis, malabsorption syndrome, hypogonadism, pernicious anemia, vitiligo, and alopecia.

(b) Isolated hypoparathyroidism

b. Iatrogenic (following surgery)

c. Functional hypoparathyroidism caused by hypomagnesemia

d. Neonatal hypoparathyroidism

(1) Maternal hyperparathyroidism

      (2) Transient neonatal hypoparathyroidism
      (3) Neonatal illness

2. Evaluation

  a. Clinical presentation. Patients with hypoparathyroidism have a decreased ability to excrete phosphate and decreased intestinal calcium absorption, bone resorption, and calcium reabsorption, resulting in hypocalcemia and hyperphosphatemia, tetany, blepharospasm, conjunctivitis, papilledema, and increased intracranial pressure. Prolonged hypocalcemia results in trophic changes of the nails and skin.

  b. Laboratory evaluation should include:

      (1) Serum calcium, phosphorus, magnesium, and alkaline phosphatase

      (2) Circulating parathyroid hormone (PTH) and circulating vitamin D metabolites

      (3) 3'-5'-Cyclic adenosine monophosphate (cAMP) clearance

3. Diagnosis

  a. The serum calcium is usually 7–8 mg/dl, with a serum phosphorus of above 5.5 mg/dl.

  b. Circulating PTH is decreased (undetectable or low normal) despite the low calcium (normally a stimulus for PTH secretion).

  c. PTH infusion. IV administration of 200 IU bovine PTH raises the serum calcium and increases the urinary excretion of phosphate and cyclic AMP, and this distinguishes hypoparathyroidism from pseudohypoparathyroidism.

4. Treatment

  a. Tetany is treated with an IV solution of 10% calcium gluconate, 2 ml/kg, given slowly with continuous electrocardiographic (ECG) monitoring. If the heart rate decreases, the infusion should be slowed or stopped.

  b. When tetany has cleared, the patient can be maintained on oral calcium gluconate (9% elemental calcium) at 200 mg/kg/day divided into four to six doses.

  c. In **chronic hypoparathyroidism,** therapy with vitamin D is recommended. Vitamin D therapy should be withheld in postsurgical hypoparathyroidism until a chronic deficiency is documented (the parathyroid function may be suppressed up to 5 days and still return to normal).

      (1) 1,25-dihydroxy vitamin D (calcitriol) in dosages of 0.25–1.0 μg per day. Each capsule contains 0.25 μg. If more than one capsule is used, 0.25 μg per day bid, or 0.5 μg bid, should be administered.

      (2) Alternatively, **dihydrotachysterol,** 0.25–0.75 mg per day. The compound exerts biologic activity for 10–14 days after the medication is withdrawn.

  d. Vitamin D therapy should be monitored with measurements of 24-hour urinary excretion of calcium and creatinine, and with frequent measurements of serum calcium. In the interest of safety, serum calcium levels are kept between 8.5 and 9 mg/dl. If the ratio of urinary calcium to creatinine exceeds 0.3, or if the serum calcium exceeds 10.5 mg/dl, the vitamin D preparation should be stopped immediately until these parameters have returned to normal. The medication should be restarted at a lower dose.

B. Pseudohypoparathyroidism is a genetic disorder resulting from an abnormality in the adenyl cyclase enzyme complex that mediates the response to PTH.

  1. Etiology. The disorder is familial, with the usual transmission appearing to be X-linked dominant.

  2. Evaluation and diagnosis

    a. Albright's hereditary osteodystrophy (obese with a round face, mental retardation, metastatic calcification especially of the basal ganglia, shortened fourth and fifth metacarpals and metatarsals) is present in many patients with this disorder. The manifestations of hypocalcemia are similar to those previously described.

    b. Laboratory findings are similar to those in hypoparathyroidism except

that circulating levels of immunoreactive PTH are elevated. **PTH infusion** is the definitive test. In pseudohypoparathyroidism, no rise in phosphate excretion or increase in serum calcium is seen.
3. **Treatment** is the same as for hypoparathyroidism.
C. **Hypercalcemia** is defined as a serum calcium > 11 mg/dl.
   1. **Etiology**
      a. **Idiopathic hypercalcemia of infancy** (Williams syndrome), when associated with supravalvular aortic stenosis, mental retardation, and "elfin" facies, presents in early infancy. Hypercalcemia **usually** resolves by 1 year of age.
      b. **Primary hyperparathyroidism** may be associated with other endocrinopathies in the patient or family members, e.g., multiple endocrine adenomatosis type 1 (**parathyroid hyperplasia or adenoma,** associated with pituitary and pancreatic islet cell tumors) or type 2a (**parathyroid hyperplasia or adenoma,** associated with medullary thyroid carcinoma and pheochromocytoma).
      c. **Secondary hyperparathyroidism** is usually caused by renal failure, but it may occur in long-term malabsorptive conditions.
      d. **Vitamin D toxicity**
      e. **Vitamin A toxicity**
      f. **Immobilization** hypercalcemia occurs predominantly in adolescents following trauma.
      g. **Familial hypercalcemic hypocalciuria (FHH)** is an autosomal dominant hereditary disorder.
   2. **Evaluation**
      a. **Presentation.** Hypercalcemia causes nausea, constipation, weight loss, headaches, personality changes, renal stones, bone pain, hypotonia, polyuria, and polydipsia.
      b. **Laboratory evaluation** should include the following:
         (1) Serum calcium, phosphorus, magnesium, CO_2
         (2) Circulating PTH and vitamin D metabolites
         (3) A 24-hour urine for calcium, phosphorus, magnesium, creatinine, cyclic AMP
         (4) Bone films, including skull and pelvis
         (5) Serum vitamin A
   3. **Diagnosis**
      a. **Hyperparathyroidism** is diagnosed by the presence of an elevated circulating PTH level, decreased serum phosphate, and bone films showing evidence of irregular surfaces and bone cysts (osteitis fibrosa cystica).
      b. **Williams syndrome** is diagnosed on the basis of clinical presentation. An echocardiogram may be helpful in establishing the diagnosis.
      c. **Vitamin A toxicity** is rare, but may occasionally be diagnosed on the basis of a careful dietary history (intake of liver) or by measurement of serum levels of retinoic acid.
      d. **Familial hypercalcemic hypocalciuria (FHH)** is characterized by elevated serum calcium with low urinary calcium and normal serum parathyroid hormone levels.
   4. **Treatment**
      a. **Acute** hypercalcemia should be treated with the infusion of 0.9% NaCl solution and with the administration of furosemide, 1 mg/kg. Hydrocortisone, 1 mg/kg q6h, is also useful in lowering serum calcium. Calcitonin, 2–8 U/kg/day divided into two doses, or etidronate, 7.5 mg/kg/day once a day for 1–5 days, may be helpful in the treatment of hypercalcemia by inhibiting bone resorption. Dietary calcium must be severely restricted.
      b. **Primary hyperparathyroidism** is treated by surgical removal of the adenoma(s); subtotal parathyroidectomy is performed for parathyroid hyperplasia.
      c. In **secondary hyperparathyroidism** due to renal failure, improvement is usually seen when the patient's calcium balance is restored. This is

accomplished by a combination of 1,25-dihydroxy vitamin D or dihydro-tachysterol therapy and lowering the serum phosphate level using a phosphate binder or dialysis.

d. Immobilization hypercalcemia resolves when weight bearing can be tolerated. In severe cases, fluid therapy in combination with furosemide or calcitonin, or both, may be needed.

D. Rickets

1. Etiology

a. **Vitamin D deficiency** may result from inadequate intake (vegetarians, breast-fed infants, infants on TPN), malabsorptive states, anticonvulsive therapy, renal disease, and inadequate renal production of 1,25-dihydroxy vitamin D (vitamin D dependency), and receptors resistant to 1,25-dihydroxy vitamin D.

b. **Excessive renal phosphate loss** also causes rickets. This is seen in X-linked hypophosphatemia (vitamin D–resistant rickets), Fanconi syndrome, and Lowe syndrome.

c. **Renal tubular acidosis** also causes rickets.

2. Evaluation

a. **Clinical presentation**

(1) Patients with vitamin D–deficient rickets present with a history of bone pain, anorexia, slowed growth, and alterations in the long bones, with widening of wrists and knees, bowed legs, and muscle weakness. A rachitic rosary (enlarged costochondral junctions) and craniotabes may be noted.

(2) Patients with hypophosphatemic syndromes usually have a family history of rickets.

b. **Laboratory evaluation** should include the following:

(1) Serum calcium, phosphorus, magnesium, alkaline phosphatase, and total CO_2

(2) Circulating vitamin D metabolites, especially 25-hydroxy vitamin D and 1,25-dihydroxy vitamin D

(3) Circulating levels of PTH

(4) Knee and wrist films

(5) Urinary calcium, phosphorus, magnesium, pH, creatinine, and amino acids

3. Diagnosis

a. **Radiologic findings** of rickets include irregular cortices and bony margins, widened metaphyses, widened growth plates, and osteopenia.

b. In **vitamin D–deficient rickets,** serum calcium is normal or low, phosphorus is low, alkaline phosphatase is elevated, and urinary phosphate excretion is not excessive. An elevated level of PTH and a decreased 25-hydroxy vitamin D level confirm the diagnosis.

c. In **hypophosphatemic rickets,** renal phosphate wastage is increased (renal tubular resorption of phosphate < 80%). Serum phosphate is usually less than 3.0 mg/dl. Serum calcium and circulating levels of PTH and vitamin D metabolites are normal, and alkaline phosphatase is elevated.

4. Treatment

a. **Vitamin D–deficiency rickets** in infants heals with 1,000–4,000 IU per day of oral cholecalciferol (vitamin D_3). The dose is reduced to 400 IU daily when the rickets has healed. When rickets is due to **intestinal malabsorption,** the dosage of vitamin D necessary to promote healing may have to be as high as 10,000 IU per day.

b. **Rickets of prematurity** cannot be prevented by vitamin D supplements alone. The diet should be supplemented with calcium and phosphorus (calcium glubionate, 60 mg elemental calcium/kg/day, and potassium phosphate, 30 mg elemental phosphorus/kg/day).

c. **Vitamin D–dependent rickets (1α-hydroxylase deficiency)** is treated with "physiologic" doses of 1,25-dihydroxy vitamin D (0.5 μg/bid).

     d. Hypophosphatemic disorders require oral phosphate supplements, given q4h, to reach a total dosage ranging from 1–5 gm per day. This is combined with 1,25-dihydroxy vitamin D, 0.25 μg per day, to maintain adequate calcium absorption and avoid hypocalcemia.

     e. To avoid the **side effects** of hypercalcemia and hypercalciuria, blood and urinary calcium concentrations should be monitored frequently.

VIII. Disorders of glucose homeostasis

    A. Hypoglycemia is defined as a plasma or serum glucose concentration < 50 mg/dl (whole blood glucose concentration < 45 mg/dl).

      1. Etiology (see Table 11-9)

      2. Evaluation

        a. Clinical manifestations are due to increased **adrenergic** activity and increased secretion of epinephrine and include: trembling, nervousness, sweating, pallor, tachycardia, hunger, nausea, vomiting, and **neuroglucopenia**, which causes drowsiness, headache, weakness, inability to concentrate, bizarre behavior, confusion, coma, and seizures.

        b. Neonatal hypoglycemia is usually transient and does not require elaborate investigation (see Chap. 6, p. 171ff).

        c. When **neonatal hypoglycemia is persistent or recurrent,** and when **hypoglycemia occurs in an infant or older child,** a blood sample should be obtained at the time of hypoglycemia for the following analyses: glucose, lactate, free fatty acids, β-hydroxybutyrate and acetoacetate, total and free carnitine, alanine, insulin, glucagon, cortisol, and GH. Urine should be tested for ketones, non–glucose-reducing substances,

---

Table 11-9. Classification of childhood hypoglycemia

Neonatal—transient
Inadequate substrate or enzyme function (prematurity, intrauterine growth retardation)
Hyperinsulinism (infant of diabetic mother, erythroblastosis fetalis)
Neonatal, infantile, childhood—persistent or recurrent
Disorders of hepatic glucose production
   Hepatic glycogenolysis, e.g., type I glycogen storage disease
   Hepatic gluconeogenesis, e.g., fructose-1, 6-diphosphatase deficiency
   Galactosemia
   Hereditary fructose intolerance
   Prolonged fasting
   Ketotic hypoglycemia (accelerated starvation)
Disorders involving production of alternative fuels
   Defects in fatty acid oxidation, e.g., long-chain fatty acyl CoA dehydrogenase
     deficiency
   Defects in ketogenesis
Hormonal abnormalities
   Hyperinsulinism
   Deficiency of counterregulatory hormones
     Growth hormone deficiency
     Cortisol deficiency (primary or secondary to ACTH deficiency)
     Glucagon deficiency
     Epinephrine deficiency
Miscellaneous
   Associated with inborn errors of metabolism (propionic acidemia, methylmalonic
     acidemia, maple syrup urine disease, tyrosinosis)
   Drugs (alcohol, propranolol, salicylates, unripe akee nut)
   Severe liver disease (fulminant hepatitis, Reye syndrome)
   Sepsis in newborn
   Cyanotic congenital heart disease

organic and amino acids, and toxins. The results may be sufficient to clarify the etiology of the hypoglycemia (Table 11-10).

   d. The patient's **response to IV glucose** provides valuable additional information about the possible cause of the hypoglycemia. Infants with hyperinsulinism typically require rates of glucose administration considerably greater than 9 mg/kg/min to maintain plasma glucose above 50 mg/dl.

   e. **If the cause of the hypoglycemia is still obscure, a formal fasting study may be necessary.** Blood glucose, metabolic substrates, and hormones are monitored at frequent intervals, and the fast is terminated when the plasma glucose concentration falls to 50 mg/dl or after 24 hours, whichever occurs first. **Glucagon (0.03 mg/kg)** is given at the end of the fast, and the **glycemic response** is monitored over the next 90 minutes. Urine is collected throughout the fasting study for measurement of ketones and organic acids.

3. **Treatment.** Hypoglycemia is an important *preventable* cause of permanent brain damage, mental retardation, and seizures. Therefore, the diagnostic evaluation should be performed in a timely fashion, and hypoglycemia must be treated aggressively.

   a. **Acute.** Glucose is given intravenously at approximately 150 percent of the hepatic glucose production rate (HGPR; newborns, 5–8 mg/kg/min; older infants and children, 3–5 mg/kg/min). High concentrations of glucose and boluses of concentrated glucose should be avoided because, in a child with hyperinsulinism, this is likely to cause severe "reactive hypoglycemia."

   b. **Hyperinsulinism.** Diazoxide, 10–25 mg/kg/day in three divided doses, is used in an effort to suppress the inappropriate insulin secretion. If no benefit is apparent within a few days, S.C. administration of a somatostatin analog (Octreotide) can be given a therapeutic trial. If unsuccessful in preventing hypoglycemia, surgery is performed and an attempt is made to locate and excise an adenoma. If a discrete lesion cannot be found, a subtotal (90–95%) pancreatectomy is performed, preserving the spleen.

   c. **Hormone deficiency** is treated by replacement of the specific hormone deficiency (see above). Neonatal hypoglycemia due to GH deficiency is treated with human growth hormone (HGH), 0.5 μg (1 U) IM **daily.**

Table 11-10. Evaluation of hypoglycemia

Test	Ketotic hypoglycemia	Excess insulin	Hormone[a] deficiency	Enzyme[b] deficiency
Glucose	Low	Low	Low	Low
Insulin	Normal	+ +−+ + +	Normal	Normal
GH	Normal	Normal	Low/normal[a]	Normal
Cortisol	Normal	Normal	Low/normal[a]	Normal
T_4/TSH	Normal	Normal	Low/normal[a]	Normal
Lactate	Normal	Normal	Normal	+ + + +
FFA	+ + + +	Low	+ +−+ + +	+ + + +
Ketones[c]	+ + + +	Low	+ +−+ + +	+ +−+ + + or low[d]
Alanine	Decreased	Normal	Normal	+ + + +

Normal = blood level is appropriate in relation to the level of blood glucose and duration of fast; + + = mildly, + + + = moderately, and + + + + = markedly elevated; FFA = free fatty acids.
[a] Deficiency of GH or ACTH may be isolated or associated with deficiency of other pituitary hormones.
[b] Deficiency of key gluconeogenic enzymes such as glucose 6-phosphatase or fructose-1,6-diphosphatase.
[c] β-Hydroxybutyrate and acetoacetate.
[d] Ketones are low in disorders of fatty acid oxidation.

   d. The treatment of **disorders of hepatic glucose production** involves avoidance of prolonged fasting by establishing a pattern of frequent feeding, which includes a bedtime snack containing protein and carbohydrate. When anorexia, nausea, and vomiting occur for any reason, the urine should be tested frequently for the presence of ketones. Ketonuria signifies the need for liquid forms of concentrated carbohydrate; if oral carbohydrate cannot be retained, glucose must be given intravenously at a rate of approximately 4–6 mg/kg/min or 10% D/W at a rate of 1,500–2,000 ml/m^2/24 hr to forestall symptomatic hypoglycemia.

   e. Treatment of **type I glycogen storage disease** involves providing a dietary source of continuous glucose. This is accomplished during the day using uncooked cornstarch with meals and 3 hours after meals. The intake of galactose and fructose, which cannot be readily converted to glucose, and which may aggravate the hyperlactatemia and hyperlipidemia, should be kept to a minimum. A source of continuous glucose is provided at night using either intermittent uncooked cornstarch or a continuous intragastric infusion of glucose via a gastrostomy or nasogastric tube.

   f. Children with **inborn errors of fatty acid oxidation and ketogenesis** must avoid prolonged fasting. Their treatment is as outlined above for disorders of hepatic glucose production. Children with these disorders cannot produce ketones normally, and ketonuria is minimal or absent despite imminent hypoglycemia. L-Carnitine is replaced in children with systemic carnitine deficiency; it may also benefit patients with secondary carnitine deficiency.

B. Diabetes mellitus

  1. Classification, etiology, and general features

   a. Virtually all children and adolescents with diabetes have **insulin-dependent (IDDM) or type I diabetes,** which is the result of an absolute deficiency of insulin. IDDM appears to be a chronic progressive autoimmune disease involving destruction of the β cells of the islets of Langerhans. By the time of clinical presentation, 90 percent of the β-cell mass has been destroyed.

     The predisposition to IDDM is at least partly determined by genetic factors. First-degree relatives of patients with IDDM have a 5 percent risk of developing diabetes, compared to 0.1–0.25 percent for the population at large. Having an affected identical twin increases the risk to about 40 percent.

   b. Non–insulin-dependent (NIDDM) or type II diabetes occurs in a minority of adolescents with diabetes. Although not ordinarily prone to ketosis, these patients may develop ketosis under conditions of stress. Most NIDDM patients are obese, and insulin resistance associated with obesity is probably the reason for their glucose intolerance.

   c. Secondary diabetes may be caused by pancreatic diseases such as cystic fibrosis, pancreatectomy, and glucocorticoid disease.

  2. Evaluation

   a. Clinical course

     (1) Onset. About 80 percent of patients present with a classic history of less than 3 weeks' duration. The most common complaints are polyuria, polydipsia, insatiable thirst, enuresis, weight loss despite polyphagia, lack of energy, increased fatigability, blurred vision, and perineal candidiasis in girls. About one third of patients have diabetic ketoacidosis at the time of presentation.

     (2) Remission. Within a few weeks or months of starting insulin treatment, about two thirds of patients enter a phase of either partial or complete remission. Partial remission is characterized by virtually normal glycemia while receiving a relatively small dose of insulin (< 0.5 U/kg/day). Approximately 3 percent of patients enter a total remission, defined as normal metabolism for at least 3 months without insulin therapy. Partial or complete remission may last from several months to 1–2 years, but is eventually replaced by increasing insulin requirements. During the remission phase stable metabolic control is easily maintained. Within 5 years of diagnosis, most patients have lost virtually all β cell function.

(3) **Intensification.** In most patients waning of the remission is a gradual process characterized by increasing insulin requirements and metabolic instability over a period of several weeks or months. In some patients, the remission may end abruptly as the result of an intercurrent infection, emotional stress, or physical trauma.

(4) **Total diabetes** refers to the complete absence of β cell function (C-peptide negative) and total dependence on exogenous insulin such that its omission for 24 hours or more results in marked hyperglycemia and ketosis.

b. **Laboratory evaluation**

(1) Most children have classic symptoms (see **2.a**). Fasting and random blood glucose levels are increased with or without ketonuria.

(2) **Transient hyperglycemia and glucosuria** occasionally occur with stress.

(a) A **glucose tolerance test (GTT)** should be performed after the child has returned to good health. Tests of glucose tolerance must be done in the morning after an overnight fast and after at least 3 days on a high-carbohydrate diet (200–300 gm/1.73 m^2/day).

(b) The **oral glucose tolerance test (OGTT)** is performed using 1.75 gm/kg glucose (maximum of 75 gm). Blood samples are obtained for measurement of glucose (and insulin in certain circumstances) in the fasting state and thereafter at 30-minute intervals for 2 hours.

(3) The presence of **anti–islet cell antibodies or insulin autoantibodies, or both,** in the patient's serum indicates a very high likelihood that IDDM will develop in the future, and loss of first-phase insulin secretion during an **intravenous glucose tolerance test (IVGTT) predicts imminent diabetes.**

3. **Diagnosis**

a. In asymptomatic individuals, the OGTT is considered diagnostic of diabetes mellitus when the fasting venous plasma glucose concentration is elevated (> 140 mg/dl) and there is a sustained elevation of the plasma glucose concentration (>200 mg/dl) at 2 hours and at an intervening time point.

b. A child is considered to have **impaired glucose tolerance (IGT) if the fasting plasma glucose concentration < 140 mg/dl but the 2-hour value exceeds 140 mg/dl.**

c. When glucosuria is not accompanied by hyperglycemia, **renal glucosuria** should be ruled out by means of an oral GTT with simultaneous testing of urine glucose.

4. **Therapy**

a. **Goals.** Treatment is aimed at relieving symptoms, promoting a state of general well-being, and ensuring normal physical, emotional, and social growth and development, including healthy family interaction.

(1) Avoidance of episodes of severe hypoglycemia and ketoacidosis is an important short-term goal of therapy while attempting to restore near normal intermediary metabolism.

(2) The long-term goal is to prevent, if possible, the micro- and macrovascular complications of diabetes. Current evidence suggests that good control of blood glucose may delay or ameliorate the long-term complications of diabetes and improve the duration and quality of life.

(3) **Intensive insulin therapy** with continuous subcutaneous infusion of insulin (CSII) or multiple daily injections (MDI) enables the conscientious patient to achieve near normoglycemia. Intensive insulin

therapy is, however, extraordinarily demanding and should be used in carefully selected children and adolescents.

b. The patient is considered to be in satisfactory **metabolic control** when the following criteria are met:
  (1) Fasting blood glucose in the range of 70–140 mg/dl
  (2) Postprandial blood glucose < 180–200 mg/dl.
  (3) At least three of four urine tests show 0–1% glucosuria.
  (4) 24-hour urine glucose excretion is less than 5–10 percent of the daily carbohydrate consumption.
  (5) Glycosylated hemoglobin (hemoglobin A_{1c}) < 1.35 times the upper limit of normal.
  (6) Ketonuria is absent.
  (7) Plasma lipids are normal.

c. **Patient education** is the foundation of successful diabetes care.
  (1) The process of educating the parents and child begins soon after the diagnosis is made. Because most parents are too upset and anxious (the *grief* reaction) to assimilate an extensive body of information, the education program should be staged; initial goals are limited to an understanding of the fundamental nature of the disease and how it is treated, and acquiring the essential "survival skills" necessary to enable the child to leave the hospital, be cared for at home, and return to school.
  (2) During the next several weeks, the basic aspects of diabetes care are consolidated by practical experience at home and frequent contact with the diabetes educator and/or physician.
  (3) Once the grief reaction has subsided, the family is usually more ready to learn the intricate details of diabetes management and to cope with intercurrent illnesses, exercise, changes in appetite, and other variations that occur in the child's daily routine.
  (4) Education involves imparting facts and teaching practical skills but should also attempt to promote desirable health beliefs and attitudes in the person who has to live with a chronic incurable disease.
  (5) The educational curriculum must be concordant with the child's level of cognitive development and the learning style and ability of the individual child and family. **Parents must be fully involved;** however, a gradual transfer of responsibility from parents to the adolescent is encouraged.

d. **Insulin**
  (1) **Preparations** are divided into three categories according to their time of onset and peak activity, and total duration of action following subcutaneous administration (Table 11-11). The onset and peak activity of human neutral protamine Hagedorn insulin (NPH) tends

Table 11-11. Insulin preparations

Type	Appearance	Action	Onset of action (hr)*	Maximum effect (hr)*	End of effect (hr)*
Regular	Clear solution	Rapid	0.5	2–4	6–8
NPH (isophane)	Cloudy suspension	Intermediate	1.5–2	4–12	18–24
Lente	Cloudy suspension	Intermediate	1–3	6–12	18–24
Ultralente	Cloudy suspension	Prolonged	0.5–3	4–20	9–36

* These figures are approximations from laboratory studies in test subjects. The times of onset, peak, and duration of effect may vary greatly among patients and are affected by many factors, including dose, species, site of injection, exercise of the injection area, and insulin antibodies.

to be earlier than that of the corresponding animal species or of human lente insulin, and the total duration of action is significantly shorter (usually no more than 18 hours; significant waning of insulin effect can occur after 12 hours).

(2) During the **remission** phase the disease can be well controlled in many children with a single injection before breakfast of intermediate-acting insulin alone or combined with a small amount of regular insulin.

(a) Persistent nocturnal hyperglycemia manifested as nocturia or enuresis, and bedtime and/or fasting hyperglycemia, signifies the need for an evening dose of insulin either before the evening meal or at bedtime if regular insulin is not required before supper.

(b) If the single morning dose of intermediate-acting insulin is substantially increased to prolong its activity through the night and early-morning hours, hypoglycemia and intense hunger usually occur during the period of maximum insulin activity in the late afternoon and early evening.

(3) **Total diabetes** can be satisfactorily controlled in most children with a twice-daily insulin regimen consisting of a mixture of rapid-acting (regular) insulin and intermediate-acting (NPH or lente) insulin mixed in the same syringe and injected subcutaneously 30 minutes before breakfast and supper.

(4) The precise **dose** of insulin is determined empirically for each patient. On an average, about 60–75 percent of the total daily dose is given before breakfast and 25–40 percent before the evening meal. Usually, about one third of each dose consists of rapid-acting insulin; however, the optimal ratio of rapid- to intermediate-acting insulin for each patient must be determined by trial and error based on the results of blood glucose monitoring before meals, at bedtime, and between 2 and 3 AM.

(5) The recommended **starting dose** of insulin in a child detected early with **moderate hyperglycemia and no ketonuria is 0.3–0.5 U/kg/day SQ**. A single dose of intermediate-acting insulin without any regular insulin will usually suffice to restore normoglycemia and relieve the symptoms within a few days.

(a) When **metabolic decompensation is more severe with ketonuria but without acidosis or dehydration,** start with **0.5–0.7 U/kg** intermediate-acting insulin and supplement with 0.1 U/kg regular insulin SQ at 4- to 6-hour intervals, aiming to achieve preprandial blood glucose levels of 80–150 mg/dl. The insulin dose is adjusted daily until satisfactory glycemic control is achieved.

(b) Once metabolic control has been established, adjustments in the insulin dose should be made by approximately 10 percent at any one time, and a minimum of 3 days is allowed to elapse after each change before further adjustments are made. Acute metabolic derangements obviously warrant more frequent adjustments.

(6) **Injection sites** should be rotated to avoid unsightly lipohypertrophy, which alters the pharmacokinetics of insulin absorption. Recommended sites include the posterior aspect of the upper extremities, anterior aspect of the thighs, buttocks, and anterior abdominal wall.

(7) The technique of drawing up, mixing, and injecting insulin is taught to parents and, when appropriate, to the child. The average child of age 12 or older can and should be encouraged to learn to give his or her own insulin injections under parental supervision.

(8) **Modification of dosage**

(a) Children's insulin requirements change during the evolution of the stages of the disease and during normal growth and pubertal development as well as with change in activity (e.g., most children are considerably more active in the spring and summer and require less insulin during these times of the year). Therefore, each child's insulin regimen must be periodically reevaluated and adjusted if necessary.

(b) During the **remission** or "honeymoon" period, the insulin requirement < 0.5 U/kg/day and a tiny minority of patients may actually require no insulin at all for a few months.

(c) During the intensification phase and in the stage of total diabetes, the total daily insulin dose in prepubertal children is in the range of 0.5–1.0 U/kg/day; in pubertal individuals it is 0.8–1.5 U/kg/day.

(d) Amounts of insulin exceeding the above ranges are rarely necessary and should raise the suspicion of overinsulinization with hypoglycemia and rebound hyperglycemia (Somogyi phenomenon). Rarely, one has to consider the extremely unusual syndromes of insulin resistance due to dysfunction of the insulin receptor.

e. Diet therapy

(1) General principles

(a) The nutritional needs of children with diabetes do not differ from those of healthy children. The total intake of calories and nutrients must be sufficient to balance the daily expenditure of energy and satisfy the requirements for normal growth.

(b) The American Diabetes Association currently recommends that carbohydrate provide 50 percent of the total calories, with protein and fat making up 20 and 30 percent, respectively.

(c) The **diet prescription** has to be adjusted periodically to achieve an ideal body weight and to maintain a normal rate of physical growth and maturation.

(d) The main objective of dietary therapy in obese non–insulin-dependent patients is to lose weight and then maintain a desirable body weight.

(e) Food consumption must be matched to the time course of action of injected insulin. Meals and snacks have to be **eaten at the same times each day,** and the total consumption of calories and the proportions of carbohydrate, protein, and fat in each meal and snack must be **consistent** from day to day. Because insulin is released continuously from the injection site, **hypoglycemia,** exacerbated by exercise, may occur if snacks are not eaten between the main meals. Hence, most children receiving twice-daily injections of insulin have a snack between each meal and at bedtime. A snack should always precede strenuous exercise unless the blood glucose is known to be very high.

(2) Exchange system

(a) The **meal plan** is formulated in consultation with a clinical nutritionist using the system of food exchanges and is individualized to meet the ethnic, religious, and economic circumstances of each family and the food preferences of the individual child.

(b) The **exchange system** is based on six food groups: milk, fruit, vegetable, bread, meat, and fat. The individual food items included in each exchange list contain approximately the same amount of carbohydrate, fat, and protein. The portion size of each item included in the six categories is given either by weight or volume. Thus, the meal plan is prescribed in terms of the number of exchanges from each food group that should be included in each meal and snack.

(c) **Prudent fat.** Because individuals with diabetes are predisposed to atherosclerosis, the amount of fat should not exceed 30 percent of the total daily calories. Dietary **cholesterol** should be reduced to no more than 300 mg per day; the amount of **polyunsaturated**

fatty acids is increased while the consumption of **saturated fat is reduced** by consuming less beef and pork, and more lean meat, chicken, turkey, fish, low-fat milk, and vegetable proteins.

(d) **Fiber.** Dietary fiber may benefit the diabetic patient by blunting the rise in blood glucose after meals. Soluble fiber can also reduce serum cholesterol levels. Unrefined or minimally processed foods, such as grains, legumes, and vegetables, should replace highly refined carbohydrates.

(e) **Fruit.** To avoid abrupt increases in blood glucose, children should eat fruit **whole** and avoid fruit juices, which should be reserved for treating episodes of hypoglycemia.

f. **Exercise.** The effects of exercise on diabetes are complex.

(1) Exercise acutely lowers the blood glucose concentration, depending on the intensity and duration of the physical activity and the concurrent level of insulinemia. Children's activities tend to be spontaneous, making exercise advice difficult, if not impossible, to implement consistently. Consequently, bursts of increased energy expenditure should be "covered" by providing an extra snack before and, if the exercise is prolonged, during the activity. A rule of thumb is to provide one bread exchange (15 gm carbohydrate) per 30 minutes of vigorous physical activity. *Strenuous exercise in the afternoon or evening should be followed by a 10–20 percent reduction in the presupper dose of intermediate-acting insulin, and a larger bedtime snack to reduce the risk of nocturnal or early-morning hypoglycemia as a result of the lag effect of exercise.*

(2) Acute vigorous exercise in the child with poorly controlled diabetes can **aggravate hyperglycemia and stimulate ketoacid production.** Therefore, **the child whose diabetes is out of control (hyperglycemia with ketonuria) should be discouraged from exercising** until satisfactory control has been restored.

(3) Exercising the limb into which insulin has been injected accelerates the rate of insulin absorption. Therefore, if exercise is planned, it is recommended that the preceding insulin injection be given in a site that is least likely to be affected by exercise.

(4) Physical training increases tissue sensitivity to insulin. Youngsters who participate in organized sports are advised to adjust their insulin dose in anticipation of sustained physical activity during a specific period of the day. The precise amounts of such reductions are determined by trial and error, but are generally in the range of 10–30 percent of the usual insulin dose.

g. **Monitoring**

(1) **Blood glucose testing**

(a) Self glucose monitoring blood (SMBG) is the preferred method of metabolic monitoring. The technique should be routinely taught to all patients with IDDM, and the ability of patients to obtain accurate results must be established. Frequent SMBG in conjunction with urine tests for ketones is essential to manage intercurrent illnesses and prevent ketoacidosis. A variety of meters with a digital display are available that enable the user to obtain measurements of blood glucose concentration within 10 percent of the value obtained in a clinical chemistry laboratory.

(b) Ideally, patients should test before each meal and at bedtime. If this is impractical or intolerable, patients should be encouraged to test before each dose of insulin, with additional tests before lunch and at bedtime at least twice each week. Alternatively, for patients who cannot tolerate such frequent monitoring, or who cannot afford the cost of the reagent strips, a period of intensive monitoring before each meal, at bedtime, and between 2 and 3 AM for several consecutive days before an office visit often provides sufficient information to confirm satisfactory control or indicate where problems lie so that appropriate adjustments in the regimen can be made.

(c) Patients can fabricate results of blood and urine testing. Inaccurate and unreliable monitoring is common and usually the result of poor technique; frequent problems include obtaining insufficient blood to cover the reagent strip with a single drop of blood, failure to time the reaction carefully, and wiping the blood off too vigorously. Newer meters have obviated some of these problems.

(2) **Urine testing**

(a) Urine glucose testing has many limitations as a method for monitoring control of diabetes. The urine glucose concentration correlates poorly with blood glucose concentrations. A negative urine test cannot distinguish between a blood glucose level that is abnormally low from one that is normal or even slightly increased. Therefore, parents fearful of a hypoglycemic reaction when their young child's urine contains no sugar, often deliberately undertreat the child to ensure that "there is always a little sugar in the urine."

(b) The urine should always be tested for the presence of ketones whenever the child is sick, when the blood glucose level exceeds 250 mg/dl, and when blood glucose levels are high before breakfast and the possibility of nocturnal hypoglycemia with rebound hyperglycemia is considered.

(3) **Glycosylated hemoglobin (hemoglobin A$_1$ or A$_1$c)**. Because assessment of glycemic control by symptoms, urine tests, or infrequently performed blood tests at home or in the office is inaccurate, quarterly determinations of glycosylated hemoglobin should be used to provide an objective measure of average glycemia during the intervening period. The level of glycosylated hemoglobin, formed when glucose is bound nonenzymatically to the hemoglobin molecule, is directly proportional to the time-integrated mean blood glucose concentration over the preceding 2–3 months.

5. **Acute complications**

a. **Hypoglycemia**

(1) Occasional episodes of **hypoglycemia** are virtually an inevitable consequence of insulin therapy. Ideally, frequency and severity of hypoglycemia should be minimized while maintaining the best possible glycemic control.

(2) The most common reasons that **hypoglycemia** occurs are bursts of physical activity without a preceding snack; prolonged or strenuous exercise without a reduction of insulin dose; meals or snacks that are delayed, omitted, or incompletely consumed; inadvertent errors in insulin dosage; and inappropriate insulin regimens.

(3) **Patients and family members must be taught to recognize the early symptoms of hypoglycemia and treat it promptly with a suitable form of concentrated carbohydrate.** Most episodes of hypoglycemia are satisfactorily treated with 10–20 gm glucose. For an infant or toddler, 5 gm is sufficient. This can be provided in the form of glucose tablets (each contains 5 gm glucose), Lifesavers, granulated table sugar, or orange or apple juice.

(4) Family members are taught to use **glucagon** (which should be kept available at home) to treat **severe hypoglycemia** when the child is unconscious or unable to swallow or retain ingested carbohydrate. Glucagon (0.02 mg/kg, maximum dose 1.0 mg) is injected IM or SQ and raises the blood glucose level within 5–15 minutes. Nausea and vomiting may follow the administration of glucagon. Oral carbohydrate to prevent further hypoglycemia should be given when consciousness has been regained after a severe insulin reaction.

(5) If the patient cannot take or retain sugar-containing solutions orally, 5–10 gm glucose is injected intravenously followed by a continuous intravenous infusion of glucose at a rate of at least 10 mg/kg/min with frequent blood glucose monitoring.

(6) A Medic Alert bracelet or necklace should always be worn to identify the patient as having diabetes mellitus.

b. Diabetic ketoacidosis (DKA)

(1) Evaluation (see also Chap. 3)

(a) Rapidly perform a clinical evaluation to establish the diagnosis and determine its cause (especially any evidence of infection) as well as the patient's degree of dehydration. Weigh the patient and measure height or length.

(b) Determine the blood glucose concentration with a reagent strip method and plasma ketones at the bedside.

(c) Obtain a blood sample for measurement of glucose, electrolytes, and total CO_2, BUN, pH, PCO_2, PO_2, hemoglobin, hematocrit, white blood cell count and differential, calcium, magnesium, and phosphorus. Calculate the anion gap $Na^+ - [Cl^- + TCO_2]$; 12 ± 2 is normal.

(d) Perform a urinalysis and obtain appropriate specimens for culture (blood, urine, throat) even if the patient is afebrile.

(e) Perform an electrocardiogram for baseline evaluation of potassium status.

(f) Determine baseline neurologic status.

(2) Supportive measures

(a) Nasogastric suction to empty the stomach is used to avoid aspiration in semiconscious or unconscious patients.

(b) Broad-spectrum antibiotics should be given to **febrile** patients after appropriate cultures of body fluids are obtained.

(c) Supplementary oxygen is given to patients who are cyanotic or in shock, and/or when the PaO_2 < 80 mm Hg.

(d) Accurately assess urine output. Bladder catheterization or condom drainage should be used, as appropriate.

(e) A flow chart should be maintained that records the patient's clinical and laboratory data, details of fluid and electrolyte therapy, administered insulin, and urine output. Successful management of diabetic ketoacidosis requires meticulous monitoring of the patient's clinical and biochemical response to treatment so that timely adjustments in the treatment regimen can be made when necessary.

(f) The severely ill child should be admitted to an intensive care unit or other facility where intensive clinical and metabolic monitoring can be carried out.

(3) Fluid and electrolyte treatment (see also Chap. 7). **All patients with DKA are dehydrated** and suffer total body depletion of sodium, potassium, chloride, phosphate, and magnesium. Patients with mild to moderate DKA are usually about 5% dehydrated, and those with severe DKA are about 10% dehydrated.

(a) The first priority is to start an intravenous infusion using a large-bore cannula and to infuse 10–20 ml/kg isotonic saline (0.9%) in 60 minutes. If hypotension or shock persists, an additional 10–20 ml/kg isotonic saline (or an equal amount of colloid) is given over the next 60 minutes.

(b) Once the circulation has been stabilized, change to half-normal saline and aim to replace half of the calculated fluid deficit in 8–16 hours; the remaining half is replenished over the next 16–20 hours.

(c) 5% dextrose is added to the infusion fluid when the blood glucose concentration reaches 250–300 mg/dl. In some instances **10% dextrose** may be needed to avert hypoglycemia.

(d) Early in the course of therapy, **continued osmotic diuresis contributes significantly to ongoing fluid losses,** and should be replaced with half-normal saline and added potassium until positive fluid balance is achieved. When the osmotic diuresis subsides, maintenance fluid is given at a rate of 1,500–2,000 ml/m²/day.

(4) Insulin. Several insulin therapy protocols are effective in managing DKA.

(a) The preferred method is **low-dose continuous intravenous administration** controlled by an infusion pump. Insulin is diluted in saline (50 U regular insulin in 50 ml saline and short tubing) and is given IV at a rate of 0.1 U/kg/hr after an IV priming dose of 0.1–0.25 U/kg. This rate of insulin infusion is sufficient to reverse DKA in the majority of patients; however, if the response is inadequate (blood glucose levels are not falling and anion gap is not decreasing) due to severe insulin resistance, the rate of insulin infusion should be increased until a satisfactory response is achieved. **A minority of patients with severe insulin resistance will not respond satisfactorily to low-dose insulin infusion and require twice or three times the usual dose.** The continuous infusion method allows the rate of insulin administration to be finely controlled, and reduces the risk of hypoglycemia and hypokalemia. The serum half-life of insulin is approximately 5 minutes, so that if insulin infusion is stopped, the serum insulin concentration decreases by 50 percent every 5 minutes. A potential **disadvantage** of low-dose continuous insulin infusion is that **inadequate insulinization rapidly occurs if the infusion infiltrates and is not promptly recognized. Therefore, low-dose insulin therapy should not be used unless it can be closely supervised.**

(b) When DKA has resolved (venous pH > 7.32, total CO_2 > 18 mEq/liter) and the change to **SQ** insulin is planned, the first SQ injection should be given at least 60–120 minutes before the infusion is stopped to allow sufficient time for the injected insulin to be absorbed.

(c) Insulin can also be effective in lowering blood glucose and reversing acidosis when given **intramuscularly,** which has the advantage of not requiring any special equipment. However, this method involves frequent IM injections and, in hypotensive patients, insulin absorption may be quite variable. Initially, 0.1–0.5 U/kg is given as an IV bolus. Thereafter, 0.1 U/kg is given IM hourly until the blood glucose reaches 300 mg/dl, and then the insulin is given SQ.

(5) Potassium replacement

(a) All patients with DKA are potassium depleted (3–10 mEq/kg) despite the fact that the initial serum potassium concentration may be normal or increased. **With the administration of fluid and insulin, serum potassium may decrease abruptly predisposing to cardiac arrhythmias. Patients whose serum potassium level is initially low are the most severely depleted** and should receive potassium early (after urinating and after insulin has been given), and their serum potassium concentration should be measured hourly.

(b) The serum potassium level should be maintained in the 4- to 5-mEq/liter range. If the laboratory has not reported the pretreatment level within an hour, **potassium should not be withheld if**

Table 11-12. Potassium replacement in diabetic ketoacidosis

Serum potassium (mEq/liter)	Infusate potassium concentration (mEq/liter)
<3	40–60
3–4	30
4–5	20
5–6	10
>6	0

insulin has already been given and the patient has urinated. Table 11-12 is a guide to initial potassium administration based on the serum concentration.

(c) Half the potassium is given as potassium chloride and the other half as potassium phosphate, thus reducing the total amount of chloride administered and partially replacing the phosphate deficit. In hyperchloremic patients, potassium acetate should be used instead of potassium chloride.

(d) The electrocardiogram can serve as a useful guide to therapy. The configuration of the T waves in standard lead II and V_2 is followed at 30- to 60-minute intervals.

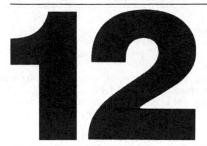

Prepubertal and Adolescent Gynecology

Marian Craighill

External genital inspection should be part of the standard physical examination. Pelvic examinations should be done routinely in sexually active adolescents. Referral of the adolescent patient to another provider to perform the pelvic examination increases the possibility that it will not be accomplished unless it is immediately available in the same setting. Because of the high prevalence of pregnancy and venereal disease in American adolescents and the need to recognize and treat pediatric gynecologic disorders as they arise, all providers of pediatric care should be familiar with gynecologic examinations, pathology, and treatment.

I. **Gynecologic examination**
  A. Typical anatomy and physiology by age
   1. From **birth to 6–8 weeks** of age
      a. Maternal estrogen effects predominate.
      b. Breast tissue is engorged and breast buds are palpable.
      c. Vaginal mucosa and introitus are bright red and plump.
      d. Genital bleeding from the uterus may occur at the end of this period as a result of the fall in maternally derived estrogen.
   2. From **8 weeks to 2 years**
      a. Maternally stimulated hormone levels (luteinizing hormone and follicle-stimulating hormone) are falling, but can do so at variable rates, resulting in **prolonged breast buds** for some girls, which may be asymmetric. Biopsy of the area can result in adolescent amastia on the biopsied side and should be avoided.
      b. **Mastitis** is possible and should be treated aggressively, usually with intravenous antibiotics.
      c. **Functional follicular ovarian cysts** may be present beginning from the fetal period and are generally asymptomatic. Most commonly they are identified as an incidental finding on ultrasound. Since spontaneous regression is the norm, treatment is generally not warranted unless the patient is symptomatic, in which case laparoscopic or ultrasound-guided aspiration is possible. Torsion is rare and laparotomy or oophorectomy should be avoided. An asymptomatic short episode of genital bleeding from the uterus can follow resolution of a functional cyst.
   3. From **2 to 8 years**
      a. Hypoestrogenic environment similar to menopause, readily susceptible to vaginitis if vaginal flora disrupted
      b. Uterus involutes to 30 percent of adult size and is palpable on rectoabdominal examination.
      c. Ratio of the size of the cervix to the size of the uterine corpus is 2 : 1.
      d. Vagina is 5 cm long with thin pink mucosa.
      e. Cervix is flush with the vagina.
      f. Hymen is thin and friable; 0.5 cm opening depending on examination technique
      g. Labia minora are prominent, thin, and pink, with minimal labia majora or vulvar fat pads.
   4. From **8 to 9 years**
      a. Estrogen stimulation begins.

    b. Cervix to corpus ratio becomes 1 : 1.

    c. Vagina lengthening to 6–8 cm, mucosa thicker

    d. Hymenal orifice 1 cm on average depending on examination technique

    e. Labia majora more prominent

    f. Breast budding generally precedes onset of menstruation by about 2 years. Tanner staging is noted (see Table 11-1).

    g. Ovaries move from abdominal to pelvic location with adult bone maturation.

  5. Adolescence

    a. Adult genital anatomy, cervix to corpus ratio 1 : 2

    b. Vaginal length is 10 cm and vaginal fornices develop.

    c. Hymenal orifice is 1 cm but redundancy with estrogenation obscures findings.

    d. Adult-appearing vulva develops in Tanner stages.

B. Age-specific gynecologic examination

  1. Birth to age 2

    a. Voluntary cooperation is not usually possible. A caretaker known to the child can either hold the child on his/her lap or the child can be held while lying on a table, with ankles drawn together in the frog-leg position.

    b. Grasp labia and give traction forward and down to inspect hymen.

      (1) Hymenal anatomy

        (a) Cresentic: most common with thin villamentous edge extending across the inferior portion of the hymenal opening. Vessels may be visible in the normal hypoestrogenic prepubertal state.

        (b) Annular: similar to crescentic but the hymen extends circumferentially. The upper border may not be appreciated without labial traction.

        (c) Redundant (also called *petal* or *tulip*). Multiple hymenal folds make vaginal inspection difficult, even with proper labial retraction.

    c. Visualization can be enhanced with an otoscope without the ear piece, providing light and magnification to evaluate pathology in the office setting.

  2. Age 2 to 5 years

    a. The child is reassured that the examination is painless. Use caretaker's lap to place child in dorsal lithotomy position, with child's feet propped on knees of caretaker if child is hesitant to assume frog-leg position on examination table when so requested.

    b. Forced examinations are remembered and are **inappropriate.**

    c. As the external genitalia are inspected, the patient is asked to hold the labia apart. This allows her to participate and have a sense of control.

    d. The knee-chest position can be used for cooperative patients (see below).

    e. Rectoabdominal examination is warranted if there is a question of a mass. The cervix feels like a small nubbin.

    f. Examination under anesthesia (EUA) is the appropriate choice when the child is unable to cooperate and there is a persistent indication to evaluate for pathology and/or a thorough intravaginal inspection is warranted.

  3. Age 5 to puberty

    a. Examine patient in frog-leg position to evaluate external genitalia for standard well child examination.

    b. If pathology is suspected add the knee-chest position to visualize the vagina and in a cooperative patient to visualize the cervix. The patient is told to "lie on her tummy with her bottom in the air." As the child takes a few deep breaths and allows her spine and stomach to "sag like an old horse," the vaginal orifice falls open. An otoscope provides the necessary light and magnification needed to visualize the cervix.

    c. Rectoabdominal examination if pathology is suspected

    d. EUA if unable to examine and persistent indication to evaluate for pathology

4. Adolescent pelvic examination (first pelvic examination)

    a. Routine (at least yearly) complete pelvic examinations including speculum examination for Papanicolaou smear and cultures for gonorrhea and chlamydia should begin when the patient is sexually active or planning to be, has been sexually active in the past, or is 18 or older. (Cultures can be deferred if the patient has never had genital contact.)

    b. Explain the rationale for the examination and the information being obtained. Describe each step to the patient.

    c. Plastic models of pelvic organs will help in demonstrating the procedure.

    d. Show the instruments, beginning with a large Graves speculum and ending with a narrow Huffman, and explain your intention to use the *smallest* size appropriate for her anatomy. This helps the patient understand that you have taken particular consideration for her first examination.

    e. Whether or not a parent remains in the room depends on the parent-adolescent relationship. In general, adolescents are better examined without parent to provide opportunity for privileged communication. Ideally, it is the patient's choice.

    f. A chaperone is mandatory for a male examiner and generally preferable for all.

    g. Examination **technique.** Ask the patient to let the legs drop apart like an open book with buttock muscles relaxed. Emphasize that the examination does not need to cause discomfort if the vaginal wall and gluteal muscles remain relaxed. Place a hand first on the knee or other nongenital location while describing motions. Next, place one finger of the examiner's nondominant hand on the gluteal fold to initiate an S2 desensitization reflex so that the next move of firm downward pressure with the forefinger of the dominant hand on the introitus is partially extinguished. With the nondominant hand remove the gluteal finger while maintaining firm introital pressure with the dominant hand and slip the speculum on top of the introital finger well into the vagina in a posteriorly angled direction as the finger is slipped out of the introitus. Note the appearance of the cervix and vaginal mucosa.

    h. Obtain a Pap smear first using wooden spatula and endocervical brush. Smear onto glass slide in a transparent layer and apply fixative immediately.

    i. Obtain gonococcal (GC) culture, with a cotton swab placed in the cervical os for 30 seconds or more, and plate *immediately* on a room-temperature Thayer-Martin plate; rapidly put in sealed CO_2 environment (sealed bag and pellet or candle jar; see also Chap. 14, p. 414).

    j. Take any other relevant samples (wet preps, etc.).

    k. The last specimen to be obtained should be a *Chlamydia* screen or culture, with a dacron swab twirled multiple times in the endocervical canal to pick up endocervical cells without picking up cervical or vaginal debris.

    l. Next, use sterile water-soluble lubricant on one or two fingers of the dominant hand placed in the vagina to elevate the uterus; with the other hand sweep down from the umbilicus toward the vagina to palpate the uterus; and then move laterally to palpate the adnexa.

      (1) With a retroverted uterus or evidence on bimanual examination of a posterior adnexal mass, a rectovaginal examination is then done *after changing gloves,* with the first finger in the vagina, the second finger in the rectum, and the same motions with the abdominal hand.

      (2) In tense or obese patients, it may be difficult to identify ovarian tissue by touch. An ultrasound can help define adnexal anatomy.

C. Breast examination. Although breast cancer will develop in 1 in 9 American women in a lifetime, it is extremely rare in children and adolescents. Adolescents should be taught to do breast self-examinations to promote healthy habits later in life and to become familiar with their breasts, so that when an unusual lump is noted, they will seek prompt medical attention. A family history of breast cancer, particularly if it occurred at a young age, increases future breast cancer risks and the importance of establishing good breast examination habits.

1. The week following menses is the best time to do the examination because physiologic lumps are least prominent.
2. The examination is done in the shower or bath, using the soapy water to help move over the breast tissue. The tips of the first two fingers on each hand are used to trap tissue, which is then rocked between the two hands in concentrically smaller circles.
3. The patient should be encouraged initially to examine her breasts with each bathing until she becomes familiar with how her breasts feel. Then, she should gradually increase the interval between examinations to once a month after her period. If periods are irregular, an arbitrary day each month is selected, e.g., the first of the month.
4. Each adolescent needs reassurance with a routine examination that her breast findings are normal. The large range of variation that is still within the "normal" limits should be stressed.
5. Benign cystic changes are found in 85 percent of women.
6. Mild asymmetry is common during development. Marked asymmetry that is present after Tanner 5 breast development has been established can only be altered with plastic surgery.
7. Accessory nipples or breasts occur in 1–2 percent of healthy patients. No therapy is indicated.
8. Periareolar follicle may drain brownish fluid for several weeks. No treatment is needed.
9. Periareolar hair is not uncommon in healthy adolescents. No treatment is indicated.

II. **Diagnostic studies**
   A. A **Papanicolaou smear** should be done on all young women who have a speculum examination. Those with a history of genital warts, hormonal therapy, abnormal Pap smears, or sexually transmitted disease (STD) may need Pap smears at more frequent intervals.
   1. With the speculum in place, an Ayer wooden spatula is scraped around the cervix, and the collected material is spread on a slide, with attention taken to cover the entire slide surface. The slide is immediately fixed with the specimen. A second specimen is taken from the endocervical canal with an endocervical brush, twirled in the endocervical canal, and streaked and fixed on a glass slide.
   2. Reporting of the results has recently been revised as follows: Specimens are designated *satisfactory* or *unsatisfactory*. Only satisfactory smears can be interpreted, and unsatisfactory smears must be repeated.
      a. No malignant cells identified (formerly class I or normal): routine follow-up indicated.
      b. Atypical cells of undetermined significance (formerly class II or IIR): indication of potential abnormality, suggesting the need for, at minimum, a repeat Pap smear in 3 to 6 months. In the face of other indications of potential pathology including a prior atypical or abnormal Pap smear, history or presence of genital warts, or partner with genital warts, immediate colposcopy is indicated. If an associated infection such as chlamydia or *Trichomonas* is present, but not one of the above indications for colposcopy, this infection should be treated and the Pap smear repeated. *Given the high rate of false-negative Pap smears, multiple repeat Paps are often appropriate in the face of the above listed indications of potential pathology* (e.g., q3mo for 1 year, then q6mo for 2 years).
      c. Low-grade squamous intraepithelial lesion (formerly class III, mild to moderate dysplasia): indication for immediate colposcopy. Colposcopically directed biopsy is needed for a definitive diagnosis. A repeat Pap smear is not appropriate because the false-negative rate is too high.

d. High-grade squamous intraepithelial lesion (formerly class IV or V, moderate to severe dysplasia or *carcinoma in situ*): indication for **immediate** colposcopy after concurrent possibility of infection is excluded.

3. Prepubertally, a **vaginal smear for estrogen** is useful for evaluating the patient's hormonal status in the absence of infection. A cotton swab moistened with saline is twirled to scrape the side wall of the vagina. The material obtained is streaked on a glass slide and fixed with Papanicolaou fixative. The maturation index gives a ratio of basal, intermediate, and superficial cells indicating degree of estrogenation.

B. Wet preparations are used in determining the cause of a vaginal discharge.
   1. In the prepubertal child, the sample is collected with a saline-moistened cotton swab or eyedropper from the introitus while the patient is supine.
   2. In the adolescent, the specimen is collected from the vaginal pool while the speculum is in place.
   3. The cotton swab is mixed with one drop saline on a slide, then is mixed with one drop 10% potassium hydroxide (KOH) on a second slide.
   4. A cover slip is promptly applied and the slides are examined under the microscope (low and high dry power).
      a. In the saline specimen, *Trichomonas* infection is indicated by the presence of lively, flagellated organisms about the size of a white blood cell.
      b. In the saline specimen, *Gardnerella vaginalis* infection is indicated by leukocytes and refractile bacteria attached to large epithelial cells ("clue cells").
      c. In the KOH specimen, *Candida albicans* infection, budding hyphae, and yeast forms are present.

C. Gram stain. In gonorrhea the smear may reveal gram-negative intracellular diplococci. However, because *Neisseria vaginalis* organisms are normal vaginal flora, only a positive culture establishes the diagnosis.

D. Cultures. Sexually active adolescents should have a routine cervical culture for gonorrhea and *Chlamydia* at the time of speculum examination or when indicated, such as after exposure to a new partner or by the patient's symptoms. The sites of culture in the symptomatic patient or contact are the urethra, cervix, rectum, and pharynx.
   1. *Gonorrhea.* Swab the area to be cultured with a cotton swab and streak directly on a plate, using a Transgrow, modified Thayer-Martin-Gembec, or Thayer-Martin medium.
   2. *Chlamydia*
      a. In a prepubertal child, or when clinical circumstances are questionable, only true cultures should be done because of the unacceptable consequences of a false-positive test, although this is labor intensive and requires a specialty laboratory.
      b. Microtrack screens identify inclusion bodies and so are technician dependent.
      c. EIA screening tests are the most cost effective and least complicated to perform, but produce both false-positive and -negative results.
   3. *Candida.* To confirm yeast vaginitis, swab the vagina and streak on Nickerson's medium. Leave the cap of the bottle with the medium partially unscrewed and incubate the tube at room temperature. The appearance of brown colonies in 3–7 days confirms the diagnosis.

E. Pregnancy tests
   1. Several 2-minute urine pregnancy tests are available. They are quick and convenient, and offer a high degree of reliability. These tests detect human chorionic gonadotropin (HCG).
   2. The **beta subunit blood** test measures HCG in serum and is positive within 5–10 days of conception. In the first trimester the value will generally double every 48 hours in a normally developing pregnancy if the specimens are processed in the same laboratory. This can be used to identify and distinguish an ectopic pregnancy, missed abortion, or threatened abortion from a normal pregnancy.

3. **False-negative and false-positive tests**

   a. **Urine.** False-negative tests occur when the pregnancy is sufficiently early to be below the test threshold. Depending on the assay, this may be less than 6 weeks of pregnancy or an ectopic pregnancy. False-positive tests are seen with detergent residue on the glassware, significant proteinuria, and some drugs (e.g., methadone, phenothiazines, and progestational agents).

   b. **Blood.** False-negative tests are obtained very early in pregnancy, generally in the first 10 days after conception, depending on the sensitivity of the assay. False-positive tests occur when a pregnancy is miscarried or terminated. The beta subunit falls by half every 48 hours and so may remain positive for several weeks after the pregnancy ends, depending on how high the titer rose initially.

F. **Buccal smear.** The patient rinses her mouth with water, and a tongue depressor is then scraped along the buccal mucosa.

   1. The material is streaked on a glass slide and placed in Papanicolaou fixative or a 3 : 1 methanol–acetic acid solution.

   2. The chromatin-positive material (Barr body) represents the second X chromosome. Normal Barr body counts vary from 10 to 49 percent. The absence of Barr bodies indicates XO or XY and a low count suggests a mosaic; XXX or XXXY causes two Barr bodies per cell.

III. **Pediatric gynecology**

A. **Common congenital abnormalities. Imperforate hymen** should be corrected before menarche. (An apparent imperforate hymen may actually be microperforate and once estrogenized may become sufficiently open that it does not require intervention.)

B. **Vaginitis**

   1. **Etiology.** Prepubertal hypoestrogenic environment with a neutral pH is susceptible to pathogens and environmental irritants.

      a. Poor perineal hygiene is likely after the age of 3, when caretakers are not directly involved with toileting.

      b. Pinworm infestation with the subsequent anal scratching can contaminate the vaginal area; an adult pinworm may migrate to the vagina and produce vaginal irritation and discharge.

      c. Bubble bath and harsh soaps further disrupt the pH and make it easier for vulvitis and secondary vaginitis to develop.

      d. Tight-fitting or nylon underpants worn with exercise or in hot weather cause maceration and promote yeast overgrowth.

      e. Masturbation or sexual abuse can play a role. Conversely, a symptomatic vaginitis will affect behavior.

   2. **Evaluation**

      a. A careful history should be traced, questioning the child about the etiologic factors listed in **1.** Ask about the quantity, duration, and type of discharge. Determine the direction in which the child wipes the anal area. Ask about the use of bubble baths, the type of soap used, symptoms of anal pruritus, and whether or not the child has had exposure to an infected adult through sexual contact or indirectly by sharing a bed, towels, and so on.

      b. Examine the child in the knee-chest position to rule out the presence of a foreign body. When indicated, obtain cultures in the frog-leg position.

      c. Culture technique (see above for age-specific examination)

         (1) Use urethral swab moistened in sterile saline.

         (2) Take all samples with a single swipe.

         (3) The best sample with least discomfort can be obtained if the vagina can be entered without touching the hymen, but an introital specimen is also acceptable.

         (4) Aerobic sample identifies most pathology. Send the swab to the laboratory in transport media for culture on blood, McConkey, and chocolate agar.

      d. Do a wet preparation for yeast and *Trichomonas*. With a persistent or severe yeast infection, check the urine for glucose to rule out diabetes. Do the Scotch Tape or pinworm paddle test to confirm the presence of pinworm infestation.

   e. Persistent discharge, particularly when recurrent after a course of treatment, suggests a possible foreign body, and EUA should be considered if an office examination does not allow good vaginal visualization.

   f. Blood-tinged discharge is more common with *Shigella* or *Salmonella* as specific pathogens or with a foreign body, but trauma must also be excluded.

3. Diagnosis. A **history of exposure** to offending agents, the presence of **symptoms** (itching, discomfort, vaginal discharge), the **character of the discharge,** a positive culture, and the **physical findings** aid in establishing the diagnosis of vulvovaginitis.

4. Therapy

   a. Nonspecific vaginitis (culture shows normal flora) is treated with the following measures:

     (1) Instruct the child to:

       (a) Improve perineal hygiene

       (b) Wear white cotton underpants

       (c) Avoid bubble baths and harsh soaps

       (d) Take sitz baths tid in plain warm water. Wash the vulvar area with mild soap (Basis, Oilatum, castile) and pat dry. Allow for further drying by lying on the back with the legs spread apart for 10 minutes.

     (2) If no improvement is seen in 3 weeks, treat the child with oral antibiotics (such as amoxicillin, ampicillin, or cephalexin) for 10–14 days or with a topical antibacterial cream (Sultrin, AVC).

     (3) If improvement still does not occur, treat the child with an estrogen-containing cream for 2–3 weeks (reversible breast tenderness and vulvar pigmentation may occur) or consider EUA.

   b. Acute severe edematous vulvitis

     (1) Sitz baths should be taken q4h, without soap and with air drying.

     (2) Witch hazel pads (Tucks) should be used instead of toilet paper.

     (3) After 2 days, sitz baths should be alternated with painting of the vulva with a bland solution, e.g., calamine lotion.

     (4) For **pruritus,** hydrocortisone cream 1%, Neo-Delta-Cortef Cream 1%, or Vioform-Hydrocortisone Cream should be applied to the vulva.

   c. Specific vaginitis

     (1) Gonococcus (see Chap. 14, p. 414)

     (2) For **group A beta-hemolytic streptococci or pneumococci:**

       (a) Amoxicillin, 25–50 mg/kg/day in three divided doses for 10 days, or

       (b) Erythromycin, 30–50 mg/kg/day PO tid

     (3) For *Trichomonas,* metronidazole (Flagyl), 125 mg tid PO for 5 days, or 1–2 gm PO in one dose

     (4) Pinworms (see Chap. 15, p. 447)

     (5) *Candida albicans.* Nystatin or other topical antifungal cream (for moist lesions) or ointment (for dry scaly lesions) should be applied to the vulva for 2 weeks. For persistent yeast infections, nystatin, 100,000 units PO qid for 2 weeks, and sitz baths in boric acid, 1 tsp per quart of warm water bid

C. Labial adhesions

   1. Etiology. The hypoestrogenic environment of the prepubertal child makes the labia susceptible to healing by agglutination after minor trauma or irritation.

   2. Evaluation. *Partial* adhesions are quite common. If they extend up progressively to involve more than half the labia, urine may collect in the vagina producing odor and discharge. *Complete* adhesions may block urine flow.

   3. Diagnosis is made by visual inspection. The labia meet in the midline along a line and the hymen cannot be visualized when the labia are retracted.

4. Treatment

  a. Partial adhesions do not usually require treatment unless they block urine flow.

  b. A small amount of estrogen cream is applied only to the line of adhesion bid for 2 weeks, then qd, and is continued to be applied to the area for at least one month after fully open. Then a bland ointment (A and D, Desitin, K-Y Jelly) is applied for several months to prevent the adhesions from reforming.

  c. If the adhesion is persistent after at least a month of estrogen cream, the same treatment is continued, but once well thinned topical 5% lidocaine ointment is applied and, once numb, the labia are gently separated. Estrogen cream is continued after manual lysis for at least one month or adhesions will recur. Spontaneous resolution at puberty is usual.

D. Genital trauma

  1. Etiology. Anatomic absence of the vulvar fat pads as well as the degree of activity make children more susceptible to genital trauma. The possibility of sexual abuse must also be considered.

  2. Evaluation

  a. The amount of bleeding correlates poorly with the degree of injury.

  b. Penetration of the hymen requires a complete EUA as injuries can extend into the peritoneal cavity. Sexual abuse should be strongly considered under such circumstances. The majority of the injury will be to the posterior fourchette, with hymenal transection or findings near the 6 o'clock position.

  c. Innocent injury such as a straddle fall will usually produce anterior labial or periurethral injury, and bruising may be extensive.

  d. Critical assessment is necessary to determine if the physical findings *are consistent with the history provided* and if the child was referred promptly for evaluation, as hymenal trauma will heal rapidly and physical findings may be gone in as little as 48 or 72 hours.

  e. Lichen sclerosus may be mistaken for trauma or abuse because subcutaneous hemorrhages can occur with minor or no history of trauma. However, the adjacent skin will generally be whitened, symptoms of itching are often present, and the involved skin is usually well demarcated.

  3. Diagnosis is made by inspection. With injury that transects the hymen at 6 o'clock and is evaluated within 72 hours of occurrence, a rape kit should be collected, generally as part of an EUA. Lichen sclerosus can be diagnosed with a skin biopsy.

  4. Treatment

  a. A vulvar hematoma can usually be treated with ice packs.

  b. A Foley catheter may be necessary if urinary retention occurs. Voiding into warm water may help.

  c. Evacuation of a hematoma is necessary only if it is expanding. In that case, broad-spectrum antibiotics should be maintained intravenously for several days to prevent secondary infection.

  d. Most injuries heal well and do not need sutures unless bleeding persists, the injury extends below the subcutaneous layer, or structures are partially avulsed and need restoration of anatomy.

  e. Lichen sclerosus is treated with topical steroids or, in very severe cases, with testosterone cream, but secondary sex changes will occur.

E. Condyloma acuminatum

  1. Etiology. Genital contact is required for transmission. Genital contact occurs in the birth canal as well as through sexual abuse. Epidemiologic evidence suggests fomites are not a source, but this is often hypothesized.

  2. Evaluation. Sexual abuse should be considered, including cultures for other STDs and an age-appropriate psychosocial evaluation. A biopsy can be evaluated both histologically and for viral DNA analysis, looking specifically for a genital subtype of the human papilloma virus, which will exclude the possibility of a common wart as etiology, but does not establish the mode of transmission. Urethral prolapse may be mistaken for condyloma but will only involve the urethra and responds to topical estrogen cream.

3. **Diagnosis** is made by visual inspection and biopsy, including histology and DNA probe.

4. **Treatment**
   a. Laser vaporization with biopsy during EUA is preferred because all lesions can be treated in one setting without conscious awareness by the child.
   b. Trichloroacetic acid and liquid nitrogen in the office setting are alternate options, but are painful and generally require multiple treatments. When sexual abuse is the etiology, this may add to the child's trauma, depending on the developmental age.

IV. **Adolescent gynecology**
   A. **Vulvovaginitis**
      1. **Etiology.** Unlike prepubertal vaginitis, which is usually nonspecific, vaginitis in the adolescent generally has a specific cause, e.g., *Neisseria gonorrhoeae, Trichomonas, Candida,* G. *vaginalis, Herpesvirus,* or *Chlamydia trachomatis,* and is often related to sexual contact. However, the most common cause of discharge in the adolescent is physiologic leukorrhea (normal desquamation of epithelial cells).
      2. **Evaluation and diagnosis.** A pelvic examination is required, with wet preparations and cultures.
         a. *Trichomonas.* A wet preparation (saline) reveals flagellated organisms dancing under the microscope. Small punctate hemorrhagic spots may be seen on the cervical and vaginal cells.
         b. *Candida.* A wet preparation (KOH) reveals budding hyphae. Nickerson's medium is used for culturing.
         c. **Nonspecific vaginitis.** A wet preparation reveals large epithelial cells coated with small refractile bacteria (clue cells). To identify G. *vaginalis,* the discharge is streaked on chocolate agar and incubated under increased CO_2 tension.
         d. **Gonorrhea.** The discharge should be cultured. See sec. **I.B.4.i.**
         e. **Leukorrhea.** A wet preparation reveals epithelial cells only and there is no itch, burn, or smell. Most common in early puberty, just before menarche.
         f. **Condyloma acuminatum.** Wart-like growths are inspected and Pap smear obtained.
         g. **Herpes vulvitis** (see Chap. 14, p. 431). Viral cultures are obtained from a fresh vesicle and set on ice. A culture from an ulcerated lesion may be negative even though active disease is present. If cultures are not available, the base of the lesion is scraped and stained with Wright stain, looking for multinucleated giant cells and inclusion bodies.
         h. *Chlamydia.* The endocervical canal should be cultured.
         i. *Pediculosis pubis* **(crabs).** Firmly attached flakes will be seen on the pubic hair. (The flakes are adult lice or nits.)
         j. **Pinworms** (see Chap. 15, p. 447)
         k. **Foreign body.** Inspect the patient for the presence of a foreign body. In the adolescent, this is often a forgotten tampon.
      3. **Treatment**
         a. For *Trichomonas* vaginitis, give metronidazole, 2 gm PO, all in one dose, or 250 mg tid for 7 days. Treat sexual partners at the same time. Instruct the patient not to drink alcohol while receiving metronidazole, because vomiting results.
         b. For **candidal (monilial) vaginitis,** a topical or intravaginal antifungal agent for 1, 3, or 7 days depending on the product and/or sitz baths with boric acid (Borax), one tbsp per quart of warm water
         c. For G. *vaginitis* (also called nonspecific vaginitis), metronidazole, 250 mg

tid PO for 7 days, for patient and partner or intravaginal metronidazole or clindamycin qd for 7 days

d. **Gonorrhea** (see Chap. 14, p. 414)

e. **Leukorrhea.** Reassure the patient and recommend good perineal hygiene and the wearing of white cotton underpants.

f. **Condyloma acuminatum**
   (1) Apply trichloroacetic acid (25% or, if resistant lesions and *carefully* applied, 85%) to lesion weekly. Initial intense burning can be lessened by immediate saline rinse or application of aloe vera gel.
   (2) If lesions do not respond, liquid nitrogen applied with a cotton swab or cryocautery probe using aqueous lubricant and freezing to ice ball
   (3) If still resistant or increasing, laser vaporization or loop electrode excision, usually under anesthesia

g. **Herpes vulvitis.** Acyclovir, 200 mg PO five doses qd, or topical cream q3h. Soothing relief may be obtained with lidocaine 2% jelly plus sitz baths. Urinating in the shower or tub may be necessary for patients with severe pain.

h. *Chlamydia.* Doxycycline, 100 mg bid PO for 10 days.

i. *Pediculosis pubis.* Lindane (Kwell) lotion should be used on all hairy areas. **Do not exceed recommended dosage; lindane can be absorbed through the skin, with potential central nervous system (CNS) toxicity.** Clothing and bedding should be washed in hot water and the partner treated simultaneously.

j. **Pinworms** (see Chap. 15, p. 447)

B. **Genitourinary infections**
   1. **Gonorrhea** (see Chap. 14, p. 414)
   2. **Pelvic inflammatory disease (PID;** see Chap. 14, p. 414)
   3. **Syphilis** (see Chap. 14, p. 415)

C. **Delayed sexual development** (see Chap. 11, p. 300)

D. **Secondary amenorrhea**
   1. **Etiology**
      a. The most common causes are pregnancy and stress produced by emotional turmoil, weight change, change in environment (camp, boarding school, college), or increased exercise.
      b. Also consider anorexia nervosa, obesity, polycystic ovary syndrome, thyroid disease, ovarian tumor, and diabetes.
   2. **Evaluation**
      a. **Pregnancy.** When a sexually active patient's period is 2 weeks late, the patient should have a pelvic examination and a pregnancy test.
      b. **Stress.** The history will elicit areas of stress in a patient's life.
      c. **Anorexia nervosa.** No specific laboratory test is available. Psychiatric evaluation is essential.
      d. **Obesity.** Determine whether or not weight gain (often rapid) is correlated with cessation of periods.
      e. **Polycystic ovary syndrome**
         (1) Hirsutism, acne, and obesity may be present.
         (2) Enlarged, cystic ovaries may be palpable on pelvic examination or identified by pelvic ultrasound.
         (3) Total serum testosterone and free testosterone are often elevated. There is an increase in the LH : FSH ratio. Urinary ketosteroids are normal to moderately elevated. DHEA-S may be elevated.
         (4) **Diabetes mellitus** (see Chap. 11, p. 325)
      f. **Thyroid disease** (see Chap. 11, p. 311)
   3. **Diagnosis**
      a. **Pregnancy** is indicated by an enlarged uterus and is confirmed by a positive pregnancy test.
      b. **Stress.** A stressful situation in the patient's life is identified and correlated with the onset of amenorrhea.

c. **Anorexia nervosa.** The classic history of prolonged weight loss secondary to poor intake, coupled with excessive activity, amenorrhea, and emotional problems, confirms the diagnosis of anorexia nervosa.

d. **Obesity.** Documentation of excessive weight gain with resultant amenorrhea is required.

e. **Polycystic ovary syndrome.** The diagnosis is considered in a patient with a history of oligomenorrhea, particularly with the physical findings of hirsutism, obesity, acne, and enlarged cystic ovaries on pelvic examination, and abnormal hormonal levels.

f. **Thyroid disease** (see Chap. 11, p. 311ff)

4. **Therapy.** Identify the cause and eliminate it when possible.

a. **Stress.** Medroxyprogesterone acetate (Provera), 10 mg PO for 10 days, to induce withdrawal bleeding, then initiate oral contraceptives to maintain bone mass.

b. **Anorexia nervosa.** Regaining sufficient weight is critical for the individual's hypothalamic suppression to cease. A greater proportion of body weight as fat is required to restore periods than to maintain them once reestablished. Oral contraceptives should be used to maintain bone mass until weight is restored.

c. **Obesity.** Loss of excessive weight initiates spontaneous periods. Provera, 10 mg qd for 10 days a month, or oral contraceptives to maintain menses and prevent PCO

d. **Polycystic ovary syndrome.** Provera, 10 mg qd for 10 days a month, will prevent endometrial hyperplasia, but oral contraceptives are the treatment of choice to protect future fertility. Treatment should be considered before full expression of the disease to prevent its occurrence.

e. **Thyroid disease** (see Chap. 11, p. 311ff)

f. **Diabetes mellitus** (see Chap. 11, p. 325ff)

E. **Dysfunctional uterine bleeding**

1. **Etiology.** One of the most common gynecologic complaints in the adolescent is irregular, prolonged menstruation.

a. In the **young adolescent** the cause is anovulatory cycles (unopposed estrogen) with incomplete shedding of the proliferative endometrium. A large amount of bleeding can occur without the menstrual lining being properly shed.

b. In the **older adolescent** it is secondary to anovulatory cycles from stress, illness, or hormonal effects.

2. **Evaluation**

a. History of drug ingestion (warfarin), birth control pills

b. Pelvic examination with cultures for *N. gonorrhoeae* and *Chlamydia*

c. Pregnancy test

d. CBC with platelet estimate

e. Tine test (in TB prevalent areas)

3. **Diagnosis.** A past history of painless bleeding with irregular intervals and particularly with irregular length suggests anovulatory bleeding. Any positive findings in the evaluation procedures suggest specific diagnoses.

4. **Treatment**

a. For irregular periods of short duration with normal hemoglobin and if the patient is not bleeding at the time of the visit, give Provera, 10 mg qd for 10 days, to bring on a proper menstrual shedding; repeat for three monthly cycles or start oral contraceptives.

b. For **persistent vaginal bleeding** without significant anemia or no response to **a,** give Lo/Ovral, one pill q6h until the bleeding stops, then one tid for 3 days, then bid for 2 days, then one qd to complete a 21-day course. Then continue Lo/Ovral or another standard low dose oral contraceptive for 3 to 6 months.

c. For **heavy vaginal bleeding** with anemia, if bleeding does not stop in 36–48 hours, consult a gynecologist.

F. **Dysmenorrhea.** Functional dysmenorrhea is very common. Organic lesions associated with dysmenorrhea include chronic PID, vaginal agenesis, rudimentary uterine horn, paramesonephric cysts, and endometriosis.
1. **Etiology.** Prostaglandins released during the menstrual flow stimulate the contractility of the endometrium. Endometriosis can also be a cause.
2. **Evaluation.** Review the menstrual history, premenstrual symptoms, timing of cramps, and how the patient deals with cramps. Patients with severe dysmenorrhea require a pelvic examination to rule out a menstrual flow obstruction.
3. **Diagnosis.** Cramping lower abdominal pain usually starts 1–4 hours before a period and lasts up to 24 hours. Some girls experience dysmenorrhea 2 days before the onset of menstrual flow, and the pain can last 4–6 days. Nausea and vomiting may accompany the cramps.
4. **Treatment**
   a. **Symptomatic relief,** first with a nonsteroidal antiinflammatory drug:
      (1) Ibuprofen (Motrin), 800 mg q6–8h
      (2) Naproxen sodium (Anaprox), 275 to 550 mg q8h
      (3) Naproxen (Naprosyn), 250 mg q8h
      (4) Aspirin, 300–600 mg q4h
   b. Bed rest, use of a heating pad, and clear fluids can be helpful.
   c. If analgesics fail, give oral contraceptives, which eliminate or substantially reduce cramps.
   d. If the cramps persist or worsen despite oral contraceptives, refer the patient for a laparoscopy to rule out endometriosis.
G. **Mittelschmerz** is the pain experienced at the time of ovulation.
1. **Etiology.** It is thought to be secondary to spillage of fluid from the rupturing follicular cyst, which irritates the peritoneum.
2. **Evaluation.** The patient usually complains of midcycle, unilateral dull and aching lower quadrant abdominal pain lasting from a few minutes to 6–8 hours. Rarely, the pain is severe, mimicking appendicitis, torsion or rupture of an ovarian cyst, or an ectopic pregnancy. Refer the patient for laparoscopy to rule out these diagnoses.
3. **Diagnosis.** The midcycle nature of the pain and absence of significant disease establish the diagnosis.
4. **Treatment**
   a. Explain the benign nature of the pain to the patient.
   b. A heating pad and mild analgesics are helpful.
   c. If persistent, use oral contraceptives.
V. **Adolescent sexuality.** The care of adolescents includes not only their physical and emotional well-being, but also their emerging sexuality. The spectrum of adolescent sexual concerns ranges from fears of homosexuality to unwanted pregnancy. To allay these concerns, the health care provider must establish a confidential, trusting relationship with the teenager, which requires time and patience. Most adolescents are reluctant to initiate discussions of sexual matters. However, sexuality introduced in the context of the system review eliminates the mutual embarrassment often felt by both provider and patient. A 15-year-old boy experiencing spontaneous erections while roughhousing with a male friend fears he is a homosexual. A 14-year-old girl missing her period after a session of heavy petting is convinced she is pregnant. A 16-year-old boy has been taught that masturbation is a sin, yet he continues, convinced he is beyond redemption. A 16-year-old girl is having unprotected intercourse in the belief that she is too young to use any type of birth control. These are but a few of the issues adolescents will raise as they progress in their normal psychosexual development. By providing respectful, nonpatronizing reassurance, the health care provider can correct most sexual misconceptions.
The decision as to whether or not sex becomes a part of a teenage relationship ultimately rests with the persons involved. Young people are influenced in such a decision by family standards, religious values, society's expectations, peer pressure, internal needs, drug and alcohol usage, and partner availability. *The provider's role is not to judge the patient's behavior, but to give sufficient information to permit the*

teenager to make a responsible decision. The issue of whose obligation it is to educate adolescents about sexuality has not been resolved. The young person has three readily available sources of information: parents, peers, and school. Some parents are uncomfortable discussing sexuality with their children. An equal number of children cannot tolerate discussing sex with their parents. Parents who hand their child a book on sex and say "Read it" have not fulfilled their role in educating their child. The feelings involved are as important as the mechanisms of sex. To understand sexuality, the "why" of sex must be explored. It is during frank discussions between parent and child that the psychology of sex can be explored. Peers as an information source are often a cause of confusion. Why then do children turn to their friends? They are available, approachable, willing to listen, and rarely make moral judgments. Their lack of expertise is rarely seen as a drawback.

Schools in general cannot provide the subtle sensitivity needed to explore adolescent sexuality. Most sex education classes are limited to the mechanics of intercourse. Many states still prohibit the schools from teaching the available methods of birth control. The feelings involved in a sexual experience, the expectations, fantasies, fulfillment, and disappointments, are virtually ignored. The dilemma of adolescent sexuality has not been resolved, which is one reason why teenage pregnancy has reached epidemic proportions in the United States. Health care providers have an opportunity and the responsibility to educate and counsel their patients on sexual issues.

VI. **Birth control.** More than half of all first sexual encounters among teenagers are unprotected. Despite the availability of contraceptives, adolescents often refrain from using them because they are not readily offered and the individuals do not necessarily plan to have sex. Patients should be questioned on their sexual activity. If asked in a direct, nonjudgmental manner, most adolescents are willing to share this information and to request a method of birth control that is most appropriate for them. **Remember that condoms are the only method of birth control that, properly used, prevent the spread of STDs** (see **F**).

A. **Oral contraceptives.** The pill, taken as prescribed, will prevent pregnancy with over 99 percent efficiency.

1. The **complications and side effects** of oral contraceptive use include the following:

   a. Nausea and bloating
   b. Breakthrough bleeding
   c. Headaches
   d. Hypertension
   e. Thrombophlebitis
   f. Fluid retention
   g. Scanty or absent periods
   h. Depression
   i. Weight gain or weight loss (statistically equally likely)
   j. Birth control pills containing 50 μg or more of estrogen or strong progestins may produce abnormal results on glucose tolerance tests in some patients. Diabetic patients who take the pill may have increased insulin requirements.
   k. The birth control pill has produced false-positive lupus erythematosus (LE) prep and arthralgias in normal patients. Both of these findings disappear when the pill is stopped. With the use of low-dose pills, these side effects have been reduced, particularly in the 15- to 25-year age group.

2. **Contraindications.** The pill is contraindicated in patients with lupus erythematosus, thrombophlebitis, and cholestatic jaundice of pregnancy.

3. **Indications for estrogen-dominant pill**

   a. Hirsutism
   b. Acne
   c. Scanty periods (on or off the pill)
   d. Increased appetite and weight gain on the pill
   e. Early-cycle spotting on the pill

4. **Indications for progesterone-dominant pill**
   a. Mucorrhea
   b. Cervical erosion
   c. Nausea or bloating on pills
   d. Fibroids
   e. Fibrocystic breast disease
   f. Cyclic weight gain
   g. Dysmenorrhea
   h. Hypermenorrhea
   i. Late-cycle spotting on the pill
5. **Changes in common laboratory values**
   a. Thyroxine (T_4) is increased, and resin T_1 is decreased. Free T_4 is unchanged.
   b. There is a slight increase in coagulation factors II, VIII–X, and XII, and a moderate increase in factor VII.
   c. Triglyceride, cholesterol, and phospholipid levels are increased in some patients using the progesterone-dominant pill.
   d. Serum folate is decreased in some patients.
   e. The erythrocyte sedimentation rate is increased slightly.
6. **Prescribing the pill**
   a. **Patient evaluation** requires the following:
      (1) A complete history and physical examination, including a pelvic examination
      (2) **Laboratory studies.** Hemoglobin and Papanicolaou smear. In patients with a family history of arteriosclerotic heart disease or stroke, cholesterol and triglyceride levels should be determined. In sexually active patients, test for syphilis and culture for gonorrhea and *Chlamydia* once a year or after contact with a new partner.
   b. **Choice of pill** (Table 12-1)
      (1) A medium-dose pill (e.g., Norinyl or Ortho-Novum 1/35) can be prescribed for patients with regular periods and no special indication for an estrogen-dominant or progesterone-dominant pill.
      (2) A low-dose pill (e.g., Brevicon, Ovcon) can also be given. Although girls receiving low- to middle-dose pills often experience midcycle breakthrough bleeding, the elimination of weight gain secondary to fluid retention is considered worth the aggravation. However, if the bleeding persists for more than three cycles, the next higher dose pill is prescribed. Because of the higher incidence of breakthrough bleeding in the low-dose pill, many girls prefer the medium-dose pill.
      (3) A progestin-dominant pill (e.g., Lo/Ovral, Loestrin) can be given if breakthrough bleeding is a problem.
      (4) An antiandrogenic pill can be given if acne or hirsutism is a problem.
      (5) Pills for 21-day and 28-day cycles are available. Since, with the latter, the teenager is taking a pill *every* day, the chances that she will forget to take it are reduced.
   c. **Follow-up.** The patient should be seen in 3 months for a blood pressure and weight check. At this visit, any problems she may be having can also be explored. Thereafter, she is seen every 6 months.
   d. **The mini-pill** is a progestogen-only pill. The pregnancy rate on this pill is higher than on combination pills (1.5–3.0 pregnancies/per 100 woman-years), and irregular menstrual bleeding occurs.
B. **Intrauterine devices (IUDs)** are available, but because infection associated with the IUD can result in permanent tubal scarring and infertility, nulliparous patients are not generally candidates for this method.
C. **Norplant,** a long-acting contraceptive, is the most effective reversible method available and does not need patient compliance for effectiveness. These are significant benefits for the adolescent who is committed to being sexually active but wants to delay childbearing for at least 5 years.

Table 12-1. Contraceptive pill activity listed according to estrogen content and endometrial potency

DRUG	ENDO-METRIAL ACTIVITY (%) Spotting and bleeding in third cycle of use[1]	ESTROGENIC ACTIVITY (mcg) Ethinyl Estradiol equivalents per day[2]	PROGESTA-TIONAL ACTIVITY (mg) Norethindrone equivalents per day[3]	ANDRO-GENIC ACTIVITY (mg) Methyltestosterone per 28 days[4]
Sub-50 mcg Estrogen				
Monophasic				
Lo-Ovral	9.6†	25	0.8	0.46
Desogen/Ortho-Cept	9.9	30	1.5	0.17
Ovcon 35	11.0	40	0.4	0.15
Levlen/Nordette	14.0†	25	0.8	0.46
Ortho-Cyclen	14.3†	35	0.3	0.18
Brevloon/Modicon/ Nelova 0.5/35	14.6	42	0.5	0.17
Genora/Nelova/ Norethin/Norinyl/ Ortho-Novum 1/35	14.7	38	1.0	0.34
Loestrin 1.5/30	25.2†	14	1.7	0.80
Loestrin 1/20	29.7†	13	1.2	0.53
Demulen 1/35	37.4†	19	1.4	0.21
Multiphasic				
Ortho-Novum 7/7/7	12.2	48	0.8	0.25
Jenest	14.1	39	0.8	0.28
Tri-Norinyl	14.7	40	0.7	0.23
Tri-Levlen/ Triphasil	15.1†	28	0.5	0.29
Tri-Cyclen	17.5†	35	0.3	0.15
Ortho-Novum 10/11	19.6	40	0.8	0.25
Progestin-Only				
Ovrette	34.9	0	0.08	0.13
Micronor/Nor-QD	42.3	1	0.12	0.13

[1] Information submitted to the United States Food and Drug Administration by the manufacturer. These rates are derived from separate studies conducted by different investigators in several population groups, and therefore, a precise comparison cannot be made.
[2] Estrogenic activity of entire tablet mouse uterine assay.
[3] Induction of glycogen vacuoles in human endometrium.
[4] Rat ventral prostate assay.
† Includes early withdrawal flow.
Source: From R. P. Dickey, *Managing Contraceptive Pill Patients* (7th ed.). Durant, OK: Essential Medical Information Systems.

D. Diaphragms. A diaphragm can only be reliably used by adolescents who are highly motivated, feel comfortable with their bodies, and are not offended by inserting a mechanical device into the vagina in anticipation of intercourse.
   1. **Fitting.** Fitting rings of various sizes are inserted into the vagina to determine the appropriate size. A correctly fitting diaphragm covers the cervix snugly without discomfort to the patient, with the posterior lip behind the cervix and the anterior rim tucked behind the pubic bone.
   2. **Instructions.** The following written instructions are given to the patient on the use and care of the diaphragm:

   a. Put 1 tbsp contraceptive cream in the cup of the diaphragm and on the rim.
   b. Insert the diaphragm no more than ½ hour before intercourse, checking that the cervix is covered.
   c. If more than ½ hour has passed since insertion, place an applicator full of contraceptive cream in the vagina with an applicator while the diaphragm is undisturbed.
   d. Leave the diaphragm in place at least 6 hours after intercourse.
   e. After removing the diaphragm, wash it with a mild soap (cornstarch can be used after washing).
   f. Check the diaphragm regularly for holes by holding it up to the light while stretching the rubber, particularly at the rim.
   g. The device should be replaced once a year and a weight change of 10 lb requires a refitting.
   E. **Foam** is a readily available form of birth control that requires no prescription, but it has a high failure rate. The adolescent is given the following instructions:
   1. Insert the contraceptive foam into the vagina 1 hour or less *before* intercourse. It is not effective after intercourse.
   2. Do not douche for 6 hours after intercourse.
   3. When possible, have the partner use a condom with foam to lessen the risk of pregnancy.
   F. **Condoms** are the only birth control devices that lessen the risk of venereal disease dissemination. Therefore, all adolescents should be strongly encouraged to use condoms with every act of intercourse **regardless of their other contraceptive method used.** Condoms containing a spermicide as lubricant are the most effective.
   G. The **contraceptive sponge (Today)** is a factor in an increased incidence of toxic shock syndrome and can produce a chemical vaginitis. It has a 15 percent failure rate.
   H. The **"morning-after" pill. High-dose estrogens** administered after unprotected intercourse are an effective means of lowering the risk of pregnancy if taken within 72 hours of intercourse. This makes it particularly useful in cases of rape or with unanticipated sex, such as after first intercourse. If there is a risk of the patient already being pregnant by previous intercourse, a discussion about whether the patient would have an abortion should be held.
   1. **Administration.** The medication is taken within 24–72 hours after intercourse.
   2. **Dosage. Ethinyl estradiol and norgestrel (Ovral),** two tablets PO bid for 48 hours. May be associated with significant nausea, requiring prochlorperazine (Compazine), 10 mg PO 1 hour before each dose, to tolerate this regimen.
VII. **Pregnancy.** Each year, more than 1 million girls 15–19 years of age become pregnant. Adolescents are psychologically very prone to denial of the possibility of pregnancy both before and after it takes place. The majority of pregnant teenagers are neither emotionally disturbed nor promiscuous, but psychological issues may precipitate the pregnancy if the baby is seen as a love object and is used to replace a recent loss by death, separation, or divorce. Threatened with punishment if she becomes pregnant, an adolescent may become pregnant to test her parents' love. Unless these complex emotional issues are resolved, another pregnancy is likely to follow the first.
   A. **Diagnosis**
   1. Many girls cannot bring themselves to express concern over a missed period, and many will deny that the possibility of pregnancy even exists. Every girl should be questioned about her menstrual cycles and sexual activity.
   2. A pregnancy test is given to confirm the suspected diagnosis (see sec. **II.E**).
   3. Pelvic examination and sizing of the uterus
   a. An 8-week pregnant uterus is the size of an orange.
   b. At 12 weeks the uterus is the size of a grapefruit at the symphysis pubis.
   c. At 16 weeks the uterus is felt midway between the umbilicus and symphysis pubis.
   d. At 20 weeks the uterus is palpable at the umbilicus.

B. Mortality, morbidity, and complications

1. The **death rate** from the complications of pregnancy, delivery, and the postpartum period is 60 percent higher for girls who become pregnant before the age of 15 years than for those who become pregnant at a later age.
2. The **causes of death** include the following:
   a. Toxemia
   b. Hemorrhage
   c. Infection
3. Pregnancy is a common cause of school dropout; 9 of 10 girls whose first delivery occurs at age 15 or younger never complete high school.
4. Couples who marry because of pregnancy have a higher divorce rate than that of the general population.

C. Abortion

1. **Methods**
   a. **Suction curettage** is done before 12 weeks in the outpatient setting and in many hospitals to 15 weeks or later depending on local factors. It can be done under local or general anesthesia. **Complications** include perforation and hemorrhage (secondary to incomplete removal of the products of conception), and infection.
   b. **Saline or prostaglandin infusion** is done at 16–24 weeks of pregnancy. **Contraindications** to saline infusion are chronic renal disease, cardiac disease, and severe anemia. **Complications** include infection, retained products of conception, and coagulopathy.
2. **Counseling.** Explore thoroughly with the pregnant teenager the options of abortion, adoption, or keeping the child. She must participate in the decision-making process. Once she has reached a decision, it should be supported by the health professionals caring for her. Health professionals must not impose their own judgment on the patient.

D. Ectopic pregnancy

1. **Etiology.** PID, prior abdominal surgery, congenital abnormalities, and diethylstilbestrol (DES) exposure in utero make ectopic pregnancy more likely because adhesions or other physical factors affect proper tubal transport of the conception to the uterus.
2. **Evaluation.** An irregular rise or fall in the quantitative blood pregnancy test should raise the suspicions of an ectopic pregnancy. Therefore, any patient with a positive pregnancy test and pain, irregular bleeding, or a uterus that does not feel pregnant on examination should receive a quantitative blood pregnancy test. If the value is more than 6,000, an abdominal ultrasound of the uterus should be done to establish whether an intrauterine pregnancy is present. (The blood value is 1,500 if a vaginal probe ultrasound is available.) In the case of a positive test and irregular bleeding at a gestation that is too small to visualize by ultrasound (value below these parameters), following the beta subunit to be sure it halves every 48 hours is an appropriate way to confirm resolution of a miscarriage rather than an ectopic pregnancy. If the values are rising, then failure to double every 48 hours suggests the need to rule out ectopic pregnancy. If the uterus is evacuated and there is no tissue of fetal origin, a laparoscopy is indicated.
3. **Diagnosis.** An ectopic pregnancy is diagnosed by finding pregnancy tissue outside the uterine cavity usually by laparoscopy.
4. **Treatment**
   a. The pregnancy is surgically removed from its location, usually by laparoscopy but occasionally by a laparotomy.
   b. Some centers use methotrexate, generally under protocol, to resolve ectopic pregnancy medically.

VIII. Rape. By definition, rape is the introduction of the penis or digits within the genitals of the victim by force, fear, or fraud. Statutory rape is intercourse with a female below the age of consent (usually 16 years). Sexual molestation is noncoital sexual contact without consent. See Chap. 3, p. 78, for the details of the evaluation and management of the acute rape victim.

Metabolic Diseases

Mark Korson

I. **General features.** Metabolic diseases are usually inherited inborn errors of metabolism that may present in infancy or later in childhood, adolescence, or adulthood. Each is due to the absent or deficient activity of a specific enzyme necessary for the metabolism of an amino acid, carbohydrate, fatty acid, or more complex intermediate compound. The clinical presentation is the consequence of toxic metabolite accumulations, lack of production of necessary intermediary products, or both. Many patients can be effectively managed using dietary modification, or vitamin or cofactor supplementation, among other therapies. With *early* diagnosis and *rapid* implementation of effective therapy, the outcome for many metabolic disorders is favorable.

II. **Clinical presentations.** The **acute presentation** of a metabolic disease either in the newborn period or thereafter constitutes a **true medical emergency.** Clinical suspicion must be high, and intensive treatment must begin **without delay** to prevent potential mortality and reduce the chance of debilitating, long-term morbidity. A careful **family history** should always be taken, with particular attention toward fetal loss, previous neonatal or infant deaths or sudden infant death syndrome (SIDS), Reye syndrome, unexplained neurologic symptoms or mental retardation in the patient or other family members, or parental consanguinity.

The possibility of a metabolic disease should be considered in an individual who has any of the following symptom complexes, especially in combination:

A. **Neonatal catastrophe.** Presentation in the newborn period is usually catastrophic after feeding has begun. **Signs and symptoms** may include the following: **hyperventilation, seizures, lethargy and coma, altered muscle tone, and hepatomegaly and jaundice,** often associated with **poor feeding and vomiting. Acute biochemical disturbances** include metabolic acidosis, hypoglycemia, and/or hyperammonemia.

B. **Biochemical disturbances.** These include metabolic acidosis, hyperammonemia, and hypoglycemia.

   1. Patients who are *chronically* acidotic are tachypneic, feed poorly, and fail to thrive.

   2. Disorders associated with *acute* metabolic decompensation are often associated with recurrent anion gap acidosis (frequently with marked ketosis), hypoglycemia, and/or hyperammonemia. At these times, patients may demonstrate an unusual odor in the urine, sweat, earwax, etc.

C. **Liver disease**

   1. Metabolic liver disease may be associated with hepatomegaly and jaundice, which may be either conjugated and/or unconjugated in nature.

   2. Hepatic dysfunction commonly occurs and may include a coagulopathy, particularly in metabolic liver disease, that presents in the neonate and young infant (e.g., galactosemia and tyrosinemia).

   3. Hypoglycemia and hyperammonemia may reflect a damaged liver as well.

D. **Neurologic disease** (see also Chap. 19)

   1. Because metabolic disorders tend to affect the central nervous system in a *diffuse* manner, neurologic symptoms are generally nonlateralizing and global, and include: altered states of consciousness, hypotonia or hypertonia, hyperreflexia, movement disorder, ataxia, and developmental delay.

2. When they occur, **seizures** are frequently multifocal in origin.

3. A genetic metabolic etiology should be considered in any child with unexplained neurologic symptoms.

E. Myopathy and/or cardiomyopathy. Metabolic disease affecting muscle may be slow and progressive in onset, or may occur suddenly during a period of acute decompensation.

   1. Symptoms may include muscle weakness, exercise intolerance with easy fatigability, or muscle tenderness with myoglobinuria following an infectious illness or period of intensive exercise.

   2. Cardiomyopathy presents with symptoms of heart failure, arrhythmia, or sudden death.

F. Storage disease

   1. Metabolic storage disorders are characterized **in early childhood** by the progressive development of coarsened facies, hepatosplenomegaly, kyphoscoliosis with joint contractures, cloudy cornea and/or retinal "cherry-red spot," and hearing loss (conductive or sensorineural). Patients follow a **neurodegenerative clinical course.**

   2. Less severe **juvenile and older-onset** forms of these disorders are much more subtle in their symptoms and may present with a learning disorder, loss of cognitive skills, or frank dementia; muscle weakness, cramping, or difficulty in walking; ataxia; seizures; or a behavioral or psychiatric disorder.

III. Diagnostic laboratory evaluation (Table 13-1)

A. Newborn blood screening

   1. Screening of newborn blood collected on a filter paper in the first few days of life ("PKU test") is routinely done in all states in the United States and Canada, and in most developed countries. Several metabolic diseases can be identified in this manner, including **congenital hypothyroidism, phenylketonuria (PKU), galactosemia, galactokinase deficiency, maple syrup urine disease (MSUD), homocystinuria, and biotinidase deficiency.** Although all states screen for PKU and congenital hypothyroidism, screening for the other disorders varies from state to state.

   2. Newborn screening allows early institution of **therapy** for a metabolic disease to occur, usually by specific dietary restriction, before the onset of clinical symptoms or irreversible neurologic damage. This is important not only for PKU and congenital hypothyroidism, but especially for disorders such as galactosemia or MSUD, in which severe morbidity or mortality can occur during the first or second week of life, either due to *gram-negative sepsis* (galactosemia) or to *acute metabolic acidosis/decompensation* (MSUD).

   3. Children with **positive newborn blood tests should be referred as soon as possible to a metabolic center** for confirmation of diagnosis and institution of therapy. Although the specific rates vary with the particular test, the degree of sensitivity and specificity for newborn screening tests is generally high. Those newborn screens obtained when a baby is less than 24 hours old will probably test positive if the child is affected. However, as a precaution, **any child whose sample is obtained during the first 24 hours of life should have another screen repeated** at the first visit to the pediatrician's office or within the first 10 days.

   4. Any neonate who is transferred from one nursery to another should have a screen test performed at both the referring and receiving hospitals to avoid those unfortunate confusing situations in which no card was ever sent, and a child was later discovered to have complications of a treatable disorder.

   5. Though a negative newborn screening result provides convincing evidence that a child does not have any of those disorders for which screening is performed, repeat definitive testing is indicated whenever a patient's clinical course is suggestive of one of these disorders.

B. Urine "spot" or color tests. The following are simple tests that can provide quick diagnostic information:

   1. Urine ketones (Acetest, Ketostix). Tests for acetoacetate and is positive in acute organic acid disorders, MSUD, and congenital lactic acidemias. An

Table 13-1. Common clinicobiochemical characteristics of some acutely presenting metabolic diseases

Disorders	Acid-base abnormalities		Hypoglycemia	Hyperammonemia	Liver dysfunction	Ketonuria		Myoglobinuria
	Primary metabolic acidosis	Primary respiratory alkalosis				Increased	Absent/decreased	
Amino acid disorders								
Urea cycle disorders	0	+		+	0			
Tyrosinemia type I			+	0	+			
Organic acid disorders								
Maple syrup urine disease	+		+			+		
Propionic acidemia	+		0	+		+		
Methylmalonic acidemia	+		0	+		+		
Multiple carboxylase deficiency (and biotinidase deficiency)	+		0	+		+		
Glutaric acidemia type I	+		0	0		+		
β-Ketothiolase deficiency	+		0	0	0	+		
Congenital lactic acidemias/mitochondrial disorders								
Pyruvate dehydrogenase deficiency	+					0		
Pyruvate carboxylase deficiency	+		0	0		+		
Respiratory chain defects	0				0			
Fatty acid β-oxidation defects								
Multiple acyl CoA dehydrogenase deficiency (glutaric acidemia type II)	0		0	0	0		+	

Long/medium/short (hydroxy-) acyl CoA dehydrogenase deficiency	O		O	O	
Primary carnitine deficiency	O		O	O	+
Carnitine palmitoyl transferase deficiency	O		O	O	+
Carbohydrate disorders					
Glycogen storage disease	+	+	+	+	
Galactosemia		O	+		GSDI
Hereditary fructose intolerance	+	+	+		
Disorders of gluconeogenesis	+	+	O		
Peroxisomal disorders					
Zellweger's disease			+	+	
Neonatal adrenoleukodystrophy			+	+	
Infantile Refsum's disease			+	O	+
Disorders of bile acid metabolism		O		O	
Disorders of metal metabolism					O
Wilson's disease			O		O

+ = feature present in most cases; O = feature present occasionally.

absent or inappropriately low ketone response to documented hypoglycemia suggests a disorder of fatty acid beta-oxidation or glycogen storage disease type I.

2. **Reducing substances** (Clinitest). Positive in galactosemia, hereditary fructose intolerance (HFI), and any disorder associated with renal Fanconi's syndrome. Since glucose is a reducing substance, untreated galactosemia (i.e., on galactose-containing formula) or HFI is characterized by a positive Clinitest response in the face of a negative dipstick for glucose.

3. **Glucose** (Clinistix; glucose oxidase method). Not positive in untreated galactosemia

4. **Ferric chloride.** Detects the phenylketones in PKU (black-green) and alpha-ketoacids in MSUD (khaki green)

5. **Cyanide-nitroprusside test.** Positive in homocystinuria and cystinuria

6. **Berry spot test.** Detects the increased excretion of glycosaminoglycans in some mucopolysaccharidoses. Very subject to false negatives

7. Other tests include the **dinitrophenylhydrazine (DNPH)** test to detect the alpha-ketoacids excreted in disorders such as MSUD, and the **nitrosonaphthol** test to detect tyrosine metabolites in the various forms of tyrosinemia.

C. **Blood tests**

1. **Amino acid determination** (HPLC) of blood (serum or plasma) should accompany urine testing for the diagnosis of amino acid, organic acid, and urea cycle disorders, as well as the lactic acidemias and mitochondrial disorders.

2. **Serum carnitine determination** should be performed when disorders of fatty acid oxidation or carnitine metabolism are suspected, and may also be indirectly helpful in the diagnosis of organic acidemias. Carnitine exists normally in a free or esterified state. Several fatty acid intermediates and organic acids bind carnitine, reducing the free fraction of carnitine and elevating the esterified fraction. A secondary carnitine deficiency is noted particularly during periods of metabolic instability, but may also be evident when an affected child is otherwise well.

3. **Blood acylcarnitines** are a useful diagnostic tool for identifying disorders of fatty acid oxidation and organic acidemias (see **C.4**). The specimen is obtained using a blood filter paper (newborn screening or "PKU card") or plasma or serum, and performed using fast atom bombardment/tandem mass spectrometry.

4. **Lactate and pyruvate determinations** should be performed when a congenital lactic acidemia or mitochondrial disorder is suspected. Other metabolic disorders may show mild increases in lactate (e.g., biotinidase deficiency). A normal lactate-pyruvate ratio is approximately 10–15 : 1 (upper limit 25 : 1). An elevated ratio is suggestive of certain disorders of energy metabolism (e.g., disorders of the respiratory chain), particularly in a normally perfused child.

5. **Peroxisomal testing** includes measurement in the blood of a combination of very long-chain fatty acids, phytanic acid, pipecolic acid, and red blood cell plasmalogens. The particular pattern of biochemical abnormalities depends on the peroxisomal disorder being considered. With the exception of very long-chain fatty acids, tests of peroxisomal function are age dependent, and false-negative results may occur. If a peroxisomal disorder is strongly suspected in the face of normal blood testing, more formal evaluation using cultured skin fibroblasts is indicated.

D. **Urine tests**

1. **Amino acid determination** can be done in urine by either paper chromatography (qualitative) or preferably by high-performance liquid chromatography (HPLC) amino acid analysis (quantitative). This test (together with blood amino acids) should be done on all patients suspected of having an amino acid, organic acid, or urea cycle disorder, as well as in those suspected of having a congenital lactic acidemia or mitochondrial disease.

2. **Organic acid determination** by gas chromatography/mass spectrometry should be performed for suspected amino acid, organic acid, fatty acid oxidation defects, and mitochondrial disorders.

3. **Orotic acid determination** is helpful in patients suspected of having a urea cycle disorder.

4. **Acylcarnitine and acylglycine determination** in urine are useful primarily for the diagnosis of defects in fatty acid oxidation and carnitine metabolism, as well as in organic acidemias. Many intermediate metabolites within these pathways conjugate with carnitine or glycine, or both, when present in excessive quantities, particularly during episodes of metabolic decompensation. However, these abnormal conjugates are also frequently detectable, though in smaller quantities, during healthy periods.

5. **Thin-layer chromatography** is a sensitive and specific screen for disorders of mucopolysaccharide, oligosaccharide, and sialic acid metabolism.

6. **Urinary bile acid** abnormalities are detected in peroxisomal diseases and other disorders of bile acid intermediate metabolism (fast atom bombardment/mass spectroscopy).

E. **Cerebrospinal fluid (CSF) tests**

1. **CSF protein** is elevated in certain storage disorders (e.g., Krabbe's disease), mitochondrial disease (e.g., Kearns-Sayre syndrome), and other demyelinating processes.

2. **Amino acids** are important for the diagnosis of an infant with nonketotic hyperglycemia (severe hypotonia, seizures, and developmental delay) in which an elevated CSF/blood glycine ratio is diagnostic. In children with mitochondrial disease, an elevation in CSF alanine may reflect an elevated lactate and pyruvate.

3. **Lactate and pyruvate** determinations are useful in the detection of mitochondrial disease in some children.

F. **When a metabolic diagnosis is being considered, it is essential that diagnostic specimens be obtained during the acute phase of illness** (see **K**). **The greatest chance of detecting unusual intermediate metabolites occurs at these times. With some disorders, even a few hours of intravenous therapy may dilute or mask a previously identifiable abnormality.** Consultation with a metabolic specialist can help direct the workup and may facilitate a quicker turnaround time when specimens are sent for specialized metabolic testing.

G. In the event that samples cannot be obtained during the acute illness, or when an initial workup is negative, **specialized stress testing or fasting studies** can be performed in a controlled hospital setting (usually a clinical research center). A metabolic specialist should be consulted before one embarks on such a workup.

H. **Diagnosis of specific enzyme deficiencies** can be confirmed using either erythrocyte, leukocyte, fibroblast, or liver specimens. The tissue necessary for diagnosis will depend on the specific enzyme to be assayed.

I. Because the above are all specialized metabolic tests done in specific reference laboratories, the laboratory performing the analysis should be contacted *in advance* regarding instructions concerning collection, preservation, and shipping of the specimens.

J. **Consumers beware! Quality control standards for most complex metabolic testing do not currently exist,** and the **reporting of inaccurate results and/or misinterpretations can occur.** Thus, care must be taken to ensure that the laboratory used for performing these tests employs a specialist with experience in clinical metabolic disease to review all test results; that it provides a written clinical interpretation for these results; and that the metabolic specialist is available to answer questions regarding abnormal results.

K. In the case of an **emergency or imminent death,** when a metabolic disorder is suspected but there is no time to determine a workup, **serum (3–5 ml minimum), plasma (3–5 ml minimum),** and **urine (10 ml minimum)** should be collected and **promptly frozen** (in smaller aliquots if possible) for later diagnostic studies. A blood specimen on filter paper (newborn screening or PKU card) is also helpful.

A **skin biopsy** should be performed and a fibroblast culture begun for future enzyme studies. The importance of a **postmortem examination** for diagnostic purposes should be impressed on the parents or family, particularly since they might be at risk for having another child with the same disease, and future reproductive decision-making may depend on the availability of prenatal diagnosis. When a complete autopsy may be denied, a partial examination is often permitted. Sections of affected tissues (particularly liver, heart, kidney, brain, and skeletal muscle) should be obtained and **quick frozen at −70° C** as soon as possible after death to preserve enzyme integrity for future testing.

IV. **Evaluation of acute metabolic disease by clinical presentation** (see Tables 13-1 and 13-2)

V. **Treatment of acutely ill patients when the possibility of a metabolic disorder cannot be ruled out**

    A. **General principles. Acute metabolic decompensation can be rapidly progressive and life threatening. Prompt institution of appropriate therapy is important, even before a specific diagnosis is made,** and should be implemented concurrently with other routine therapies.

        1. **Discontinue all oral feedings** while the child is acutely ill and thereafter until a specific diagnosis is made and a special diet prepared if necessary.

        2. Provide adequate respiratory and circulatory support, **with correction of metabolic acidosis** (see B) or hyperammonemia, or both (see E), when present.

        3. Begin the **collection of all necessary specimens** for diagnosis (see Table 13-2).

        4. Attempt to reduce the ongoing catabolic process (and subsequent endogenous production of toxic substrate) by providing **IV 10% dextrose** at a flow rate greater than maintenance.

            a. Insulin therapy promotes anabolism and may be required, especially since the renal threshold for glucose may be altered during a period of decompensation.

            b. Keep glucose levels higher than normal (> 100–120 mg/dl) during the presenting phase of illness.

            c. Use intralipid with caution and only when a disorder of fatty acid oxidation is not possible.

            d. Avoid the use of any solution containing lactate.

        5. Facilitate the removal or excretion of toxic intermediate compounds. This may involve a trial of **vitamin cofactors** in organic acidemias (see C), **carnitine** in organic acid and fatty acid oxidation defects (see D), and intravenous **urea cycle medications** for hyperammonemia < 500 μg/dl (see E). However, in cases of intractable acidosis, severe hyperammonemia (> 500–600 μg/dl), or deteriorating mental or neurologic status in a patient with a metabolic disorder or the strong likelihood of having a metabolic disorder, **dialysis is indicated. Hemodialysis** is likely superior to peritoneal dialysis; exchange transfusions are not adequate. Transfer to a more specialized center should **not be delayed** to institute a trial of a less effective mode of therapy.

        6. Because acute metabolic crises can be precipitated by stress or infection, **evaluation and prompt treatment for sepsis or infection, or both,** should be instituted promptly.

            a. Up to 20–25 percent of untreated neonates with **galactosemia** may develop gram-negative sepsis. Therefore, sepsis must be ruled out if any suspicious symptoms are noted in a newly diagnosed infant with galactosemia.

            b. Some **organic acidemias** (e.g., propionic and methylmalonic acidemia) are associated with significant **neutropenia and thrombocytopenia** during acute crises or periods of inadequate metabolic control.

        7. **Careful monitoring** of intake/output, electrolytes, blood pH, total CO_2, ammonia, glucose, neurologic status, and other relevant clinical parameters is necessary.

Table 13-2. Initial laboratory evaluation of acutely presenting metabolic disease

	Blood test	Urine test	Other

All patients	Blood gas
	Bicarbonate
	Electrolytes
	BUN
	Glucose
	Calcium phos-
	  phate
	Ammonia
	AST/ALT
	Lactate
	Amino acids
	CBC
		Urinalysis
		Ketones
		Reducing sub-
		  stances
		Amino acids
		Organic acids	

When considering more specific groups of metabolic disease, add the following studies:

	Blood test	Urine test	Other
Amino acid disorders	PT, PTT		CSF amino acids
Organic acid disorders	Carnitine Acylcarnitines		

Congenital lactic acidemias/mitochondrial disease	Lactate and
	  pyruvate
	CK
			CSF lactate and
			  pyruvate

Fatty acid oxidation defects	Uric acid CK Carnitine Acylcarnitines	Acylglycines	
Carbohydrate disorders	PT, PTT Triglycerides, cholesterol Uric acid		

Peroxisomal disorders	PT, PTT
	Very long-chain
	  fatty acids
	Phytanic acid
	Pipecolic acid
	Red blood cell
	  plasmalogens
		Bile acids	

Disorders of bile acid metabolism	PT, PTT Bile acids	Bile acids	

AST/ALT = Aspartate aminotransferase (AST)/Alanine aminotransferase (ALT); PT = prothrombin time; PTT = partial thromboplastin time; CK = creatine kinase; CBC = complete blood count with differential and platelets; BUN = blood urea nitrogen.

B. Metabolic acidosis (see also Chap. 7, p. 200)

1. Distinguish between a *primary metabolic acidosis* (i.e., *low* pH, *low* PCO_2, *low* bicarbonate) and a *primary respiratory alkalosis with compensatory metabolic acidosis* (i.e., *high* pH, *low* PCO_2, *low* bicarbonate).

   a. The first case suggests an **organic acidemia**, congenital lactic acidemia, or mitochondrial disorder and requires therapy with sodium bicarbonate or other alkali.

   b. The second scenario occurs in many individuals with **severe hyperammonemia;** ammonia is a primary respiratory stimulant. In such a situation, correction with bicarbonate is not indicated.

2. Acidosis should be treated, particularly when the blood pH drops below 7.22 and the bicarbonate below 14 mEq/liter. Below these levels, effective physiologic compensation may not occur.

3. **IV bicarbonate or acetate** solutions can be used for correction of acidosis. Following a bolus, continue with an infusion. In severe metabolic crises, as much as 1 mEq/kg/hr alkali may be required.

4. **Monitor acid-base status** carefully so that overcorrection does not occur. Rapid correction of blood pH may cause a paradoxical rise in central pH and worsening of CNS symptoms.

5. **As a rule, do not use a solution containing lactate** (which may aggravate the status of a child with a congenital lactic acidemia or mitochondrial disorder).

C. Vitamin/cofactor therapy

1. When an organic acidemia cannot be ruled out, a trial of vitamin/cofactor therapy is indicated to potentially stimulate any residual enzyme activity and thereby enhance the degradation of the accumulated (toxic) substrate.

2. Consider the use of the following vitamins or cofactors (they can be administered simultaneously): **biotin** when propionic acidemia, multiple carboxylase deficiency, or pyruvate carboxylase deficiency is a consideration (10 mg/day); **vitamin B_{12} (preferably hydroxocobalamin over cyanocobalamin)** when methylmalonic acidemia is a possibility (1 mg/day); **riboflavin** when glutaric acidemia is being considered (100 mg/day); and **thiamine** when a congenital lactic acidemia is contemplated (20 mg/day).

3. The patient's abnormal biochemical parameters should be monitored (urine organic acids, blood lactate, etc.) to determine whether or not cofactor therapy is effective.

D. Carnitine therapy

1. Any individual with a potential organic acidemia or fatty acid oxidation defect (including cardiomyopathy) warrants a trial of carnitine PO or IV. A baseline quantitative carnitine level (as well as all the diagnostic laboratory tests) should be obtained before the onset of therapy.

2. The oral preparation is commercially available; the dose is 100 mg/kg/day in two or three divided doses.

3. The IV preparation is currently available on an experimental protocol basis from Sigma-Tau Pharmaceuticals. The dosage should begin at 25 mg/kg/day and increase to 100 mg/kg/day as tolerated.

E. Hyperammonemia

1. Perhaps the most common reason for an elevated ammonia level is improper technique or handling of the specimen. A *free-flowing specimen* (especially arterial in a patient with diminished perfusion) should be obtained. Specimens should generally be kept on ice, and transported and processed immediately by the laboratory to avoid artifactual elevations.

2. **Severe hyperammonemia** (> 500–600 μg/dl) should be managed with dialysis, preferably hemodialysis.

3. Significant and prolonged hyperammonemia may be associated with **increased intracranial pressure.** Appropriate intervention should be started when indicated, although steroids should be avoided because of their catabolic potential (which may aggravate the hyperammonemia).

4. When hyperammonemia is less severe (< 500 μg/dl), **pharmacologic therapy**

to facilitate waste nitrogen excretion is indicated. This includes intravenous sodium benzoate (250 mg/kg/day) and sodium phenylacetate (250 mg/kg/day) given as a continuous infusion. These medications are available on an experimental protocol basis from Dr. Saul Brusilow at Johns Hopkins Hospital (410-955-0885). The oral form for these medications (marketed as Ucephan) is commercially available through Kendall-McGaw Pharmaceuticals.

5. When hyperammonemia is associated with low levels of arginine, **arginine** should be supplemented intravenously (170 mg/kg/day).

6. Once a specific urea cycle diagnosis is made, adjustments in the doses of these intravenous medications may be required (e.g., IV arginine at 650 mg/kg/day for citrullinemia and argininosuccinic aciduria).

7. **Ammonia levels must be monitored regularly,** every 4–6 hours, until they have normalized. Given the composition of the urea cycle medications, electrolytes and gases should be monitored closely as well.-

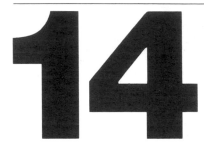

Antibiotics and Infectious Disorders

Edward J. O'Rourke

I. **Principles of antimicrobial therapy.** Whenever possible, a single antimicrobial agent should be used, and the antimicrobial spectrum should be kept as narrow as possible. The use of multiple or broad-spectrum antimicrobials is associated with an increased likelihood of colonization and superinfection by drug-resistant organisms and is usually far more expensive. However, when severely ill patients or those whose defenses are impaired are suspected of being infected, they should be given broad-spectrum therapy pending the definitive results of cultures.

   A. **Identification of the infecting pathogen.** The most probable infecting pathogen(s) can often be determined from various host factors, the site of infection, the results of rapid diagnostic procedures, the patient's underlying illness, and local epidemiologic factors.

   1. **Host factors**

      a. **Age.** In the neonatal period the most common pathogens are *Escherichia coli*, other gram-negative enteric bacilli, group B streptococci, and staphylococci. *Haemophilus influenzae* type B, pneumococci, and meningococci are common and serious pathogens between the ages of 2 months and 5 years. Incidence of serious infections caused by *H. influenzae* type B appears to be declining rapidly since the introduction of effective vaccines.

      b. **Defects of humoral immunity** (see also Chap. 17, p. 504ff). Patients with congenital or acquired hypogammaglobulinemia or defects of certain complement components, particularly C3, have an increased incidence of infections with encapsulated pyogenic organisms, such as pneumococci, meningococci, *H. influenzae* (type B and nontypable strains), and *Staphylococcus aureus*. Infants and children with acquired immunodeficiency syndrome (AIDS) also have a higher incidence of infection with these organisms.

      c. **Defects in cellular immunity.** The T lymphocytes and their effector cells are probably important in the defense against intracellular bacteria, *Listeria, Nocardia,* fungi, certain viruses, and *Pneumocystis carinii*. Human immunodeficiency virus (HIV) infection is an important acquired cause of defects in cellular immunity.

      d. **Granulocytopenia and granulocyte disorders** (see Chap. 16, p. 480ff)

      e. **Miscellaneous defects conferring increased risk**

         (1) Patients with **splenic hypofunction** may have fulminant infections, most commonly due to the pneumococcus, meningococcus, and *H. influenzae* type B.

         (2) Patients with severe **hepatic dysfunction** have an increased frequency of bacteremias with *E. coli,* other enteric gram-negative bacilli, and occasionally the pneumococcus.

         (3) Patients with **nephrotic syndrome** have an increased incidence of infections (especially peritonitis) caused by pneumococci, gram-negative bacilli, and *H. influenzae* type B.

         (4) Primary peritonitis occurs almost exclusively in patients with ascites associated with cirrhosis or nephrosis.

   2. **Site of infection.** Table 14-1 lists the bacterial and fungal pathogens that cause acute infections at various sites. The common pathogens are those

Table 14-1. Bacterial and fungal causes of acute infections in various sites

Site	Common organisms	Less common organisms	Comments
Skin (primary)	Group A streptococcus *Staphylococcus aureus*	*Haemophilus influenzae* type B Gram-negative enteric bacilli *Candida*	Face, periorbital Impaired host Paronychia, intertriginous skin, diaper dermatitis
Skin (trauma)	*Staph. aureus*	Group A streptococcus	Burns and surgical wounds (early)
		Pseudomonas aeruginosa	Burns (late), puncture wounds of foot
		Anaerobes	Severe trauma and abdominal wounds
		Clostridium spp.	Severe trauma and abdominal wounds
		Gram-negative enteric bacilli	Severe trauma and abdominal wounds
		Erysipelothrix *Pasteurella multocida*	Animal products Animal bites
Conjunctiva	*Haemophilus* species *Staph. aureus* Pneumococcus	Gonococcus *Chlamydia trachomatis* *P. aeruginosa*	Neonates, sexual history Neonates

Table 14-1 (continued)

Site	Common organisms	Less common organisms	Comments
Middle ear	Pneumococcus H. influenzae (nontypable and type B) Branhamella catarrhalis Group A streptococcus	Gram-negative enteric bacilli Mycobacterium tuberculosis	Neonates Chronic drainage
Sinuses	H. influenzae (nontypable) Pneumococcus Oral anaerobes	Staph. aureus Gram-negative enteric bacilli Pseudomonas Group A streptococcus Aspergillus Phycomycetes	Chronic infection Impaired hosts Impaired hosts, diabetics
Cervical adenitis	Group A streptococcus Staph. aureus Oral anaerobes	Toxoplasma, cat-scratch fever agent Nontuberculous mycobacteria M. tuberculosis	Cats Children <4 years Contact history, abnormal chest x ray
Mouth and pharynx	Group A streptococcus	Gonococcus Candida Oral anaerobes Corynebacterium diphtheriae Mycoplasma pneumoniae	Sexual history Antibiotic therapy, impaired host Vincent's infection Gray membrane School-aged children
Epiglottis	H. influenzae type B	C. diphtheriae Pneumococcus	Gray membrane

Lower respiratory tract	Pneumococcus	
	M. pneumoniae	
	H. influenzae type B	Children <8 years
	Staph. aureus	Influenza, impaired host, neonate
	Group A streptococcus	Pharyngitis, large pleural effusions
	Group B streptococcus	Respiratory distress in neonates
	Klebsiella and other gram-negative bacilli	Impaired hosts
	Oral anaerobes	Aspiration, lung abscess
	Bordetella pertussis	Characteristic cough
	M tuberculosis	Exposure history
	C. trachomatis	Infants <12 weeks
Endocardium	Viridans streptococci	
	Staph. aureus	
	Enterococcus	
	Staphylococcus epidermidis, diphtheroids, etc.	Prosthetic valves
	P. aeruginosa	Addicts
	Candida and other fungi	Large emboli
Gastrointestinal tract	Shigella	
	Salmonella	
	Yersinia enterocolitica	Symptoms of appendicitis
	Vibrio parahaemolyticus	Shellfish ingestion
	Campylobacter	
	Vibrio cholerae	Foreign travel
	Escherichia coli	Foreign travel
	Aeromonas hydrophila	Waterborne
	Entamoeba histolytica	Foreign travel
	Giardia lamblia	Foreign travel, day care center
	Clostridium difficile	Antibiotic therapy

Table 14-1 (continued)

Site	Common organisms	Less common organisms	Comments
Urinary tract	E. coli and other enteric gram-negative bacilli	Enterococcus	Chronic recurrent infections
		P. aeruginosa	Chronic recurrent infections
		Staphylococcus saprophyticus	Adolescent and school-aged girls
		Staph. aureus	Bacteremia, kidney abscess
Bone	Staph. aureus	Salmonella	Sickle cell disease
		Pseudomonas	Foot puncture
		Streptococcus groups A and B	
		H. influenzae type B	
		M. tuberculosis	
Joints	Staph. aureus	Gram-negative bacilli	Neonates
	H. influenzae type B	Gonococcus	Neonates, sexually active adolescents
	Group A streptococcus	Pneumococcus	
		Staphylococcus epidermidis	Prostheses
		M. tuberculosis	
Meninges	H. influenzae type B	Enteric gram-negative bacilli	Neonates, surgery
	Meningococcus	Group B streptococcus	Neonates
	Pneumococcus	Staph. aureus	Surgery and shunts
		Staph. epidermidis	Shunts
		Listeria monocytogenes	Impaired hosts, neonates
		Cryptococcus	Impaired hosts
		M. tuberculosis	

responsible for the majority of infections at a given site. The uncommon pathogens are rare or associated only with specific clinical situations, which are indicated. The list is not exhaustive. Further discussion of specific sites of infection is found in sec. **IV.**

3. Rapid diagnostic procedures
   a. A **Gram stain** is an extremely valuable, rapid, and inexpensive test, and should be performed on all body fluids and exudates from suspected sites of infection. Two common pitfalls include:
      (1) **Underdecolorization.** This problem is recognized by the blue staining of cell nuclei and can be avoided by repeating the decolorization step of the Gram stain.
      (2) **Gram-stained artifacts** most commonly resemble "sheets of gram-positive cocci." This problem is avoided by the use of fresh stains and gentle heat fixing. An experienced observer should review questionable findings.
   b. **Methylene blue** will demonstrate fetal leukocytes in diarrheal stools.
   c. **Microbial antigen detection.** Rapid immunologic techniques for the detection of microbial antigens in serum, urine, cerebrospinal fluid (CSF), and other body fluids may allow early etiologic diagnosis of hepatitis type B, cryptococcal meningitis, and infections with *H. influenzae* type B, meningococci, pneumococci, K-1 *E. coli,* group B streptococci, group A beta-hemolytic streptococci, and other organisms.
   d. **Serology.** Classically, a fourfold titer rise or two-tube dilution difference in antibody titer is required to diagnose an acute viral infection. Two serum samples are needed, one taken during the acute phase of the illness and a second drawn 10–21 days later. However, many recent antibody tests are done by the enzyme-linked immunosorbent assay (ELISA) method and are not reported out as titers but as optical density units that require reference to the internal controls for that test. Additionally, the following serologic tests can be performed on a single serum specimen:
      (1) **A single positive ELISA test for HIV,** when confirmed by Western blot, is accepted as documentation of HIV infection (although children < 15 months old may have passively acquired antibody without being infected).
      (2) Tests for **heterophil antibody,** which become positive during the second week of infectious mononucleosis. The test usually reverts to negative within 6 months of acute mononucleosis.
      (3) When immunoglobulin M (IgM) titers are available, or when antibody to various viral components has been demonstrated to appear at different times following acute infection, as with Epstein-Barr virus or hepatitis B virus, a single serum specimen can be tested against a panel of antigens to determine whether an infection has occurred recently or in the past.
      (4) **Cold agglutinins,** which are found in 75 percent of patients with *Mycoplasma* pneumonia during the second week of illness. A simple bedside test, described below, can give a clue to the presence of a *Mycoplasma* infection. Bedside cold agglutinin titers must be confirmed with formal cold agglutinin or *Mycoplasma* complement fixation titers, or both, due to the large number of false-positive tests. Various other infectious agents can produce positive results. To perform the bedside test, add three or four drops of whole blood to an oxalate or sodium citrate tube and place on ice for 30 seconds. Tilt the tube, hold it up to a light source, allowing the blood to run down the side of the tube, and observe for agglutination that disappears after warming the tube in your hand (37° C).
   e. All microbiologic specimens should be plated on appropriate media as promptly as possible. Urine specimens may, however, be refrigerated overnight, if necessary.
      (1) Specimens that contain cold-labile organisms, such as the meningo-

coccus or gonococcus, should be aspirated into a syringe, sealed, and promptly taken to the laboratory. Many organisms, especially anaerobes, **will not survive on swabs that are allowed to dry.** On the other hand, group A beta-hemolytic streptococci will survive at least 24 hours on a dry swab. If this organism is specifically sought, the swab need not be placed in a liquid medium. Thus, irrelevant organisms may not survive, permitting a better yield of streptococci.

(2) *Shigella* and many *Salmonella* species do not survive cooling and storage of stool specimens. Therefore, the stool must be cultured promptly, or a buffered transport medium should be used. *Salmonella* (but not *Shigella*) survives drying on rectal swabs.

B. Choice and dosage of antimicrobial agents

1. **Antibiotic susceptibility.** The recommended choice and dosage of antimicrobials for specific pathogens are outlined in Tables 14-2 and 14-3.

   a. Frequently, the likely pathogen(s) is (are) susceptible to several antimicrobials. A rational choice is then based on drug toxicity, pharmacologic factors relating to the patient (age, renal and hepatic function), and pharmacologic factors relating to the infection (antimicrobial penetration and activity at the site of infection). Cost of a course of therapy should also be considered, especially when several antibiotics are likely to be effective against the pathogen.

   b. Agents with potentially serious side effects should be used only when they offer a definitive advantage over less toxic agents.

2. **Combinations of antimicrobial agents.** Although a single antimicrobial agent should provide adequate therapy for the majority of infections, combination therapy is recommended for specific organisms or certain clinical situations. These include **endocarditis** (see sec. **IV.M.1**) caused by enterococci or by viridans streptococci relatively resistant to penicillin, **severe *Pseudomonas* infection** (an aminoglycoside [gentamicin or tobramycin] and an antipseudomonal penicillin [mezlocillin or piperacillin]), **active tuberculosis** (see sec. **O**), **cryptococcal** meningitis and disseminated infections caused by other yeasts (amphotericin B and 5-fluorocytosine, provided the organism is sensitive to 5-fluorocytosine), and empiric antibiotic therapy for severely ill patients. The regimen most commonly used for suspected bacterial sepsis in neonates is ampicillin and gentamicin. For **suspected bacterial sepsis** in older infants and children, ampicillin with sulbactam (if meningitis is unlikely) or ampicillin with chloramphenicol or a third-generation cephalosporin is acceptable, while the combination of an antipseudomonal penicillin and gentamicin is standard empiric coverage for immunosuppressed patients or patients with suspected nosocomial sepsis.

3. **Monitoring antimicrobial dosage.** When treating a serious illness or when using an antibiotic with a narrow therapeutic–toxic ratio, antibiotic levels should be monitored. Table 14-4 gives the recommended therapeutic levels of such antimicrobials.

   a. Peak levels should be measured 1 hour after an intramuscular dose, 30 minutes after the end of a 30-minute intravenous infusion, or immediately after a 1-hour infusion. Trough levels should be measured just before the next dose. Antibiotic levels in the serum can also be measured indirectly as bactericidal activity against the patient's pathogen (serum bactericidal level).

   b. In certain infections such as **endocarditis** and **osteomyelitis,** the level and bactericidal power of antibiotics in the patient's serum against the pathogen can be monitored during therapy. The peak bactericidal level should be at least 1 : 8 and the trough at least 1 : 2. Serum bactericidal levels are useful in monitoring compliance and absorption of oral antibiotics when they are given to treat bone and joint infections outside the hospital.

4. **Antimicrobial activity at the site of infection**

   a. Antimicrobial penetration into the central nervous system (CNS)

Table 14-2. Choice of antimicrobial agents for specific pathogens[a]

Organism	Infection	Drug of choice	Pediatric dose[a]
Gram-positive cocci			
Group A streptococcus	Pharyngitis,[b] impetigo	Penicillin G	25,000 U/kg/day PO or IM
	Cellulitis	(Alt.: erythromycin, ceph-	50,000–100,000 U/kg/day PO,
	Pneumonia, empyema, bacter-	alosporin, vancomycin)	IM, or IV
	emia		100,000 U/kg/day IV or IM
	Meningitis		300,000 U/kg/day IV
Viridans streptococci	Subacute bacterial endocarditis	Penicillin G plus gentamicin until sensitivity to penicillin is established	250,000 U/kg/day IV
		(Alt.: cephalothin, vancomycin)	
Enterococcus	Urinary tract	Ampicillin (or amoxicillin)	50–100 mg/kg/day PO (20–40
		(Alt.: nitrofurantoin)	mg/kg/day PO)
	Subacute bacterial endocarditis	Ampicillin or penicillin G plus gentamicin	300 mg/kg/day (ampicillin) IV
			250,000 U/kg/day (penicillin G) IV
		(Alt.: vancomycin and gentamicin)	180 mg/m² or 4.5–7.5 mg/kg/day (gentamicin) IV
Pneumococcus	Pneumonia	Penicillin G	50,000 U/kg/day (penicillin G)
		(Alt.: erythromycin, cephalosporin, chloramphenicol, vancomycin)	PO, IM, or IV
	Meningitis, complications (empyema)		300,000 U/kg/day IV
Staphylococcus aureus (penicillin-resistant)[c]	Mild infection	Semisynthetic penicillin	50–100 mg/kg/day PO or IM
	Systemic infection	(Alt.: cephalothin,[d] clindamycin, vancomycin), amoxicillin-clavulanate	200 mg/kg/day IV
Staphylococcus epidermidis[e]	Endocarditis	Semisynthetic penicillin[d]	200 mg/kg/day IV
	Shunt infection	(Alt.: cephalothin,[d] vancomycin)	

Table 14-2. (continued)

Organism	Infection	Drug of choice	Pediatric dose[a]
Gram-positive bacilli			
Clostridium perfringens	Gas gangrene	Penicillin G (Alt.: chloramphenicol)	200,000 U/kg/day IV
Clostridium tetani	Tetanus	Penicillin G (Alt.: tetracycline) Human antitoxin (see Table 14-6)	100,000 U/kg/day IV
Listeria monocytogenes	Meningitis	Ampicillin ± gentamicin (Alt.: trimethoprim-sulfamethoxazole, erythromycin, tetracycline, chloramphenicol)	300–400 mg/kg/day IV For newborn dosages, see Table 6-1
Corynebacterium diphtheriae *bull neck*	Diphtheria	Procaine penicillin G (Alt.: erythromycin) Horse antitoxin (see Table 14-6)	25,000–50,000 U/kg/day IM
Gram-negative cocci			
Meningococcus	Meningitis Meningococcemia	Penicillin G (Alt.: chloramphenicol, cefuroxime, cefotaxime, sulfonamide)	300,000 U/kg/day IV 150,000 U/kg/day IV
Gonococcus (see Table 14-9)	Gonorrhea	See Table 14-9	
Gram-negative bacilli			
E. coli	Urinary tract	Sulfisoxazole (Alt.: ampicillin, amoxicillin, trimethoprim-sulfamethoxazole, amoxicillin-clavulanate, cephalexin)	100 mg/kg/day PO
	Surgical wound, pneumonia, sepsis	Gentamicin (Alt.: ampicillin, cephalosporins, chloramphenicol, amikacin)	180 mg/m² or 4.5–7.5 mg/kg/day IV

Organism	Infection	Drug of choice	Dosage
E. coli	Meningitis	Ampicillin and gentamicin (Alt.: third-generation cephalosporins, amikacin)	For newborn dosages, see Table 6-1
Klebsiella	Urinary tract	Trimethoprim-sulfamethoxazole (Alt.: cephalexin, tetracycline, amoxicillin-clavulanate)	8 mg/kg/day trimethoprim 40 mg/kg/day sulfamethoxazole PO
	Pneumonia, sepsis	Gentamicin (Alt.: cephalosporin, amikacin)	180 mg/m² or 4.5–7.5 mg/kg/day IV
Proteus mirabilis	Urinary tract	Ampicillin (or amoxicillin) (Alt.: cephalexin, trimethoprim-sulfamethoxazole, chloramphenicol)	50–100 mg/kg/day PO (20–40 mg/kg/day PO)
	Systemic	Gentamicin (Alt.: ampicillin, cephalosporins, amikacin, chloramphenicol)	180 mg/m² or 4.5–7.5 mg/kg/day IV
Proteus, indole positive	Urinary tract	Trimethoprim-sulfamethoxazole (Alt.: chloramphenicol, ticarcillin, tetracycline)	8 mg/kg/day trimethoprim 40 mg/kg/day sulfamethoxazole PO
	Systemic	Gentamicin (Alt.: cefoxitin, amikacin)	180 mg/m² or 4.5–7.5 mg/kg/day IV
Pseudomonas aeruginosa	Urinary tract	Carbenicillin (indanyl) (Alt.: tetracycline with acidification)	50–65 mg/kg/day PO
	Systemic	Gentamicin (Alt.: tobramycin, amikacin) plus (Alt.: azlocillin, piperacillin, ceftazidime)	180 mg/m² or 4.5–7.5 mg/kg/day IV 200–300 mg/kg/day IV
Salmonella	Systemic	Chloramphenicol (Alt.: ampicillin, trimethoprim-sulfamethoxazole)	50–100 mg/kg/day PO, IV

Table 14-2 (continued)

Organism	Infection	Drug of choice	Pediatric dose[a]
Serratia		Gentamicin (Alt.: cefoxitin, trimethoprim-sulfamethoxazole, ticarcillin, amikacin)	180 mg/m² or 4.5–7.5 mg/kg/day IV
Shigella		Trimethoprim-sulfamethoxazole (Alt.: ampicillin, chloramphenicol, tetracycline)	10 mg/kg/day trimethoprim 50 mg/kg/day sulfamethoxazole PO
Bacteroides	Respiratory infections Abdominal abscess, bacteremia	Penicillin G Clindamycin (Alt.: chloramphenicol, cefoxitin, metronidazole)	100,000 U/kg/day IV 25 mg/kg/day IV
Pasteurella multocida		Penicillin G (Alt.: amoxicillin-clavulanate, erythromycin)	50,000 U/kg/day PO
H. influenzae	Otitis media	Ampicillin or amoxicillin (Alt.: erythromycin plus sulfonamide, trimethoprim-sulfamethoxazole, cefaclor), amoxicillin-clavulanate	
	Bacteremia Epiglottitis Pneumonia Meningitis	Chloramphenicol *plus* ampicillin initially (Alt.: cefuroxime, ceftriaxone)	100 mg/kg/day IV 300 mg/kg/day IV

[a] See Table 14-3 for maximum doses and Chap. 6 for doses in neonates. [b] Always treat for 10 days to prevent postinfection sequelae. [c] In life-threatening staphylococcal infections gentamicin can be added for initial therapy. [d] Cephalosporins are not predictably active in vivo against penicillin-resistant staphylococci, regardless of the results of in vitro susceptibility tests. [e] May be resistant to semisynthetic penicillins. Usually sensitive to vancomycin, aminoglycosides, and rifampin. [f] Since sensitivity patterns vary, antibiotic choice should be based on specific sensitivity determination whenever possible.

Table 14-3. Doses of antimicrobial agents[a]

Antimicrobial	Daily dose	Frequency	Route	Usual maximum adult dose
A. Penicillins				
1. Oral penicillin G[a,b]	25,000–100,000 U/kg	q6h	PO	6.4 MU
Phenoxymethyl penicillin (V)[b]			PO	6.4 MU
2. Parenteral				
a. Aqueous penicillin G	25,000–400,000 U/kg	q2–4h	IV	24 MU
b. Procaine penicillin G	25,000–50,000 U/kg	q12–24h	IM	4.8 MU
c. Benzathine penicillin G[b]	600,000–1,200,000 U	Single dose	IM	1.2 MU
3. Penicillinase resistant				
a. Methicillin, oxacillin, nafcillin	100–200 mg/kg	q4–6h	IV or IM	12 gm
b. Cloxacillin[b]	50–100 mg/kg	q6h	PO	4 gm
c. Dicloxacillin	25–50 mg/kg	q6h	PO	4 gm
4. Broad spectrum				
a. Ampicillin	50–100 mg/kg	q6h	PO	4 gm
	50–400 mg/kg	q4h	IV or IM	12 gm
b. Amoxicillin	20–40 mg/kg	q8h	PO	3 gm
c. Amoxicillin-clavulanate	20–40 mg amoxicillin component	q8h	PO	3 gm
d. Carbenicillin	400–600 mg/kg	q2–4h	IV	40 gm
e. Ticarcillin	200–300 mg/kg	q4h	IV or IM	30 gm
f. Mezlocillin	100–300 mg/kg	q4–6h	IV or IM	18 gm
g. Piperacillin	100–300 mg/kg	q4–6h	IV or IM	18 gm
h. Azlocillin	100–300 mg/kg	q4–6h	IV or IM	18 gm (up to 24 gm with cystic fibrosis)

Table 14-3 (continued)

Antimicrobial	Daily dose	Frequency	Route	Usual maximum adult dose
B. Cephalosporins				
1. Cephalothin	80–160 mg/kg	q4–6h	IV	12 gm
2. Cefazolin[b]	50–100 mg/kg	q6–8h	IV or IM	6 gm
3. Cephalexin[b]	25–50 mg/kg	q6h	PO	4 gm
4. Cefamandole	50–150 mg/kg	q4–6h	IV or IM	12 gm
5. Cefuroxime	75–150 mg/kg	q8h	IV or IM	12 gm
6. Cefoxitin	80–160 mg/kg	q4–6h	PO	4 gm
7. Cefaclor	40 mg/kg	q8h	IV	8 gm
8. Moxalactam	150–200 mg/kg	q6–8h	IV or IM	8 gm
9. Cefotaxime	100–200 mg/kg	q6h	IV or IM	4 gm
10. Ceftriaxone	50–100 mg/kg	q12–24h	IV or IM	6 gm
11. Ceftazidime	100–150 mg/kg	q8–12h	PO	4 gm
C. Erythromycins[b]	30–50 mg/kg	q6h	IV[c]	4 gm
	15–50 mg/kg	q6h	PO	
D. Clindamycin[b]	10–25 mg/kg	q6h	IV or IM	1.8 gm
	10–40 mg/kg	q6h	PO	4.8 gm
E. Sulfonamides[b]	150 mg/kg	q6h	IV	8 gm
	100 mg/kg	q6h	PO	
Trimethoprim (TMP)-sulfamethoxazole (SMZ)	8–20 mg TMP/kg	q12h	IV	960 mg TMP
	40–100 mg SMZ/kg			4.8 gm SMZ
	150 mg TMP/m²/dose[d]	>10 yr: q12h <10 yr: q8h		

	Dose	Interval	Route	Maximum
F. Aminoglycosides				
1. Streptomycin[b]	20–30 mg/kg	q12h	IM	2 gm
2. Kanamycin	600 mg/m^2 or 15–22.5 mg/kg	q8h	IM	1.5 gm
3. Gentamicin[e]	180 mg/m^2 or 3–7.5 mg/kg	q8h	IV or IM	5 mg/kg/day
4. Tobramycin	150 mg/m^2 or 3–7.5 mg/kg	q8h	IV or IM	5 mg/kg/day
5. Amikacin	600 mg/m^2 or 15–22.5 mg/kg	q8h	IV or IM	1.5 gm
G. Nitrofurantoin[b]	5–7 mg/kg	q6h	PO	400 mg
H. Chloramphenicol	50–100 mg/kg	q6h	PO or IV	4 gm
I. Tetracycline,[b,e] chlortetracycline,[b,e] oxytetracycline[b,e]	20–40 mg/kg	q6h	PO	2 gm
	10–20 mg/kg	q12h	IV or IM	2 gm
1. Doxycycline[b,e]	5 mg/kg	q12h	PO or IV	200 mg
2. Minocycline[b,e]	4 mg/kg	q12h	PO	200 mg
J. Vancomycin	50 mg/kg	q6h	PO	2 gm
	40 mg/kg	q6h	IV	2 gm

[a] 1 mg = 1,600 units.
[b] Not recommended for newborns.
[c] Can be given in continuous drip.
[d] Loading dose is 250 mg TMP/m^2 if no trimethoprim-sulfamethoxazole has been given in the past 24 hr.
[e] Not recommended for children <8 years of age.

Table 14-4. Therapeutic and toxic serum levels of antimicrobials with a narrow toxic-therapeutic ratio

Antimicrobial	Therapeutic peak levels (μg/ml)	Probably toxic peak levels (μg/ml)	Probably toxic trough levels (μg/ml)
Gentamicin	4–8	>12	>2
Tobramycin	4–8[a]	>12	>2
Kanamycin	15–35	>35	>10
Amikacin	15–35	>35	>10
Streptomycin	15–35	>35	>10
Chloramphenicol (free)	5–25	>25[b] >50[c]	
Vancomycin	25–40	>40	
5-Fluorocytosine	50–100	>100	
Trimethoprim	5–10	>10	

[a] 6–10 in cystic fibrosis.
[b] Reversible marrow suppression.
[c] Gray syndrome.

(1) Chloramphenicol, the sulfonamides, and most antituberculous agents penetrate normal meninges well.

(2) The penicillins penetrate effectively, but only in the presence of inflamed meninges. Large doses must be given **parenterally and maintained throughout therapy.**

(3) Some cephalosporins, including cephalothin, cefazolin, cefaclor, cefamandole, and cefoxitin, **do not penetrate the CSF** in therapeutic amounts. As a result, meningitis due to sensitive organisms may develop during parenteral treatment of bacteremic infections with cephalosporins of poor penetration. Cefuroxime penetrates the meninges, but delayed sterilization of CSF in *H. influenzae* meningitis, possibly related to inadequate CSF drug level, has limited the use of cefuroxime when meningitis is suspected. All third-generation cephalosporins have good penetration of inflamed meninges.

(4) The levels of aminoglycoside antibiotics in the CSF after parenteral therapy are unpredictable and are often inadequate for the therapy of gram-negative meningitis.

b. **Antimicrobial activity in the urinary tract** (see sec. IV.K). In patients with normal renal function, many antimicrobials reach much higher concentrations in urine than in serum. As a result, routine sensitivity tests based on achievable serum concentrations are not always reliable predictors of antibiotic efficacy. **Therefore, a report of antibiotic resistance should prompt a repeat urine culture** rather than a change in regimen, unless the patient's symptoms have failed to respond. An effective regimen should sterilize the urine within 12–24 hours.

(1) **Acidification** enhances the activity of the tetracyclines, nitrofurantoin, and the penicillins and cephalosporins. **Alkalinization** markedly enhances the activity of the aminoglycosides and erythromycin, and extends the spectrum of the latter to include many gram-negative rods.

(2) Because of ionic partitioning into acid secretions, **trimethoprim** may be particularly useful in treating recurrent urinary tract infections in females (anterior urethra) and prostatitis in males.

c. **Antimicrobial penetration into the eye.** Most antibiotics have poor penetration into the aqueous and vitreous humor. For this reason, both parenteral and intraocular antibiotics are usually necessary for the treatment of endophthalmitis. Subconjunctival or intravitreal injection of antibiotic should be done by an ophthalmologist. Trimethoprim-sulfamethoxazole (TMP-SMZ) and chloramphenicol are the only antibiotics that penetrate the eye well when given systemically.

5. Failure of therapy. There is variation in the rate of resolution of infections. Causes for failure of treatment should be considered when fever and signs of infection are prolonged. These include inadequate antibiotic therapy, complication of original infection, complications of treatment, and host factors (immune deficiency, anatomic defect, presence of a foreign body).

6. Pharmacologic considerations

   a. Use of antimicrobial agents in infants and young children

   (1) In **neonates,** antibiotic dosage must be individualized, and serum levels should be monitored, particularly when using toxic drugs. Guidelines for initial antibiotic dosage in neonates can be found in Chap. 6.

   (2) In general, dosage intervals are **longer** in younger infants than in older infants. Drug half-lives in premature infants are longer than in full-term infants. Similarly, decreases in renal function are associated with long half-lives of aminoglycoside antibiotics. Therefore, doses and intervals near the lower limits of the ranges given in Chap. 6 should be chosen in these groups.

   (3) To achieve a given blood level, older infants and children less than 10 years of age usually require higher doses of antimicrobials (based on weight) than do older children and adults.

   (4) Dosage of toxic antibiotics should be adjusted according to the age of the patient. For **gentamicin** the usually recommended dosage is 2.5 mg/kg q8h in children under 5 years of age, 2 mg/kg in children 5–10 years old, and 1.5 mg/kg in children over 10. However, these recommendations rarely produce levels above the therapeutic range, and levels may be subtherapeutic. A single gentamicin dosage of 60 mg/m^2 q8h produces reproducible peak levels in all age groups regardless of body habitus.

   b. Use of antimicrobial agents in renal failure. The routes of metabolism and excretion of antimicrobials are summarized in Table 14-5.

   (1) Antimicrobials handled mainly by the kidneys

   (a) Antibiotics excreted primarily by renal mechanisms are best avoided in patients with severe renal failure. If used, drug levels must be obtained before repeat doses.

   (b) Adjustment in dosage is based on estimates of renal function as described for the aminoglycosides (see below). Analogous calculations can be made for other drugs handled mainly by the kidneys (Table 14-6).

   (i) Interval extension. The standard dose of the antibiotic is given, and the dosage interval is prolonged in direct proportion to the increase in serum creatinine concentration, as in the following equation.

   $$\text{New interval} = \text{standard interval (q8h)} \times \frac{\text{patient's creatinine}}{\text{normal creatinine}}$$

   Peak and trough levels with this method are similar to those obtained in patients with normal renal function. However, this approach may lead to relatively long periods of subtherapeutic levels before the next dose.

   (ii) Dosage adjustment. The standard dose is given (loading dose), and the standard interval is maintained. Subsequent doses (maintenance doses) are reduced in proportion to increases in the serum creatinine, as in the following equation.

Table 14-5. Metabolism and excretion of commonly used antimicrobial agents

Mainly renal	Renal and nonrenal	Nonrenal
Antibacterial agents — systemic		
Aminoglycosides	Penicillins	Chloramphenicol
	Tetracycline[b]	Erythromycin[a]
	Clindamycin	
Vancomycin	Imipenem	Doxycycline
		Minocycline
Polymyxins		
Polymyxin B		Metronidazole
Colistin		
Antibacterial agents — urinary tract		
Methenamine[b]	Nitrofurantoin[a,b]	Nalidixic acid[b]
	Sulfonamides[b]	
	Trimethoprim	
Antituberculous agents		
Ethambutol	Para-aminosalicylic	Rifampin
	acid[a,b]	Isoniazid
Antifungal agents		
5-Fluorocytosine		Amphotericin B
		Ketoconazole
Antiviral agents		
	Acyclovir	
	Ara-A	

[a] Should be avoided in severe hepatic failure.
[b] Should be avoided in severe renal failure.

$$\text{Maintenance dose} = \text{standard dose} \div \frac{\text{patient's creatinine}}{\text{normal creatinine}}$$

Levels can be maintained within a narrower range with less chance of subtherapeutic levels. However, this method may result in higher peak and trough levels than in (i) and may predispose the patient to greater toxicity.

(c) **The serum creatinine is unreliable in acute or unstable renal disease, in severe uremia, and in intermittent dialysis. Thus, serum antibiotic levels should be measured frequently and directly to ensure therapeutic levels** (see Table 14-4).

(2) **Antimicrobials handled by both the kidney and extrarenal mechanisms** can be used in standard doses in patients with mild or moderate renal failure (creatinine clearance > 30 ml/1.74 m^2 or serum creatinine < 3 mg/dl). The dosage interval should be increased if renal failure is moderate or severe. **Nitrofurantoin and all tetracyclines except doxycycline are contraindicated in severe renal failure.** In addition, sulfonamides and para-aminosalicylic acid (PAS) should be avoided in severe renal failure.

(3) **Antimicrobials handled by nonrenal mechanisms.** When these agents are used in patients with renal failure, the dosage need not be adjusted.

c. **Use of antimicrobials in hepatic failure.** Among antimicrobials metabolized by the liver (see Table 14-5), metabolic and execretory pathways differ. Specific guidelines for dosage modifications in liver failure therefore cannot be formulated. Antimicrobials with a narrow toxic-therapeutic ratio (e.g., **nitrofurantoin**) or with a high risk of hepatotoxicity (e.g., **PAS**) are **contraindicated** in cases of severe liver failure. When possible, **clindamycin, erythromycin, chloramphenicol, tetracyclines, isoniazid (INH)**, and **rifampin** should be avoided in patients with severe liver failure. If any of these agents is used, serum levels should be monitored.

II. **Other aspects of therapy and prevention**
  A. **Treatment of fever** (see Chap. 2, p. 33)
  B. **Surgery.** The need for adequate drainage of loculated pus, removal of necrotic tissue, relief of obstruction, and removal of foreign bodies should always be considered.
  C. **Immune globulin.** Passive immunization is useful in the prevention and treatment of certain infections (Table 14-6). The use of immunoglobulin preparations for hepatitis B is covered in Table 14-13. Additional considerations for hepatitis A and varicella prevention follow.
    1. IM immune globulin (IG) is recommended for prophylaxis of **hepatitis A** for all household and sexual (heterosexual or homosexual) contacts of persons with hepatitis A; for staff, attendees, and, if there is epidemiologic evidence of hepatitis A transmission in a day care center, all members of households whose diapered children attend; for close contacts if there is a school- or classroom-centered outbreak; for residents and staff in certain institutions for custodial care when outbreaks occur; and for common-source exposure. The dose of IG is 0.02 ml/kg IM once. For travelers to high-risk areas outside the usual tourist routes, IG may be beneficial for preexposure prophylaxis of hepatitis A. For such travelers, a single dose of IG (0.02 ml/kg IM) is recommended for up to 3 months of travel; for more prolonged stays, 0.06 ml/kg should be given every 5 months (*M.M.W.R.* 39[RR-2], 1990).
    2. **Varicella-zoster immune globulin (VZIG)** is indicated after significant exposure to **chickenpox** or **zoster** for susceptible children with primary immunodeficiency disorders or neoplastic disease (leukemia or lymphoma), recipients of immunosuppressive therapy, and newborns of mothers in whom varicella develops within 5 days before or 48 hours after delivery. Premature infants and infants less than one month of age should be evaluated on an individual basis.
    3. Human IV gamma globulin is indicated in therapy of Kawasaki syndrome (*N. Engl. J. Med.* 315:341, 1986) and for some children with HIV infections. Other uses in therapy or prevention of infectious diseases are under active study.
  D. **Isolation procedures.** Guidelines for hospital precautions and periods of contagiousness of common communicable diseases of childhood can be found in *Pediatrics* 53:663, 1974, and updated in *Infection Control* 4:249, 1983 (Centers for Disease Control [CDC] Guideline for Isolation Precautions in Hospitals).
  E. **Antimicrobial prophylaxis.** Indications for antimicrobial prophylaxis are summarized in Table 14-7.
III. **Specific antimicrobial agents.** Table 14-2 summarizes the drugs of choice and dosages for specific bacterial pathogens. Modification of drug dosage for neonates is discussed in sec. I.B.6.a and in Chap. 6, and modifications in renal failure in sec. I.B.6.b. Penetration of antimicrobial agents in the tissues and CSF is discussed in sec. I.B.4.a. The antituberculous agents are summarized in Table 14-8. Antifungal agents are discussed in **B**, and antiviral therapy and agents in sec. **V.B.**
  A. **Antimicrobial agents**
    1. **The penicillins** inhibit cell wall synthesis and kill growing bacteria by lysis.
      a. **Penicillin**
        (1) **Spectrum and indications.** Penicillin is the drug of choice for infections due to pneumococci, streptococci (except enterococci), *Clostridia, Neisseria,* oral anaerobes, and spirochetes. It is also used in treatment

Table 14-6. Immune globulin prophylaxis and therapy

Disorder	Value	Purpose	Dose (IM)	Comment
Standard human immune globulins				
Measles	Proved	Modification	0.05 ml/kg	Rarely indicated
		Prevention	0.25 ml/kg	Given immediately after exposure to unvaccinated children
			0.50 ml/kg (maximum 15 ml)	For immunosuppressed patients
Varicella	Limited	Modification	0.6–1.2 ml/kg	Give immediately after exposure if VZIG is not available. See indications for use in the text.
Hepatitis A	Proved	Prevention	0.2 ml/kg	See text.
Special human immune globulins[a]				
Tetanus (TIG)	Proved	Prevention	250–500 U	See text, sec. **IV.B.4** for indications.
		Treatment	3,000–6,000 U	
Rabies (RIG)	Proved	Prevention	20 IU/kg	See text, sec. **IV.B.3** for indications.
Varicella-zoster (VZIG)	Proved	Prevention	1 complete vial/10 kg (maximum 5 vials)	See text, sec. **II.C.2** for indications. Give within 72 hr after exposure.
Hepatitis B (HBIG)	Proved	Prevention	See Table 14-11	
Special animal immune serums[a]				
Botulism (trivalent ABE)	Proved	Treatment		As soon as possible after testing for sensitivity to serum
Diphtheria	Proved	Treatment	20,000–120,000 U	As soon as clinical diagnosis is made; higher doses for more extensive disease
Intravenous human immune globulin[b]				
Kawasaki syndrome	Proved	Prevention of coronary artery aneurism	400 mg/kg/day IV for 4 days	

VZIG = varicella-zoster immune globulin;
[a] Detailed information about indications, source of supply, and dosage can be obtained from the Centers for Disease Control (404) 329-3311 (8:00 AM–5:00 PM weekdays) and (404) 329-3644 (off-duty hours).[b] Monomeric functionally intact gamma globulin.

Table 14-7. Antimicrobial prophylaxis

Disease	Indication	Antimicrobial and dosage
Preexposure		
Rheumatic fever[a]	History of acute rheumatic fever; lifetime for patients with heart disease; to age 21 in patients without heart disease	*Parenteral* Benzathine penicillin G, 1.2 mg IM monthly *Oral* Sulfadiazine, 500 mg PO qd (< 30 kg), 1 gm PO qd (>30 kg) Penicillin G or V, 200,000–250,000 U PO qd-bid Erythromycin, 250 mg PO bid, in patients sensitive to both sulfonamides and penicillin
Endocarditis[b]	*Dental and upper respiratory procedures* including bronchoscopy, in patients with valvular heart disease, prosthetic heart valves, congenital heart disease (but not uncomplicated secundum atrial septal defect), idiopathic hypertrophic subaortic stenosis, and mitral valve prolapse	*Oral* Penicillin V >60 lb: 2 gm 1 hr before procedure and 1 gm 6 hr later <60 lb: half adult dose at each time Penicillin allergy: erythromycin, 20 mg/kg 1 hr before procedure and 10 mg/kg 6 hr later *Parenteral*[c] Ampicillin, 50 mg/kg IM or IV 30 min to 1 hr before procedure and repeat once 8 hr later *or* aqueous penicillin G, 50,000 U/kg IM or IV 30 min to 1 hr before procedure and repeat once 8 hr later *plus* gentamicin, 2 mg/kg IM or IV 30 min to 1 hr before procedure and repeat once 8 hr later Penicillin allergy: vancomycin, 20 mg/kg IV infused over 1 hr, beginning 1 hr before procedure and repeat once 8 hr later
	Gastrointestinal and genitourinary procedures in patients with valvular heart disease, prosthetic heart valves, congenital heart disease (but not uncomplicated secundum atrial septal defect), idiopathic hypertrophic subaortic stenosis, and mitral valve prolapse	*Parenteral*[c] Ampicillin, 50 mg/kg IM or IV 30 min to 1 hr before procedure and repeat once 8 hr later *plus* gentamicin, 2 mg/kg IM or IV 30 min to 1 hr before procedure and repeat once 8 hr later Penicillin allergy: vancomycin, 20 mg/kg IV infused over 1 hr, beginning 1 hr before procedure and repeat 8 hr later

Table 14-7 (continued)

Disease	Indication	Antimicrobial and dosage
		plus gentamicin, 2 mg/kg IM or IV 30 min to 1 hr before procedure and repeat once 8 hr later
		Oral[d]
		Amoxicillin
		>60 lb: 3 gm 1 hr before procedure and 1.5 gm 6 hr later
		<60 lb: half adult dosage at each time
Postexposure		
Tuberculosis	Household exposure to active disease[e] Recent or prior tuberculin conversion not previously treated Tuberculin-positive child or adolescent in circumstances favorable to reactivation[f]	Isoniazid, 10 mg/kg/day to 300 mg/day for 1 year
Meningococcal disease[g]	Persons in intimate contact with index case, including household members, day care center contacts, medical personnel	Rifampin <1 mo: 5 mg/kg PO bid × 2 days ≥1 mo: 10 mg/kg PO bid × 2 days (max. 600 mg/dose) Sulfadiazine (if strain susceptible) <1 yr: 500 mg PO qd × 2 days 1–12 yr: 500 mg PO bid × 2 days ≥12 yr: 1 gm PO bid × 2 days
Haemophilus influenzae type B disease	Household contacts if child ≤4 yr lives in home; possible day care center contacts	Rifampin, 20 mg/kg/day PO once/day × 4 days
Pertussis	Contacts not previously immunized	Erythromycin, 50 mg/kg/day PO × 10 days
Gonorrhea	Neonates Contact of known case	Erythromycin ophthalmic ointment See Table 14-9
Syphilis	Contact of known case	Benzathine penicillin G, 2.4 mg IM

[a] Modified from M. Markowitz, Rheumatic Fever. In R. E. Behrman and V. C. Vaughn, *Nelson Textbook of Pediatrics*. Philadelphia: Saunders, 1983. P. 593.[b] *Med. Lett. Drugs Ther.* 26:3, 1984.
[c] Oral regimen is safer and preferred for most patients. Parenteral regimens are recommended for those with prior endocarditis and those on continuous oral penicillin prophylaxis.[d] Parenteral regimens are more likely to be effective.[e] A PPD test should be performed after 3 months; if negative, prophylaxis can be discontinued if no further contact takes place.[f] Circumstances include corticosteroid or immunosuppressive therapy (INH for the duration of therapy); measles vaccine administration (1 month); illness with measles, pertussis, or influenza (1 month); and surgery with general anesthesia (1 month).[g] If serogroup A or C, immunization with meningococcal A or C vaccine may be helpful, since half the secondary cases occur more than 5 days after the index case. *M.M.W.R.* 30:113, 1981.

Table 14-8. Drug therapy in tuberculosis

Drug	Daily dose per kilogram body weight[a]	Route and mode of administration of daily dose	Major adverse reactions
Isoniazid	10–20 mg (max. 600 mg)	PO in 1–2 divided doses	Hepatotoxicity,[b] peripheral neuropathy[c] Rash, fever
Rifampin	10–20 mg (max. 600 mg)	PO in 1–2 divided doses	Hepatotoxicity,[b] GI disturbance, thrombocytopenia (rarely)
Streptomycin	20–40 mg (max. 1 gm)	IM in 1–2 divided doses	Eighth cranial nerve toxicity (primarily vestibular), rash, fever, nephrotoxicity
Para-aminosalicylic acid	200–300 mg (max. 12 gm)	PO in 2–4 divided doses	GI irritation (10%) Rash, fever
Ethambutol[d]	10–15 mg (max. 1,500 mg)	PO in 1 dose	Optic neuritis (especially with higher doses — ophthalmologic monitoring recommended) Rash, fever

[a] The high dose is recommended for critically ill patients and the low dose for prophylaxis and long-term therapy after improvement. [b] Hepatotoxicity is rare in children. Therapy should not be stopped because of mild abnormalities in liver function tests unless the patient has clinical symptoms. [c] Pyridoxine is unnecessary in most children, but is important in adolescents, whose diets may be inadequate, or in malnourished children. [d] Not recommended by manufacturer for children under 13.

of anthrax, diphtheria, actinomycosis, leptospirosis, and rat-bite fever. Penicillin G is more active than penicillin V.

(2) Pharmacology

(a) Oral preparations are penicillin G and penicillin V (phenoxymethyl penicillin). Because penicillin G is acid labile, its absorption is **variable.** Penicillin V is well absorbed, especially when given 1 hour before meals.

(b) Parenteral preparations differ in their peak serum level and half-life.

(i) Aqueous penicillin G results in rapid attainment of high blood levels after IM or IV administration. Its rapid excretion in patients (except newborns) with normal renal function requires that it be administered frequently (usually q4h) for optimal therapy. It is prepared as a potassium or sodium salt (1.7 mEq/106 units).

(ii) Procaine penicillin G is absorbed slowly from IM injections and produces relatively low but prolonged serum concentrations. It should thus be used only in infections due to highly susceptible organisms or in large dosage.

(iii) Benzathine penicillin G produces even lower blood levels, which last for as long as 3–4 weeks. It is used primarily against group A streptococci and *Treponema pallidum,* prophylactically in patients with rheumatic heart disease, and therapeutically when adherence to a program of oral penicillin is questionable.

b. Penicillinase-resistant penicillins

(1) Spectrum and indications. These agents are resistant to hydrolysis by the beta-lactamase produced by staphylococci and are therefore the drugs of choice for penicillin-resistant staphylococcal infections. They are approximately 10 times less active than penicillin G against penicillin-sensitive organisms.

(2) Pharmacology. The only clinically significant difference between preparations is in their routes of administration. Because **methicillin, oxacillin,** and **nafcillin** are not well absorbed after oral administration, they are used only parenterally. **Cloxacillin** and **dicloxacillin** are well absorbed orally.

c. Ampicillin and amoxicillin

(1) Spectrum and indications

(a) Ampicillin has the gram-positive spectrum of penicillin and is more active against enterococci and *Listeria.* Like penicillin, **it is inactive against penicillinase-producing staphylococci.** It is also active against many gram-negative organisms, including most *H. influenzae* strains, *Salmonella, Proteus mirabilis, Branhamella catarrhalis* and some *E. coli* and *Shigella.*

(b) The spectrum of **amoxicillin** is very similar to that of ampicillin.

(2) Pharmacology. The major difference between ampicillin and amoxicillin is that the latter is better absorbed after oral administration, even when given with meals. Amoxicillin is therefore given in lower dosage and may produce fewer gastrointestinal side effects than ampicillin. Because amoxicillin can be given q8h rather than q6h as with ampicillin, compliance may be approved.

d. Amoxicillin and clavulanic acid

(1) Spectrum and indications. Clavulanic acid binds irreversibly to the active site of many beta-lactamases, inactivating the enzyme. The combination of amoxicillin with clavulanic acid extends the spectrum of amoxicillin to include beta-lactamase–producing strains of *Staph. aureus, H. influenzae, B. catarrhalis, E. coli, Proteus, Klebsiella pneumoniae,* and gonococci. This combination is not active against *Pseudomonas aeruginosa* or many amoxicillin-resistant strains of

Enterobacter and *Serratia*. Amoxicillin-clavulanate is effective in otitis media, sinusitis, urinary tract infections (UTIs), skin and soft tissue infections, and both human and animal bite wounds. Because of its higher cost and the side effect of diarrhea, we reserve this drug combination for second- or third-line therapy (after amoxicillin and TMP-SMZ), except for treatment of bite wounds.

    (2) Pharmacology. Both components are rapidly absorbed and they are excreted at similar rates in the urine. Probenecid delays renal excretion of amoxicillin but not of clavulanic acid.

e. Ampicillin and sulbactam

    (1) Spectrum and indications. Sulbactam is a penicillin-like compound that, like clavulanate, binds irreversibly to most beta-lactamases, inactivating the enzyme. When combined with ampicillin, sulbactam acts to protect the ampicillin from beta-lactamases and effectively extends the antimicrobial spectrum of ampicillin to include beta-lactamase–producing organisms, such as *H. influenzae, M. catarrhalis,* many *E. coli, K. pneumoniae,* anaerobes including *Bacteroides fragilis,* and all methicillin-sensitive *Staph. aureus.* This combination of a well-proven and safe antibiotic (ampicillin) with a beta-lactamase inhibitor that has virtually identical pharmokinetics and tissue penetration as ampicillin has proved to be a useful alternative to combination therapy or third-generation cephalosporins in the empiric therapy of pneumonia, cellulitis, UTI, and other community-acquired infections, especially in young children at risk for *H. influenzae.* It is not used to treat meningitis and has no activity against organisms that are resistant to ampicillin by mechanisms other than production of beta-lactamase (e.g., *Pseudomonas*).

    (2) Pharmacology. Ampicillin and sulbactam have very similar pharmacokinetic profiles. Dosing is based on the ampicillin component (not to exceed 200 mg/kg/day) and administration is intravenous.

f. Carbenicillin and ticarcillin

    (1) Spectrum and indications. These agents extend the spectrum of ampicillin to include *P. aeruginosa* and some *Proteus* species. Some strains of *Enterobacter* and *Serratia* may also be sensitive. Ticarcillin is more potent than carbenicillin against *P. aeruginosa* and is therefore used in lower dosage. Both have in recent years been supplanted by newer antipseudomonal penicillins (see **g**), although oral indanyl carbenicillin remains useful as the only oral anti-pseudomonal antibiotic available for use in children.

    (2) Pharmacology. Oral indanyl carbenicillin attains therapeutic levels only in urine and is indicated only for UTIs caused by gram-negative organisms resistant to ampicillin and other oral agents.

g. Azlocillin, mezlocillin, and piperacillin

    (1) Spectrum and indications. These uride (azlocillin and mezlocillin) and piperazine (piperacillin) derivatives of ampicillin retain the activity of ampicillin to enterococci and *H. influenzae,* and are more active than carbenicillin or ticarcillin against aerobic gram-negative bacilli, including *P. aeruginosa* and *Klebsiella* species. Like ticarcillin and carbenicillin, they are not active against penicillinase-producing strains of *Staph. aureus* or *H. influenzae.* In vitro studies demonstrate synergy with aminoglycosides against *P. aeruginosa.* Combination therapy with an aminoglycoside is advised for any serious infection. These agents have replaced ticarcillin and carbenicillin for most indications.

    (2) Pharmacology. Mezlocillin, azlocillin, and piperacillin are monosodium salts (1.8 mEq Na$^+$/gm), whereas carbenicillin and ticarcillin are disodium salts (5 mEq Na$^+$/gm). These drugs are administered only by the IV route.

h. Ticarcillin–clavulanic acid. Spectrum and indications. The combination of ticarcillin with clavulanic acid, a beta-lactamase enzyme inhibitor, extends the spectrum of activity of ticarcillin to include beta-lactamase–producing strains of *Staph. aureus, H. influenzae, E. coli, Klebsiella,* and some other gram-negative bacilli. Strains of *P. aeruginosa* and gram-negative bacilli that produce the Richmond-Sykes type 1 beta-lactamases, which are resistant to ticarcillin, are still resistant to ticarcillin–clavulanic acid. Ticarcillin–clavulanic acid has limited use because of its cost and lack of demonstrated superiority over less expensive antibiotic regimens.

i. **Side effects of the penicillins**
(1) **Immediate allergic reactions** include anaphylaxis, angioneurotic edema, and urticaria. **A previous maculopapular rash due to ampicillin does not signify an increased risk of immediate reactions.** Because penicillins share the same chemical structure, patients who are allergic to one preparation may react to others and occasionally may react to the cephalosporins.

(a) **Patients suspected of having a penicillin allergy** can be skin tested with two types of materials: penicilloyl-polylysine (PPL, available commercially as Pre-Pen) and a "minor determinant" mixture. Patients with a positive reaction to PPL are likely to have an allergic reaction to therapeutic doses of penicillin. Patients with a positive reaction to minor determinants are likely to have an immediate reaction such as anaphylaxis.

(b) **Intradermal skin testing with aqueous penicillin G** may cause severe reactions in the highly allergic patient. Therefore, a scratch test with a dilute solution (5 U/ml in saline) should first be performed (together with a saline control). If no local reaction occurs within 20 minutes, a second scratch test is performed with a more concentrated solution (10,000 U/ml). If this is negative, a small skin bleb is raised by intradermal injection of the concentrated solution. A negative intradermal test suggests that an anaphylactic reaction to therapeutic penicillin G is unlikely, **but does not absolutely exclude this possibility. Appropriate drugs and equipment for respiratory and circulatory assistance should be at the bedside during the skin-testing procedure and the first doses of penicillin.**

(2) **Aqueous procaine penicillin G** may produce **a nonallergic immediate reaction** simulating anaphylaxis, especially when it is mistakenly injected into the intravascular space.

(3) **Delayed reactions** include fever, eosinophilia, hemolytic anemia, serum sickness, and urticaria. Interstitial nephritis may occur with all penicillins but has been most often described with methicillin. Neutropenia and anicteric hepatitis occur rarely. The most common delayed reactions are maculopapular rashes, which occur during 8 percent of all treatment courses with ampicillin (50–100% in the presence of infectious mononucleosis); they are less common with other penicillins. When indications are clear, antibiotic therapy can be continued because the rash usually disappears. Very rarely, it may progress to erythroderma and exfoliative dermatitis.

(4) **Dose-related effects** include CNS toxicity, hypokalemia, and coagulation disorders. The last of these is most typical with carbenicillin, but may also occur with penicillin, especially in patients with renal failure. Diarrhea from oral preparations may also be dose related. The sodium or potassium contained in aqueous penicillin preparations can contribute to congestive heart failure (CHF) or hyperkalemia.

2. **Cephalosporins.** The mechanism of action of the cephalosporins is similar to that of the penicillins. There are now three generations of cephalosporins, with multiple representatives of each generation currently on the market. This class of drug has gained in popularity because of its broad-spectrum

activity and relative lack of toxicity. To limit the confusion and subsequent misuse of cephalosporins in our hospital, we limit the choices to one representative per generation, except for special indications. In the discussion below, most members of each generation are discussed. However, The Children's Hospital formulary includes only cephalexin (first generation, PO), cefazolin (first, parenteral), cefoxitin (second, parenteral, used when enhanced anaerobic coverage is needed), cefprozil (second, PO), cefixime (third, PO), ceftriaxone (third, parenteral), and ceftazidime (third, parenteral, enhanced activity against *P. aeruginosa*).

a. **Cephalothin and its analogues**
   (1) **Spectrum and indications.** Cephalothin and its analogues, **cefazolin, cephalexin, cephapirin,** and **cephradine,** have similar antimicrobial spectra. They are active against gram-positive cocci, including penicillinase-producing *Staph. aureus*, and against gram-negative rods, including many community strains of *E. coli, Klebsiella,* and *P. mirabilis*. Generally, they have poor activity against enterococci or *H. influenzae*, and, despite disk sensitivity tests indicating activity against methicillin-resistant staphylococci, the cephalosporins are usually ineffective clinically against these organisms. Cephalothin and cefazolin are more resistant to staphylococcal penicillinase than other cephalosporins and are therefore the cephalosporins of choice for serious staphylococcal infections.
   (2) **Pharmacology.** Cephalothin and its analogues differ in their pharmacologic properties, especially with respect to routes of administration. Cephalothin, cefazolin, and cephapirin are available only for IM or IV administration. Cephalothin is painful when administered IM and should be given IV. Cephradine can be given parenterally or PO; cephalexin and cefadroxil are given PO only. The half-life in blood of most of these agents is very short (30–60 minutes), and parenteral therapy should therefore be given at 4-hour intervals except for cefazolin (q6–8h). Cefadroxil has an extended half-life and can be dosed once or twice a day. **With the exception of third-generation agents, the cephalosporins penetrate poorly into the CNS and should therefore not be used to treat meningitis or when meningitis may ensue as a complication of a bacteremic condition.**

b. **Second-generation cephalosporins**
   (1) **Spectrum and indications.** Cefamandole, cefuroxime, and cefoxitin extend the spectrum of the older cephalosporins to many strains of resistant gram-negative bacteria. Cefamandole and cefuroxime are more active against *H. influenzae* type B (including ampicillin-resistant strains). Cefaclor is two to eight times more active than cephalexin against *H. influenzae* type B. However, some strains, including some beta-lactamase–producing strains, are resistant to cefaclor. Cefprozil has antimicrobial activity similar to that of cefaclor but has a longer serum half-life. In general, aerobic gram-negative enteric organisms are more likely to be sensitive to gentamicin or tobramycin, anaerobes to clindamycin, or ampicillin/sulbactam.
   (2) **Pharmacology.** Cefamandole, cefuroxime, and cefoxitin are given IV q6–8h. Cefprozil can be given PO bid. Because they are excreted unchanged into the urine, the dosage should be reduced in patients with renal insufficiency. None of the second-generation cephalosporins should be used to treat meningitis. In general, the second-generation cephalosporins are being replaced by third-generation compounds for use in pediatrics.

c. **Third-generation cephalosporins**
   (1) **Spectrum and indications.** Cefotaxime, ceftriaxone, cefixime, moxalactam, cefoperazone, and ceftazidime have broad-spectrum activity against gram-negative enteric bacteria, many of which are resistant

to the older cephalosporins and aminoglycosides. These agents are also highly active against *H. influenzae* type B (including beta-lactamase–producing strains), and *Neisseria* species. Activity against anaerobes is good but not better than that of cefoxitin. Third-generation cephalosporins generally have less activity against gram-positive cocci than do first-generation drugs, and like all cephalosporins they are inactive against enterococci and *Listeria monocytogenes*. Cefixime has no antistaphylococcal activity at all. Antipseudomonal activity is only fair except for ceftazadime, which has excellent activity. Because of their high cost, these agents should be used only when they offer a clear advantage. One advantage of ceftriaxone and cefixime is a long half-life, which allows q24h dosing, and makes outpatient management possible in selected cases.

(2) Pharmacology. Most third-generation drugs are excreted primarily by the kidney; ceftriaxone has both renal and hepatic excretion, and cefoperazone is excreted primarily in bile. Ceftriaxone and cefixime have a serum half-life of 4–6 hours, allowing q12–24h dosing. All others have a 1- to 2-hour half-life and q6–8h dosing. CSF penetration is good through inflamed meninges.

d. Side effects of the cephalosporins. Side effects include: allergic reactions, nephrotoxicity, thrombocytopenia, granulocytopenia, dose-related encephalopathy, and anicteric hepatitis. Moxalactam and cefoperazone may cause bleeding, because of an increase in prothrombin time, which is reversible with vitamin K; moxalactam may also induce platelet dysfunction.

3. Aminoglycosides inhibit protein synthesis.

a. Spectrum and indications. The aminoglycosides are bacterial against a broad range of enteric gram-negative bacilli and *Staph. aureus,* but the various analogues differ in their antimicrobial spectra. Aminoglycosides are valuable and proven antibiotics; however, they have a narrow therapeutic index and careful attention must be given to proper dosing and drug level monitoring. Despite the recent popularity of cephalosporins, aminoglycosides remain a mainstay of antimicrobial therapy in the neonate and young infant as well as in hospitalized children.

(1) They are not effective against streptococci, pneumococci, anaerobes, and spirochetes.

(2) Many gram-negative bacilli, especially in hospitals, have become resistant to **streptomycin** and **kanamycin.** In addition, neither agent is active against *P. aeruginosa.* **Streptomycin** is now used only as an antituberculosis agent.

(3) Gentamicin is active against most gram-negative rods, including *P. aeruginosa,* and is the aminoglycoside of choice for the empiric treatment of gram-negative infections, in which resistant gram-negative bacilli are common.

(4) Tobramycin is more active than gentamicin against *P. aeruginosa* (2–4 times).

(5) Amikacin is active against many enteric gram-negative bacilli that are resistant to gentamicin. Unless such organisms are common, this agent should be reserved for infections that have proved resistant to the other aminoglycosides or in settings where gentamicin-resistant organisms are common.

(6) Netilmicin is an aminoglycoside with antibacterial activity similar to that of tobramycin. Netilmicin may be associated with less ototoxicity than other aminoglycosides, but it has not gained wide use in pediatrics.

b. Pharmacology

(1) The aminoglycosides are poorly absorbed from the GI tract. However, they may reach toxic levels after oral administration in patients with a damaged gut or with renal failure.

(2) Because the aminoglycosides have a narrow toxic-therapeutic ratio, dosage must be adjusted to obtain safe, effective serum levels (see Table 14-4).

(3) Aminoglycoside levels should be monitored to minimize the risk of ototoxicity and nephrotoxicity. We routinely monitor pre- and post-dose levels every 2–3 days in critically ill patients and in all patients who are receiving prolonged courses of therapy. However, in otherwise healthy children with normal renal function who are started on standard-dose aminoglycoside therapy empirically with the intention of stopping therapy within 48–72 hours (a usual time for culture results to become available), measuring levels is of limited use. If therapy is continued beyond 48–72 hours, levels should be monitored. Aminoglycoside-related ototoxicity and nephrotoxicity are most likely to occur with prolonged administration or improper dosing.

(4) Aminoglycosides are excreted almost entirely by the kidneys. The dosage must be adjusted when there is even a minor degree of renal impairment.

c. **Side effects**

(1) **Nephrotoxicity** due to renal tubular damage is enhanced by the concurrent use of cephalothin and diuretics (especially when sodium depletion occurs) and by preexisting renal disease. It is usually reversible. **The serum creatinine should be monitored in all patients receiving aminoglycoside therapy.**

(2) Ototoxicity (both vestibular and auditory) is enhanced by preexisting ear disease, concurrent administration of diuretics, and preexisting renal disease. **It may be irreversible** unless recognized early. Patients should be examined daily for symptoms of "fullness" in the ears, tinnitus, or vertigo. Ability to hear a watch tick provides a simple but sensitive bedside screening test for the high-tone hearing loss characteristic of aminoglycoside toxicity.

(3) **Neuromuscular blockade** with respiratory paralysis has been described, usually after peritoneal irrigation with high concentrations of aminoglycoside or in association with botulism.

4. **Newer antibiotics: carbapenems, monobactams, and quinolones**

a. **Imipenem-cilistatin.** Imipenem, a carbapenem, has the widest spectrum of any lactam antibiotic yet released and is available only in combination with cilistatin, an enzyme inhibitor that is important in achieving effective urinary concentrations. Activity includes nearly all gram-positive organisms, including enterococci but excluding methicillin-resistant staphylococci. It is highly active against most Enterobacteriaceae species and anaerobes, including *B. fragilis*. Although highly active, it is not usually used as monotherapy against *Pseudomonas* because resistance can develop while a patient is undergoing therapy. Its use in pediatrics is currently limited to very specific infections with organisms resistant to other antibiotics.

b. **Aztreonam.** This first monobactam antibiotic has no significant gram-positive or anaerobic activity, but is highly active against most Enterobacteriaceae and *P. aeruginosa*. Although combination therapy will often be needed, aztreonam has the potential to replace aminoglycosides in many gram-negative infections.

c. **Quinolones.** As synthetic agents based on the structure of naladixic acid, quinolones are highly active against gram-negative bacteria in addition to many gram-positive organisms. Quinolones are well absorbed after oral administration. Their use in pediatrics is limited because they have been shown to damage cartilage in growing animals. Limited data do not show evidence of similar toxicity in children; however, the data are insufficient currently to recommend use of quinolones for children except in special circumstances.

5. **Erythromycin,** a macrolide antibiotic, inhibits bacterial protein synthesis by binding to ribosomes.

    a. Spectrum and indications. Erythromycin is bacteriostatic at low concentrations against *Mycoplasma pneumoniae*, spirochetes, and most gram-positive organisms. It is commonly used as an alternative drug in penicillin-allergic patients with group A streptococcal and pneumococcal infections. It is only moderately active against *H. influenzae* and can be used with a sulfonamide in treating otitis media. Erythromycin is the drug of choice for *Legionella* and *M. pneumoniae* infections, pertussis, the diphtheria carrier state, *Campylobacter* infections, and chlamydia pneumonia. Clarithromycin and azithromycin, newer macrolides, have recently been licensed and have the advantage of being more active as well as better tolerated than erythromycin. There has been only limited use of clarithromycin or azithromycin in pediatrics to date.

    b. Pharmacology. Erythromycin base is acid labile and poorly absorbed. Erythromycin estolate is well absorbed, even in the presence of food, but must be hydrolized to the active base by the liver. A variety of parenteral preparations are also available. Active erythromycin is excreted in low concentrations in urine and in higher concentrations in bile.

    c. Side effects include nausea, vomiting, and diarrhea. Erythromycin estolate occasionally causes a cholestatic jaundice in adults. However, in children, the estolate form rarely causes hepatitis, is better absorbed, and is more effective than the ethylsuccinate form.

  6. Clindamycin inhibits bacterial protein synthesis.

    a. Spectrum and indications

      (1) Clindamycin has a spectrum similar to that of erythromycin, except that it is inactive against *M. pneumoniae*, *Neisseria gonorrhoeae*, *Neisseria meningitidis*, and *H. influenzae*. It is quite active against nonenterococcal gram-positive organisms and most anaerobes.

      (2) Clindamycin is often used for serious anaerobic infections due to *B. fragilis* and is popular as part of the "triples" regimen with ampicillin and gentamicin to provide empiric coverage for perforated appendix or other forms of peritonitis. It is an alternative to penicillin for infections due to group A streptococci and pneumococci, and to penicillinase-resistant penicillins for staphylococcal infections. However, resistance to clindamycin may emerge during therapy, and staphylococcal endocarditis may relapse after clindamycin treatment.

    b. Pharmacology. Absorption is not decreased by the presence of food. Clindamycin is metabolized by the liver.

    c. Side effects

      (1) GI side effects (nausea, vomiting, abdominal cramps, diarrhea) are common. **Pseudomembranous colitis,** which is also associated with many other antibiotics, may develop and become severe if treatment is continued. Assays for the enterotoxin *Clostridium difficile* in the stool may confirm the diagnosis; oral vancomycin or oral metronidazole is the treatment of choice for pseudomembranous colitis.

      (2) Uncommon side effects include rash, anaphylaxis, and hepatitis. **Rapid IV infusion may produce syncope or cardiopulmonary arrest.**

  7. Chloramphenicol inhibits bacterial protein synthesis at the ribosomal level.

    a. Spectrum and indications

      (1) Chloramphenicol is active against most gram-positive organisms, most gram-negative bacilli (except *P. aeruginosa*), anaerobes (including *B. fragilis*), and *Rickettsia*. At low concentrations it is bacteriostatic for most organisms and bactericidal for highly sensitive organisms such as *H. influenzae*; at high concentrations it is bactericidal for sensitive organisms.

      (2) It is still a drug of choice for serious *Salmonella* infections (including typhoid fever) and rickettsial infections (including Rocky Mountain spotted fever). Although the role of chloramphenicol in pediatrics has increasingly been suppla‑ ted by third-generation cephalosporins, it remains a drug of choice for serious *H. influenzae* infections.

(3) As a well-tolerated antibiotic with near complete bioavailability after oral administration, chloramphenicol is useful for oral outpatient continuation therapy of many infections due to susceptible organisms. Serum concentrations after oral administration are equivalent to levels obtained with parenteral dosing.

b. Pharmacology. Chloramphenicol is well absorbed from the GI tract and diffuses well into tissues and the CSF. Most of the drug is conjugated in the liver and excreted in the urine.

c. Side effects.

(1) Aplastic anemia is a rare (1 in 50,000 courses of treatment) but serious side effect unrelated to either dose or plasma level. There are inadequate data to suggest that the oral preparation is more likely to cause this side effect than is parenteral administration.

(2) Dose-related bone marrow suppression is common and reversible, occurring regularly when plasma-free chloramphenicol levels exceed 25 μg/ml or with prolonged therapy. Manifestations include increased serum iron, decreasing reticulocyte counts, and a falling hematocrit. Thrombocytopenia and leukopenia also occur. The bone marrow shows the characteristic vacuolation of erythroblasts. Free erythrocyte protoporphyrin may be elevated.

(3) In neonates in whom high serum levels of chloramphenicol (> 50 μg/ml) develop, a shock-like syndrome ("gray baby syndrome") may occur. Dosage should be reduced and serum levels monitored (see Table 14-4). This syndrome has been very rare since appropriate dosing and monitoring of chloramphicol have been used in neonates.

8. The tetracyclines inhibit bacterial protein synthesis and are not used commonly in early childhood because of their side effects.

a. Spectrum and indications

(1) The tetracyclines have broad-spectrum bacteriostatic activity against gram-positive organisms, enteric gram-negative bacilli, anaerobes, mycoplasms, spirochetes, and rickettsiae. *Serratia, Proteus,* and *P. aeruginosa* are almost always resistant.

(2) Tetracyclines are the drugs of choice for brucellosis, cholera, Q fever, relapsing fever, Rocky Mountain spotted fever (in children older than 8 years), psittacosis, lymphogranuloma venereum, and nonspecific urethritis. They are second-line drugs for *Mycoplasma* pneumonia, tularemia, gonorrhea, syphilis, melioidosis, granuloma inguinale, and eradication of the meningococcal carrier state (minocycline).

b. Pharmacology. The absorption of tetracycline is impaired by concurrent food intake and the presence of divalent cations (calcium, iron). The serum half-life is relatively short (6 hr). Doxycycline and minocycline are absorbed more completely then tetracycline, and have a longer half-life (14–20 hr). Most tetracyclines are excreted mainly by the kidney, but also reach high concentrations in bile. **Doxycycline,** which is eliminated mainly by nonrenal mechanisms, **is the only tetracycline that can be safely used in renal failure.**

c. Side effects

(1) Tetracyclines may produce **permanent yellow discoloration of the deciduous teeth** (when given during the second and third trimester of pregnancy and the first 3 months of life) and of permanent teeth (when given to children 3 months–8 years of age). Tetracyclines should therefore be avoided during these periods. Other side effects include upper and lower **GI symptoms,** candidal superinfection, and dose-related **hepatitis.**

(2) Preexisting renal dysfunction is exacerbated by all the tetracyclines except doxycycline.

(3) Rare side effects include allergy, photosensitivity (dimethyl chlortetracycline), benign intracranial hypertension, and reversible vestibular disturbance (minocycline).

9. **Vancomycin** inhibits bacterial cell wall synthesis.
   a. **Spectrum and indications.** Vancomycin is bactericidal for most gram-positive organisms but is only bacteriostatic for enterococci. It is active against staphylococci, beta-hemolytic streptococci, viridans streptococci, pneumococci, *Corynebacterium,* and *Clostridium.*
      (1) Vancomycin is useful in the treatment of serious infection caused by methicillin-resistant staphylococci.
      (2) Vancomycin and gentamicin combined are the treatment of choice for enterococcal endocarditis in patients with allergy to penicillin.
      (3) Oral vancomycin is effective treatment for staphylococcal enterocolitis and antibiotic-induced colitis associated with enterotoxin-producing *Clostridium.*
   b. **Pharmacology.** Vancomycin is not absorbed after oral administration. After parenteral administration it enters tissues well, but diffuses poorly across inflamed meninges. It is excreted primarily by the kidneys, and dosage must be adjusted in renal failure and serum levels must be followed (see Table 14-4). **It is not eliminated by hemodialysis** (see Table 14-6). To avoid a histamine-like reaction (red man syndrome), vancomycin is infused over at least 30 minutes and can be preceded by antihistamine administration if necessary.
   c. **Side effects include:**
      (1) Fever, phlebitis, and maculopapular and urticarial rashes. Anaphylaxis is rare.
      (2) **Ototoxicity** and **nephrotoxicity** may occur with high serum levels and may be enhanced when aminoglycosides are used concurrently. Renal function should be monitored as with aminoglycosides (see **3**).
10. **The sulfonamides** block the synthesis of dihydrofolic acid from para-aminobenzoic acid in bacterial cells.
    a. **Spectrum and indications**
       (1) Sulfonamides have a broad bacteriostatic spectrum, including most gram-positive cocci (but not enterococci); gram-positive bacilli; most gram-negative organisms, including *H. influenzae, Chlamydia, Actinomyces,* and *Nocardia;* and protozoa (malaria, *Toxoplasma,* and *Pneumocystis*).
       (2) The **major indications** for sulfonamides include uncomplicated UTI, *Nocardia* infections, and, together with other drugs, toxoplasmosis and *P. carinii* pneumonia.
       (3) Erythromycin with a sulfonamide is a second-line regimen for otitis media. Trimethoprim combined with sulfamethoxazole is an important drug in pediatrics and is discussed below.
       (4) Sulfonamides provide effective rheumatic fever prophylaxis, but cannot be relied on for the treatment of group A streptococcal infections.
    b. **Pharmacology** (e.g., sulfisoxazole). Must sulfonamides are well absorbed orally. They are metabolized by the liver, and both active drug and metabolites are excreted primarily by the kidney. Products of tissue necrosis inhibit the action of sulfonamides. Therefore, these agents should not be used for severe suppurative infections.
    c. **Side effects**
       (1) **Allergic reactions** include fever, rash (usually maculopapular, occasionally urticarial, rarely exfoliative or the rash of Stevens-Johnson syndrome), systemic vasculitis, myocarditis, and pulmonary eosinophilia. Patients who have experienced rash with sulfa drugs should not receive any sulfa-containing compounds subsequently.
       (2) Rare **hematologic effects** include reversible agranulocytosis and aplastic anemia. Acute hemolytic anemia may occur in patients with glucose-6-phosphate dehydrogenase (G-6-PD) deficiency.
       (3) Sulfonamides compete with bilirubin for albumin-binding sites, thereby increasing the risk of **kernicterus** in neonates. **They are**

contraindicated in pregnancy near term and in jaundiced infants or infants at risk of developing severe jaundice (e.g., ABO incompatibility).

11. **Trimethoprim-sulfamethoxazole.** Both drugs inhibit folic acid synthesis.
   a. **Spectrum and indications**
      (1) The antimicrobial spectrum includes most gram-positive cocci, *H. influenzae*, *M. catarrhalis* and *P. carinii*, and many enteric gram-negative bacilli.
      (2) The **major indications** include treatment and prophylaxis of otitis media, UTIs, and *P. carinii* pneumonia. It is a very effective and inexpensive drug in the treatment of acute otitis media, especially after amoxicillin failure, and is useful in the treatment of shigellosis, *Salmonella* infections, and infections caused by susceptible gram-negative bacilli.
      (3) As a well-tolerated antibiotic with near complete bioavailability after oral administration, TMP-SMZ is useful for oral outpatient continuation therapy of many infections due to susceptible organisms. Serum concentrations after oral administration are equivalent to levels obtained with parenteral dosing.
   b. **Pharmacology.** The dosage should be decreased in patients with severe renal dysfunction. IV usage for *P. carinii* is discussed in Chap. 15.
   c. **Side effects** (see also **10**)
      (1) Rash, nausea, vomiting, and thrombocytopenia are the most common side effects. Hematologic suppression due to weak inhibition of folic acid metabolism may be reversible with folinic acid. **The drug should be used with caution in patients with preexisting hematologic disease, in patients receiving immunosuppressive therapy, or in patients who are dehydrated.**
      (2) Mild, reversible renal impairment may occur.
12. **Nitrofurantoin** may inhibit bacterial carbohydrate metabolism.
   a. **Spectrum and indications**
      (1) Nitrofurantoin is active against most gram-positive cocci (including enterococci) and gram-negative urinary pathogens. Sensitive organisms usually do not become resistant during therapy.
      (2) The only indications for nitrofurantoin are the treatment and prophylaxis of UTIs.
   b. **Pharmacology.** The drug reaches therapeutically effective levels only in the urine, which is its major route of excretion.
   c. **Side effects**
      (1) **GI side effects** (nausea, vomiting, abdominal cramps) occur frequently and are dose related. They are less common with the macrocrystalline form, which is more slowly absorbed but equally effective. Serious systemic toxicity may occur in renal failure.
      (2) Other adverse reactions include allergy (rashes, fever, eosinophilia, hepatitis, asthma, and acute pneumonitis), dose-related peripheral neuritis, pulmonary fibrosis, and hemolytic anemia in patients with G-6-PD deficiency.
13. **Metronidazole** is reduced by enzymes in anaerobic bacteria. These reduction products disrupt DNA and inhibit nucleic acid synthesis.
   a. **Spectrum and indications**
      (1) Most aerobic organisms are resistant, but metronidazole is bactericidal for almost all anaerobic organisms, including *B. fragilis* and *Clostridium*.
      (2) Metronidazole is probably the drug of choice only for endocarditis due to *B. fragilis* (because of its bactericidal activity) and for *B. fragilis* infections that are resistant to other drugs. It is equally effective as oral vancomycin in treatment of *C. difficile* pseudomembranous colitis. Metronidazole is also useful in the treatment of trichomoniasis and amebiasis and is an alternative drug for giardiasis (see Chap. 15).

b. Pharmacology
   (1) Metronidazole is well absorbed from the GI tract and enters into all tissues, including the CSF. Serum concentrations after oral dosage are similar to those achieved with equal IV doses.
   (2) The drug is largely metabolized in the liver and excreted by the kidney. No alteration in dosage is necessary for renal insufficiency; however, the dosage in patients with hepatic disease should be decreased and serum levels monitored.
c. Side effects
   (1) Nausea, dry mouth, and metallic taste are most frequent.
   (2) Uncommon neurologic reactions include reversible peripheral neuropathy, vertigo, ataxia, and convulsions. Reversible neutropenia and rash have also been reported.
   (3) The package insert contains a warning that metronidazole is carcinogenic in rodents. No human tumors have ever been attributed to metronidazole therapy.
14. Mupirocin inhibits RNA and protein synthesis by binding to isoleucyl transfer RNA synthetase.
   a. Spectrum and indications
      (1) A topical agent highly active against staphylococci, including methicillin-resistant strains. Also active against streptococci except enterococci. Useful as an alternative to oral antibiotic therapy for impetigo. May also prove useful for eradicating nasal carriage of *Staph. aureus.*
      (2) The unique mechanism of action may explain the limited cross-resistance with other antibiotics.
   b. Pharmacology. Exclusively a topical agent with minimal systemic absorption and rapid clearance of any absorbed drug.
   c. Side effects. Very low incidence. Intranasal use of topical preparation may be associated with itching and stinging.
B. Antifungal agents
   1. Amphotericin B and nystatin. Both bind to a sterol constituent in the fungal cell membrane, thereby increasing its permeability.
      a. Spectrum and indications
         (1) Both drugs are active against *Candida* species, *Cryptococcus neoformans, Sporotrichum schenckii, Blastomyces dermatitidis, Histoplasma capsulatum, Coccidioides immitis, Aspergillus* species, and Phycomycetes.
         (2) These drugs are the antimicrobials of choice for fungal infections on the skin and mucosal surfaces (nystatin) or disseminated to other organs (amphotericin B). Severe mucosal infections may require systemic amphotericin B.
      b. Pharmacology. Both drugs are poorly absorbed after oral administration.
         (1) Nystatin is available only for topical use on the skin, on the mucosal surfaces, and in the GI tract. **Amphotericin** is given by slow (2–4 hr) IV infusion in 5% dextrose. Premedication with an antihistamine, antipyretic, and meperidine, and the addition of 10–50 mg hydrocortisone to each 500 ml of 5% dextrose in water (D/W) of the infusate, may minimize systemic reactions. If possible, dosage should be increased gradually, beginning with a dose of 1 mg on the first day. However, in serious systemic fungal infections it is important to increase dosage quickly to full therapeutic levels.
         (2) Amphotericin B has a half-life of approximately 20 hours and can therefore be given in increased dosage every other day when prolonged treatment is necessary, especially on an outpatient basis.
      c. Side effects
         (1) Immediate side effects during infusion of amphotericin B are very common and include fever, chills, headache, nausea, vomiting, and,

rarely, hypotension. Reversible **nephrotoxicity** and **normochromic normocytic anemia** also occur.

(2) Rare adverse reactions include allergic reactions, peripheral neuropathy (with intrathecal administration), and cardiotoxicity with rapid infusion.

2. **5-Fluorocytosine (5-FC)** may be converted to the antimetabolite 5-fluorouracil within the fungal cell and thereby interfere with nucleic acid synthesis.

a. **Spectrum and indications**

(1) 5-FC is active against *Cryptococcus neoformans,* most species of *Candida albicans,* and *Torulopsis glabrata.* All these organisms may become resistant during therapy, particularly when 5-FC is used alone in low dosage. Sensitivity must be confirmed before this agent is used alone for *Candida* infections.

(2) The **major indication** for 5-FC is its use together with amphotericin B for cryptococcal meningitis. This combination may also be useful for severe disseminated infections with sensitive *Candida* species and possibly *Aspergillus.*

b. **Pharmacology.** 5-FC is well absorbed orally, is not metabolized significantly, and is excreted almost entirely by glomerular filtration. In patients with renal dysfunction, the dosage should be adjusted and serum levels monitored frequently (see Table 14-4).

c. Side effects include bone marrow suppression and, rarely, hepatitis, GI side effects, and skin rashes.

3. **Ketoconazole,** an imidazole, impairs the synthesis of ergosterol, thus affecting fungal cell membrane permeability.

a. **Spectrum and indications**

(1) Ketoconazole is active against *Candida* species, *C. immitis, H. capsulatum, B. dermatitidis, Paracoccidioides brasiliensis,* and the dermatophytes.

(2) The drug is approved for the **oral** treatment of certain systemic fungal infections, including candidiasis, candiduria, chronic mucocutaneous candidiasis, oral thrush, histoplasmosis, coccidioidomycosis, chromomycosis, and paracoccidioidomycosis. Because it penetrates poorly into the CSF, it should not be used for fungal meningitis. Few controlled studies of the efficacy of ketoconazole have been done in infants and children, and there are limited toxicity data for children under 2 years of age. It is not used to treat serious fungal infections.

b. **Pharmacology.** Ketoconazole has the advantage of oral administration. It is metabolized by the liver and excreted in bile.

c. **Side effects.** The frequently reported adverse effects have been nausea and vomiting, and these symptoms may be minimized by taking the drug with meals. Liver dysfunction is a possible serious adverse effect.

4. **Fluconazole,** a new imidazole, inhibits the P-450 cytochrome system of fungi, impairing the synthesis of ergosterol and affecting fungal cell membrane permeability. Fluconazole is more active than ketoconazole for *Candida* and *Cryptococcus.* Although experience with pediatric patients is limited, it appears to be both efficacious and safe for children.

a. **Spectrum and indications**

(1) Fluconazole is highly active against *Candida* species, *C. neoformans, C. immitis, H. capsulatum, Bl. dermatitidis, P. brasiliensis,* and the dermatophytes.

(2) Effective in oropharyngeal, esophageal, urinary, and systemic candidiasis. Useful for maintenance therapy of cryptococcal meningitis.

b. **Pharmacology.** Once-daily dosing is possible based on a half-life of 30 hours and good oral absorption. Fluconazole penetrates well into most tissues and body fluids including CSF. Excretion is primarily renal.

     c. Side effects. Fluconazole is generally well tolerated. Nausea (3.7%) is the most common adverse reaction. Headache, skin rash, vomiting, abdominal pain, and diarrhea are less commonly reported.

    5. Clotrimazole, like the other imidazoles, interferes with synthesis of the fungal cell wall. It is active against dermatophytes, most species of *Candida*, *C. neoformans,* and most filamentous fungi.

    Only topical forms of clotrimazole are currently available as an effective alternative for cutaneous dermatophyte and candidal infections and for vaginal candidiasis.

IV. Treatment of infectious diseases

  A. Skin infections

    1. Bullous impetigo, scalded skin syndrome, and **staphylococcal scarlet fever** represent a spectrum of dermatologic manifestations of staphylococcal infection resulting from release of soluble toxins by *Staph. aureus.*

      a. Etiology. The infecting organism is *Staph. aureus* (usually bacteriophage group II).

      b. Evaluation

        (1) Cultures of the skin, nose, throat, and blood should be made (exceptions include children with only localized bullous impetigo and older children who are afebrile and nontoxic).

        (2) Gram stain of the denuded skin or bullous fluid, or both, will differentiate direct staphylococcal skin invasion from the more common toxin-mediated skin changes. The fluid aspirated from intact bullae will be sterile in scalded skin syndrome, but may contain *Staph. aureus* in bullous impetigo.

      c. The **diagnosis** is established by the clinical picture in association with recovery of *Staph. aureus* from the patient. Nikolsky's sign (gentle rubbing of the skin results in sloughing of the epidermis) is usually indicative of the scalded skin syndrome; its absence does not exclude the diagnosis.

      d. Therapy

        (1) A 7- to 10-day course of a penicillinase-resistant penicillin or first-generation cephalosporin generally is sufficient. Except in mild bullous impetigo, the antibiotic is usually given parenterally (e.g., oxacillin, 100–200 mg/kg/day divided q4h IV, or cefazolin, 150 mg/kg/day divided q8h IV).

        (2) After a good clinical response has been achieved, therapy can be completed with oral dicloxacillin or cephalexin.

        (3) Contact precautions are indicated until the lesions have resolved.

        (4) Corticosteroids have not been demonstrated to be beneficial.

        (5) In patients with extensive skin losses, hydration and maintenance of normal body temperature are important. Avoid unnecessary skin trauma (e.g., adhesive from tape).

    2. Cellulitis (including erysipelas)

      a. Etiology. *Staphylococcus aureus,* group A streptococci, and, in children under age 5, *H. influenzae* type B. In infants, group B streptococcal infection should be considered.

      b. Evaluation

        (1) A blood culture and antigen detection studies (e.g., counterimmunoelectrophoresis or latex agglutination) should be done in patients with severe cellulitis, fever, generalized toxicity, or impaired host defenses.

        (2) Needle aspiration of the advancing border of an active lesion should be carried out for Gram stain and culture.

        (3) Sinus x-rays should be done in patients with periorbital cellulitis.

      c. The **diagnosis** is usually established by the characteristic warm, erythematous, tender, and indurated skin.

        (1) Streptococcal cellulitis (erysipelas) is suggested by advancing, well-demarcated, heaped-up borders; facial involvement may assume a butterfly distribution.

(2) *H. influenzae* **type B** is suggested by a fever higher than 38.9°C (102° F) and sometimes by a purple discoloration of the skin. Most patients with *H. influenzae* type B cellulitis are bacteremic, and additional sites of infection should be considered (e.g., septic arthritis or meningitis).

d. Therapy

(1) Application of local heat, e.g., warm compresses, 10–20 minutes qid or more

(2) If feasible, immobilization and elevation of the affected extremity

(3) Incision and drainage of any primary suppurative focus

(4) Antibiotics

(a) Localized cellulitis without fever can be treated with oral antibiotics. However, if evidence of systemic toxicity is present, parenteral antibiotics should be given until sustained clinical improvement has occurred. It is important to note that the cellulitis, with advancing erythema, does not halt immediately once effective therapy has been given. It is common for the cellulitis to appear to spread over the first 24–36 hours after starting effective therapy. Clinical judgment and evidence of toxicity should be considered before changing antibiotics.

(b) Initial therapy for the child over 5 years of age with extremity cellulitis includes a penicillinase-resistant penicillin or first-generation cephalosporin if *H. influenzae* type B is not suspected, or an agent such as cefuroxime, or ampicillin-sulbactam, which provides broad coverage for the possible infecting organisms.

(c) *H. influenzae* type B is a common cause of periorbital (preseptal) or cheek cellulitis, and therefore the empiric antibiotic regimen should cover that organism.

(d) For therapy in immunocompromised patients, an antibiotic that is effective against gram-negative enteric organisms and *Pseudomonas* should be included.

(e) Streptococcal disease or erysipelas usually responds to benzathine penicillin G, 0.6–1.2 MU IM in one dose, or oral penicillin V, 125–150 mg qid. More severely ill patients may initially require IV penicillin, 100,000 U/kg/day q4h. Treatment should be continued for 7–10 days.

(f) Staphylococcal cellulitis is usually treated with a penicillinase-resistant penicillin or cephalosporin (nafcillin or oxacillin, 100–200 mg/kg/day IV q4h, or cefazolin, 150 mg/kg/day IV q8h) for severe infections or with oral dicloxacillin or cephalexin for milder infections.

(g) *H. influenzae* cellulitis, in view of the high incidence of positive blood cultures in this disease, is treated parenterally with ampicillin in combination either with sulbactam or choramphenicol. Alternatively, cefuroxime, cefotaxime, or ceftriaxone can be used pending ampicillin sensitivity testing.

(h) Orbital cellulitis. Hospitalization and high doses of antibiotics given IV are indicated. The initial choice should include a penicillinase-resistant penicillin and, in children, an antimicrobial that is effective against *H. influenzae*. Computed tomographic (CT) studies of the orbit are useful to determine if an abscess or sinusitis is present.

B. Bites

1. Animal bites

a. Etiology. Potential pathogens include *Staph. aureus*, anaerobic and microaerophilic streptococci, other anaerobic cocci, *Clostridium* species (including *C. tetani*), *Pasteurella multocida*, *Streptobacillus moniliformis*, and *Spirillum minus* (the latter two cause the two types of rat-bite fever).

b. Evaluation includes an assessment of the patient's immunity to tetanus as well as the extent of the wound.

c. A bacterial complication of an animal bite is suggested by the finding of cellulitis.

d. Therapy. Besides cleansing, local antisepsis, and surgical care of the bite, including irrigation and debridement if necessary, prophylactic measures for rabies or tetanus, or both, should be considered. Antibiotics are used when the bite is on the face or hands and when a puncture wound (e.g., cat bite) is present. Ampicillin-clavulanate is useful for oral therapy; ampicillin-sulbactam or the combination of penicillin and oxacillin is useful for parenteral administration.

2. **Human bites,** especially those occurring on the palmar surface of the hand, may result in extensive, rapidly developing infection.

   a. Etiology. Infections are usually mixed and are caused by a variety of organisms, including staphylococci, gram-negative anaerobes and spirochetes from the mouth, and aerobic streptococci.

   b. Evaluation. The principles of management are similar to those for management of animal bites, but irrigation, debridement, and provision for drainage assume much greater importance. Because of the potential for anaerobic infection, these wounds are usually not sutured.

   c. Therapy with a penicillinase-resistant penicillin or a cephalosporin, begun prophylactically at the time of the bite, will cover the usual causative organisms.

3. **Rabies prophylaxis.** The recommendations are based on those of the CDC (*M.M.W.R.* RR-33:1–19, 1991).

   a. Evaluation. Consider the following before administering antirabies treatment:

   (1) Species of biting animal

   (a) Carnivorous wild animals (especially skunks, raccoons, foxes, coyotes, and bobcats) and bats are more likely to be infective than are other animals. Postexposure prophylaxis should be initiated after the bite of one of these animals unless the animal is tested and shown not to be rabid. Local epidemiology of rabies should also figure in decisions to give prophylaxis.

   (b) Domestic dog or cat bites sometimes require prophylaxis, depending on local epidemiology, but bites of rodents and lagomorphs rarely do. The state or local health department should be consulted in questionable cases.

   (2) Vaccination status of the biting animal. An adult animal immunized properly with one or more doses of rabies vaccine has only a minimal chance of having rabies and transmitting the virus.

   (3) Circumstances of the biting incident. An unprovoked attack is more likely to indicate that the animal is rabid than is a provoked attack. Bites sustained during attempts to feed or handle an apparently healthy animal should generally be regarded as provoked.

   (4) Type of exposure. The likelihood that rabies infection will result from a bite varies with its extent and location. A nonbite exposure (scratches, abrasions, open wounds, or mucous membrane contamination with saliva or other potentially infectious material from a rabid animal) may rarely result in rabies virus transmission. Casual contact, such as petting a rabid animal without sustaining a bite, may not be an indication for prophylaxis.

   b. Postexposure prophylaxis

   (1) Local wound treatment includes thorough cleansing with soap and water along with measures to prevent bacterial infection and tetanus (see **4**).

   (2) Immunization. If prophylaxis is indicated, both rabies immune globulin (RIG), one dose of 20 IU/kg (up to half a dose infiltrated in the wound and the rest given IM), and human diploid cell rabies vaccine (HDCV) or rabies vaccine, absorbed (RVA) should be given IM at a different site. Five doses of HDCV or RVA, 1 ml IM, are given on days 0, 3, 7, 14, and 28.

4. Tetanus immunization

   a. Tetanus toxoid, 0.5 ml IM (DT in children 6 years old) is indicated in the following:

   (1) Clean minor wounds if the fully immunized child (3 or more previous doses) has not received a booster dose in the last 10 years, or if the child is incompletely immunized (< 3 previous doses of toxoid).

   (2) Contaminated wounds (tetanus-prone wounds) if the fully immunized child has not received a booster dose in the last 5 years, or if the child is incompletely immunized.

   (3) All wounds neglected for more than 24 hours.

   b. Human tetanus immunoglobulin (TIG), 250–500 units IM in a separate injection site, should also be given in the following situations:

   (1) Contaminated wounds if the child is incompletely immunized

   (2) All wounds neglected for more than 24 hours

   c. If tetanus immunization is incomplete at the time prophylaxis for a wound is given, the recommended series should be completed.

C. Otitis media. Eustachian tube dysfunction causes inadequate ventilation of the middle ear, resulting in a negative middle ear pressure. Persistent negative pressure produces a sterile transudate within the middle ear. Concurrent or subsequent contamination of the middle ear with infected nasopharyngeal contents occurs by aspiration and insufflation during crying and nose blowing

1. Acute otitis media

   a. Etiology

   (1) *Streptococcus pneumoniae, H. influenzae* (nontypable), *M. catarrhalis,* and group A streptococci are the most common causative organisms; *Staph. aureus* and enteric gram-negative bacilli (in neonates) are less frequent causes.

   (2) Viruses and *M. pneumoniae* have been isolated from middle ear fluid infrequently; their significance is uncertain.

   (3) Of *Haemophilus* isolates, the nontypable *H. influenzae* (nonencapsulated) species comprise the majority of middle ear isolates, are not associated with invasive infection, and are responsible for a small but significant proportion of infections in older children and adults. *H. influenzae* type B is uncommon.

   b. Evaluation

   (1) Pneumotoscopy

   (2) Tympanometry

   (3) **Tympanocentesis.** Middle ear aspiration should be performed on children who are seriously ill, have a poor response to antibiotics, or have a complication of acute otitis media. It is also useful in newborns and immunocompromised children. Diagnostic tympanocentesis should be performed under semisterile conditions with the aid of an operating microscope or otoscope with operating head; a spinal needle is inserted through the anteroinferior segment of the tympanic membrane.

   c. Diagnosis. A bulging, opacified, discolored eardrum through which the landmarks are poorly visualized, together with decreased mobility of the drum, defines acute otitis media.

   d. Treatment

   (1) Antibiotics PO are prescribed for all patients, generally for 10 days. Amoxicillin is the first drug of choice as it is safe and inexpensive. Recurrent otitis shortly after amoxicillin therapy or amoxicillin failure is reason to use alternative antibiotics. In some areas with high levels of beta-lactamase–producing *H. influenzae* or *B.*

catarrhalis, alternative antibiotics might be given initially. We generally use TMP-SMZ as a second-line drug, as it is inexpensive, well tolerated, and very likely to cover pathogens that are resistant to amoxicillin. Direct comparisons of alternative antibiotics are limited, but suggest that amoxicillin-clavulanate is superior to cefaclor as a third-line agent. Cefixime, cefprozil, cefaclor, amoxicillin-clavulanate, and erythromycin-sulfisoxazole cost three to five times as much as amoxicillin or TMP-SMZ.

(a) Amoxicillin, 20–40 mg/kg/day q8h

(b) TMP-SMZ, 8 mg/kg/day of TMP component divided q12h

(c) Amoxicillin-clavulanate, 20–40 mg/kg/day q8h of amoxicillin component

(d) Cefprozil, 30 mg/kg/day q12h

(e) Cefixime, 8 mg/kg/day q24h

(f) Erythromycin-sulfisoxazole, 30–50 mg/kg/day q6h of erythromycin component

(2) **Analgesics** (acetaminophen, codeine) may be indicated.

(3) **Antihistamines** and **decongestants** are not indicated in otitis media except to relieve coryza symptoms.

(4) The patient should be reevaluated within 30 days after starting therapy to determine whether effusion persists. If complete resolution has occurred, the patient is discharged. Periodic monitoring is required for patients with repeated episodes of otitis media. If effusion persists after 4 weeks, treatment is the same as that for chronic otitis media.

(5) Repeated episodes of otitis media with clearing of middle ear effusion between attacks can be managed by the use of prophylactic antibiotics including TMP-SMZ (4 mg and 20 mg, respectively/kg/day) or sulfisoxazole (50 mg/kg/day) in a single daily dose.

2. **Subacute and chronic otitis media**

a. **Etiology.** Persistent negative intratympanic pressure results in a sterile transudate within the middle ear. Persistence of fluid within the middle ear space for 4–8 weeks after acute otitis media defines subacute otitis media, and thereafter the condition is referred to as chronic otitis media. A low-grade inflammatory reaction may lead to an exudate "glue" secretion. Bacteria are present in up to 50 percent of glue effusions; their exact role is unclear.

b. **Evaluation**

(1) Pneumotoscopy is essential.

(a) The tympanic membrane is classically thickened with a gray or amber fluid in the middle ear. Sometimes, a fluid meniscus, air bubbles, or bluish fluid may appear in the middle ear.

(b) The mobility of the tympanic membrane is always impaired.

(c) Protracted eustachian tube dysfunction may lead to the development of a cholesteatoma if it is not reversed by restoring normal middle ear ventilation.

(2) Tympanometry can be performed when the findings are equivocal.

(3) Audiometry can be performed on children over 3 years of age.

(4) Anatomic defects may be present.

c. **Diagnosis.** An immobile tympanic membrane with diminished mobility and fluid can be seen on pneumotoscopy.

d. **Treatment**

(1) Attempts can be made to improve ventilation of the middle ear by the Valsalva maneuver, blowing up a balloon, etc.

(2) The efficacy of decongestants, antihistamines, and adenoidectomy has not been proved.

(3) An effusion that is present for longer than 12 weeks can be removed by myringotomy with insertion of ventilation tubes, especially if it is associated with a hearing deficit.

(4) Prolonged administration of oral antibiotic such as amoxicillin is sometimes effective and may avert the need for myringotomy.

3. **Chronic suppurative otitis media with perforation or cholesteatoma** is a sequela of acute suppurative infection, and the patient should be referred to an otolaryngologist for evaluation and management.

D. **Oropharyngeal infections**
1. **Streptococcal pharyngitis (tonsillitis)**
   a. **Etiology.** Group A beta-hemolytic streptococci
   b. **Evaluation** must include a properly obtained throat culture (vigorous swabbing of both tonsillar areas and the posterior pharynx, which, if done properly, usually induces a gag reflex).
      (1) The disease should be suspected in any patient with a sore throat and fever. In infants, streptococcal infection is more likely to present as persistent nasopharyngeal discharge, with fever and excoriation of the nares.
      (2) Any history in the patient or family of recent streptococcal pharyngitis, scarlet fever, rheumatic fever, or penicillin allergy should be noted.
   c. The **diagnosis** is supported by a positive throat culture or rapid antigen detection and confirmed by a rising antistreptolysin O titer (500 Todd units as an absolute value on a single specimen, or a two-tube rise in serial specimens analyzed simultaneously). Other causes of exudative pharyngitis include viruses, gonococci, and groups C and G streptococci. *Corynebacterium diphtheriae* may produce a gray-to-black fibrinous exudate (membrane) in the posterior pharynx. Oral anaerobes sometimes cause painful, deep, punched-out ulcerations on an erythematous base that is covered by a poorly adherent pseudomembrane.
   d. **Therapy**
      (1) **Penicillin.** Prevention of rheumatic fever requires either benzathine penicillin G given IM or a 10-day course of oral penicillin. The parenteral route ensures treatment for a sufficient length of time, while oral therapy is dependent on the cooperation of the patient. Treatment schedules are as follows:
         (a) **Intramuscular penicillin (benzathine).** Children should be given a single injection of 600,000–1,200,000 units. The larger dose is preferable for children over 60 lb.
         (b) **Oral penicillin.** Children and adults are given 125 or 250 mg tid–qid for a full 10 days. Therapy must be **continued for the entire 10 days,** even though the temperature returns to normal and the patient is asymptomatic.
      (2) For patients with documented penicillin allergy, oral erythromycin, 40 mg/kg/day in four divided doses, or clindamycin, 10–20 mg/kg/day in four divided doses for 10 days, is recommended. Cephalosporins are also effective. Sulfonamides, while effective in the prophylaxis of streptococcal infection, are ineffective in their treatment.
      (3) Bed rest is not necessary. After 24 hours of antibiotic therapy, children are no longer contagious and can return to school.
      (4) Throat cultures are indicated for symptomatic family members, but are not necessary for others unless recurrent streptococcal pharyngitis occurs in the family. Such recurrences may necessitate antibiotic treatment of the entire family.
2. **Vincent's angina**
   a. **Etiology.** Mixed oral anaerobic bacteria are the causative organisms.
   b. **Evaluation.** Culture of the ulcerated lesion is necessary to rule out diphtheria and group A streptococcus.
   c. **Diagnosis.** Painful, deep, punched-out ulcerations on a red, edematous base are present, covered by a poorly adherent gray pseudomembrane. Involvement may include the tonsillar fossa, soft palate, and pharynx; inflammatory neck nodes are present. Culture and microscopic examination may confirm the diagnosis.

d. Treatment
  (1) Antibiotics. Penicillin V, 50 mg/kg/24 hr in four divided doses, is given for 10 days.
  (2) Local hygiene. 3% Hydrogen peroxide mouthwash and gargles q2h, with normal saline gargles at alternate hours. Cepacol or Chloraseptic mouthwashes may be soothing.
  (3) Analgesics are given as necessary: acetaminophen or codeine, or both; viscous lidocaine; or diclonine HCl mouthwashes and gargles q2–3h.
3. Abscesses involving the peritonsillar, retropharyngeal, or parapharyngeal spaces may complicate infections in and around the oropharynx.
  a. Peritonsillar abscesses commonly occur in children over 10 years of age.
    (1) Etiology. Group A streptococci and oral anaerobes
    (2) Evaluation. The soft palate and uvula may be swollen and displaced toward the unaffected side. The patient complains of severe throat pain and may speak with a muffled, "hot-potato" voice.
    (3) Diagnosis. Surgical drainage of the abscess usually yields the organism.
    (4) Therapy
      (a) Surgical drainage is the cornerstone of effective therapy and should be performed under general anesthesia using a cuffed endotracheal tube to minimize the chances of aspiration and/or mediastinitis.
      (b) After effective surgical drainage, the antibiotic treatment of choice is a 10-day course of penicillin, initially IV until acute manifestations have subsided and then continued PO.
  b. Retropharyngeal or parapharyngeal abscesses commonly occur in children younger than 3 years.
    (1) Etiology. Group A streptococci, *Staph. aureus*, and oral anaerobes
    (2) Evaluation. Abscesses in these locations should be suspected with displacement of structures or a mass in the posterior pharynx. A lateral neck x-ray will corroborate the former, but a submental vertex view may be required to demonstrate the latter. The possibility of an embedded foreign body should never be overlooked.
    (3) Diagnosis. Culture of aspirated surgical drainage may yield the organisms.
    (4) Therapy. Because of the high incidence of mixed infections at these sites, a penicillinase-resistant penicillin should be given in addition to penicillin G. Alternatively, ampicillin-sulbactam can be used. Clindamycin is an alternative drug for the penicillin-allergic patient. Surgical drainage is the mainstay of treatment.
E. Cervical adenitis. Lymph nodes often enlarge in response to localized or systemic infection. Marked enlargement (3 cm or more) associated with tenderness and erythema indicates progressive infection within the node.
  1. The etiology varies with the location of the infected neck glands:
    a. Tonsillar nodes (at the angle of the jaw) are likely to be infected by throat pathogens.
    b. Submandibular node infection follows oral or facial disease. Unilateral "cold" submandibular nodes, in the absence of orofacial infection, suggest infection with atypical (nontuberculous) mycobacteria.
    c. Posterior cervical node infection suggests an adjacent skin infection.
    d. Bilateral cervical node enlargement of marked degree indicates infectious mononucleosis, acute toxoplasmosis, secondary syphilis, a phenytoin reaction, or infiltrative node disease.
    e. Recurrent episodes of adenitis should raise the suspicion of chronic granulomatous disease or IG deficiency.
  2. Evaluation and diagnosis. The history, examination of the area drained by affected lymph nodes, and laboratory data (including antistreptolysin O, Monospot, complete blood count and differential, and VDRL as indicated) may reveal the likely cause of adenitis.

a. Needle aspiration of the node offers a simple, safe means of diagnosis. Gram and acid-fast stains of aspirates may provide immediately helpful information. Aspirates should be cultured for aerobes, anaerobes, and mycobacteria.

b. Although *Mycobacterium tuberculosis* adenitis is now uncommon, tuberculin testing is prudent. A positive tuberculin skin test mandates a chest x-ray. Atypical mycobacterial adenitis is commonly associated with a mildly positive tuberculin test; a Mantoux skin test with greater than 15 mm of induration should raise suspicion of *M. tuberculosis,* however.

c. Surgical drainage or excisional biopsy is appropriate for infected nodes that are fluctuant ("pointing") or refractory to broad-spectrum antibiotic therapy. The therapy of choice for atypical mycobacterial adenitis is excisional biopsy.

d. Cervical adenitis is a common cause of torticollis in children.

3. **Therapy**

a. Unless stains of the node aspirate suggest another organism, a penicillinase-resistant penicillin or first-generation cephalosporin should be given as initial therapy, because the most likely organisms are *Staph. aureus* and group A streptococci. Oral anaerobes can be isolated from some nodes but other pathogens, such as *H. influenzae* type B, are seen only rarely.

b. **Streptococcal adenitis.** Penicillin G, either IM or IV in severe cases, is given until the fever and localized inflammation have subsided. This response should occur within 2–3 days, after which a 10-day course of oral penicillin (penicillin G, 50,000 U/kg/day, or penicillin V, 50 mg/kg/day) can be completed. Hot compresses and antipyretics also are prescribed.

c. **Staphylococcal adenitis.** Since the organism is often penicillin resistant, one of the penicillinase-resistant semisynthetic penicillins or a first-generation cephalosporin is given. Severity of the illness determines whether the IV route and hospitalization are necessary.

(1) **Recommended preparations:**

(a) **IV.** Nafcillin, oxacillin, or methicillin, 100–200 mg/kg/day q4h, or cefazolin, 80 mg/kg/day q8h

(b) **PO.** Dicloxacillin, 25 mg/kg/day qid, or cephalexin, 25–50 mg/kg/day qid

(2) The duration of treatment is determined by the patient's response, but a 10- to 14-day course is usually sufficient.

d. **Tuberculous adenitis.** Antituberculous drugs are given (see Table 14-8).

e. **Nontuberculous mycobacterial adenitis.** Although the natural history of this disease is variable, the adenopathy will often resolve spontaneously. The nontuberculous mycobacteria are not communicable from human to human, and the patient presents no danger to siblings or classmates.

(1) Because nontuberculous strains are frequently resistant in vitro to the usual antituberculous drugs, observation is usually the preferred management.

(2) When increasing adenopathy or related symptoms indicate more aggressive management, complete surgical excision of the involved nodes is recommended. Antituberculous therapy should be given postoperatively until culture reports demonstrate that *M. tuberculosis* is not present.

F. **Impetigo**

1. **Etiology. Nonbullous impetigo** is characterized by crusted lesions caused primarily by streptococci and sometimes secondarily infected by staphylococci. Glomerulonephritis may result from impetigo caused by **streptococci M, type 49 or 55.**

2. **Evaluation**

a. **Gram stain** is rarely helpful due to frequent secondary infection.

b. **Laboratory evaluation.** If nephritogenic strains are suspected, throat and skin cultures should be done on close contacts.

3. Diagnosis
   a. Subjective findings. The patient may have a history of antecedent minor trauma, insect bites, or exposure to other infected children. The lesions are usually relatively asymptomatic, but occasionally pruritus is a prominent feature.
   b. Objective findings
      (1) Nonbullous impetigo. Multiple lesions, most numerous on the face and extremities, are characterized by a thick, adherent, yellowish-brown crust. Involved areas spread centrifugally and coalesce into large, irregularly shaped lesions with no tendency for central clearing. Regional lymphadenopathy is common.
      (2) Bullous impetigo (see **A.1**)
4. Treatment
   a. Minimal disease. Local cool water soaks can be used to remove crusts. The area is washed with Betadine or Hibiclens, and a topical antibiotic (mupirocin, Bacitracin, or Ilotycin) is applied two to three times a day. However, if the lesions do not resolve quickly with topical care, systemic antibiotic therapy is indicated.
   b. Moderate or extensive disease. Mupirocin, cephalexin, dicloxacillin, or erythromycin (see Tables 14-1 and 14-2) usually is effective therapy. Although impetigo is often caused by penicillin-sensitive organisms, the presence of *Staph. aureus* is common enough to justify empiric anti-staphylococcal therapy.

G. Infestations
   1. Scabies
      a. Etiology. Scabies is caused by infestation with the mite, *Sarcoptes scabiei*. Transmission is usually by direct personal contact; however, fomite transmission (bedclothes, towels) is possible.
      b. Evaluation. Put a drop of oil on a suspected burrow and on a glass slide. Scrape the top from a burrow tract with a No. 15 blade. Place the scraping in the oil on the slide, cover with a cover slip, and examine under low power for adult mites, ova, and feces.
      c. Diagnosis
         (1) Subjective findings include intense pruritus of patients and persons with whom they are in contact. Incubation time for first infection after contact is a minimum of 3 weeks.
         (2) Objective findings. The most frequent areas involved are the interdigital webs of the fingers, hypothenar eminences, volar surface of the wrist, elbows, periareolar skin, anterior axillary folds, intergluteal fold, penis, scrotum, and, in infants, palms, soles, head, and neck.
            (a) A fresh burrow is a 2-mm flesh-colored, linear papule with a black dot at one end.
            (b) On the genitalia, lesions are firm, 0.5-cm red nodules.
            (c) Lesions in infants are often pustular, especially on palms, soles, and scalp.
            (d) A generalized dry, red, scaly rash may accompany infestation, obscuring burrows.
      d. Therapy
         (1) For nonpregnant women, children, and adults without severely excoriated skin, apply a scabicide lotion, 1% gamma benzene hexachloride (Kwell), to affected skin for 12 hours. Rinse off. Reapply once 7 days later in the same way.
         (2) Wash bedclothes, towels, and clothes in hot water, dry clean, or isolate them daily between the two treatments.
         (3) Treat close contacts.
         (4) Antihistamines are indicated for intense pruritus.
         (5) For severely excoriated skin, use compresses to dry out the lesions, then treat as in **(1)** above.

(6) For female infants and pregnant women, use 6–10% precipitated sulfur applied at night for 3 successive nights.

2. Pediculosis

a. Etiology. Pediculosis is caused by *Pediculus humanus,* the body louse, or *Phthirus pubis,* the pubic "crab" louse, or both. *P. humanus capitis* is transmitted via hats, combs, hairbrushes, and the backs of theater seats; *P. humanus corporis* transmission is via shared clothing and bedding. Although *P. pubis* transmission is most commonly through sexual contact, infestation is possible via clothing, bedding, and towels.

b. Evaluation. Look for the lice.

c. Diagnosis

(1) Subjective findings include intractable pruritus and positive history of close contacts.

(2) Objective findings

(a) Pediculosis capitis. Oval egg capsules (nits) appear along the hair shafts as highlights that are fixed in position and do not brush away easily. Adult lice are seen on the scalp. Purulence and matting of the hair often occur over the occiput and nape of the neck. Occipital and posterior cervical adenitis may be present.

(b) Pediculosis corporis. Excoriated papules, parallel linear excoriations, and, in chronic cases, scaling, lichenification, and hyperpigmentation are seen across the shoulders, in the interscapular area, and around the waist. The initial lesion is a red pinpoint macule. After 7–10 days, the time required for sensitization to the louse salivary antigens, the bites become urticarial and papular. Lice and ova are found in the seams of clothing.

(c) Pediculosis pubis. Pruritus usually dominates the clinical picture, but there may be no symptoms. The yellow, translucent, 1- to 3-mm adult louse is seen on close examination of the skin. Oval egg capsules (nits) are firmly attached to hair shafts 1–2 cm above the skin surface. Reddish-brown, particulate accumulations of excreted heme pigment, deposited on the skin about hair shafts, are the most apparent clinical sign. Discrete, round, bluish-gray macules (maculae caeruleae), measuring 0.5–1.5 cm in diameter, are occasionally seen on the lower abdomen and inguinal areas.

d. Therapy

(1) Apply pediculicidal agent (pyrithrin) to affected area for 12 hours. Rinse off. Repeat once, 8 days after first application. Gamma benzene hexachloride (Kwell) can be used in the same manner, but has more reported toxicity.

(2) If eyebrows and eyelashes are involved, petrolatum should be applied until the infestation is eliminated.

(3) If secondary bacterial infection is prominent, prescribe an appropriate antibiotic directed against gram-positive organisms (see Table 14-1).

(4) Wash towels, bedclothes, caps, and head scarves in hot water.

(5) Treatment of family members and close contacts is indicated.

(6) Although topical agents kill adult lice and nits, the nits do not fall off the hairs spontaneously. Applications of a 1 : 1 solution of white vinegar and water, followed by a shower, will help dissolve the nits cemented to the hairs and wash off their remains.

H. Pneumonia

1. Etiology

a. Neonates. Gram-positive cocci, particularly group B streptococcus and occasionally *Staph. aureus,* and gram-negative enteric bacilli cause most neonatal bacterial pneumonias.

b. Children 1 month–5 years of age. Respiratory viruses cause the majority of pediatric pneumonias. *Chlamydia trachomatis* causes an afebrile pneumonia in infants under 16 weeks of age, in whom a history of conjunctivitis is present in 50 percent, eosinophilia is common, and the chest x-ray shows hyperinflation and diffuse interstitial or patchy infiltrates. The major bacterial pathogens in this age group are *Strep. pneumoniae* and *H. influenzae* type B. Pneumococci commonly cause lobar or segmental consolidation, but bronchopneumonia is not infrequent. *H. influenzae* type B can mimic pneumonia caused by a number of organisms and is not infrequently associated with extrapulmonary infection. *Staph. aureus* is suggested by rapidly evolving respiratory distress, empyema, and the characteristic radiologic features of rapid progression, lobular ectasia, and pneumatoceles in a child less than 3 years old. Even in an extremely ill child, however, the initial x-ray film may demonstrate only faint local mottling.

   c. **Children 5 years of age and older.** The pneumococcus is the major cause of bacterial pneumonia in this age group. *M. pneumoniae* is a common cause of pneumonia in school-aged children, adolescents, and young adults.

   d. **Immunocompromised hosts** are subject to pneumonia caused by any organism, but gram-negative organisms, *P. carinii,* cytomegalovirus, and fungi are frequently found in pneumonia in these patients.

   e. **Anaerobic bacteria,** especially penicillin-sensitive oral anaerobes, may cause pneumonia and lung abscess in patients who aspirate.

   f. After viral infections, *Staph. aureus,* group A. streptococcus, and *Strep. pneumoniae* may cause bacterial pneumonia. Group A streptococcal pneumonia may occur in children without prior illness and usually has a sudden onset, with high fever, chills, dyspnea, and pleuritic pain. Bacteremia and a serosanguineous pleural effusion are often associated.

   g. **Tuberculosis** should always be considered as a possible cause of infectious pneumonia, especially in the child who responds slowly or not at all to antibiotic therapy.

2. Evaluation
   a. Chest x-ray (posteroanterior and lateral)
   b. Tuberculin skin test
   c. Sputum or deep tracheal aspirate for Gram stain and culture. Cultures for bacteria from the nasopharynx should be interpreted with great caution.
   d. Cultures for respiratory viruses (which are rarely found in asymptomatic persons) and fluorescent antibody techniques for rapid diagnosis of certain viruses (e.g., respiratory syncytial virus) are now more widely available.
   e. Blood culture(s) in the patient who appears toxic
   f. A diagnostic thoracentesis if pleural fluid is present
   g. Serologic titers (acute and convalescent) are not very satisfactory for most pathogens, but for *Mycoplasma* (cold agglutinin titer $> 1 : 64$, or complement fixation titers), group A streptococcus (antistreptolysin O titer), *Chlamydia, Legionella,* and *Rickettsia* (Q fever) may be the most useful means to make a presumptive diagnosis.
   h. Rapid diagnostic techniques for detecting bacterial antigens in body fluids
   i. Bronchoscopy with bronchoalveolar lavage and protected brush biopsy or open lung biopsy in critically ill children to establish the etiologic diagnosis to guide antimicrobial therapy
   j. Leukocyte and differential counts are occasionally helpful, but, in general, should not be relied on to distinguish bacterial from other causes.

3. The **diagnosis** is usually established by the chest x-ray and physical signs of consolidation. An etiologic diagnosis is usually made from the clinical features described, the cultures, antigen detection studies, and, in the case of a few organisms, by serology.

4. Therapy
   a. **Antibiotics**
      (1) Children who are mildly ill with features suggestive of viral disease can be managed without antibiotics, provided the patient can be followed closely.

(2) Infants and hospitalized patients should receive antibiotics when pneumonia is diagnosed.

(3) The choice of specific antibiotics is based on interpretation of available gram-stained specimens, the patient's age, and other suggestive clinical features.

(4) Specific recommendations before etiologic diagnosis

(a) Neonates should receive both a penicillinase-resistant penicillin and an aminoglycoside IV.

(b) The toxic, hospitalized child aged 1 month–5 years should be treated with both a penicillinase-resistant penicillin (200 mg/kg/day q4h) and chloramphenicol (75 mg/kg/day q6h). Alternatively, a second- or third-generation cephalosporin or ampicillin-sulbactam will provide appropriate empiric coverage.

(c) The nontoxic child aged 1 month–5 years should be given an antibiotic that is effective against both *Strep. pneumoniae* and *H. influenzae* type B, such as amoxicillin. Trimethoprim-sulfamethoxazole is an alternative and also provides staphylococcal and ampicillin-resistant *H. influenzae* coverage. If the clinical syndrome clearly suggests *Chlamydia*, erythromycin (30–50 mg/kg/day q6h) should be administered.

(d) In the older child, suspected *Mycoplasma* pneumonia is treated with oral erythromycin (30–50 mg/kg/day in four daily doses for 10 days).

(e) Identification of the pathogen or failure to respond to these regimens necessitates reevaluation of the choice of antibiotics.

(f) The **duration** of antimicrobial therapy is based on the individual patient's clinical response, but, in general, staphylococcal pneumonia requires 3 weeks of parenteral therapy followed by 1–3 weeks of oral therapy. *H. influenzae* and streptococcal pneumonia usually respond to 1–2 weeks of therapy, and pneumococcal pneumonia will resolve with only 7 days of therapy.

b. Indications for hospitalization include the following: significant respiratory distress or toxicity, cyanosis, age under 6 months, empyema or pleural effusion, possible staphylococcal pneumonia, and inadequate home care.

c. In the case of empyema, **drainage** by repeated aspiration or insertion of a chest tube may be necessary. (Loculated pleural fluid may explain persistent fever in the face of seemingly adequate antibiotic therapy.)

d. Symptomatic care should include oxygen, maintenance of adequate hydration, high humidity (such as the use of a humidifier in the home), bronchodilators if bronchospasm is present, and deep tracheal suction in patients with an ineffectual cough.

e. Postural drainage and **physiotherapy** may be helpful, particularly with underlying bronchiectasis.

f. Initial follow-up of the ambulatory patient should be on a day-to-day basis until definite clinical improvement has occurred.

g. Although radiologic resolution may lag behind clinical improvement, persistence of radiologic abnormalities without improvement for more than 4–6 weeks should alert the physician to possible underlying pulmonary disease (e.g., tuberculosis, foreign body, cystic fibrosis).

I. Infections of the central nervous system

1. Meningitis

a. Etiology. Meningitis is a complication of bacteremia. *H. influenzae* type B (60–65%), meningococci, and pneumococci account for most cases of acute bacterial meningitis in children over 2 months of age. Infrequently involved organisms are streptococci, *Staph. aureus*, and gram-negative enteric bacteria, except in neonatal meningitis. Since the introduction of protein-conjugated *H. influenzae* type B vaccines, the incidence of meningitis has dropped dramatically.

b. Evaluation

(1) In infants, the **presenting symptoms and signs** are nonspecific and include a high-pitched cry, irritability, anorexia, vomiting, lethargy, and/or a full fontanel. Meningeal signs are uncommon, and fever is not invariably present. The closest attention must be paid to alterations in consciousness if an early diagnosis is to be made. Convulsions may be an early manifestation of meningitis. Thus, convulsions associated with fever in infancy are generally an indication for CSF examination.

(2) In older children, meningeal signs are more reliable. Brudzinski's sign (flexion of the neck with the patient supine causes involuntary flexion of the hips) can be helpful in determining the need for lumbar puncture (LP).

(3) Patients with evidence of bacteremia should be carefully assessed for meningitis.

(4) An **LP** should be performed as soon as the diagnosis is suspected. **Before** the LP is performed, a blood glucose level should be obtained for comparison with the CSF glucose.

(5) **Papilledema is a relative contraindication to LP,** and, if it is present, a neurosurgical consultation should be considered before proceeding. (Papilledema is rare in **acute** bacterial meningitis, and its presence may suggest other diagnostic possibilities, e.g., brain abscess.)

(6) Other diagnostic procedures include blood culture, smears and cultures from any purpuric lesions, cultures of other body fluids (e.g., stool, urine, joint, abscess, middle ear), blood urea nitrogen (BUN), serum and urine electrolytes and osmolarity, chest x-ray, and tuberculin test. In infants the head circumference should be carefully measured.

c. The **diagnosis** can be established only by LP.

(1) In bacterial meningitis the CSF is characteristically cloudy and under increased pressure, usually with > 100 white blood cells (WBC)/mm^2, predominantly neutrophils, elevated total protein, low glucose (less than one half of the pre-LP blood glucose concentration), and organisms in the CSF gram-stained smear. However, some of these findings are often absent, and any of these abnormalities must be viewed with suspicion, particularly the presence of **any** neutrophils. The CSF culture usually confirms the diagnosis.

(2) Rapid etiologic diagnosis of bacterial meningitis may be possible by using methods to detect capsular polysaccharide antigens.

d. Therapy. IV antibiotic therapy should be initiated immediately after bacteriology specimens have been obtained. The initial choice of antibiotics usually is based on the gram-stained smear of CSF and the patient's age. Dexamethasone therapy should be considered for infants and children 2 months and older with strong evidence for bacterial meningitis. Dexamethasone therapy probably reduces the risk of hearing impairment following *H. influenzae* type B meningitis.

(1) In children over 2 months of age in whom there is no reason to suspect an unusual organism, either ampicillin (300–400 mg/kg/day q6h) and chloramphenicol (100 mg/kg/day q6h), or cefotaxime (150 mg/kg/day q8h) or ceftriaxone (75–100 mg/kg/day q12–24h), are equally acceptable. If *H. influenzae* is recovered, and sensitivity is confirmed in vitro, ampicillin can be used to complete therapy. If the culture discloses meningococci or pneumococci, penicillin G is the drug of choice. Alternative therapy with a third-generation cephalosporin is reasonable. We still favor the ampicillin-chloramphenicol combination because of its established record of safety and efficacy. Additionally, no regimen has proved superior.

(2) **Infants less than 2 months old** (see Chap. 6, p. 181ff)

(3) The duration of therapy depends on the infant's clinical course, but antibiotics should generally be administered 7–10 days for *H. influenzae*, 5–7 days for meningococcus, and 10–14 days for pneumococcal meningitis.

(4) Other aspects of management

(a) If indicated, dexamethasone should be administered with or immediately after the initial dose of antibiotics. The regimen is 0.6 mg/kg/day given q6h IV for the first 4 days of therapy.

(b) All patients should be carefully evaluated for evidence of hypotension, abnormal bleeding, and the syndrome of inappropriate secretion of antidiuretic hormone (SIADH), which usually occurs within the first 72 hours of therapy. Although fluids should generally be restricted to three-quarters maintenance until it is documented that SIADH is absent, it is very important to avoid dehydration. As most patients presenting with meningitis have been ill and febrile for 12–24 hours before diagnosis, they are typically dehydrated on admission. Rehydration to restore a euvolemic state should precede any fluid restriction. Maintenance of blood pressure and cerebral perfusion pressure takes priority over SIADH prophylaxis.

(c) During treatment, frequent observation of vital signs and daily neurologic examinations, measurement of head circumference, and transillumination of the head (if the fontanel is open) should be performed.

(d) LP should be repeated after 24–48 hours of therapy only in patients whose disease is severe or who respond poorly to treatment. Cultures and stains are usually negative after 24–48 hours if treatment is effective.

(e) Fever during therapy most commonly results from phlebitis, drugs, nosocomial infection, subdural effusion (which may occur in up to 50% of infants and children during the acute illness, usually without producing symptoms or fever), or coexisting viral infection. Unless an obvious cause is found, prolonged (greater than 7 days) or secondary fever during therapy should prompt a repeat CSF examination and a search for localized infection in the subdural space, bones, joints, pericardium, or pleural spaces. Computed tomography is useful to document subdural effusions, but we do not routinely perform scans on all patients.

(f) Because relapse of bacterial meningitis rarely occurs within the first 3 days following completion of antibiotic therapy, we do not routinely repeat LP or observe patients in the hospital after completion of therapy. In addition, selected children with uncomplicated cases of bacterial meningitis can finish therapy with oral chloramphenicol (same dose as IV; check levels) or ceftriaxone, 50–75 mg/kg q24h, given IM once a day.

(g) Close household and day care center contacts of children with meningitis are at increased risk of secondary disease caused by *H. influenzae* type B (for household contacts < 6 years, the risk is about 0.5%) and *N. meningitidis* (for all persons, the risk is about 0.5%). Close observation is mandatory, and prophylaxis should be considered for persons at risk.

(h) Currently, it is recommended that all children with invasive disease due to *H. influenzae* type B receive rifampin therapy (once a day for 4 days in a 20 mg/kg dose; maximum dose, 600 mg/day) before discharge to eradicate carriage from the nasopharynx (*Red Book*, American Academy of Pediatrics, 1991).

2. For a discussion of **neonatal meningitis**, see Chap. 6, p. 181ff.

3. Brain abscess. Normal brain tissue is resistant to bacterial infection.

However, ischemic brain injury (e.g., cyanotic heart disease), parameningeal infection (sinusitis, mastoiditis, skull osteomyelitis), and skull trauma increase the risk of brain abscess.

a. Etiology. Causative bacteria are usually derived from the upper airway or mouth. Mixtures of aerobes (streptococci, *Staph. aureus*, diphtheroids, *Haemophilus*) and anaerobes (*Peptococcus, Bacteroides*) are common. Unusual agents are occasionally responsible, especially in immunocompromised patients.

b. Evaluation. Brain abscess must be considered in patients with evidence of a rapidly progressive intracranial mass.

(1) The **history** should focus on possible predisposing causes. Headache and seizures are common. Fever is seldom prominent.

(2) In the **physical examination,** attempts should be made to uncover extracranial infection and localize the neurologic lesion. An assessment should be made for elevated intracranial pressure (ICP).

(3) Laboratory examination includes blood cultures and a CT scan and may require skull x-rays and an electroencephalogram (EEG). **CSF examination should be avoided in patients with increased ICP.** It seldom adds to the evaluation (CSF changes are neither universally present nor pathognomonic for brain abscess). Leukocytosis may or may not be present.

c. The **diagnosis** is made by confirmation of an intracranial mass by CT scan. Even small abscesses can be localized by skilled personnel and generally make an arteriogram unnecessary.

d. Therapy

(1) Classically, treatment for cure of brain abscess has been surgical excision or drainage. Although surgical drainage is still an option, many cases can be managed medically with antibiotic therapy, ideally following aspiration for culture. Careful monitoring by CT scan and neurologic examination is necessary to assess the efficacy of empiric therapy in this setting.

(2) Initial empiric antibiotic therapy usually includes chloramphenicol (100 mg/kg/day IV q6h) and penicillin (300,000 U/kg/day IV q4h). This can be modified after bacteriologic evaluation of the abscess contents.

(3) To reduce brain swelling, fluids should be restricted moderately to keep the patient "dry." Hyperosmotic agents, such as mannitol, and dexamethasone may also help to reduce cerebral edema (see Chap. 3, p. 71ff).

(4) Follow-up CT scans are used to monitor resolution of the abscess and to help determine the duration of antibiotic therapy.

(5) Parameningeal foci of infection responsible for brain abscess may also require surgical drainage (sinus, mastoid).

J. Gastrointestinal infections: Bacterial gastroenteritis. See Chap. 10 for viral and Chap. 15 for parasitic infections.

1. Etiology

a. Bacterial agents cause diarrhea less frequently than do viruses. The principal bacterial agents in the United States are *Salmonella, Shigella,* and in some areas, *Campylobacter fetus* subspecies *jejuni.* Other agents include *Yersinia enterocolitica, Aeromonas hydrophila,* and *Vibrio parahaemolyticus* (which causes shellfish poisoning). Enteropathogenic *E. coli* (EPEC) organisms are uncommon in the United States.

b. Traveler's diarrhea, a self-limited disease that lasts for several days, is usually caused by enterotoxigenic *E. coli* (ETEC), although *Shigella* and *Salmonella,* other bacteria, viruses, and *Giardia* have been implicated.

c. Pseudomembranous colitis (antibiotic-associated colitis) is caused by *C. difficile* toxin, produced as the organism overgrows the residual gut flora of antibiotic-treated patients.

d. Food poisoning can be caused by several bacteria (usually toxin producing), including staphylococci, *Clostridium perfringens, Clostridium botulinum* (botulism), *V. parahaemolyticus,* and *Bacillus cereus.*

2. **Evaluation** includes an epidemiologic history, assessment of the character and duration of the abnormal stools, and careful assessment of the patient's state of hydration.

   a. The demonstration of sheets of fecal leukocytes in diarrheal stools is well correlated with inflammatory (usually bacterial) disease.

   b. Indications for stool cultures are bloody stools, toxicity, severe diarrhea, chronic disease or impaired host defenses, and epidemic diarrhea (see Chap. 10, p. 274ff).

   c. In hospitalized patients with fever and diarrhea, one or more blood cultures should be taken.

3. **Diagnosis**

   a. Stool cultures handled routinely will identify only *Salmonella* and *Shigella.* If *Campylobacter, Yersinia,* or *Vibrio* is suspected, the laboratory should be alerted. **Toxin-producing** *E. coli* (ETEC) is reliably identified only by special assay for enterotoxin. The toxin of *C. difficile* can be identified directly in stool samples from patients with pseudomembranous colitis.

   b. For *Yersinia,* a fourfold rise in serologic titer is diagnostic.

   c. In **food poisoning** the contaminating organism can be inferred from the incubation period (time from ingestion to onset of symptoms)—for *Staph. aureus,* 3–6 hours, but as early as 30 minutes; for *C. perfringens,* 1–25 hours, usually 8–12 hours; and for *Salmonella,* 12–18 hours, up to 72 hours—or from careful epidemiologic history and the physical signs as with botulism.

4. **Therapy and prevention.** Therapy is directed primarily toward fluid and electrolyte management.

   a. *Salmonella.* Because antibiotics may prolong the carrier state, most patients with *Salmonella* in the stool are not treated.

      (1) **Indications for treatment** are infection in young infants, impaired host defenses, sickle cell anemia, chronic inflammatory bowel disease, severe toxicity, and enteritis with bacteremia if fever and toxicity persist by the time the positive blood culture is obtained.

      (2) Serious *Salmonella* infections can be treated with ampicillin (100 mg/kg/day), chloramphenicol (50–100 mg/kg/day), or TMP-SMZ (10 mg TMP/kg/day). Ciprofloxacin may be effective for multiple resistant organisms but is rarely used in pediatrics.

   b. *Shigella sonnei* are likely to be resistant to ampicillin. Thus, TMP-SMZ (10 mg TMP/kg/day q12h for 5 days) should be given when *Shigella* is isolated before susceptibility is known. Susceptible strains can be treated with ampicillin (100 mg/kg/day q6h for 5 days). Amoxicillin is ineffective, and antidiarrheal drugs may prolong the course of disease.

   c. Enteritis caused by *Campylobacter* can be successfully treated with erythromycin (40 mg/kg/day PO q6h for 5–7 days) if symptoms have not resolved by the time the culture result is available.

   d. **Traveler's diarrhea**

      (1) Drinking only boiled or carbonated water or other processed beverages and avoiding unpeeled fruits, salads, and ice may prevent infection.

      (2) Several drugs, including doxycycline, bismuth subsalicylate, and TMP-SMZ may help prevent infection. Because the disease is usually self-limited, no specific prophylactic therapy is generally recommended.

   e. **Pseudomembranous colitis** is treated by withdrawal of the implicated antibiotic (may be a penicillin or cephalosporin as well as clindamycin) and institution of oral vancomycin (40 mg/kg/day in four divided doses) or oral metronidazole (35 mg/kg/day in four divided doses) when the presence of *C. difficile* toxin in the stool has been confirmed. Vancomycin or metronidazole therapy should be continued for 7–10 days or until follow-up stools are negative for toxin.

K. Genitourinary infections

1. Urinary tract infections

a. **Etiology.** First infections are most commonly caused by *E. coli.* Other pathogens include *Proteus, Klebsiella, Pseudomonas, Streptococcus faecalis, S. saprophyticus,* and *Staph. aureus.*

b. **Evaluation and diagnosis.** Clinical manifestations of UTI vary with age. UTI must be considered in any acutely ill or nonthriving infant.

(1) **Pyelonephritis** is suggested by high fever, toxicity, flank pain, and costovertebral angle tenderness and is commonly associated with ureteral reflux. **Cystitis** is associated with suprapubic pain, dysuria, frequency, urgency, and enuresis. Localization of the site of infection may be very difficult, especially in young children.

(2) At any age, UTI may be asymptomatic (asymptomatic bacteriuria) and persist without treatment, seldom becoming overtly symptomatic. Up to two thirds of preschool and school-aged girls may be symptom free with their first UTI.

(3) **Physical examination** should include blood pressure measurement, a search for congenital malformations, and a careful examination of the abdomen, genitalia, and perineum.

(4) **Laboratory studies**

(a) **Urine microscopy** can provide an accurate provisional diagnosis of UTI if used to quantitate the concentration of bacteria in a fresh, clean sample: One or more bacteria per oil field in gram-stained, **uncentrifuged** urine is equivalent to 105 colonies/ml. The presence of numerous bacteria per high-power field in the centrifuged urine sediment does not necessarily indicate infection.

(b) Pyuria is not specific for bacterial infection but is usually present in UTI. Proteinuria and gross hematuria are uncommon with UTI. Microscopic hematuria is common.

(c) Urine culture provides proof of infection, but its value in young children is reduced by specimen collection errors.

(i) Infected urine will contain > 105 colonies/ml (except in some neonates, in whom > 104 colonies may indicate infection). Negative cultures of voided samples are of value in ruling out infection.

(ii) Repetition of cultures increases diagnostic precision in all age groups. A single midstream, clean-catch specimen will accurately predict the presence of UTI 80 percent of the time; two consecutive positive cultures increase the accuracy to 95 percent.

(iii) Diagnostic precision is greatest with urine obtained by suprapubic bladder aspiration, for which any growth of bacteria should be considered significant, or sterile catheterization, for which > 104 colonies/ml are significant. In skilled hands, both procedures are safe. They are most appropriately used to resolve urgent or difficult diagnostic problems in younger children and are preferred over "bagged" urine specimens for culture in any infant who will be started on antibiotic therapy before culture results are available.

(iv) Note that contamination of samples may provide > 105 colonies/ml of a single species. More typically, contaminated cultures contain several species in concentrations < 105 colonies/ml. Urine specimens should be refrigerated at 4°C and cultured promptly to avoid growth of contaminants.

(d) A **blood culture** should be obtained in patients with pyelonephritis and in neonates or young infants with UTI.

(e) We prefer to study all patients with well-documented UTI approximately 3 weeks after the infection with a voiding cystourethrogram and renal ultrasound.

(f) Contributing factors to recurrent infections include poor perineal hygiene, vulvovaginitis, pinworm infestations, constipation, and vesicoureteral reflux.

c. **Therapy**

(1) Most initial and uncomplicated UTIs respond to oral sulfonamides such as sulfisoxazole (120–150 mg/kg/day PO qid). Effective alternatives are amoxicillin (25 mg/kg/day PO tid), TMP-SMZ (8 mg/kg/day trimethoprim PO bid), cefixime (8 mg/kg/day PO qd), and nitrofurantoin (5 mg/kg/day PO qid). The usual duration of therapy is 10 days.

(2) Children with **pyelonephritis** require parenteral antibiotics, hydration, and hospitalization. Ampicillin (100–200 mg/kg/day q6h IV) is effective against many urinary tract pathogens, but is generally combined with sulbactam or an aminoglycoside for initial therapy of suspected pyelonephritis. Alternatively, aztreonam, a second- or third-generation cephalosporin, or parenteral TMP-SMZ can be used. A previous history of pyelonephritis or infection with a resistant organism indicates the need for broad-spectrum coverage. The recommended duration of therapy is usually 10–14 days, but clinical improvement should be evident within 48–72 hours. Once the patient is afebrile and has a sterile repeat urine culture, therapy can be switched to oral antibiotics.

(3) Infants, especially newborns, with UTI should have prompt urologic evaluation as well as aggressive antibiotic treatment.

(4) Ongoing antimicrobial therapy is based on the clinical response of the patient and the results of subsequent urine cultures.

(a) A culture should be obtained 24–48 hours after therapy has been initiated, and at this time the urine should be sterile.

(b) A Gram stain of the unspun specimen should not show organisms, and the sediment should be clear of leukocytes 24–48 hours after therapy.

(c) Adequate clinical responses may be seen despite in vitro resistance of the organism isolated, because of the high concentrations of antimicrobials in the urine (see sec. **I.B.4.b**).

(d) Failure to respond should increase suspicion of an underlying anatomic abnormality or abscess.

(5) Adequate **hydration** of the patient is important.

(6) Continuous bladder drainage by an indwelling catheter should be done only when absolutely necessary and discontinued at the earliest possible time; a **closed drainage system is mandatory.** On removal of the catheter, a urine culture should be obtained.

d. **Follow-up** of a UTI should be carefully organized, because infection tends to recur, often in asymptomatic form. Recurrence is most likely during the first 6–12 months after an infection.

(1) After therapy is discontinued, urine cultures are indicated 1 week later, every month during the subsequent 3 months, every 3 months during the next 6 months, and then twice a year.

(2) Among patients with **significant vesicoureteral reflux,** recurrent infection is prevented by prophylactic antibiotic therapy, which is continued until reflux resolves or is repaired.

(3) Some normal girls experience **multiple recurrences** of UTI. They should be carefully assessed for correctable contributing factors. When infections are frequent, socially distressing, or associated with renal scarring, prophylactic antibiotic therapy is often prescribed for 6–12 months. TMP-SMZ (2 mg TMP/kg/day PO in one dose) or nitrofurantoin (2 mg/kg/day in one dose) can be used.

(4) Home screening can improve the follow-up of UTI, using simple,

inexpensive tests such as the nitrate chemical test for bacteria and agar-coated dip slides.

2. **Gonorrhea.** The infecting organism is *N. gonorrhoeae.* The disease is seen with increasing frequency in children under 12 years of age.
   a. **Evaluation**
      (1) In males, urethral specimens can be obtained by "stripping" the penis.
      (2) In females, pelvic examination allows the physician to evaluate cervical and adnexal tenderness as well as obtain culture material from the cervix. In prepubertal girls, gonococcal infection may present as purulent vulvovaginitis rather than cervicitis.
      (3) In both males and females, the rectum and pharynx should be cultured for *N. gonorrhoeae.*
      (4) *N. gonorrhoeae* is relatively fastidious, and specimens should be cultured promptly and placed in a high CO_2 atmosphere (e.g., candle-jar) or in a special packet with a CO_2 generating pellet. Transgrow medium is an excellent transport medium for *N. gonorrhoeae* and should be used when direct cultures are not practical.
      (5) **A serologic test for syphilis should be performed in all patients with gonorrhea** (see **4.a**) and repeated 2 months after treatment if an agent other than penicillin is used. Coexisting sexually transmitted diseases such as *Chlamydia* infection should be considered.
   b. **Diagnosis.** *N. gonorrhoeae* is identified by demonstration of gram-negative diplococci on gram-stained smears of urethral discharge or by culture of appropriate specimens on Thayer-Martin media. Smears of cervical mucus are not reliable.
   c. **Treatment.** Treatment is outlined in Table 14-9. Case contact finding, as well as sex education and counseling, is as important as the drug therapy. Child abuse must be investigated in cases involving young children.
      (1) Patients should abstain from sexual relations for 7 days and return for repeat cultures 7–14 days after treatment.
      (2) Contacts of the patient should be cultured and treated.

3. **Pelvic inflammatory disease (PID)**
   a. **Etiology.** *N. gonorrhoeae* can be cultured from the cervix in about 50 percent of cases of PID. Pathogens that cause nongonococcal PID include *C. trachomatis,* gram-positive and gram-negative anaerobes, gram-negative aerobic bacilli, *Mycoplasma hominis,* and *Actinomyces israelii.*
   b. **Evaluation**
      (1) A **history** of acute lower abdominal pain with vaginal discharge, fever, and chills suggests the diagnosis. The menstrual period is often a precipitating factor.
      (2) **Pelvic findings** include pain on cervical motion, adnexal tenderness, and sometimes a mass.
      (3) **Laboratory abnormalities** include a normal to elevated WBC count and an elevated erythrocyte sedimentation rate (ESR) (75–85%). Culture of the endocervix and rectum or pharynx for *N. gonorrhoeae* and *Chlamydia*—and intraoperative cultures if surgical drainage is required—should be obtained.
      (4) **Ultrasound** examination may help to delineate the extent and foci of infection within the pelvis.
      (5) **Laparoscopy** is occasionally necessary to establish the diagnosis.
   c. **Diagnosis**
      (1) Gram stain of cervical drainage may or may not reveal gram-negative intracellular diplococci; nevertheless, the diagnosis must be confirmed by culture.
      (2) When cultures for *N. gonorrhoeae* are negative and the response to therapy for gonococcal PID is poor, the diagnosis of nongonococcal PID becomes more likely.

Table 14-9. Recommended treatment schedules for gonococcal infections

Type	Drugs of choice	Dosage	Alternatives
Urethritis/cervicitis or anal — women	Amoxicillin *plus* probenecid, followed by tetracycline HCl	3 gm PO once 1 gm PO once 500 mg PO × 7 days	Penicillin G procaine, 4.8 million U IM[a] once, *plus* probenecid, 1 gm PO once Spectinomycin, 2 gm IM once Cefoxitin, 2 gm, *or* cefuroxime, 1.5 gm, IM once Cefotaxime, 1 gm IM once, *or* ceftriaxone, 250 mg IM once
Anal — men	Penicillin G procaine *plus* probenecid	As for urethritis	Spectinomycin, 2 gm IM once Ceftriaxone, 250 mg IM
Pharyngeal	Tetracycline HCl[b] *or* penicillin G procaine *plus* probenecid	As for urethritis As for urethritis	Trimethoprim-sulfamethoxazole, 9 tablets[c] PO qd for 5 days, *or* ceftriaxone, 250 mg IM
Pelvic inflammatory disease	See text, sec. **IV.K.3.**		
Ophthalmia (adults)	Penicillin G crystalline *plus* saline irrigation	10 million U IV daily for 5 days	Cefoxitin, 1 gm, *or* ceftriaxone, 1 gm IM qd, *or* cefotaxime, 500 mg, IV qid for 5 days *plus* saline irrigation
Bacteremia and arthritis	Penicillin G crystalline followed by amoxicillin	10 million U IV daily for 3 days 500 mg/PO qid for 4 days	Tetracycline, 500 mg PO qid[b] for 7 days Erythromycin, 500 mg PO qid for 7 days Cefotaxime, 500 mg, *or* cefoxitin, 1 gm, IV qid for 7 days Ceftriaxone, 1 gm IM qd for 7 days

Table 14-9. (continued)

Type	Drugs of choice	Dosage	Alternatives
Meningitis	Penicillin G crystalline	At least 10 million U IV daily for at least 10 days	Cefotaxime, 2 gm IV q4h for at least 10 days Ceftriaxone, 1 gm IM qd for 10 days
Endocarditis	Penicillin G crystalline	At least 10 million U IV daily for at least 3 to 4 weeks	
Neonatal			
Ophthalmia	Penicillin G crystalline *plus* saline irrigation	50,000 U/kg/day IV in 2 doses for 7 days	
Arthritis and septicemia	Penicillin G crystalline	75,000–100,000 U/kg/day IV in 4 doses for 7 days	
Meningitis	Penicillin G crystalline	100,000 U/kg/day IV in 3 or 4 doses for at least 10 days	
Children (<45 kg)—urogenital, anal, and pharyngeal	Amoxicillin *plus* probenecid, *or* penicillin G procaine *plus* probenecid	50 mg/kg PO once 25 mg/kg (max. 1 gm) once 100,000 U/kg IM once 25 mg/kg (max. 1 gm) once	Ceftriaxone, 125 mg IM
Arthritis	Penicillin G crystalline	150,000 U/kg/day IV for 7 days	Ceftriaxone, 125 mg IM
Meningitis	Penicillin G crystalline	250,000 U/kg/day IV in 6 divided doses for at least 10 days	Ceftriaxone, 125 mg IM

[a] Divided into two injections at one visit. [b] Or doxycycline, 100 mg PO bid. [c] Each tablet contains trimethoprim, 80 mg, and sulfamethoxazole, 400 mg.
Source: Modified from *Med. Lett. Drug Ther.* 26:5, 1984.

(3) Differential considerations include: acute appendicitis, ectopic pregnancy, ruptured ovarian cyst, ovarian abscess, and endometriosis.

d. Therapy

(1) **Indications for admission** to the hospital include toxicity, uncertain diagnosis, suspected pelvic abscess, signs of peritonitis, pregnancy, inability to take oral medications, failure of response to outpatient therapy, and poor follow-up arrangements.

(2) **Inpatient therapy** must be individualized, and surgical drainage may be necessary. Some regimens for PID follow.

(a) Cefoxitin, 2.0 gm IV qid, plus doxycycline, 100 mg IV bid. Continue for at least 4 days and at least 48 hours after the patient's condition improves. Then continue doxycycline, 100 mg PO bid, to complete 10–14 days total therapy.

(b) Clindamycin, 600 mg IV qid, plus gentamicin, 2 mg/kg IV, followed by 1.5 mg/kg tid, plus doxycycline, 100 mg IV bid. Continue IV drugs for at least 4 days and at least 48 hours after the patient's condition improves. Then continue doxycycline, 100 mg PO bid, to complete 10–14 days total therapy.

(3) **Outpatient therapy**

(a) Cefoxitin, 2 gm IM; amoxicillin, 3 gm PO; or ceftriaxone, 250 mg IM. Each of these regimens except ceftriaxone is accompanied by probenecid, 1 gm PO. Each regimen is followed by doxycycline, 100 mg PO bid for 10–14 days.

(b) Patients should be reevaluated in 48–72 hours; those who do not respond favorably should be hospitalized.

4. **Syphilis.** The infecting organism is *T. pallidum.*

a. **Evaluation and diagnosis** (see also Chap. 6)

(1) Dark-field examination of skin lesions (chancre or rash). The material is infectious and should be handled with care.

(2) Serologic tests for syphilis are usually nonreactive when the chancre first appears, but become reactive during the following 1–4 weeks. A biologic false-positive test with nonspecific antigens (VDRL, RPRCT, Wasserman, Hinton, Kolmer) may be caused by a variety of other illnesses and should be confirmed by tests specific for *T. pallidum* (FTA-ABS, TPI).

(3) **Congenital syphilis.** Although a positive serologic test for syphilis in the neonate may represent passively acquired maternal antibody, these infants should be treated if a definite history of adequate maternal treatment cannot be obtained.

b. **Therapy for syphilis** is outlined in Table 14-10. Case contact finding, as well as sex education and counseling, is as important as the drug therapy. Child abuse must be investigated in cases involving younger children.

5. **Toxic shock syndrome (TSS)**

a. **Etiology.** Toxic shock syndrome is a multisystem illness caused by a toxin produced by *Staph. aureus.*

b. **Evaluation.** The illness most often occurs in menstruating women, especially in women using tampons, but it has been seen in children of both sexes who have nonvaginal foci of infection.

(1) TSS typically begins suddenly with high fever, vomiting, and watery diarrhea and sometimes with sore throat, headache, and myalgias. Within 48 hours the disease may progress to hypotensive shock with the appearance of a diffuse scarlatiniform rash and nonpurulent conjunctivitis. The rash later desquamates. Alterations in consciousness may be present, and renal, cardiac, and pulmonary dysfunction may develop.

(2) Laboratory findings may include elevated BUN, creatinine, bilirubin, serum glutamic oxaloacetic transaminase (SGOT), and creatine phosphokinase (CPK). A leukocytosis with a left shift and a low to normal

Table 14-10. Recommended treatment schedules for syphilis

Stage	Drugs of choice	Dosage	Alternatives
Early (primary, secondary, or latent less than 1 year)	Penicillin G benzathine	2.4 million U IM once	Tetracycline HCl, 500 mg PO qid for 15 days Erythromycin, 500 mg PO qid for 15 days
Late (more than 1 year's duration, cardiovascular)	Penicillin G benzathine	2.4 million U IM weekly for 3 doses	Tetracycline HCl, 500 mg PO qid for 30 days Erythromycin, 500 mg PO qid for 30 days
Neurosyphilis	Penicillin G crystalline *or* Penicillin G procaine *or* Penicillin G benzathine	2 to 4 million U IV q4h for 10 days 2.4 million U IM qd *plus* probenecid, 500 mg PO qid, both for 10 days 2.4 million U IM weekly for 3 doses	Tetracycline HCl, 500 mg PO qid for 30 days Erythromycin, 500 mg PO qid for 30 days

Congenital
  CSF normal
  CSF abnormal
	Penicillin G benzathine
	Penicillin G crystalline
	or
	Penicillin G procaine
		50,000 U/kg IM once
		25,000 U/kg IM or IV bid for at least 10 days
		50,000 U/kg IM daily for at least 10 days	

Source: Modified from *Med. Lett. Drugs Ther.* 26:5, 1984.

platelet count are usually present. The urinalysis may reveal pyuria and proteinuria.

(3) Cultures of the blood (although bacteremia is not part of this syndrome), vagina, nasopharynx, anus, and any wound should be obtained in suspected cases.

c. The presumptive **diagnosis** can be established by recovery of *Staph. aureus* from a mucosal site in a patient with a clinically compatible illness.

d. **Therapy**

(1) Adequate volume replacement with colloid-containing fluids and blood pressure support with pressors may be required.

(2) Penicillinase-resistant penicillin therapy should be given parenterally (e.g., oxacillin, 200 mg/kg/day in divided doses q4h).

(3) Menstruating patients should be advised about the possible recurrence of TSS if tampons are used.

L. **Infections of the bones and joints**

1. **Septic arthritis**

a. **Etiology.** Usually *Staph. aureus*, *H. influenzae* type B, or group A streptococci. Penetrating injuries or skin infections are associated with *Staph. aureus* infections. Suppurative arthritis, sterile inflammatory arthritis, and tenosynovitis may be associated with gonococcal disease in sexually active adolescents, sometimes with characteristic skin lesions. Gram-negative enteric bacteria, pneumococci, and *N. meningitidis* are less commonly involved. Tuberculous arthritis is uncommon. Lyme disease may mimic septic arthritis.

b. **Evaluation**

(1) Careful **examination** of the patient for other foci of infection

(2) **X-ray films** of the joint(s) and adjacent bones

(3) Multiple **blood cultures** and examination of blood and joint fluid by rapid immunologic techniques for microbial antigen detection (see sec. **I.A.3.c**).

(4) **Arthrocentesis.** Analysis of the joint fluid includes Gram stain, culture (including plating on prewarmed chocolate agar if *H. influenzae* or *Neisseria* is suspected), WBC and differential, total protein, and joint/blood glucose ratio.

(5) Joint infection may be overlooked in the toxic, prostrate patient with bacteremia. **Delayed diagnosis may result in extensive damage to growth cartilages.**

(6) Hip involvement is common in children, and this joint is difficult to assess. **Repeated examination of the hips and all other joints** is an important aspect of managing bacteremic patients.

c. **Diagnosis.** The presence of bacteria in the synovial fluid establishes the diagnosis. Joint or blood cultures, or both, are positive in most but not all patients with septic arthritis. Ultrasound examination of the hip can be helpful to establish the presence of an effusion. Lyme disease should be considered for both acute and chronic arthritis in endemic areas.

d. **Therapy**

(1) **Drainage.** Prompt aspiration of the affected joint is both diagnostic and therapeutic, because adequate drainage is critical to the prevention of sequelae. Whether open surgical drainage or repeated needle aspiration is chosen depends on the **joint involved** (the hip and shoulder require surgical drainage), **age** (infants and young children usually require surgical drainage), **viscosity** of the synovial exudate, the offending **pathogen** (staphylococcal disease usually necessitates surgical drainage, whereas meningococcal or gonococcal arthritis may require only needle aspiration), and the **response** of the patient to antibiotics.

(2) **Antibiotics.** The initial choice of antibiotics is based on the gram-stained smear of the synovial fluid and the patient's age.

(a) In the absence of a diagnostic Gram stain, the initial choice should include a penicillinase-resistant penicillin (e.g., oxacillin, 200 mg/kg/day q4h IV, up to 12 gm/day). For children 2 months–5 years of age, an agent effective against *H. influenzae* should be added (chloramphenicol, 75 mg/kg/day q6h IV). Cefuroxime is an alternative administered in a dosage of 150 mg/kg/day q8h IV. Ampicillin-sulbactam can also be used, based on a dose of 200 mg/kg/day q6h IV of the ampicillin component.

(b) Once the pathogen is identified, therapy may require modification to provide the most effective drug with the least toxicity.

(c) Because antibiotics diffuse well into synovial fluid, local instillation is not necessary.

(d) Antibiotic therapy for 2–3 weeks is usually sufficient for septic arthritis. After an initial period of IV antibiotic therapy, when the clinical condition has stabilized, we finish therapy with oral antibiotics. Care must be taken to choose an oral drug based on in vitro sensitivities and pharmacokinetics that is tolerated at two to three times the normal oral dose. Serum bactericidal levels obtained 1–2 hours after oral dosing should have a titer of 1 : 8 or better for continuation of oral therapy to be confidently recommended. Dosing can be adjusted or probenecid added to the regimen (for penicillins and cephalosporins) to achieve desired serum levels (*J. Pediatr.* 92:485, 1978).

(3) Other therapeutic measures include early immobilization of the joint and physical therapy when the inflammation subsides.

2. **Acute osteomyelitis**

   a. **Etiology**

   (1) *Staph. aureus* is the organism responsible in 75–80 percent of cases.

   (2) Other organisms include group A streptococci, pneumococci, and *H. influenzae*. Special associations include *Salmonella* in sickle cell anemia, gram-negative enteric pathogens and group B streptococci in neonates, and *P. aeruginosa* following a penetrating injury of the foot or in drug addicts. Mycobacteria are rare causes.

   b. **Evaluation**

   (1) **A careful search for metastatic infection in other bones and soft tissues is indicated.**

   (2) Multiple blood cultures, cultures of other sites, x-ray films, and radionuclide scans of suspected bony sites

   (3) In the presence of localized bony tenderness or a positive bone scan, needle aspiration or open biopsy of the bone for Gram stain and culture is indicated.

   c. The **diagnosis** is based on the characteristic clinical picture and results of needle aspiration or bone biopsy. Although the classic radiologic findings of disease may not appear until 10 or more days, deep soft tissue swelling **in conjunction with local bone tenderness** is good evidence of osteomyelitis. Bone scans may provide early confirmation.

   d. **Therapy.** Prevention of chronic osteomyelitis and other sequelae depends on early diagnosis and treatment.

   (1) Administration of a penicillinase-resistant penicillin (e.g., oxacillin, 200 mg/kg/day q4h IV, up to 12 gm/day) is started as soon as the appropriate cultures have been obtained.

   (2) A second antibiotic is chosen if an organism other than *Staph. aureus* is suspected (e.g., chloramphenicol in the child < 5 years of age or when *H. influenzae* is a possibility).

   (3) Patients with sickle cell anemia require appropriate coverage for both staphylococcus and salmonella. Ampicillin-sulbactam, cefuroxime, or oxacillin with chloramphenicol would provide both.

   (4) *Pseudomonas* osteomyelitis always requires excellent surgical drain-

age and only brief antibiotic therapy with tobramycin and ticarcillin or ceftazidime for 1–2 weeks.

(5) Surgical drainage should be considered for most long bone infections unless the history before diagnosis is short and the response to antibiotic therapy is prompt.

(6) Antibiotic therapy is usually given for 4–6 weeks. In patients who respond promptly, therapy can be completed with oral antibiotics (e.g., cephazolin, 100 mg/kg/day q6h PO; dicloxacillin, 100 mg/kg/day q6h PO), provided the organism is known, compliance is certain, and serum inhibitory and bactericidal titers are monitored [*J. Pediatr.* 92:485, 1978; see **1.d.(2)(d)**].

M. Infections of the cardiovascular system

1. Infective endocarditis

a. Etiology. In children, congenital heart disease is present in most cases of bacterial endocarditis. Predisposing lesions including tetralogy of Fallot, ventricular septal defect, patent ductus arteriosus, aortic stenosis, and coarctation. Cyanotic children with shunts (Blalock, Waterston, Potts) are also at risk.

(1) A prior event leading to bacteremia (e.g., dental manipulation or infection, or manipulation of the GI or genitourinary tracts) or prior cardiac surgery (e.g., prosthetic valve implantation or creation of an aortopulmonic shunt) is frequently implicated as a precipitating factor. *(Strep viridans)*

(2) Alpha-hemolytic streptococci and *Staph. aureus* are most commonly involved.

(3) *Haemophilus* species, *Staph. pneumoniae*, group A streptococci, and anaerobes rarely cause endocarditis in children; enterococci cause it infrequently. When infection complicates cardiac surgery, *Staphylococcus epidermidis*, gram-negative bacilli, and fungi should be considered.

b. Evaluation includes the following:

(1) A **history,** with special attention to fever (particularly its duration, height, and time of onset), malaise, and symptoms of embolism (to the brain, kidneys, or spleen).

(2) **Physical examination,** with attention to cardiac auscultation for new or changing murmurs; cutaneous manifestations, such as petechiae, splinter hemorrhages, Osler's nodes, Janeway lesions; splenomegaly; and, if indicated, needle marks from illicit drug use.

(3) **Laboratory studies,** including a complete blood count (CBC), ESR, and urinalysis, should be obtained. Urine culture, multiple microscopic examinations of fresh urine sediment for red blood cells and red cell casts, cultures of possible noncardiac foci, chest x-ray, serum complement, serum protein analysis, and rheumatoid factor are recommended. A baseline electrocardiogram should be obtained.

(4) **Cultures of blood** (three to six sets over a 48-hour period) from different sites should be obtained before therapy is started in subacute bacterial endocarditis. In the seriously ill child who requires immediate therapy, three sets of blood cultures should be obtained.

(5) Because bacteremia is continuous in endocarditis, there is no advantage to culturing only with temperature spikes or to drawing blood for culture from arteries rather than veins.

(6) Once isolated, the causative organism should be saved. After appropriate antibiotics have been started, serum bactericidal levels can be determined [see **d.(4)**].

(7) **Echocardiographic evaluation** can be helpful in establishing a presumptive diagnosis.

c. The **diagnosis** is established by positive blood cultures in association with a compatible clinical picture:

(1) Typically, the bacteremia is low grade and continuous. Consequently, the majority (85–90%) of blood cultures is positive.

(2) Splenomegaly is common.

(3) The development of a new regurgitant murmur and extracardiac findings indicating systemic emboli or vasculitis are significant.

(4) **Laboratory abnormalities** include anemia, leukocytosis with a shift to the left, elevated ESR, microscopic hematuria, and hyperglobulinemia.

(5) When the blood cultures are negative, a presumptive diagnosis is based on the typical clinical syndrome.

d. **Therapy**

(1) If the diagnosis is clinically evident, initiation of antibiotics should begin while the results of the blood cultures are still pending.

(2) In acute bacterial endocarditis, therapy with penicillinase-resistant penicillin and gentamicin **should be initiated within several hours of the patient's admission to the hospital.**

(3) Once the pathogen has been identified, recommended antibiotics are as follows (see Table 14-2):

(a) **Viridans streptococci.** Aqueous penicillin G, 250,000 U/kg/day q4h IV, up to 20 MU daily.

(b) *Staph. aureus.* A penicillinase-resistant penicillin (e.g., oxacillin, 200 mg/kg/day q4h IV) should be given. In severely ill patients, gentamicin (4.5–7.5 mg/kg/day q8h IV) can be added for the first 7–10 days. Vancomycin (40 mg/kg/day q6h IV) is an alternative in penicillin-allergic patients.

(c) **Enterococci.** Give ampicillin, 300 mg/kg/day q6h IV, and gentamicin, 3.0–7.5 mg/kg/day q8h IV.

(4) Drug therapy is individualized on the basis of the organism's in vitro sensitivities and the results of serum bactericidal tests. A serum bactericidal level of 1 : 8 or greater at the time of peak antibiotic concentration is desirable. Although subjective improvement (e.g., in appetite) may be prompt, fever can remain elevated for several days after initiation of antibiotic therapy.

(5) In general, the duration of antibiotic therapy is 4–6 weeks.

(6) In addition to a daily physical examination, the ESR and urinalyses are useful variables to follow.

(7) Recurrent manifestations attributed to embolization and associated vasculitis do not necessarily indicate failure of antibiotic therapy.

(8) Fever may persist for 5–7 days despite adequate antibiotic therapy.

(9) **Surgical replacement** of the infected valve, when indicated, may be lifesaving. The indications for surgery in endocarditis include congestive heart failure refractory to medical therapy, more than one major embolic episode, worsening valve function, ineffective therapy (as in fungal endocarditis), mycotic aneurysm, and most cases of prosthetic valve endocarditis.

e. **Prevention of endocarditis.** Prophylactic antibiotic regimens are outlined in Table 14-7. The choice of regimen should be individualized according to both the risk of the underlying heart disease and the risk of the procedure. The regimens that require parenteral administration of potentially toxic antibiotics should be reserved for high-risk situations.

(1) Patients with prosthetic heart valves or grafts are at highest risk; patients with rheumatic heart disease are also at high risk. Patients with congenital heart diseases, such as ventricular septal defect, atrial septal defect, patent ductus arteriosus, and the "click-murmur" syndrome, are at lower risk.

(2) High-risk procedures are dental manipulations, especially surgery and tooth extractions in patients with poor oral hygiene, and manipulations of the infected genitourinary tract, especially when entero-

cocci are present. Procedures such as bronchoscopy, endoscopy, proctosigmoidoscopy, barium enemas, and liver biopsies may be associated with bacteremia but have a lower risk.

2. Acute rheumatic fever

a. Etiology. Acute rheumatic fever (ARF) is a sequela of pharyngeal infection with a group A streptococcus, but the exact pathogenesis is still unknown. It has been proposed that the disease may be (1) a direct reaction to streptococcal extracellular or cellular substances, (2) an immunologic process stimulated by *Streptococcus,* or (3) a persistent infection by *Streptococcus* or one of its variants.

b. Evaluation should include the following:

(1) **A history,** with emphasis on antecedent infections, fever, arthralgia, and previous RF, as well as familial and social history

(2) **Physical examination,** with attention to joints, skin (rashes and subcutaneous nodules), and the cardiovascular system

(3) **Laboratory studies** should include ESR, C-reactive protein, CBC, ECG, chest x-ray, streptococcal antibodies (antistreptolysin O, anti-DNase B, anti-NADase, antihyaluronidase), and throat culture.

c. Diagnosis

(1) No single laboratory test, symptom, or sign is pathognomonic, although several combinations are suggestive of ARF.

(2) According to the revised Jones criteria, RF is likely in the presence of one major and two minor criteria [see **(4)** and **(5)**], or two major criteria plus evidence of a preceding streptococcal infection. Chorea alone may be sufficient for a diagnosis.

(3) **ARF may not fulfill the revised Jones criteria,** especially early in the disease. Conversely, other diseases, such as rheumatoid arthritis, systemic lupus erythematosus, Schönlein-Henoch purpura, serum sickness, sickle cell hemoglobinopathy, and septic or postinfectious arthritis, may occasionally fulfill the criteria at certain points in their natural history.

(4) **Major criteria**

(a) **Carditis**

(b) **Polyarthritis.** Tenderness, usually with heat, swelling, and redness, involving more than one joint especially, but not exclusively, and involving the larger joints, especially the knee, ankle, elbow, wrist, and hip

(c) **Subcutaneous nodules** usually occur only in children with severe carditis of several weeks' duration.

(d) **Erythema marginatum** is an uncommon finding in RF and is not specific to the disease.

(e) **Chorea** is often associated with emotional instability.

(5) **Minor criteria**

(a) **Fever.** Rarely above 40°C (104°F); associated with shaking chills

(b) **Arthralgias.** Joint point without objective findings

(c) **Prolonged P-R interval on the ECG** (not in and of itself diagnostic of carditis)

(d) **Increased ESR, C-reactive protein, leukocytosis**

(e) **Previous history of ARF or rheumatic heart disease**

(6) **Other criteria** include epistaxis, abdominal pain, and rheumatic pneumonia.

d. Treatment

(1) **Eradication of streptococci** (see Table 14-2)

(2) **Antiinflammatory agents**

(a) **Aspirin** is indicated for arthritis without carditis and possibly in children with mild cardiac involvement. The dosage of acetylsalicylic acid is 100 mg/kg/day in four to six divided doses for 3–4 weeks. The optimal serum level is about 20–25 mg per day.

Although salicylates undoubtedly give symptomatic relief, there is no proof that they alter the course of the myocardial damage.

(b) Corticosteroids have been controversial in the therapy of ARF since their introduction.

(i) Corticosteroids are almost mandatory in patients with severe carditis and CHF. Prednisone, 2 mg/kg/day for 4–6 weeks, is given, with tapering over the next 2 weeks. Corticosteroids reduce inflammation promptly, but there is no conclusive evidence that they prevent residual valvular damage.

(ii) In patients with carditis without cardiomegaly or CHF, the use of corticosteroids instead of salicylates remains controversial and more a matter of personal preference.

(3) Anticongestive measures, including digitalis (see Chap. 9, p. 245ff), should be used in patients with ARF in the same fashion as in other patients with CHF, despite possible increased sensitivity in the inflamed myocardium.

(4) Bed rest is accepted during the acute phase when CHF is present. In the absence of objective data, we think it is prudent to keep children on limited activity, if not on bed rest, until the ESR returns to normal.

(5) Children with chorea should be moved to a quiet environment with understanding nurses and should be protected against self-inflicted injury due to uncontrollable movements. Drug treatment with phenobarbital, chlorpromazine, diazepam, and haloperidol has been tried, with varying success.

(6) Prevention of rheumatic recurrences

(a) All children with documented RF with or without carditis—and all those with rheumatic heart disease—should receive prophylaxis against a second attack (see Table 14-7).

(b) Any of the following approaches is acceptable, provided compliance is assured. If severe residual heart disease is present or the patient is unreliable, the first alternative is preferable.

(i) Benzathine penicillin, 1.2 million U every 28 days

(ii) Penicillin G or V, 200,000–250,000 U PO qd–bid

(iii) Sulfadiazine, 0.5 mg per day for those weighing under 30 kg; 1 gm per day for those weighing over 30 kg

(iv) Erythromycin, 250 mg PO bid, in patients sensitive to both sulfonamides and penicillin

3. Myocarditis (see Chap. 9, p. 241ff)

N. Lyme disease

1. Etiology. *Borrelia burgdorferi* is the tick-borne spirochete that causes Lyme borreliosis (Lyme disease). Humans are usually infected after prolonged (> 24 hour) attachment of an infected tick of the *Ixodes ricinus* complex. *Ixodes dammini* (deer tick) is the most common member of this tick group in the northeastern US.

2. Evaluation

a. Clinical manifestations of Lyme borreliosis vary according to the stage of infection. Recent classification schemes divide Lyme disease manifestations into stage 1: early localized, stage 2: early disseminated, and stage 3: late persistent phases. Clinical findings include the following.

(1) Erythema chronicum migrans (ECM), the characteristic rash seen in early Lyme infection, occurs in about 60–80 percent of cases. The lesion characteristically begins as a red macule, which expands to form an annular erythema with central clearing. Lesions vary in size but usually expand to greater than 5 cm in diameter if untreated. In some patients ECM never develops and therefore it is virtually impossible to diagnose early Lyme disease clinically, as other manifestations are nonspecific and accompanied by only minor constitutional symptoms. Additional skin findings are often noted days to weeks after initial infection and may resemble the primary ECM lesion or present as malar, urticarial, or diffuse erythematous rash. Acrodermatitis chronica atrophicans, a chronic localized scleroderma-like rash, may occur years after the primary infection and represents persistent disease.

(2) **Arthritis** along with **arthralgia** and **myalgia,** often fleeting and migratory, are common findings of the second stage of Lyme disease. More chronic forms of arthritis generally reflect the persistent infection of the third stage.

(3) **Neuritis** and **meningitis** may occur as either acute findings related to the second stage of disease or as chronic conditions occurring in the persistent third stage. Bell's palsy is common a few weeks to months after infection, reflecting the early disseminated stage. Meningitis is also fairly common and may present as classic summertime "aseptic" meningitis except for its prolonged course. Less commonly, peripheral neuropathies are found in both the second and third clinical stages. Chronic neurologic involvement, including encephalomyelitis, ataxia, and polyradiculitis, is generally a manifestation of late-stage Lyme disease and may occur years after initial infection and persist for years.

(4) Carditis has been found in 4–8 percent of patients with Lyme disease within several weeks of infection. Atrioventricular blocks of varying types are reported. Less commonly, pericarditis and myocarditis occur. Cardiac manifestations are usually brief.

3. **Diagnosis.** Lyme disease is primarily a clinical diagnosis. Serology is the only practical laboratory aid presently and should not be used without clinical correlation. If ECM is present, serologic confirmation is unnecessary. ELISA tests, both indirect and capture IgM types, are useful but considerable interlaboratory variation exists. Current recommendations are to send ELISA studies, for both IgG and IgM antibodies, at least 3 weeks after tick bite without giving "presumptive" antibiotic therapy before serologies are drawn. IgG and IgM ELISA titers need to be interpreted with reference to the clinical stage of disease suspected. Patients with symptoms of persistent infection or with more than 2–3 months of "early" symptoms may have negative IgM titers; alternatively, a patient with very early symptoms may have only IgM antibodies. As antibody is first detectable after 2–4 weeks of illness, a basic problem with serologic testing is that some patients may be antibody negative at the time ECM is present and early treatment may ablate the expected antibody response. False-positive tests are also a problem, both in normal individuals with asymptomatic seroconversion and in patients with other inflammatory conditions. For difficult cases with borderline ELISA serology, Western blot studies in a reference laboratory should be ordered.

4. **Therapy**
   a. **Early infection (ECM).** Amoxicillin, 40 mg/kg/day divided tid for 14–21 days, or doxycycline (children > 8 yr), 100 mg bid for 14–21 days. Retreatment is sometimes necessary and is based on clinical response.
   b. **Arthritis or isolated facial palsy.** Amoxicillin, 40 mg/kg/day divided tid for 20–30 days, or doxycycline (children > 8 yr), 100 mg bid for 20–30 days. If treatment fails, do not repeat oral therapy, but switch to a full course of parenteral therapy (see below).
   c. **Late manifestations, meningitis or carditis, or failure of oral therapy.** Ceftriaxone, 50 mg/kg/day (up to 2 gm) given as single IV or IM dose for 14 days. Alternatively, penicillin G, 200,000 U/kg/day IV in six divided doses daily for 14 days.
   d. **Prophylaxis for tick bite is not recommended,** as complications of antibiotic therapy are approximately equal to the risk of Lyme disease from any given tick bite.

O. **Tuberculosis (TB)**
   1. **Etiology.** *M. tuberculosis* is the infecting organism. Rarely, *Mycobacterium bovis* is the etiologic agent, especially with nonpulmonary TB.

2. **Evaluation**
   a. **Clinical manifestations** of childhood TB include:
      (1) Persistent cough, pulmonary infiltrates, and pleural effusion or enlarged hilar nodes
      (2) Chronic draining otitis media, cervical adenopathy
      (3) Aseptic meningitis
      (4) Occult fever, failure to thrive, weight loss, and anemia or hepatosplenomegaly
      (5) Aseptic pyuria
      (6) Monoarticular arthritis, dactylitis, back pain, or bony tenderness
   b. **Screening.** The tuberculin skin test is the best means of identifying infected children. Serious tuberculous disease (e.g., meningitis, miliary disease) will almost never develop in the child with primary tuberculosis who receives isoniazid (INH) prophylaxis for a year. An annual or biennial tuberculin test is recommended by the American Academy of Pediatrics for the office or outpatient clinic, unless local circumstances necessitate more frequent testing. For screening of low-risk populations, the tine test is adequate, but an intermediate-strength purified protein derivative (PPD), 5-TU, is indicated for patients whose tine tests are positive or who are suspected of having TB.
   c. When TB is suspected, a detailed inquiry into possible contacts with persons with active TB, an intermediate-strength PPD (5 U), and a chest x-ray are essential.
   d. Atypical (nontuberculous) mycobacteria can cause cervical adenitis or (uncommonly) pulmonary infection. These strains are often resistant to conventional TB therapy. Nontuberculous strains may cross-react with intermediate-strength PPD, but the reaction is usually less than 10 mm unless infection is recent.
   e. In the presence of a positive skin test and chest x-ray, the following should be done:
      (1) Obtain and culture three **gastric** aspirates in the morning, immediately on the patient's awakening.
      (2) Culture three **first-voided** morning urine collections.
      (3) **Liver function tests.** A liver biopsy, or bone marrow biopsy, may be necessary if miliary disease is suspected. A pleural biopsy may be diagnostic in patients with pleural effusions.
   f. In the presence of neurologic abnormalities, **CSF examination,** including culture and acid-fast stain, is necessary. Infants under 6 months should have a CSF examination even without abnormalities.
   g. In proved cases of TB, **skin tests and chest x-rays of family members and contacts** are indicated.
3. **Diagnosis**
   a. The demonstration of acid-fast bacilli in exudate or tissue is the most direct method of diagnosis. The judicious use of needle biopsy specimens of pleura, liver, or bone marrow often yields the diagnosis.
   b. The culture may not become positive for 3–6 weeks, but a presumptive diagnosis of TB is often made on the basis of the clinical presentation, epidemiologic history, and skin test reactivity to tuberculin antigen. Induration ≥ 10 mm from an intermediate-strength PPD generally indicates prior infection with the tuberculosis bacillus (symptomatic or asymptomatic).
4. **Therapy** (see also Table 14-8)
   a. **Asymptomatic converter** (positive skin test with a negative chest x-ray). Oral INH, 10 mg/kg (maximum of 300 mg) once a day for 9 months. Follow-up chest x-rays are obtained at 3- to 6-month intervals and again on completion of therapy.
   b. **Primary nonprogressive pulmonary TB (including an effusion) and cervical adenitis.** Oral INH, 10 mg/kg/day q24h, plus rifampin, 10 mg/kg/day q24h, or PAS, 0.2–0.3 gm per day. Ethambutol, 15 mg/kg/day,

is given in place of PAS for patients over 13 years of age. The major side effect of ethambutol is optic neuritis (blurred vision, color blindness, visual field alteration), which is difficult to monitor in young children.

c. **Tuberculous meningitis, progressive pulmonary disease, and miliary TB.** INH (20 mg/kg/day) and rifampin (10 mg/kg/day) for 12–24 months plus streptomycin (20–40 mg/kg/day to 1 gm/day) for the first 4 weeks of therapy.

d. **Nonpulmonary primary disease, skeletal TB, and urinary tract TB.** Treatment is as described in **b** for 12–24 months.

e. If the isolated *M. tuberculosis* is resistant in vitro to INH, a number of other agents are available. When possible, in vitro susceptibility testing should guide their selection. In patients from areas where resistance is endemic, initial therapy for most forms of TB should include three first-line agents.

f. **Household contacts**
   (1) Household exposure to an adolescent or adult with active TB requires isoniazid prophylaxis (10 mg/kg/day). If the child's PPD is still negative at 3 months, and if the person with active TB is under regular treatment or has left the home, the child's treatment can be discontinued. Periodic tuberculin tests should be followed. Documented exposure of a young infant to TB requires initiation of antitubercular therapy. Therapy should continue pending negative skin tests 3 months or more following exposure.
   (2) The infant born to a woman with active tuberculosis should be separated from the mother until she is considered noncontagious. Bacillus Calmette-Guérin (BCG) may be helpful when close medical supervision of the infant in the first year of life cannot be guaranteed. INH for 1 year is probably effective prophylaxis, but its potential neurotoxicity must be considered.

g. Pyridoxine, 25–50 mg once a day, is unnecessary in children under 10 years of age unless nutrition is inadequate.

h. Corticosteroids given in conjunction with antimicrobial therapy may lessen the inflammatory complications of tuberculous pericarditis and pleuritis. They may also be indicated when large hilar lymph nodes are obstructing the passage of air and when severe respiratory distress complicates diffuse pulmonary tuberculosis. In meningitis, corticosteroids may reduce increased ICP.

i. INH treatment commonly causes a transient asymptomatic elevation of liver enzymes during the first 3 months of therapy. Routine monitoring for hepatotoxicity is unnecessary, but if overt hepatotoxicity occurs, the drug should be discontinued.

P. **Fungal diseases**
 1. **Candidiasis**
    a. **Etiology.** *Candida albicans* is the most common pathogen, but other species, including *C. tropicalis, C. krusei, C. parapsilosis,* and *C. guilliermondi,* may also cause invasive disease.
    b. **Evaluation**
       (1) **Cultures** of the blood, urine, oropharynx, and stool
       (2) **Gram stain** and potassium hydroxide (KOH) prep of mucosal lesions
       (3) If esophageal involvement is suspected, a **barium swallow** and **esophagoscopy** (with biopsy and culture of lesions) are most helpful.
       (4) If disseminated disease is suspected, the ocular fundi and skin should be carefully examined. Cardiac ultrasound and LP may be indicated.
    c. **Diagnosis.** The demonstration of yeasts and pseudohyphae in scrapings of skin or mucosal lesions or tissue specimens is diagnostic. Repeated isolation of *Candida* from the blood suggests endocarditis, an infected intravascular device (e.g., a hyperalimentation line), or disseminated candidiasis. Recovery of > 103 organisms/ml suggests UTI.

d. Treatment. The duration of therapy depends on severity of disease and speed of response.

  (1) **Esophagitis** in immunocompromised hosts can be treated with amphotericin B, usually 0.25 mg/kg/day, but up to 1 mg/kg/day for 7–10 days. Alternatively, fluconazole, 6 mg/kg/day PO qd, can be used.

  (2) **Disseminated infection, endocarditis, and meningitis** should be treated with full doses of amphotericin B (1 mg/kg/day). 5-Fluorocytosine (150 mg/kg/day q6h) can be added in seriously ill patients, but only if the organism is sensitive to this agent.

  (3) Candidal infection restricted to the bladder may respond to continuous irrigation with amphotericin B (50 mg/1,000 ml; maximum dose, 1 mg/kg/day in sterile **distilled water**). Infection restricted to the bladder or kidney can also be treated with 5-fluorocytosine alone, 50–100 mg/kg/day PO q6h for 7 days, or with fluconazole, 6 mg/kg/day PO qd for 7 days.

  (4) **Chronic mucocutaneous candidiasis** has been successfully treated with oral ketoconazole. Fluconazole should be at least as efficacious.

2. Cryptococcosis

  a. Etiology. The causative organism is *C. neoformans*.

  b. Evaluation

   (1) **History.** Respiratory symptoms and subtle neurologic symptoms, including headache and diplopia.

   (2) **CSF** examination, including India ink preparation, culture for fungus, and cryptococcal antigen test. Culture yields are improved by culturing a large volume of CSF.

   (3) Sputum and urine culture for fungus

   (4) Cryptococcal antigen test on the serum and urine

   (5) Chest x-ray; occasionally, a lung biopsy is necessary.

  c. Diagnosis. The presence of cryptococcal antigen in the CSF, serum, or urine or a "positive" India ink smear strongly suggests the diagnosis. The diagnosis is established by the growth of cryptococci from CSF or lung tissue. India ink results should be confirmed with an antigen test.

  d. Treatment

   (1) **Cryptococcal meningitis** can be treated with a combination of amphotericin B, 0.3 mg/kg/day, and 5-fluorocytosine, 150 mg/kg/day PO divided q6h for at least 6 weeks. Patients with severe marrow impairment in whom further marrow suppression from 5-fluorocytosine may develop can be treated with amphotericin B alone (1 mg/kg/day) to a total dose of 2 or 3 gm. Fluconazole is effective therapy of cryptococcal meningitis in adults.

   (2) Treatment should be monitored with weekly examination of the CSF by culture and India ink smear and for cryptococcal antigen concentration. Cultures should become sterile promptly. Microscopy should show a decrease in the number of organisms, and antigen testing should show at least a fourfold decrease in level during treatment.

   (3) After completion of treatment, the CSF should be examined q2–3 months for 1 year to detect relapses. Immunocompromised patients can be maintained on a regimen of fluconazole to prevent relapse.

  e. Cryptococcal pneumonia, in the absence of dissemination to the CNS, may not require therapy unless it is progressive. Close observation for at least 1–2 months is necessary if treatment is not given.

3. Invasive aspergillosis

  a. Etiology. A variety of *Aspergillus* species are pathogenic in humans, the most common being *A. fumigatus*.

  b. Evaluation

   (1) Careful examination for sinusitis, necrotic nasal lesions, pneumonia, pleuritic pain, and necrotizing skin lesions

   (2) X-ray or CT scans of the sinuses and chest

   (3) **Direct microscopic examination and culture of sputum and biopsy**

specimens from suspected sites. Early diagnosis is essential, and biopsies should be performed promptly.

   c. Diagnosis

     (1) Demonstration of septate hyphae 3–4 μm in diameter with an acute (45-degree) angle branching in tissues is diagnostic of invasive aspergillosis.

     (2) A chest x-ray showing a ball within a cavity is suggestive of aspergilloma.

   d. The **treatment** for invasive aspergillosis is amphotericin B, 0.75–1.0 mg/kg/day (for a total dosage of 30–35 mg/kg over a period of 6 weeks or longer), and surgical debridement of cutaneous and sinus lesions. In severely ill patients, rifampin can be added.

V. Antiviral therapy

  A. Principles

   1. Viruses are obligate intracellular parasites that depend on the host cell for growth and replication. Clinically useful antiviral agents must act at stages of infection or replication involving virus-specific metabolic activities.

   2. The **toxicity** of antiviral drugs depends on the degree to which the metabolic apparatus of the host cell is able to utilize the drug.

  B. Antiviral agents in clinical use

   1. Amantadine has a mechanism of action that is not fully understood. It may interfere with penetration and uncoating of virus.

     a. Antiviral spectrum. Active against all influenza A strains but not against influenza B.

     b. Pharmacology. Rapidly absorbed from the GI tract, with peak blood levels 2–4 hours after an oral dose. Of an orally administered dose of amantadine, 90 percent is excreted unchanged in the urine and has a serum half-life of 20 hours.

     c. Adverse effects. Amantadine is well tolerated in children. In 3–7 percent of healthy adults, there are CNS symptoms, such as difficulty in thinking, confusion, light-headedness, hallucinations, anxiety, and insomnia.

     d. Clinical indications. Amantadine is useful in chemoprophylaxis of influenza A in unvaccinated persons at high risk and provides 70 percent protection against clinical illness. It is also useful in chemotherapy of infection, if begun in the first 24 hours of illness, and results in a diminution of fever and a 50 percent reduction in the duration of illness.

   2. Adenine-arabinoside (vidarabine, Ara-A, Vira-A) blocks DNA synthesis by inhibiting the activity of the virus-specific DNA polymerase. Since the introduction of acyclovir and trifluridine, the indications for vidarabine have diminished to the point that it is not a drug of choice for any viral infection. We no longer use vidarabine.

     a. Antiviral spectrum. Ara-A has activity against the herpesvirus, pox viruses, and vaccinia.

     b. Pharmacology. Ara-A is rapidly deaminated to arabinosyl hypoxanthine and excreted in the urine. The plasma half-life is 4 hours. The drug is poorly soluble and must be given parenterally in large volumes of fluid. The 3% ophthalmic ointment has poor ocular penetration.

     c. Adverse effects. In small numbers of patients, nausea, vomiting, and diarrhea develop at doses less than 15 mg/kg/day. At 20 mg/kg/day, tremors, weight loss, and bone marrow megaloblastosis are seen. Doses of 30 mg/kg/day produce thrombocytopenia and leukopenia. There is occasional neurologic toxicity consisting of tremors, ataxia, painful paresthesias, encephalopathy, or abnormal EEG findings.

     d. Clinical indications. Ara-A is currently approved for use in herpes simplex encephalitis, neonatal herpes, and topically in acute herpetic keratoconjunctivitis and recurrent epithelial keratitis. However, systemic acyclovir is preferred for therapy of encephalitis and neonatal disease, and topical trifluridine is favored for opthalmologic indications.

3. **Acyclovir (acycloguanosine)** acts as an inhibitor of the virus-specific DNA polymerase after being converted to the phosphorylated active form by a virus-specific thymidine kinase.
   a. **Antiviral spectrum.** Acyclovir is active against herpes simplex types 1 and 2 and varicella-zoster, and has some activity against Epstein-Barr virus.
   b. **Pharmacology.** Acyclovir is distributed widely in the body with therapeutic levels detected in CSF and in vesicles. Oral absorption is incomplete and variable with 20 percent bioavailability. Serum half-life is 2.5 hours and excretion is primarily renal.
   c. **Adverse effects.** Toxicity has proved to be minimal. Some patients may have a reversible mild rise in creatinine. It is important to ensure good urine output to avoid crystallization and obstructive uropathy.
   d. **Clinical indications.** Acyclovir has proved to be a very useful drug in management of herpes simplex and varicella-zoster virus infections. It is now the drug of choice for herpes simplex virus (HSV) encephalitis and for neonatal herpes infections. Acyclovir is effective in varicella-zoster infections of normal or immunocompromised patients. Prophylactic acyclovir has been used successfully in patients undergoing bone marrow transplants and in leukemia patients to prevent reactivation of herpes simplex infections. In primary herpes genitalis, oral or parenteral therapy decreases duration of symptoms and new lesion formation. Topical acyclovir is of little benefit for recurrent orofacial or genital lesions, except in decreasing viral shedding. Given orally, acyclovir effectively suppresses recurrent herpes genitalis, but the condition recurs at the pretreatment frequency when acyclovir is discontinued.
   e. **Dosage**
      (1) **Herpes simplex encephalitis:** 30 mg/kg/day or 1,500 mg/m^2/day IV divided q8h for 10 days
      (2) **Neonatal herpes simplex:** 30 mg/kg/day or 1,500 mg/m^2/day IV divided doses q8h for 10–14 days
      (3) **Varicella-zoster infections in immunocompromised patients:** 30 mg/kg/day or 1,500 mg/m^2/day IV divided q8h for 7 days
      (4) **Primary herpes simplex genitalis:** 200 mg PO five times a day for 10 days
      (5) **Recurrent herpes simplex genitalis:** 400 mg PO two times a day for up to 12 months as prophylaxis
      (6) **Herpes simplex prophylaxis in immunocompromised patients:** 15 mg/kg/day or 750 mg/m^2/day IV divided q8h or 30 mg/kg/day PO five times a day during periods of severe immunosuppression
4. **Ribavirin** (virazole) has antiviral inhibitory activity against many RNA and DNA viruses. The mechanism of action is not precisely known and may vary between viruses.
   a. **Antiviral spectrum.** Ribavirin is active in vitro against over 20 viruses. Current clinical use is limited to respiratory syncytial virus, but clinical studies to measure its effectiveness against other viruses including influenza and HIV are in progress.
   b. **Pharmacology.** The pharmacology of ribavirin is not yet fully detailed. Administration of aerosolized drug results in high respiratory secretion levels and some systemic absorption with low plasma levels. Oral drug is absorbed with 35–50 percent bioavailability.
   c. **Adverse effects.** Few side effects have clearly been related to ribavirin aerosol administration. Precipitation of drug within the ventilatory apparatus can cause significant problems in patients on respirators. Use of ribavirin aerosol in patients requiring assisted ventilation should be done only with extreme caution.
   d. **Clinical indications.** The only approved indication at this time is for severe respiratory syncytial virus infections. Treatment is moderately effective when administered by continuous aerosol early in the course of

severe lower respiratory tract infection. Treatment is carried out for 12–18 hours per day for up to 7 days with the drug (6 gm/day) delivered to an oxygen hood from an SPAG-2 aerosol generator. Some immunosuppressed patients do not clear respiratory syncytial virus during initial therapy and may benefit from a second course of ribavirin aerosol. Patients with underlying cardiac or pulmonary disease may benefit most from early therapy.

C. Treatment of specific viral diseases
  1. Hepatitis
    a. Etiology. Hepatitis can be caused by a wide range of viruses. The most common agents are hepatitis A (infectious hepatitis), hepatitis B (serum hepatitis), and hepatitis C (which accounts for most of what was formerly called non-A, non-B hepatitis). Other viruses that can cause hepatitis include Epstein-Barr virus, cytomegalovirus, and Coxsackie viruses A and B. Neonatal hepatitis may be the result of infection with herpesvirus, cytomegalovirus, echoviruses, or toxoplasmosis.

    b. Diagnosis. The common hepatitis viruses cannot be cultured in clinical laboratories, and diagnosis is made primarily by serology. Tests include the following:
      (1) Hepatitis A antibody. An IgM antibody rise to hepatitis A indicates acute hepatitis.
      (2) Hepatitis B surface antigen (HBsAg), formerly called Australia antigen (HAA) can be present both in acute disease and in the carrier state.
      (3) Antibody to HBsAg (anti-HBs) develops after an infection and is indicative of immunity.
      (4) Hepatitis B e antigen (HBeAg) is a soluble antigen that correlates with a high titer of hepatitis B virus in the serum and a high degree of infectivity.
      (5) IgM antibody to the hepatitis B virus (HBV) core antigen (IgM anti-HBc) is highly specific for acute or recent HBV infection and may be present when neither HBsAg nor anti-HBs is detectable.
      (6) Heterophil or Monospot, or viral capsid antigen (VCA) IgM and IgG for Epstein-Barr virus
      (7) Serology for toxoplasmosis
      (8) Viral cultures if cytomegalovirus or enteroviruses are suspected

    c. Treatment
      (1) There is no specific therapy for viral hepatitis. Interferon alpha appears to be useful in management of chronic hepatitis B or C. Preexposure vaccination for hepatitis B is now recommended for all infants (universal immunization). Promising hepatitis A vaccines are under study but are not yet available for routine use.
      (2) Prophylactic immune globulin should be given to contacts. (See sec. **II.C.1** and Table 14-6 for IG for hepatitis A immunization.)
        (a) Hepatitis A immune globulin in a dose of 0.02 ml/kg should be given to household, sexual, and day care contacts as soon as possible after exposure.
        (b) Hepatitis B. Percutaneous inoculation by needle stick or transfusion, exposure of contact's mucous membranes, or newborn exposure to infectious material requires prophylaxis with either immune globulin or high-titer hepatitis B immune globulin (HBIG) and vaccination according to Table 14-11.
        (c) Hepatitis C. Although studies of postexposure prophylaxis have been equivocal, immune globulin (0.06 ml/kg) may be useful.

  2. Herpes simplex infections
    a. Genital herpes
      (1) Etiology. Usually involves HSV type 2; HSV type 1 occurs less frequently.
      (2) Evaluation may include a Tzanck preparation of vesicle base scrapings (not vesicular fluid) to look for multinucleated giant cells,

Table 14-11. Hepatitis B immune globulin and vaccine prophylaxis

Exposure	HBsAg testing	Recommended prophylaxis*
HBsAg-positive person	—	HBIG (0.06 ml/kg IM) within 24 hr and 1 month later*
HBsAg status unknown High risk for positivity Acute hepatitis Institutionalized Down syndrome patients Hemodialysis IV drug user Male homosexual Person of Asian origin	Yes (if results can be obtained within 7 days of exposure)	IG (0.06 ml/kg) immediately, and, if HBsAg is positive: HBIG (0.06 ml/kg) immediately *and* 1 month thereafter;* if HBsAg is negative, no further therapy needed
Low risk for positivity Average hospital patients	Yes	Nothing or IG (0.06 ml/kg)
Source unknown	Yes	Nothing or IG (0.06 ml/kg)
Exposure of a newborn to an HBsAg-positive mother (especially those mothers who are also HBeAg positive)		HBIG (0.5 ml IM) within 12 hr of birth and hepatitis B vaccine*

* For use of hepatitis B vaccine, see *M.M.W.R.* 34:313, 1985.Source: Adapted from the recommendations of the Immunization Practices Advisory Committee. *M.M.W.R.* 30:423,1981 and 33:285, 1984.

immunofluorescent staining of vesicle base scrapings, and/or viral culture of a vesicle swab.

(3) **Therapy**

    (a) Oral acyclovir shortens both duration of symptoms and shedding of virus in primary genital herpes infections in adults, but does not affect the risk or severity of subsequent recurrent genital lesions. Topical therapy is less effective.

    (b) Recurrent genital lesions may be effectively suppressed by oral acyclovir therapy; however, lesions will develop at the pretherapy recurrence rate after discontinuation of prophylactic acyclovir. Prophylaxis for an adult-sized patient is 400 mg acyclovir PO bid for up to a year.

b. **Herpes simplex encephalitis**

    (1) **Etiology.** Usually, HSV type 1; rarely, HSV type 2

    (2) **Evaluation**

        (a) The **history** often includes fever, seizures, headache, and confusion.

        (b) **Physical examination** may reveal focal neurologic signs.

        (c) A brain scan, EEG, and CT or magnetic resonance imaging (MRI) will usually reveal a focal defect, most often in the temporal lobe(s). Radiographic findings may not be present early in the course of encephalitis.

        (d) The gold standard for **diagnosis** requires isolation of virus from a brain biopsy specimen; however, brain biopsy is rarely performed in our institution for this purpose, as empiric therapy with acyclovir is considered to be less risky for the patient. With improved cranial imaging techniques (CT and MRI), the exclusion of other treatable diseases, such as brain abscess, tumor, or hemorrhage, is more reliable than in the past. Even so, it is important to carefully consider alternative diagnoses even after beginning acyclovir, as other potentially treatable diseases may mimic HSV encephalitis.

(e) **Immunofluorescence assays** for HSV antigen or frozen brain sections are less sensitive than viral cultures, but can result in an earlier diagnosis.

(f) Orofacial HSV infection or rising antibody titers are not diagnostic.

(3) **Therapy**

(a) Careful management of increased ICP

(b) Acyclovir is the drug of choice. The dosage is 30 mg/kg/day IV in three divided doses for 10–14 days.

(c) When started empirically, without confirming HSV as the etiology of encephalitis, it is necessary to reconsider the need for therapy several days into the clinical course. We often stop therapy if characteristic EEG, CT, or MRI studies fail to show abnormalities or if the clinical course is not consistent with HSV encephalitis even after treating with acyclovir for a few days.

c. **Disseminated herpes simplex**

(1) **Etiology.** Usually HSV type 1 in older children and HSV type 2 in neonates

(2) **Evaluation**

(a) The **history** will usually include evidence of immunosuppression as the result of immunodeficiency or chemotherapy.

(b) The **physical examination** should include careful inspection of evidence of complications such as bacterial superinfection, tenderness of the liver, or pneumonia

(3) Acyclovir in a dose of 30 mg/kg/day IV divided q8h is the drug of choice for neonatal disseminated herpes. Ara-A is an alternative agent with an efficacy similar to that of acyclovir in preliminary data; however problems with administration of Ara-A make acyclovir the preferred drug at this time.

3. **Infectious mononucleosis syndromes** are most commonly the result of infection with Epstein-Barr virus but can also be due to cytomegalovirus or toxoplasmosis.

a. **Epstein-Barr virus (EBV)**

(1) **Evaluation**

(a) The **history** includes sore throat, malaise, and fever.

(b) The **physical examination** may reveal fever, lymphadenopathy, splenomegaly, hepatomegaly, jaundice, periorbital edema, and/or rash, with or without an exudative pharyngitis.

(c) **Laboratory findings** include lymphocytosis with 10 percent or more atypical lymphocytes, a positive Monospot after the second week of illness, and/or a heterophil titer of over 1 : 32. Children under 5 years may not have a positive Monospot or heterophil titer, but will have positive serology for EBV viral capsid antigen (IgG and/or IgM).

(d) **Interpretation of serologic tests.** Antibodies to the EB VCA of both IgG and IgM classes appear early in infection. After several weeks, antibody to the EBV early antigen (EA) appears. Antibodies to EA and IgM antibodies to VCA usually fall to undetectable levels within several months, although antibody to EA persists in a number of patients. With resolution of infectious mononucleosis, antibodies to antinuclear antigen (EBNA) appear and, along with VCA IgG antibodies, persist for life. Titers measured by ELISA methods are sometimes difficult to interpret, as each laboratory has its own standards for positivity. If necessary, these tests can be repeated on a fresh specimen to determine if titers are rising.

(2) **Treatment**

(a) **Primarily supportive.** The illness usually lasts 5–20 days, with a prolonged convalescence.

(b) For airway compromise or marked splenomegaly, prednisone, 1–2 mg/kg/day PO for 5–7 days, is recommended.

(c) Avoid ampicillin; it may cause rashes.

(d) To avoid splenic rupture, strenuous activity and contact sports should be prohibited while the spleen is enlarged.

b. Cytomegalovirus (CMV)

(1) Evaluation

(a) The physical findings and history are similar to those for EBV.

(b) Monospot and EBV serology are negative.

(c) Diagnose by a rise in antibody to cytomegalovirus or by culture of the virus. Be aware that CMV excretion in the urine occurs occasionally following a remote infection, and therefore the isolation of CMV from urine is often not sufficient proof of causality.

(2) Treatment is supportive. In life- or sight-threatening cytomegalovirus infections, therapy with DHPG (ganciclovir, Syntex), can be considered. Only immunocompromised hosts generally require ganciclovir therapy.

c. Toxoplasmosis (see Chap. 15, p. 455ff)

4. Varicella-zoster

a. Etiology. Herpes zoster and varicella (chickenpox) are caused by varicella-zoster virus (VZV). The reactivation of VZV months or years after chickenpox occurs in a dorsal spinal or cranial nerve ganglion, with spread to the appropriate cutaneous dermatome and occasionally to distant sites. The spread of infection to visceral organs (disseminated zoster) is usually due to underlying immunodeficiency.

b. Evaluation and diagnosis

(1) In zoster patients, the **history** should exclude other causes of localized vesicular disease.

(2) The **physical examination** should include careful inspection for the number and character of vesicles and for evidence of complications, such as bacterial superinfection, cutaneous dissemination, tenderness in the abdomen or liver, and paresis of the muscles in the involved area (e.g., urinary retention). When cranial nerve V is involved, vesicles on the tip of the nose (innervated by the nasociliary branch) suggest the possibility of keratoconjunctivitis or uveitis, or both.

(3) A Tzanck preparation can be done to look for multinucleated giant cells. Alternatively, immunofluorescent staining of infected cells scraped from the base of a fresh vesicle is more specific and a fairly sensitive means of diagnosing VZV infection. Without a viral culture or IFA, the diagnosis of herpes zoster is not completely reliable, since herpes simplex virus can also cause dermatomal involvement.

(4) In immunosuppressed persons, the tempo of disease and extent of viral spread should be determined by periodic pox counts, serial chest x-rays, serum liver enzyme analyses, and CNS examinations.

c. Treatment

(1) Wet-to-dry soaks are applied to involved dermatomes tid, using Burow's solution to facilitate debridement. Superinfection is treated with a penicillinase-resistant oral penicillin or cephalosporin and topical antibiotics.

(2) Pain symptoms are treated appropriately. Because postherpetic neuralgia is not a problem in children, systemic corticosteroids are not indicated.

(3) When **cranial nerve V** is involved, referral to an ophthalmologist is indicated.

(4) Scopolamine eye drops (0.3%) are used to produce **mydriasis** and **cycloplegia.** Corticosteroid drops are indicated when **interstitial keratitis** or **uveitis** is present (in the absence of dendritic keratitis).

(5) Disseminated skin vesicles may occur in 10 percent of previously healthy persons. This does not indicate an adverse prognosis, and they need not be treated.

(6) In the immunosuppressed person the presence of fever, rapidly increasing numbers of new vesicles, failure of vesicle maturation, elevation of serum liver parenchymal enzymes, and onset of respiratory or CNS symptoms are indications for treatment with acyclovir, 30 mg/kg/day, in three divided doses for 7 days. **There is no indication for the use of zoster immune globulin or plasma in the therapy of established disease.**

(7) Although oral acyclovir has recently been approved for use in therapy of early primary varicella infections (chickenpox) in children over the age of 2 years, we do not routinely administer this therapy. In certain situations, such as patients with chronic illness, those receiving low-dose oral steroid therapy, or those with other risk factors for severe varicella (but not high enough risk for parenteral therapy), we make exceptions and treat. The dose is 20 mg/kg PO four times a day for one week and should only be used if it can be started within 24 hours of onset of varicella.

(8) Hospital contacts of patients with zoster or chickenpox who have no history of prior chickenpox or whose VZV immunofluorescent antibody tests are negative must be isolated in the hospital, discharged, or kept away from work from the 8th to 21st day after exposure.

(9) Immunosuppressed children who have not had chickenpox should receive VZIG (0.2 ml/kg) following close exposure to zoster or chickenpox. If patients remain hospitalized following varicella exposure and prophylactic therapy with VZIG, they should be placed on respiratory precautions from the 7th until the 28th day following exposure.

(10) Varicella-zoster vaccine may be available in the near future.

5. **Acquired immunodeficiency syndrome (AIDS)**
   a. **Etiology.** The human immunodeficiency virus was isolated from AIDS patients in 1983 and is now well established as the etiologic agent. HIV is an RNA cytopathic human retrovirus. A viral enzyme, reverse transcriptase, allows the viral genome to be integrated into the infected cells' DNA. Viral infection may lead to cell death or to a latent infection, which may be reactivated subsequently. Destruction of T-helper (CD4) lymphocytes and monocytes contributes to the immunodeficiency syndromes. Although antibodies to the viral protein are capable of neutralizing HIV, the gene encoding the protein shows a high degree of variability between strains, and variant viruses may evade the immune system, contributing to viral persistence. At the time of this writing, over 4,000 pediatric AIDS cases have been reported to the CDC. Many more children with HIV infection (but not the full AIDS) are not included in the CDC statistics.
   b. **Evaluation**
      (1) History
         (a) Pediatric HIV infections now occur primarily in infants born to infected mothers. Children exposed in utero or perinatally have a 20–30 percent chance of acquiring the infection. The median age at onset of symptoms in HIV-positive infants is 8–12 months. Over 80 percent of HIV-infected children will be symptomatic by 2 years of age.
         (b) Both symptomatic and asymptomatic women can transmit HIV to their infants. HIV infection should be considered in infants of IV drug abusers, women who are sexual partners of IV drug abusers, or prostitutes, or if the father is a hemophiliac or known to be HIV positive.

(c) Recipients of any blood products, except gamma globulin, between 1979 and 1985 are at risk. Most hemophiliacs treated with factor VIII concentrate before 1985 have antibody to HIV.

(d) Adolescents may become infected by needle sharing during IV drug abuse or through sexual activity.

(2) **Clinical features**

(a) As in the adult disease, weight loss, failure to thrive, hepatosplenomegaly, lymphadenopathy, persistent oral candidiasis, diarrhea, fever, malaise, progressive neurologic disease, and unusual infections are common.

(b) The most common presentation in children is *P. carinii* pneumonia.

(c) Features of AIDS unique to the pediatric population include the high incidence of **diffuse persistent parotitis, recurrent unexplained serious bacterial infections, and lymphoid interstitial pneumonitis (LIP).**

(d) Kaposi's sarcoma and other malignancies are unusual in pediatric AIDS patients.

(e) Developmental delay is very common in HIV-infected children. HIV encephalopathy occurs in some children and is manifested by spasticity, loss of developmental milestones, microcephaly, seizures, and atrophy with basal ganglion calcifications on cranial imaging studies.

c. **Diagnosis**

(1) The CDC periodically updates its classification system for HIV infection in children and this should be used as a reference (*M.M.W.R.* 36:225,1987).

(2) Initial laboratory evaluation of suspected pediatric AIDS patients includes **serologic testing** with an ELISA screen for HIV antibody and Western blot confirmation of positive tests.

(a) Evaluation of HIV antibody status may be complicated by the presence of maternal antibody in infants of seropositive mothers. It is therefore necessary to repeat any positive antibody tests until the child is 15 months of age to eliminate false-positive results due to passively acquired antibody.

(b) Viral culture, polymerase chain reaction testing for proviral DNA, and p24 antigen detection may have a role in early diagnosis.

(3) Further laboratory evaluation includes, in addition to HIV antibody tests, a CBC, quantitative immunoglobulin assays, liver function studies, and chest x-ray. Detailed lymphocyte studies including T-cell enumeration, T_4/T_8 ratio, and in vitro response to mitogens are useful to follow known HIV-infected children, but are not generally done as screening tests.

(4) **Evaluation of pneumonia** requires aggressive efforts to identify the pathogen(s). Bronchioloalveolar lavage and transbronchial biopsy may be useful, but **open lung biopsy** should be done if no clear pathogen is demonstrated and the patient fails to respond to empiric therapy for *P. carinii*. Viral as well as bacterial cultures should be sent when evaluating pneumonitis.

d. **Therapy**

(1) There is currently no definitive therapy for HIV infection.

(a) Medical management includes treatment of AIDS-associated infections and general support of the patient.

(b) Clinical trials of intravenous gamma globulin and antiviral agents such as zidovudine (AZT) and ddI are in progress to determine efficacy in the pediatric population and to refine criteria for use. AZT is prescribed for symptomatic HIV-infected children regardless of CD4 counts and in asymptomatic seropositive children with less than 500 CD4 lymphocytes/mm^3. For children who cannot tolerate AZT or who have disease progression while receiving AZT, ddI can be prescribed.

(c) Intravenous gamma globulin appears to be of benefit to some patients. We generally begin monthly IVIG therapy in HIV-positive patients who have had at least one serious bacterial infection or an episode of bacteremia.

(2) Acute or recurrent *Pneumocystis* **pneumonia** is treated with either TMP-SMZ or pentamidine (see Chap. 15, p. 456).

(a) Prophylactic therapy with TMP-SMZ (8 mg/kg trimethoprim with 40 mg/kg sulfamethoxazole given either three times/wk or daily in one or two divided doses) or, for patients who do not tolerate TMP-SMZ, dapsone (1 mg/kg/day as single daily dose) is recommended for all children who have had an episode of PCP, who have CD4 lymphocyte percentages less than 20, or who have fewer than an age-dependent minimum absolute number of CD4 lymphocytes ranging from 1,500/mm^3 in infants less than 1 year old to 200/mm^3 in 6-year-olds.

(b) There are currently no pediatric trials of aerosolized pentamidine prophylaxis.

(3) The use of diphtheria-pertussis-tetanus (DPT), pneumococcal, *H. influenzae* B-conjugate, inactivated polio (IPV), and influenza vaccines is potentially beneficial to HIV-positive children who are capable of responding to the antigens. The measles-mumps-rubella (MMR) vaccine is recommended for both symptomatic and asymptomatic HIV-infected children (*M.M.W.R.* 37:181, 1988). **Oral polio (OPV) should be avoided, as an inactivated alternative is available (IPV).**

(4) Varicella-zoster immune globulin should be administered after exposure to varicella. Clinical varicella and severe herpes labialis can be treated with acyclovir (see sec. **V.B.3**).

(5) Despite aggressive medical management, AIDS in the pediatric population appears to have no better prognosis than in adults. Children should remain with their families and, if possible, be managed out of the hospital with medical and social supports. As the disease is uniformly fatal, appropriate judgment must be used when considering use of life support systems.

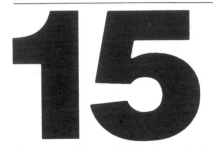

Parasitic Infections

Craig Wilson

Infections with protozoa and helminths are subject to rational principles of diagnosis and therapy. Most parasitic infections occur in temperate as well as tropical environments. Their incidence varies with climate, sanitation, and socioeconomic conditions. The frequency with which the clinician in temperate areas encounters parasitic infections is increasing, both as a result of intercontinental travel and the use of immunosuppressive agents. This chapter is limited in scope to the parasitic diseases most commonly encountered by pediatricians in the United States. Diseases not discussed include schistosomiasis, filariasis, trypanosomiasis, and leishmaniasis, despite their impact as major world health problems. Discussions of babesiosis, trichomoniasis, and balantidiasis have also been omitted because of their low impact on the general pediatric population. Standard parasitology or tropical medicine texts should be consulted for more information on these topics.

I. **Principles of diagnosis.** The diagnostic features of common parasitic infections are summarized in Table 15-1.

A. **General**

1. **The diagnosis of parasitic infection can rarely be made on clinical grounds alone.** The clinical picture in many parasitic infections may be identical, and different clinical presentations may be produced by a single parasite. In addition, parasitic infections are often asymptomatic or produce only mild symptoms. Commonly, a diagnosis of parasitic infection is suspected only because of an abnormal, unexpected laboratory finding.

2. **The diagnosis of most helminthic or protozoal infections requires the demonstration of the parasite in body excreta, fluids, or tissue.**

3. Many parasites have an intricate route of migration through the human host and affect several organs successively or simultaneously. The choice of appropriate diagnostic techniques and materials thus rests on some understanding of the life cycles of the possible infecting agents.

4. Knowledge of the **geographic distribution** of parasitic infections and their **mode of acquisition** and **means of spread** often aids diagnosis and therapy. Detailed information is available from standard parasitology texts.

5. **Patients commonly harbor several parasites.** This is particularly true of intestinal protozoa and/or helminthic infections. A complete evaluation must be made to avoid overlooking the most important infecting species in each clinical setting.

B. **Hematologic changes in parasitic infections**

1. **Erythrocytes.** Anemia is an inconstant and nonspecific finding in most parasitic infections. It reflects the general nutritional status of the patient rather than any direct effect of the infecting parasite. Iron deficiency anemia in hookworm disease and hemolytic anemia in malaria and babesiosis are exceptions.

2. **Eosinophils**

a. Eosinophilia is often the first clue to the presence of **helminth** infection and reflects the tissue migratory phase of these infections. **Protozoa,** conversely, generally do *not* evoke an eosinophilia. The finding of eosinophilia in amebiasis, malaria, toxoplasmosis, or giardiasis suggests an additional helminth infection.

Table 15-1. Diagnostic features of commonly encountered parasitic infections

Disease	Mode of spread	Location in humans	Clinical features	Laboratory diagnosis	Eosinophilia*	Remarks
Roundworms (nematodes)						
Ascariasis	Fecal-oral	Adult: small intestine Larvae: lung	Vague abdominal distress; cough and pneumonia during lung migration	Eggs in feces	Usually mild; moderate to marked during migration	Aberrant wanderings may cause clinical disease
Hookworm	Larvae in soil; skin penetration	Small intestine	Vague abdominal distress; anemia in severe infections	Eggs in feces	Mild to moderate	Distinguish infection from disease
Whipworm	Fecal-oral	Large intestine	Rarely symptomatic	Eggs in feces	Absent to mild	
Strongyloidiasis	Larvae in soil; skin penetration	Upper small intestine	Duodenitis; hyperinfection syndrome rarely	Larvae in *fresh stool*; duodenal aspirate	Moderate to marked	
Pinworm	Fecal-oral	Large intestine, perianal area	Perianal pruritus	Scotch-tape swab for eggs; gross examination of area for worms	Absent	Very common; usually asymptomatic
Creeping eruption (cutaneous larva migrans)	Larvae in soil; skin penetration (larvae from dog, cat feces)	Skin	Intensely pruritic, serpiginous skin lesions	Physical examination	Variable	
Visceral larva migrans	Fecal-oral, via pica (eggs from dog, cat feces)	Liver, lung, muscle, eye	Fever, hepatosplenomegaly	Clinical diagnosis, serology	Marked	

Table 15-1. (continued)

Disease	Mode of spread	Location in humans	Clinical features	Laboratory diagnosis	Eosinophilia*	Remarks
Trichinosis	Ingestion of undercooked pork	Striated muscle	Fever, diarrhea, periorbital edema, muscle pain	Biopsy of muscle, skin; serologic tests	Marked	
Tapeworms (cestodes)						
Beef tapeworm	Ingestion of undercooked beef	Small intestine	Asymptomatic	Proglottid segments passed with feces	Absent	
Pork tapeworm	Ingestion of undercooked pork	Small intestine	Asymptomatic; rare autoinfection with CNS symptoms (cysticercosis)	Proglottid segments passed with feces, serology	Absent	
Fish tapeworm	Ingestion of raw or undercooked fish	Small intestine	Asymptomatic; rarely, vitamin B_{12} deficiency	Eggs in feces	Absent	
Hydatid disease	Fecal-oral (eggs from carnivore feces)	Liver, lung, bone, brain	Usually asymptomatic; occasionally, pressure symptoms in affected organ	Removal of cyst; skin and serologic tests	Variable	
Flukes (trematodes)						
Schistosoma mansoni	Cercarial in streams; skin penetration	Venules of large intestine	Fever, colitis, hepatomegaly, portal hypertension	Eggs in feces; rectal biopsy	Moderate to marked	Africa, S. America; common in Puerto Ricans
Schistosoma haematobium	Same	Venules of urinary bladder	Fever, malaise, hematuria	Eggs in urine; bladder or rectal biopsy	Moderate to marked	Africa

Schistosoma japonicum	Same	Venules of small intestine	Fever, malaise, abdominal pain, diarrhea, hepatomegaly	Eggs in feces; rectal biopsy	Moderate to marked	S.E. Asia
Protozoa Intestinal amebiasis	Fecal-oral	Lumen and wall of large intestine	Bloody diarrhea, fever, abdominal pain; mild, intermittent GI symptoms	Trophozoites in *fresh stool* or proctoscopic material, cysts in stool	Absent	
Extraintestinal amebiasis	Hematogenous dissemination from intestinal sites	Liver, lung	Hepatomegaly, fever	Trophozoites from abscess or sputum; serologic tests	Absent	
Giardiasis	Fecal-oral	Upper small intestine	Diarrhea, abdominal pain, malabsorption	Cysts and trophozoites or antigen in *fresh stool*; duodenal aspirate	Absent	
Toxoplasmosis	Congenital, raw meat, cat feces (?)	CNS, eye, reticuloendothelial system—potentially any organ	Congenital; acute mononucleosis-like illness; asymptomatic; disseminated in immunosuppressed host	Biopsy; serologic tests	Absent	

Table 15-1. (continued)

Disease	Mode of spread	Location in humans	Clinical features	Laboratory diagnosis	Eosinophilia*	Remarks
Malaria	Bite of infected *Anopheles* mosquito; transfusion or congenital acquisition rarely	Erythrocytes, hepatocytes	Fever, splenomegaly, anemia, thrombocytopenia; shock, encephalopathy with *Plasmodium falciparum*	Repeated blood smears	Absent	Important to distinguish *P. falciparum* from relapsing malarias
Pneumocytosis	Unknown	Lungs	Fever, cough, hypoxia, lung infiltrates in compromised host	Sputum; bronchial brushings; lung biopsy	Absent	Compromised host
Babesiosis	Bite of tick; transfusion	Erythrocytes, reticuloendothelial system	Resembles malaria	Repeated blood smears	Absent	Severe in asplenics; certain areas in US
Cryptosporidiosis	Fecal-oral	GI tract, intracellular	Explosive diarrhea, abdominal pain, flatulence	Oocysts or antigen in stool	Rare	Progressively severe in immunocompromised host

* Mild, 5–10%; moderate, 10–20%; marked, >20%.

b. The level of eosinophilia is of diagnostic aid. In general, tissue migratory helminths evoke a profound eosinophilia, and those that exist within the lumen of the bowel evoke a mild eosinophilia or none at all (see Table 15-1).

C. Direct identification of parasites. Many techniques are available to identify parasites in excreta, fluids, and tissue. Examination of specimens is usually done by hospital, public health, or private laboratories. However, several simple procedures, which require little equipment, are available that the physician can perform when the patient is seen. It is helpful to have charts of diagnostic stages of helminths and protozoa available for accurate interpretation. If more sophisticated procedures are needed, standard texts of parasitology can be consulted.

1. Blood

a. The **thin dry smear** is useful in detecting and speciating malarial parasites. The technique is identical to routine blood smears used for hematologic studies. Wright or Giesma stain is used in the usual fashion, and parasites are seen within red blood cells (RBCs). Species differentiation is of therapeutic importance once malaria parasites have been identified.

b. The **thick dry smear** for the detection of malaria parasites yields a much higher concentration of parasites than the thin smear and thus is useful when the parasites are few and thin smears are negative. However, the thick smear is harder to interpret, because the erythrocytes are lysed, and the parasites are seen on a background of stained proteinaceous debris, platelets, and residual nuclei of white blood cells (WBCs).

c. A recent adaption of the office-based complete blood count (CBC) technique with microcapillary tubes containing acridine orange (QBC tube, Becton-Dickinson, Franklin Lakes, NJ) could offer the rapid diagnosis of malaria (or filariasis) in an office/hospital setting with a minimum of expertise. However, fluorescence illumination is necessary for this procedure.

2. Stool. Examine feces as soon after passage as possible and before barium or cathartics are given. While helminth ova and protozoal cysts can be easily identified in preserved or older specimens, the identification of free-living, motile forms of most protozoa requires the examination of liquid stool within 30 minutes or same-day examination of formed stool.

a. **Direct examination** of stool enables the rapid identification of intestinal parasites. Free-living, motile forms and ova and cysts can be identified, particularly if there is a heavy infestation. The procedure takes a few minutes and makes use of supplies found in all laboratories.

(1) Examine the specimen grossly for flecks of blood and mucus. If present, take a sample from these areas.

(2) Place a match head–sized sample on each of two microscope slides with a wooden applicator.

(3) Mix one sample with two drops of saline and cover with cover slip.

(4) Add two drops of dilute iodine solution to the other sample, mix, and cover similarly.

(5) Observe for the presence of erythrocytes and leukocytes. **Erythrocytes** suggest amebic colitis, and **leukocytes** suggest bacterial infection or inflammatory bowel disease and *not* parasitic infection. A Wright stain may be indicated.

(6) Examine the stained slide for the presence of helminth eggs under low power and for protozoal cysts under high power and oil immersion.

(7) Examine the unstained slide under low and high power for the presence of motile organisms (amebas, trophozoites, larvae).

b. **Concentration.** Two commonly used procedures for concentration of specimens are the formalin-ether sedimentation or zinc sulfate flotation methods. A useful reference is D. M. Melvin and M. M. Brooke, *Laboratory Procedures for the Diagnosis of Intestinal Parasites* (3rd ed.), U.S.

Dept. of Health, Education, and Welfare, Public Health Service, publication (#CDC 82-8282, 1982).

   c. **Preservation of specimens.** Polyvinyl alcohol (PVA) or formalin-based fixatives are readily available for specimens that cannot be examined promptly. PVA is particularly useful when protozoan parasites are suspected or permanent stains are desired.

   d. **Scotch-tape examination** is a useful and simple technique for the demonstration of pinworm eggs.

   (1) Evert a strip of Scotch tape, gummed side outward, on the edge of a tongue blade.

   (2) Dab the perianal area first thing in the morning.

   (3) Place on a microscope slide, sticky side down, on a drop of toluene.

   (4) Examine under low power for characteristic eggs.

   e. **Coproimmunodiagnostic tests** are now commercially available for *Giardia* and *Cryptosporidium*. Both are based on detection of parasite antigens in stool specimens and appear to offer increased sensitivity over standard microscopic methods.

D. Serologic tests in parasitic diseases

   1. Immunodiagnostic tests are helpful in several parasitic infections. They are to be used and interpreted **in conjunction with** clinical and laboratory evaluation and should not be solely relied on for diagnosis.

   2. Serologic tests are specifically helpful in invasive amebiasis, **Toxocara** infection, cysticercosis, trichinosis, toxoplasmosis, and possibly echinococcosis.

   3. The serologic tests referred to in Table 15-1 are performed at the Centers for Disease Control (CDC), Atlanta, GA, and by some local health departments.

II. Principles of treatment

A. In general all protozoal or helminth infections are treated. For specific treatment regimens, see sec. III, where the drug of choice is listed, followed by alternatives (other ref: *Med. Let. Drugs Ther* 30:15–24, 1988). All regimens are to be administered PO unless otherwise indicated. The availability and efficacy of therapeutic agents and their expected side effects and toxicity are listed in Table 15-2. Exceptions to treatment are usually in highly endemic areas with low parasitic burden and in patients with minimal or no symptomatology. Also, certain protozoa are considered commensals and are not usually treated. These include *Trichomonas tenax* and *hominis*; *Enteromonas hominis*; *Chilomastix mesnili*; *Entamoeba coli, hartmani,* or *polecki*; *Endolimax nana*; and *Iodamoeba bütschlii*. However, if the patients are **symptomatic** (usually chronic gastrointestinal complaints) and no other etiology is identified, treatment should be considered.

B. Follow-up clinical and laboratory assessment is always indicated to determine if treatment has been effective. Stools should be examined several weeks after the treatment of intestinal parasites is completed, and retreatment given if a cure has not been achieved. In general, retreatment with the same drug is more desirable than proceeding to an alternative agent that is more toxic, less efficacious, or both. The exception to this rule is treatment of *Plasmodium falciparum* infections, in which drug resistance is an increasing problem.

C. Patient education. The physician should always combine treatment with patient education aimed at prevention of future parasitic infection. Attention should be given to the environmental circumstances that resulted in the child's acquisition of infection.

III. Specific parasites

A. Roundworms (nematodes)

   1. *Ascaris*

   a. **Etiology.** Fecal-oral passage of infective ova of *Ascaris lumbricoides*. The human is the only susceptible host. The infection is worldwide in distribution.

   b. **Evaluation.** Two distinct clinical phases occur:

   (1) **Transient tissue migration phase of the larvae.** This is marked by

Table 15-2. Adverse effects of antiparasitic drugs

Drug	Frequent	Infrequent
Chloroquine phosphate (Aralen Phosphate)	Anorexia, nausea, visual disturbances	Retinopathy—only with prolonged, high dosage
Dehydroemetine	Diarrhea, nausea, vomiting, myalgias, ECG changes	Hypotension
Diiodohydroxyquine, USP		Rash, acne, slight thyroid enlargement, nausea, diarrhea, cramps, anal pruritus, optic atrophy and vision loss in children after prolonged use in high dosage for months
Diloxanide furoate (Furamide)	Flatulence	Nausea, vomiting, diarrhea, urticaria, pruritus
Furazolidone (Furoxone)		Anorexia, nausea, hypersensitivity reactions*
Mebendazole (Vermox) **contraindicated in pregnancy**		Diarrhea, abdominal pain
Metronidazole* (Flagyl) **contraindicated in first trimester**	Anorexia, nausea, vomiting, metallic taste	Peripheral neuropathy, ataxia, neutropenia
Niclosamide (Yomesan)		Nausea
Paromomycin (Humatin)	Anorexia, nausea, vomiting	Nephrotoxicity
Pentamidine isethionate	Dizziness, tachycardia, headache, vomiting, hypotension, pancreatitis	Nephrotoxicity, hepatotoxicity
Piperazine citrate (Antepar)		Anorexia, rash, ataxia
Primaquine phosphate	Anorexia, nausea	Hemolytic anemia in G-6-PD deficiency, methemoglobinemia
Pyrantel pamoate (Antiminth)	Anorexia, nausea	
Pyrimethamine (Daraprim) **contraindicated in pregnancy**		Folate-deficient macrocytic anemia
Pyrvinium pamoate (Povan)	Anorexia, nausea, red-colored stool	
Quinacrine HCl (Atabrine Hydrochloride)	Nausea, vomiting, dizziness	Psychoses, exfoliative dermatitis, hepatic necrosis, yellowing of skin
Quinine sulfate	Tinnitus, nausea, vomiting, vertigo	Hypotension, hemolytic anemia
Thiabendazole (Mintezol)	Anorexia, nausea, vomiting, dizziness	Tinnitus, drowsiness, shock
Trimethoprim-sulfamethoxazole (Bactrim, Septra)		Rash, hemolytic anemia, bone marrow suppression

G-6-PD = glucose 6-phosphate, dehydrogenase.

*Carcinogenic in rats and mutagenic in bacteria (see *Med. Lett. Drugs Ther.* 17:53, 1975). Significance for humans not known.

focal hypersensitivity reactions, peripheral eosinophilia, and hyper-
-immunoglobulin E (IgE). Intensity of host reactions, and therefore
symptoms, vary greatly, but in general are proportional to worm
burden. The reactions are usually greatest in the pulmonary/alveolar
phase. When present, the symptoms vary from slight cough to severe
seasonal pneumonitis.

(2) **Prolonged intestinal phase of the adults.** The patients, when symptomatic, generally have vague abdominal pain, or peptic ulcer–like
symptoms occur. The most common, although rare, complication is
intestinal obstruction.

c. The **diagnosis** is confirmed by detection of characteristic ova in feces by
direct examination or concentration techniques or by regurgitation or
stool passage of adult worms.

d. **Treatment.** The occasional aberrant wanderings of individual worms and
subsequent serious consequences require that **all** *Ascaris* infections be
treated.

(1) *Ascaris* **pneumonitis.** Symptomatic treatment

(2) **Intestinal ascariasis**

(a) Pyrantel pamoate, 11 mg/kg in one dose (maximum 1 gm), or

(b) Mebendazole, 100 mg bid for 3 days for children 2 years old or
older, or

(c) Piperazine citrate, 75 mg/kg/day for 2 days (maximum 3.5 gm-
/day)

e. **Prevention.** Sanitary disposal of feces

2. **Hookworm**

a. **Etiology**

(1) Human hookworms belong to two genera, *Necator* and *Ancylostoma*.
The former is prevalent in the southern United States, South and
Central America, Asia, and Africa. The latter is rarely seen in the
United States.

(2) Infections spread by skin penetration of soil-living larvae hatched
from eggs passed in infected feces.

b. **Evaluation.** Three clinical phases of hookworm infection are recognized:

(1) **Penetration of the skin by larvae.** A local papulovesicular dermatitis
lasting 7–10 days is common, as is secondary bacterial infection of the
lesions.

(2) **Transient tissue migration by larvae.** A generally mild pneumonitis
with peripheral eosinophilia is rarely recognized except in experimental infections.

(3) The **prolonged intestinal phase** results from the attachment of
blood-feeding adult worms to the small intestinal mucosa of the host.
Symptomatology is generally related to worm burden.

(a) **Light hookworm infestations** are usually asymptomatic; when
they are symptomatic, epigastric discomfort is the most common
complaint. Infection is confirmed by demonstrating hookworm
ova in feces.

(b) **Heavy hookworm infestations.** Large numbers of worms are
present, and significant blood loss occurs. The most common
symptoms are those of chronic iron deficiency anemia (lassitude,
dyspnea, growth retardation), hypoproteinemia (edema), and
protein-losing enteropathy.

c. **Diagnosis.** The demonstration of large numbers of hookworm ova in the
feces (>400 eggs per gram of stool) by any standard concentration
method. Species differentiation can be difficult and is usually made by
geographic area of acquisition.

d. **Treatment**

(1) **Drugs**

(a) Mebendazole, 100 mg bid for 3 days for children $\geq$ 2 years old

(b) Pyrantel pamoate, 11–20 mg/kg in one dose (maximum 1 gm)

(c) Thiabendazole, 50 mg/kg/day in divided doses bid for 2 days (maximum 3 gm/day)

(2) Iron supplementation should be given to patients with hookworm disease.

e. **Prevention.** Sanitary disposal of feces and wearing of shoes to prevent contact of bare feet with contaminated soil

3. **Whipworm**
   a. **Etiology.** Fecal-oral spread of *Trichuris trichiura*. The infection is worldwide, and the human is the natural reservoir and only susceptible host. The adult localizes to the cecum and lives in continuous intimate tissue contact.
   b. **Evaluation and diagnosis**
      (1) When present, symptoms are usually those of colitis. Severity of symptoms is usually related to chronicity and worm burden. Occasionally, patients present with acute dysentery-like symptoms or rectal prolapse.
      (2) The presence of typical ova in feces by direct fecal smear or concentration techniques is diagnostic.
      (3) Eosinophilia is not associated with trichuriasis, and its presence should suggest another parasitic infection.
   c. **Treatment.** Mebandazole, 100 mg bid for 3 days, to children ≥ 2 years old.
   d. **Prevention.** Sanitary fecal disposal and wearing of shoes to prevent skin penetration by the larvae.

4. **Pinworm**
   a. **Etiology.** Fecal-oral spread of *Enterobius vermicularis*, a 4-mm worm just visible to the naked eye and the most common helminth found in humans in the United States. Autoinfection is quite common. Humans are the only known hosts.
   b. **Evaluation and diagnosis**
      (1) Perianal itching, vulvitis, and vaginitis in young children suggest the presence of pinworms. Symptoms may be intense enough to cause insomnia, restlessness, hyperactivity, and nocturnal enuresis.
      (2) Adult worms may be seen in the perianal area and on the surface of freshly passed feces, particularly in the early morning.
      (3) Characteristic ova are demonstrated by Scotch-tape swab (see sec. **I.C.2.d.**). Examination should be made first thing in the morning and repeated on consecutive days if necessary. *A single swabbing reveals only about 50 percent of infections*; three swabbings will uncover 90 percent; and, although uncommonly done in practice, five examinations are required to exclude the possibility of infection. Scrapings from beneath the fingernails may show eggs in 30 percent of infected children.
      (4) If diagnostic procedures fail to reveal pinworms, a therapeutic trial is reasonable in markedly symptomatic children.
   c. **Treatment.** Initial treatment of single infected members in a household is most reasonable. If reinfection occurs or if more than one member is infested, all members of a household should be treated simultaneously.
      (1) Mebendazole, 100 mg in one dose for children ≥ 2 years old; repeat after 2 weeks, or
      (2) Pyrantel pamoate, 10–20 mg/kg in one dose (maximum 1 gm); repeat after 2 weeks
      (3) Recurrence after treatment is not uncommon. Some regimens include routine retreatment after 2 months.
   d. **Prevention.** Boiling of sheets, undergarments, pajamas, and the like is of little or no value. Hand washing and fingernail cleanliness may reduce transmission and autoinfection. Simply changing and washing sheets and undergarments is reasonable, as is morning showering or washing of the perianal area.

5. Strongyloides
   a. Etiology. Skin penetration of *Strongyloides stercoralis* larvae passed in infected feces. Autoinfection may occur.
   b. Evaluation and diagnosis. Most children are asymptomatic.
      (1) The most common symptoms are cutaneous (urticarial eruptions) and gastrointestinal (abdominal pain, diarrhea).
      (2) Larvae (not ova) are found in freshly passed feces or by aspiration of duodenal contents.
      (3) Infections are associated with a moderate to marked eosinophilia.
      (4) Fatal, overwhelming disseminated infection may occur in children who harbor this parasite and who are undergoing immunosuppression.
   c. Treatment. Thiabendazole, 25 mg/kg bid for 2 days (maximum 3 gm/day). All patients should have a repeat stool examination in 6–12 months.
   d. Prevention. Sanitary disposal of feces and wearing of shoes.
6. Visceral larva migrans
   a. Etiology. Ingestion of the ova of dog and cat ascarids, *Toxocara canis,* and *Toxocara cati.* Larvae emerge in the intestine and migrate extensively throughout the body.
   b. Evaluation and diagnosis
      (1) Most infections are asymptomatic. The most common presenting symptom is fever. Other signs include wheezing or coughing, hepatomegaly, and occasional pulmonary infiltrates. Rare fatal cases involve myocardial or central nervous system invasion. Ocular involvement (endophthalmitis or retinal granulomas) is not uncommon, is usually seen in older children, and rarely occurs with other systemic symptoms.
      (2) Hypergammaglobulinemia, marked elevation of isohemagglutinins, marked eosinophilia (20% or more), and leukocytosis are present.
      (3) The parasite is rarely demonstrated; stool examination and tissue biopsy are useless. Serologic testing (enzyme-linked immunosorbent assay [ELISA]) by the CDC, Atlanta, GA, is sensitive and specific.
   c. Treatment
      (1) The disease is often mild and self-limited, lasting several weeks. Specific treatment is usually unnecessary.
      (2) In severe cases, or in patients with ocular involvement, antihelminthic therapy may be beneficial.
         (a) Thiabendazole, 50 mg/kg/day in divided doses bid for 5 days (maximum 3 gm/day), **or**
         (b) Diethylcarbamazine, 6–12 mg/kg/day in divided doses tid for 7–10 days
      (3) Antiinflammatory therapy with corticosteroids or antihistamines, or both, may offer relief of severe symptoms. Corticosteroids should be used in conjunction with antihelminthics in treating ocular disease.
      (4) Thiabendazole (for 2 days) can be used for treating cutaneous larva migrans.
      (5) Eosinophilia may persist for months despite therapy.
   d. Prevention. Avoidance of contamination of play and work areas by dog and cat feces. Periodic deworming of puppies and kittens is an important control measure.
7. Trichinosis
   a. Etiology. Ingestion of raw meat containing encysted larvae of *Trichinella spiralis* (pork is the principal source of human infection). The infection is more common in temperate than in tropical environments.
   b. Evaluation and diagnosis
      (1) A history of ingestion of uncooked or undercooked pork or carnivorous game. Homemade sausage is a common source of infection.
      (2) The clinical picture may suggest the diagnosis, but is often unclear until the second or third week of infection. At this time the full-blown

picture of fever, facial and periorbital edema, headache, photophobia, conjunctivitis, and severe muscle pain and tenderness may develop. Signs of encephalitis, meningitis, and myocarditis may appear later in the illness.

(3) A muscle biopsy specimen may reveal the characteristic larvae. Histologic examination of tissue for the presence of an inflammatory reaction is essential to confirm **recent** infection. A negative biopsy does not rule out the diagnosis.

(4) Marked peripheral eosinophilia (in 20–80%) after the third week of infection, which may persist for months

(5) Agglutination or flocculation reactions with rising titer demonstrated on paired samples are an important confirmatory test (tests turn positive in the third week of infection and may remain positive for months to years).

  c. **Treatment**

(1) Thiabendazole in a dose of 25 mg/kg/dose given bid for 5 days (maximum 3 gm/day)

(2) Corticosteroids may ameliorate severe symptoms.

  d. **Prevention.** Consumption of only well-cooked pork. Pork is *not* inspected for trichinosis in the United States.

B. **Tapeworms (cestodes)**

1. **Beef tapeworm**

  a. **Etiology.** The disease is transmitted by the ingestion of undercooked beef containing *Taenia saginata* larval cysts. The infection is worldwide in distribution; the human is the definitive host, and cattle are the intermediate host.

  b. **Evaluation and diagnosis.** Most patients are asymptomatic, and the infection is noted only when migrating proglottids pass through the anus. Observation of gravid proglottids is diagnostic.

  c. **Treatment**

(1) **Niclosamide** achieves a 90 percent cure rate.

    (a) No prior bowel preparation is required, but tablets should be chewed thoroughly. The dosage is as follows:

    (b) 34–50 kg, 1.5 gm in one dose

    (c) >50 kg, 2 gm in one dose

    (d) The worm will be macerated, and search for the scolex (head) is thus unprofitable.

    (e) Retreat if proglottids reappear in subsequent months.

(2) **Praziquantel,** 10–20 mg/kg once

  d. **Prevention.** Thorough cooking of beef

2. **Pork tapeworm, adult worm infection**

  a. **Etiology.** Ingestion of undercooked pork containing larval cysts (cysticerci) of *Taenia solium*

  b. **Evaluation and diagnosis.** Adult worms rarely produce symptoms. The passage of gravid motile proglottids through the anus raises the suspicion of infection. Confirmation is obtained by laboratory examination of the proglottid.

  c. **Treatment.** Same as for beef tapeworm (see above)

  d. **Prevention.** Thorough cooking of pork

3. **Pork tapeworm, cysticercosis**

  a. **Etiology.** Ingestion or autoinfection with eggs of *T. solium* from food or water contaminated with human feces results in systemic infection by the larval stage of the organism involving muscle, subcutaneous tissues, eye, and brain. The larvae form cysts (cysticerci), which remain viable for at least 3–5 years. Symptoms of infection do not occur until death of the cysticerci invokes an inflammatory response. Clinical presentation of cerebral cysticercosis is often focal seizures years after infection.

  b. **Evaluation and diagnosis.** Unexplained seizures in persons from endemic areas should raise suspicion. A computed tomographic (CT) scan may reveal single or multiple calcified or enhancing space-occupying lesions. Serologic studies can be done at the CDC, Atlanta.

c. **Treatment.** Medical therapy, once limited to anticonvulsants, now is aimed at speeding the resolution of noncalcified lesions and minimizing neurologic signs and symptoms. Both praziquantel and albendazole are superior to no therapy as monitored by CT resolution of active neurocysticercosis. Dexamethasone is usually administered simultaneously to minimize deleterious effects of the inflammatory response, which is increased after administration of praziquantel or albendazole. Of note, cerebrospinal fluid (CSF) concentrations of praziquantel are decreased, whereas the CSF concentration of albendazole appears to increase by simultaneous administration of dexamethasone. The role of surgical therapy has traditionally been alleviation of obstruction or mass effect. Surgical excision is no longer common and is limited to lesions that are easily accessible.

d. **Prevention.** Avoid contact with infected human feces. Avoid undercooked meat.

4. **Hydatid disease**
   a. **Etiology.** Humans are infected by ingesting the eggs of *Echinococcus granulosus* passed in the feces of carnivores.
   b. **Evaluation and diagnosis.**
      (1) A slowly growing, usually asymptomatic cyst in the proper epidemiologic setting suggests the diagnosis. Two thirds occur in the liver and one fourth in the lung, and the remainder are widely scattered.
      (2) The **x-ray** appearance (of a mass with a calcified rim) is typical but not pathognomonic.
      (3) Serologic tests are positive in the majority of cases.
      (4) Demonstration of the characteristic gross and histolic appearance on removal of the cyst. **(Aspiration is dangerous and should not be done.)**
   c. **Treatment.** Easily accessible cysts are removed surgically. Most cysts are asymptomatic and can, in fact, be left untreated. Freezing of the cyst and subsequent surgical removal have given favorable results (*N. Engl. J. Med.* 284:1346, 1971). When surgery is contraindicated or if cysts rupture spontaneously during surgery, albendazole may also be useful, 10 mg/kg/day for 28 days, repeated as necessary.
   d. *Echinococcus multilocularis* has a life cycle similar to that of *E. granulosus,* but adult worms reside in foxes. The larvae reside in small wild rodents. Infected dogs and other sources of egg contamination represent the link to occasional human infection. *E. multilocularis* is found mainly in Alaska, Canada, Siberia, and central Europe. In humans, larvae form irregular, alveolar cysts. The germinative tissues spread rapidly to produce neoplasm-like growths that are difficult to manage surgically. However, surgical excision is the only reliable means of therapy. Albendazole or mebendazole may have some benefit (*Am. J. Trop. Med. Hyg.* 37:162, 1987; *Bull. WHO* 64:383, 1986). Prevention is focused on keeping dogs free of infection.

5. **Fish tapeworm**
   a. **Etiology.** The disease is transmitted by the ingestion of undercooked or raw fish containing *Diphyllobothrium latum* larvae. The infection is worldwide, but it is concentrated in the cool lake regions of the major continents (e.g., in the Great Lakes region).
   b. **Evaluation and diagnosis.** Most patients are asymptomatic, although, rarely, a vitamin B_{12} deficiency state may occur, caused by the adult worms' capacity to take up vitamin B_{12} in the upper small intestine. Mild abdominal symptoms may occur. Characteristic eggs are passed in the stool.
   c. **Treatment.** Give niclosamide as in **B.1.c.(1).**
   d. **Precaution.** Fish should be cooked properly.

C. Protozoa
1. Amebiasis
   a. **Etiology.** Fecal-oral passage of cysts of *Entamoeba histolytica*. Amebiasis is worldwide in distribution, and the human is the only known host. Sporadic localized epidemics occur in the United States, and the disease is endemic in many institutionalized populations. Recent studies suggest that there are at least two morphologically indistinct species of *E. histolytica*, which can be distinguished by monoclonal antibodies, growth phenotyes, and DNA probes as *pathogenic* and *nonpathogenic* forms.
   b. **Evaluation and diagnosis**
      (1) **Intestinal amebiasis**
         (a) Intestinal amebiasis varies in presentation from the asymptomatic carrier state (by far the most common) to fulminant colonic disease.
            (i) **Mild colonic infection** is characterized by alternating diarrhea and constipation.
            (ii) **Amebic dysentery** presents most frequently as subacute illness. Mild tenderness, bloody diarrhea, low-grade fever, weakness, and malaise are characteristic. The tempo of the illness may clinically distinguish it from more acute, bacillary dysentery. Abdominal tenderness is common, particularly over the sigmoid and cecal areas; appendicitis is sometimes erroneously diagnosed.
         (b) Confirmation in acute cases is obtained by demonstrating motile amebic trophozoites in **fresh stool**, or cysts in the carrier state. Proctoscopy may be useful if multiple stool samples are negative.
         (c) Erythrocytes are plentiful and leukocytes are minimal in the stool, which is helpful in distinguishing between amebic and bacillary dysentery.
         (d) Eosinophilia is *not* found.
      (2) **Extraintestinal amebiasis** most commonly affects the liver.
         (a) Disease may occur without the signs or symptoms of intestinal infection. Fever, chills, or enlarged tender liver, elevated right diaphragm, minimal liver function abnormalities, and the finding of a filling defect on liver scan are highly suggestive. Of all amebic abscesses, 95 percent are single and situated in the upper part of the right lobe of the liver.
         (b) Serologic tests for invasive amebiasis (indirect hemagglutination, counter immunoelectrophoresis, complement fixation) are extremely accurate.
         (c) Percutaneous liver aspiration is recommended in large abscesses only. Aspirated material may show amebas. However, their absence does not rule out hepatic infection, since organisms tend to be located at the margins of the abscess.
         (d) A therapeutic trial is an accepted diagnostic measure **in a severely ill patient.**
   c. **Treatment**
      (1) **All stages** of amebiasis are treated at the present time.
         (a) **Asymptomatic carrier state**
            (i) Diiodohydroxyquin, 30–40 mg/kg/day in divided doses tid for 20 days (maximum 2 gm/day), or
            (ii) Diloxanide furoate, 20 mg/kg/day in divided doses tid for 10 days (maximum 1.5 gm/day)
         (b) **Intestinal infection**
            (i) Metronidazole, 35–50 mg/kg/day in divided doses tid for 10 days (maximum 2.25 gm/day)
            (ii) As a second choice, paromomycin, 25–30 mg/kg/day in divided doses tid for 5–10 days, can be used alone.
            (iii) In severe cases, use metronidazole, 35–50 mg/kg/day in

divided doses tid for 10 days (maximum 2.25 gm/day), **and** diiodohydroxyquin as above. For alternative therapy, use dehydroemetine hydrochloride, 1.0–1.5 mg/kg/day intramuscularly for 5 days (maximum 90 mg/day), **and** diiodohydroxyquin as above.

   (c) Hepatic infection
      (i) Metronidazole, as in **(b)**, and
      (ii) Diiodohydroxyquin, as in **(a)**, or
      (iii) Dehydroemetine, as in **(b)**, followed by
      (iv) Chloroquine phosphate, 10 mg base/kg/day for 21 days (maximum 300 mg base/day), **and**
      (v) Diiodohydroxyquin, as in **(a)**
  (2) In addition to specific amebicidal therapy, **supportive care** is important in invasive amebiasis. Hospitalization, bed rest, and good nutritional intake may contribute to rapid recovery.
  (3) Follow-up stool examinations should be done at 1- and 2-month intervals to ensure that a cure has been achieved.
  (4) Once tests for a pathogenic/nonpathogenic species are more widely available, treatment recommendations for asymptomatic carriers will probably change.
 d. Prevention. Sanitary disposal of feces and treatment of asymptomatic cyst passers

2. Giardiasis
 a. Etiology. Fecal-oral spread of *Giardia lamblia*. Infection is worldwide and is common in institutionalized and day care populations.
 b. Evaluation and diagnosis
  (1) Most infestations are asymptomatic. Abdominal discomfort, a bloated feeling, and diarrhea are the most common complaints, usually lasting 7–10 days but, not uncommonly, longer. The diarrhea is not bloody; stools may be bulky and offensive. Steatorrhea and malabsorption, including lactose intolerance, may occur.
  (2) The diagnosis is confirmed by the demonstration of characteristic motile trophozoites in **fresh diarrheal stool** or **duodenal aspirate** by direct examination. Cysts may be seen in formed stools by direct or concentration methods.
  (3) A coproimmunodiagnostic kit is available that is generally more sensitive than stool examination (Alexon Inc., Mountain View, CA).
 c. Treatment
  (1) Specific therapy is highly effective.
    (a) Furazolidone suspension, 5 mg/kg/day in divided doses qid for 7–10 days.
    (b) Metronidazole, 15 mg/kg/day in divided doses tid for 5–10 days (maximum 750 mg/day)
    (c) Quinacrine, 6–9 mg/kg/day in divided doses tid for 5–7 days (maximum 300 mg/day)
  (2) Supportive measures and restoration of nutritional status are important in patients with malabsorption.
 d. Prevention. Sanitary disposal of feces

3. Malaria
 a. Etiology. Malaria, among the most *lethal* of worldwide human infections, is transmitted by the bite of an *Anopheles* mosquito infected with *Plasmodium*. Four species of *Plasmodium* infect humans: *P. falciparum, P. vivax, P. ovale,* and *P. malariae. P. falciparum* is the most lethal of the four and also presents the problem of drug resistance.
 b. Evaluation and diagnosis
  (1) The most important factor when considering the diagnosis of malaria is the patient's immune status with respect to malaria. *P. falciparum* malaria in a nonimmune patient is a much more rapidly fatal disease.
  (2) The clinical manifestations of malaria infection are protean. Fever,

rigors, malaise, headaches, myalgias, and arthralgias commonly occur in acute infections. **Splenomegaly** is the most consistent physical finding. In children, GI complaints, including loss of appetite, vomiting, or diarrhea, may predominate particularly in nonimmunes. In infants, pallor or jaundice is also seen.

(3) Fever in a nonimmune individual with *P. falciparum* is rarely periodic. The fever pattern may become periodic *after* infection is well established (patients from endemic areas): q48h in *P. vivax* and *P. ovale* infections, q72h in *P. malariae* infections, and q36–48h in *P. falciparum* malaria. Typically, the patient appears well between fever paroxysms.

(4) **It is exceedingly important in a nonimmune individual to distinguish between relapsing malaria *(vivax and ovale)* and falciparum malaria** (Table 15-3). Documented malarial infections in nonimmune individuals should be treated as falciparum malaria. Mixed infections do occur, and one should be aware of this possibility. Textbooks of parasitology should be consulted to aid in species differentiation.

(5) The complications of *P. falciparum* infection include cerebral malaria (presenting as coma, delirium, and convulsions), massive hemolysis, disseminated intravascular coagulation, renal failure, pulmonary edema, and cardiovascular collapse.

(6) A history of residence or travel in an endemic area is almost always elicited.

(7) **The diagnosis rests on the demonstration of malaria parasites in the peripheral blood.**

(8) Nonimmune individuals are usually symptomatic with very low parasitemias. Therefore, a single negative blood smear **does not rule out malaria.** Serial smears over 48–72 hours should be done if no other source of fever or symptoms can be identified.

c. **Treatment.** The choice of antimalarial drugs depends on the infecting species and the geographic area of acquisition in infection.

(1) *P. falciparum* **infections in nonimmune individuals, even when the level of parasitemia is low, should be treated immediately. The patient should be observed in the hospital until clinical improvement or a decrease in parasitemia is noted.** *P. falciparum* infections in individuals from indigenous areas can be treated on an outpatient basis, based on clinical symptoms with follow-up blood smears at 7 and 28 days. Malaria, other than that caused by *P. falciparum*, can be treated on an outpatient basis.

(2) **Falciparum infections** acquired anywhere **except** the Caribbean, north of the Panama Canal, and most Middle Eastern countries are

Table 15-3. Differentiation of malarial parasites.

Falciparum	Relapsing
Small monotony of ring forms	Large ring forms
No (rare) late trophozoites	
Pathognomonic, crescent-shaped gametocytes	Late trophozoite and schizonts common
Rings frequently with two chromatin dots	Rings rarely with two chromatin dots
No Schüffner's dots	Schüffner's dots (*Plasmodium vivax* and *P. ovale*)
Parasites at margins of red blood cells	Parasites usually central
More than one parasite per red blood cell	Usually only one parasite per red blood cell

potentially chloroquine resistant. Alternative drugs should be given, as outlined in **(5)(b)**.

(3) In **relapsing malaria**, therapy must be directed against both the erythrocytic and exoerythrocytic parasites to prevent relapse. There is no resistance to chloroquine, but relapse may occur if this agent is used alone.

(4) In addition to vigorous antimalarial therapy, the complications of falciparum malaria require intensive supportive measures. Transfusions with packed RBCs are given in severe hemolytic anemia. Mannitol can be used in renal failure, and dialysis may be necessary. Careful attention to fluid and electrolyte balance is essential. Anticonvulsants are often required in cerebral malaria.

(5) **Recommended treatment regimens.** Given the rapidly evolving problem of drug resistance in malaria, the CDC maintains a 24-hour-a-day service for treatment and prophylaxis recommendations: 404-639-1610.

   (a) **Relapsing malaria**

     (i) Chloroquine phosphate, 10 mg base/kg (16.6 mg/kg salt) PO (or IM if necessary), followed by 5 mg/kg 6 hours later, then 5 mg/kg/day for 2 days, **and**

     (ii) Primaquine, 0.3 mg/kg/day for 14 days (maximum 15 mg base/day). **All patients at risk for glucose 6-phosphate dehydrogenase deficiency should be screened before therapy with primaquine.**

   (b) **Falciparum malaria**

     (i) **Nonchloroquine-resistant area**

     Chloroquine phosphate, as in **(a)**

     (ii) **Chloroquine-resistant area**

     Quinine sulfate, 25 mg/kg/day in divided doses tid for 3 days (maximum 2 gm/day), **and**

     Pyrimethamine

     < 10 kg, 6.25 mg per day for 3 days

     10–20 kg, 12.5 mg per day for 3 days

     20–40 kg, 25 mg per day for 3 days

     >40 kg, 50 mg per day in divided doses bid for 3 days, **and**

     Sulfadiazine, 100–200 mg/kg/day in divided doses qid for 5 days (maximum 2 gm/day)

     If the patient is critically ill and unable to take medication PO, use quinine dihydrochloride intravenously in a dosage of 25 mg/kg/day. Give one-half dose over 1 hour, then one-half dose 6–8 hours later if oral therapy still cannot be started. (Dilute medication to a concentration of 0.5–1.0 mg/ml in normal saline, and infuse at a rate of 0.5–1.0 mg/min with electrocardiographic [ECG] and blood pressure monitoring; maximum 1,800 mg/day.) Protocols using IV quinidine have also been established.

     (iii) **Multiply resistant areas.** Should standard therapy fail in areas with multiply resistant strains of *P. falciparum* (currently limited to eastern Thailand), the combination of quinine (as above) and tetracycline (5 mg/kg qid for 7 days) is recommended.

(6) Response to therapy is followed by dramatic clinical improvement. Repeated blood smears show disappearance of parasitemia. **Pyrimethamine and primaquine are contraindicated in pregnancy.**

  d. **Prevention.** Barrier protection from mosquitoes should be practiced whenever possible, especially between dusk and dawn. Persons traveling through or residing in malarious areas should receive prophylactic suppressive therapy as follow ·.

   (1) **Chloroquine-sensitive area**

(a) Chloroquine phosphate, 5 mg base/kg (8.3 mg salt/kg; maximum 300 mg base) once a week, to be started 1 week before travel and continued for 4 weeks after the last exposure

(b) To prevent relapsing malaria, a 14-day course of primaquine should be taken concurrently with the final 2 weeks of chloroquine therapy.

(2) **Chloroquine-resistant area.**

(a) For children $\geq$ 15 kg, weekly mefloquine can be used for prophylaxis (15-19 kg, ¼ tablet; 20-30 kg, ½ tablet; 31-45 kg, ¾ tablet).

(b) For children $\geq$ 9 years of age, doxycycline (2 mg/kg;day; maximum 100 mg/day) can be used.

(c) For smaller and younger children, recommendations are more complex and should be done in consultation with a Traveler's Clinic or the CDC.

4. **Toxoplasmosis**

a. **Etiology.** *Toxoplasma gondii,* an obligate intracellular parasite, is responsible for this infection. Congenital transmission has been clearly established. The mode of acquisition of postnatally acquired infection remains obscure. Transmission by meat ingestion and spread by cat feces are strong possibilities.

b. **Evaluation and diagnosis**

(1) Infection is largely asymptomatic. Serologic evidence of prior infection is demonstrated in 25-40 percent of the population of the United States. Several symptomatic forms are recognized:

(a) **Congenital infection** is always the result of acute infection in a previously seronegative mother. The clinical symptoms at birth vary from asymptomatic to severely affected (TORCH syndrome), usually dependent on the timing of the in utero infection. A number of subclinically infected infants, asymptomatic at birth, may be found to have chorioretinitis, mental retardation, or learning problems later in life.

(b) **Acquired infection** shows clinical variations ranging from a mild virus-like illness with lymphadenopathy to chorioretinitis without systemic illness. Fatal, usually focal, disease (pneumonia and encephalitis), which is nearly always reactivation disease, can occur in the compromised host.

(2) Demonstration of **rising antibody titers** by complement fixation (CF), hemagglutination (HA), indirect fluorescent antibody tests (IFA), and the Sabin-Feldman dye test establishes the diagnosis. Newborn infections can be diagnosed by demonstration of IgM *Toxoplasma* antibodies or the persistence of high titers of CF, HA, or IFA beyond 4 months of age.

(3) Rarely, in special circumstances, the diagnosis may be established by the demonstration of organisms in tissue sections or smears of body fluids. Intraperitoneal mouse inoculation is required for isolation. To determine if an infection is recent, however, rising serologic titers are still required.

c. **Treatment**

(1) **Congenital infection.** Protocols for length of therapy are presently being evaluated. The current recommendation is for a one-year course of therapy.

(a) Pyrimethamine, 1 mg/kg/day for the initial few weeks, then change to qod

(b) Sulfadiazine, 85 mg/kg/day divided bid

(c) Supplementation with folinic acid is recommended (5 mg every 3 days).

(d) Consider additional corticosteroid therapy for active inflammatory overt congenital disease.

(e) For a concise discussion of therapeutic regimens, see J. S. Remington and G. Desmonts, Toxoplasmosis. In J. S. Remington and J. O. Klein (Eds.), *Infectious Diseases of the Fetus and Newborn Infant* (3rd ed.). Philadelphia: Saunders, 1990.

(2) Acquired infection. Treatment depends on the clinical severity of the illness. Dosagae for pyrimethamine is the same as for congenital infection. Dosage for sulfadiazine should be increased to 100–200 mg/kg/day (maximum 6 gm/day). Duration is 3–4 weeks.

(3) Reactivation disease in immunocompromised host. Pyrimethamine and sulfadiazine in the above suggested doses are the initial recommended therapy. Obtain an infectious disease consultation if alternative therapies are necessary.

d. Prevention. Because the mode of spread of infection remains unknown, preventive measures are speculative. However, avoidance of ingestion of raw meat and areas of cat feces contamination, particularly during pregnancy, is prudent.

5. *Pneumocystis* **pneumonia**

  a. Etiology. *Pneumocystis carinii,* an organism of uncertain classification, is the causative agent. Little is known of the route of infection or the pathogenesis of disease, but the almost exclusive pulmonary focus suggests a respiratory portal of entry.

  b. Evaluation and diagnosis

    (1) *P. carinii* generally produces a diffuse interstitial pneumonia in immunologically compromised hosts. The symptoms are usually insidious in onset. The diagnosis must be considered when pneumonia develops in patients with leukemia, lymphoma, hypogammaglobulinemia, and acquired immunodeficiency syndrome (AIDS), and in those receiving immunosuppressive therapy. This is an opportunistic infection seen in malignancy in **remission** and in malnutrition states as well. Bacterial pathogens should be ruled out by appropriate sputum studies.

    (2) Diagnosis requires the demonstration of the parasite in bronchoalveolar lavage, lung biopsy tissue sections, or induced sputum.

  c. Treatment

    (1) *P. carinii* pneumonia (PCP) develops in patients with severe underlying illness.

    (2) Oxygen and other respiratory supportive measures are of great importance.

    (3) Vigorous attempts should be made to confirm the diagnosis before therapy is instituted. In a desperately ill patient in whom this is impossible, therapy can be started when the disease is suspected.

    (4) Trimethoprim (TMP)-sulfamethoxazole (Bactrim), 20 mg TMP and 100 mg sulfamethoxazole/kg/day in four divided doses IV or PO for 14–21 days, is the drug of choice for therapy of *P. carinii* pneumonia.

    (5) Pentamidine isethionate, 4 mg/kg IV daily in one dose for 14–21 days, is a more toxic alternative. It is rarely justified to give pentamidine empirically.

    (6) Many other therapies have proved effective or are being evaluated for PCP. Obtain an infectious disease consult for recommendations beyond initial therapy.

    (7) Corticosteroids (prednisone, 1 mg/kg/day) should strongly be considered as adjunctive therapy in any PCP that requires oxygen therapy.

  d. Prophylaxis. The efficacy of preventive prophylaxis has been established in nearly every clinical setting where PCP is seen.

    (1) The use of TMP and sulfamethoxazole (Bactrim) for prophylaxis, 5 mg TMP and 20 mg sulfamethoxazole/kg/day in two divided doses, has been successful in preventing *P. carinii* pneumonia in immunocompromised patients. Every other day or thrice weekly regimens have been established in many clinical settings.

(2) Pentamidine, either aerosolized or IV, given at 2-week to monthly intervals, has also proved to be effective prophylaxis.

6. Cryptosporidiosis

   a. Etiology. *Cryptosporidium* is a gastrointestinal intracellular coccidian parasite that is increasingly being recognized as a common cause of diarrhea worldwide, particularly in children. As in giardiasis, *Cryptosporidium* appears to lack host specificity and thus zoonotic reservoirs are likely. It is increasingly being recognized as common infection in the day care setting.

   b. Evaluation and diagnosis. Most infections are probably asymptomatic.

   (1) In **normal hosts** the disease is characterized by explosive-onset GI symptoms (watery diarrhea and abdominal pain), with a varying clinical course lasting 10–14 days (not uncommonly longer).

   (2) In **immunocompromised patients** the disease often escalates with the degree of immunocompromise and is one of the common etiologies of chronic debilitating diarrhea in this setting.

   (3) Mucus is often present in feces but blood and leukocytes are uncommon. Malabsorptive phenomena are common in the chronic setting.

   (4) Oocysts can be detected in fecal smears using modifications of acid-fast staining techniques. Because of intermittent shedding, particularly in immunocompetent individuals, at least two specimens should be examined. A more specific and sensitive coproimmunodiagnostic technique has recently been commercially released (Meridian Diagnostics, Cincinnati, OH).

   c. Treatment. There presently is no recommended specific form of therapy. The newer azolide antibiotics appear to have some efficacy, but have not been extensively evaluated in children. Supportive measures are the present mainstay of therapy.

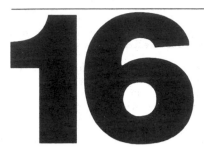

Hematologic Disorders

Alan S. Wayne

I. Red blood cells (RBCs)

A. Normal RBC values vary with age and between populations (e.g., altitude). The count is highest at birth, falling gradually until a point at which erythropoiesis is stimulated. This "physiologic nadir" occurs at around 1–3 months in preterm and 2–4 months in full-term infants. RBC size is also largest at birth, decreasing gradually over the first years of life (Table 16-1).

B. Anemia is usually defined as a count below the 95th percentile. The incidence of anemia in the first years of life is significant in all populations, ranging from 3–30 percent. Consequently, screening should occur at or before one year of age.

1. **Etiology.** There are four basic causes: loss, destruction, sequestration, and hypoproduction. Anemia can be further classified by RBC size (i.e., micro-, macro-, normocytic), RBC shape (e.g., sickle cell), or etiology.

2. **Evaluation.** The initial evaluation should include patient and family history, physical examination, and complete blood count (CBC) with indices, smear, and reticulocyte count. Notably, since the mean corpuscular volume (MCV) determined by electronic methods represents an average RBC volume, the presence of subpopulations of different size can lead to a "false" MCV determination. Consequently, the peripheral smear and RDW are essential components of the workup of anemia.

3. **Microcytic, hypochromic anemias** account for the vast majority of anemias in early childhood (Table 16-2).

   a. Iron deficiency is the most prevalent form of childhood anemia.

   (1) The **etiology** is usually multifactorial:

   (a) Inadequate iron stores at birth

   (b) High requirements due to growth and expanding blood volume

   (c) Low dietary availability of iron and impaired absorption

   (d) On occasion, blood loss, most frequently due to microscopic fecal hemorrhage from excessive intake of cow's milk in the first years of life and menstruation during adolescence. The source of loss may be difficult to detect.

   (2) **Evaluation and diagnosis**

   (a) **History.** Children are usually between 3 months and 2 years of age (>6 months in full-term infants). Low-birth-weight and premature infants are especially prone. Dietary risk factors include limited breast feeding (<6 months) or extended exclusive breast feeding (>1 yr), early institution of solids, excessive whole milk intake (>1 qt/day), tea, and the absence of iron supplements.

   (b) **Physical examination** may reveal a pale and pudgy child, the so-called "milk baby," with edema, glossitis, stomatitis, and/or spoon nails.

   (c) **Laboratory evaluation** often reveals hypochromia, microcytosis, anisocytosis, thrombocytosis, and pale serum. Free erythrocyte protoporphyrin (FEP) is elevated. Hemoglobin (hgb) A_2 (electrophoresis) may be low, and stool or urine guaiac may be positive. Transferrin saturation < 16% and serum ferritin < 15 ng/m. A common and cost-effective approach in the proper clinical setting

Table 16-1. Normal RBC parameters*

Age	Hemoglobin (gm/dl)	Hematocrit (%)	MCV (fl)
Birth	16.5 ± 3	51 ± 9	108 ± 10
1 mo	14 ± 4	43 ± 12	104 ± 19
6 mo	11.5 ± 2	35 ± 6	91 ± 17
1 yr	12 ± 1.5	36 ± 3	78 ± 8
2–6 yr	12.5 ± 1	37 ± 3	81 ± 6
6–12 yr	13.5 ± 2	40 ± 5	86 ± 9
12–18 yr	14 ± 2	42 ± 6	89 ± 11

MCV = mean corpuscular volume; fl = femtoliters
* Data are reported as means ± 2 standard deviations and are adapted from B. H. Lubin, Reference Values in Infancy and Childhood. In D. G., Nathan, F. A. Oski (Eds.), *Hematology of Infancy and Childhood* (Vol. 2). Philadelphia, Saunders, 1987. P. 1680.

is to provide a diagnostic and therapeutic trial with 3 mg/kg/day elemental iron. An hgb rise of >1 gm/dl at 1 month is usually seen. Reticulocyte peak should occur at 10–14 days.

(3) **Therapy.** Elemental iron, 3–6 mg/kg/d divided tid for 4–6 months, should be adequate to achieve a normal hgb and to replenish marrow stores. Lower doses may be required to avoid gastrointestinal (GI) intolerance. Ferrous sulfate (20% elemental iron by weight) is effective and inexpensive. Oral supplements should **not** be given with food since this may impair absorption. Rarely, deficiency may be severe enough to warrant parenteral therapy or transfusion.

(4) **Prevention**
   (a) Supplementation with iron drops (1 mg/kg/day at 4 months for full-term and 2–4 mg/kg/day at 2 months for preterm infants)
   (b) Iron-fortified cereal or formula
   (c) Avoidance of risk factors
b. **Lead poisoning** (see Chap. 4)
c. **Thalassemia**
   (1) **Etiology.** The thalassemia syndromes are genetic disorders of hgb synthesis involving beta- or alpha-chain production that are transmitted by autosomal recessive pattern. β-Thalassemia is most frequent in populations originating in the Mediterranean, Middle East,

Table 16-2. Findings in microcytic anemias

	Iron deficiency	Thalassemia Trait	Thalassemia Major	Plumbism	Chronic disease
RDW	↑	NL	↑	↑	NL
MCV	↓	↓	↓	↓	NL ↓
RBC no.	↓	NL	↓	↓	↓
FEP	↑	NL	NL	↑ ↑	↑
hgb A$_2$	↓	β- ↑	β- ↑	NL	NL
		∝-NL	∝-NL		
Iron	↓	NL	↑	NL	↓
TIBC	NL ↑	NL	NL ↑	NL	NL ↓
% saturation	↓	NL	↑	NL	↓
Ferritin	↓	NL	↑	NL	NL ↑

FEP = free erythrocyte protoporphyrin; hgb = hemoglobin; TIBC = total iron-binding capacity; ↑ = increased; ↓ = decreased; NL = normal.

and India, and α-thalassemia in those of African, Southeast Asian, Mediterranean, and Middle Eastern descent.

(2) β-Thalassemia trait (heterozygous condition) presents as a mild microcytic, hypochromic anemia. History is unremarkable except possibly for ethnic background and parental microcytic anemia. Physical examination is unrevealing. The diagnostic laboratory feature is an increased hgb A_2 on electrophoresis. (Concurrent iron deficiency results in falsely low hgb A_2 and may confound the diagnosis.) Notably, microcytosis and elevated hgb A_2 are present in the affected parent as well. No therapy is necessary for thalassemia trait, but families should be instructed regarding the genetic significance in relation to homozygous disease.

(3) β-Thalassemia major (homozygous condition) results in severe manifestations due to hemolysis and ineffective erythropoiesis. Although there is some variation in the degree of anemia, most are RBC transfusion dependent. Historically life-threatening β-thalassemia major was known as Cooley's anemia. Thalassemia intermedia refers to homozygous patients with more mild stigmata.

(a) Evaluation

(i) History and physical examination. The ethnic and family history are often obvious. β-Thalassemia major is clinically silent in the early months of life due to the presence of large amounts of fetal hgb (hgb F). Signs and symptoms typically develop between 6 and 9 months of age, although somewhat later in those with elevated hgb F or less severe disease. Progressive anemia, failure to thrive, hepatosplenomegaly, and abnormal bone growth due to marrow expansion, most notably macrocephaly and facial deformities, are common.

(ii) Laboratory evaluation. In addition to severe microcytic, hypochromic anemia, the smear reveals prominent reticulocytosis, polychromasia, nucleated RBCs, target cells, and basophilic stippling. hgb electrophoresis reveals decreased or absent hgb A_1 and increased hgb A_2 (and often hgb F). Elevated iron is common due to associated increased GI absorption. Radiographs reveal characteristic features including medullary expansion and cortical thinning, especially of the craniofacial bones. Finally, both parents have microcytic anemia and elevated hgb A_2.

(b) Therapy. Without treatment, severe β-thalassemia major is invariably fatal. Chronic RBC transfusions result in improved survival. However, iron overload eventually ensues, causing damage to the liver, endocrine glands, and heart. Without chelation therapy, iron toxicity leads to death in the second or third decade of life.

(i) Packed, leukodepleted RBC transfusion (10–20 ml/kg) should be given at sufficiently frequent intervals (every 3–5 weeks) to maintain the hematocrit (Hct) above 30%. This regimen should eliminate the increased erythropoietic drive, allowing normal linear growth and bone development.

(ii) Deferoxamine (DF) chelation should be instituted when transferrin becomes fully saturated and a chelatable iron pool is demonstrated by DF challenge (see Chap. 4, p. 108). With the usual quantity and frequency of transfusion, this generally requires a cumulative burden >500 ml/kg of RBCs. The standard dose of DF is 30–50 mg/kg/night given over 10–12 hours by subcutaneous infusion pump. The dose can be titrated by following indices of iron overload, excretion, and/or binding capacity generated by DF. Such therapy has been shown to dramatically reduce iron-induced organ damage and improve survival. **Iron supplements are strictly prohibited.**

(iii) **Splenectomy** is usually performed to decrease transfusion requirements in those with splenic enlargement. If at all possible, this should be delayed until after age five to decrease risk of septicemia. Pneumococcal, *Haemophilus influenzae* type B, and meningococcal vaccination and postsplenectomy antibiotic prophylaxis should be provided to all such children (see Tables 14-2 and 14-11). Furthermore, episodes of fever warrant close medical attention to evaluate and treat for potential life-threatening bacterial sepsis.

(iv) **Folic acid** (1 mg/day) supplementation should be prescribed to those not maintained on chronic transfusion (i.e., thalassemia intermedia) to prevent folate deficiency and megaloblastic crisis caused by increased erythropoiesis.

(v) **Bone marrow transplantation** is curative. Due to associated morbidity and mortality, this procedure is currently performed in few centers and only using HLA-matched sibling donors.

(4) α-**Thalassemia trait.** "Silent carriers" have normal function of three of the four α genes (-α/αα) and no hematologic findings. Those with only two normal genes (-α/α or —/αα) display mild microcytosis and hypochromia, most often without anemia. History and physical examination are unrevealing except possibly for ethnic background. The hgb electrophoresis is normal. Diagnosis is one of exclusion, "confirmed" by documenting parental microcytosis. Although rarely performed, molecular studies (e.g., DNA sequencing, globin synthetic ratio) are available. As in β-thalassemia trait, no therapy is necessary.

(5) α-**Thalassemia (hgb H disease).** In this form of thalassemia, only one of four α genes functions normally (—/-α), resulting in significant anemia and hgb H (β_4) on electrophoresis. Loss of function of all four α genes (—/—) results in **hgb Bart's disease** (γ_4), a fatal cause of hydrops fetalis. α-Thalassemia can be diagnosed at birth and is most frequent in Southeast Asians. Laboratory findings include severe anemia and the characteristic abnormal bands on hgb electrophoresis. DNA analysis or α/β synthetic ratios can be used for confirmation. **Principles of therapy** are the same as for β-thalassemia. The need for transfusion (and, consequently, chelation) will depend on the severity of the anemia.

(6) Prevention. Genetic counseling and prenatal detection have proved to be effective in decreasing the birth rate of children affected with severe thalassemia (β and α).

d. **Hemoglobin E (heterozygous and homozygous conditions).** This hemoglobinopathy is extremely common in Southeast Asians. In heterozygotes, anemia is absent and the predominant feature is mild microcytosis. Homozygotes display mild anemia and more severe microcytosis. Compound heterozygotes (hgb E/β-thalassemia) are phenotypically similar to β-thalassemia major. Diagnosis is confirmed by hgb electrophoresis. Treatment depends on the severity of anemia. Oxidant medications should be avoided since hgb E is unstable.

e. **Sideroblastic anemias** are inherited or acquired disorders characterized by impaired iron or heme utilization during erythroid maturation. Extremely rare in childhood, they are manifested by iron-deficient red cells in the face of adequate or excessive iron stores. **Evaluation** is notable for hypochromia and microcytosis (often severe), reticulocytopenia, elevated iron with full transferrin saturation, and on occasion tissue iron overload (i.e., hemochromatosis). **Diagnosis** is confirmed by bone marrow

iron staining, which reveals ring sideroblasts. Treatment includes pyridoxine (some forms are responsive), transfusion, and iron chelation.
4. **Macrocytic anemias.** An elevated MCV is most commonly due to an increase in the percentage of young RBCs (i.e., reticulocytes). Consequently, the smear should be closely scrutinized for the presence of such large, polychromatophilic cells before the differential diagnosis of macrocytosis is pursued further. Macrocytic anemias are frequently associated with megaloblastic changes in the bone marrow. Peripheral manifestations seen on smear include ovalocytes, neutrophils with hypersegmented nuclei ($\geq$5/cell), nucleated RBCs, basophilic stippling, and Howell-Jolly bodies. Intramarrow hemolysis (i.e., ineffective erythropoiesis) results in elevations in serum lactic dehydrogenase (LDH), direct bilirubin, and iron. Those most severely affected may have additional cytopenias due to impaired myelopoiesis or megakaryopoiesis, or both.
   a. **Etiology.** Macrocytic anemias can be subdivided according to the presence or absence of megaloblastosis.
      (1) Causes of **megaloblastic anemia** include vitamin B_{12} and folate deficiencies, drugs that interfere with folate metabolism (e.g., phenytoin, methotrexate, trimethoprim), metabolic disorders (e.g., orotic aciduria, methylmalonic aciduria, Lesch-Nyhan syndrome), and thiamine-responsive anemia.
      (2) **Isolated macrocytic anemia** (i.e., without megaloblastosis) can be associated with liver disease, bone marrow failure syndromes, drugs (e.g., valproic acid, carbamazepine), and hypothyroidism.
   b. **Evaluation and diagnosis.** A thorough medication history and neurologic examination are essential. Bone marrow examination is usually required. Notably, coexistent nutritional deficiencies may exist, complicating diagnosis and treatment. It is imperative to correctly diagnose B_{12} deficiency, since treatment with folate may result in hematologic improvement while allowing progressive neurologic deterioration.
      (1) **Vitamin B_{12} deficiency** may be due to pernicious anemia, intestinal malabsorption (generalized or selective), drug-induced or dietary deficiency, liver disease, or metabolic disorders. Symptoms and signs, may include malaise, anorexia, diarrhea, glossitis, splenomegaly, paresthesias, and peripheral neuropathy. Neurologic evaluation for defects including dorsolateral spinal degeneration is critical. Specific findings may include low vitamin B_{12}, abnormal Schilling test, and response to a trial of B_{12}.
      (2) **Folic acid deficiency.** Since folate stores are relatively small, deficiency may develop within 1 month and anemia within 4 months of deprivation. Etiologies include dietary inadequacy, malabsorption, drug-induced antagonism or deficiency, inborn errors of metabolism, and conditions associated with high folate demand (e.g., rapid growth, chronic hemolysis, malignancy, hyperthyroidism). The dietary history may be suggestive (e.g., breast or goat's milk). Specific symptoms are often absent, although malaise, anorexia, poor growth, and recurrent infection may be seen. Neurologic signs are not associated. Essential laboratory findings include **low folate and normal B_{12} levels.**
   c. **Therapy**
      (1) **Vitamin B_{12} deficiency.** To replenish body stores, B_{12} replacement should begin with 25–100 μg per day intramuscularly for 10–14 days. Maintenance therapy with 50–1,000 μg per month IM is effective in preventing recurrence. (Massive doses are required for certain metabolic defects.) The hematologic response should be rapid, with marrow megaloblastosis improving within hours, reticulocytosis appearing by day 3, and anemia resolving within 1–2 months. Patients should be monitored for hypokalemia and hyperuricemia during the first few weeks of treatment.
      (2) **Folic acid deficiency.** Initial treatment with 20–200 μg per day of

folic acid IM for 10–14 days should suffice. Except in the event of malabsorption, the standard approach is to treat with 1–5 mg per day PO. This dose given for 1–2 months is usually adequate to replenish body stores even in patients with malabsorption. In the event that maintenance therapy is required (e.g., chronic hemolytic conditions), 1 mg per day is more than sufficient. Clinical response is rapid, following a time course similar to that of B_{12} deficiency.

5. **Normocytic anemias.** Common causes of normocytic anemia include hemorrhage, hemolysis, and hypoproduction.

   a. **Hemorrhage.** Acute bleeding is associated with a proportionate loss of plasma and cells, and no consequent change in hgb or Hct. Anemia ensues only on reequilibration of the total blood volume (TBV), which may take up to 3 days. **Evaluation** should focus on sites of bleeding. Reticulocytosis is often seen within 6–12 hours due to mobilization of marrow stores; however, full response takes up to 5–10 days. Nucleated RBCs are also seen during marrow recovery. Chronic hemorrhage eventually leads to iron deficiency, with resultant microcytosis and diminished reticulocyte response. **Treatment** should be directed toward the underlying cause of hemorrhage. Restoration of TBV with crystalloid is often beneficial in the initial therapy of severe bleeding. Iron replacement may be necessary.

   b. **Hemolytic anemias** result from premature destruction of red cells and include a large, diverse group of disorders. **Etiologies** are found in Table 16-3.

      (1) **Evaluation.** (a) History of pallor and jaundice, sometimes acute in onset, family history, and exposures to precipitating agents, such as toxins, infection, drugs, or foods, may suggest a diagnosis. (b) **Laboratory features** may include elevated serum LDH, direct hyperbilirubinemia, decreased serum haptoglobin, and, with severe hemolysis, hemoglobinemia and hemoglobinuria. RBC morphologic abnormalities, in particular fragments such as bites, helmets, spherocytes, and schistocytes; elevated reticulocyte count; and in certain disorders, pathognomonic shapes (e.g., sickle forms), may be revealing. In *chronic* hemolytic conditions, anemia may be *mild* or *absent* due to compensatory erythropoiesis. Such patients may come to medical attention only during an aplastic crisis from erythroid hypoplasia (most commonly due to parvovirus B19). Since reticulocytosis is absent in this situation, the underlying diagnosis of hemolysis may not be suspected. (c) Further *diagnostic evaluation* should be pursued as indicated, including direct and indirect Coombs test, glucose 6-phosphate dehydrogenase (G-6-PD) screen, hgb electrophoresis, Heinz body preparation, and family CBCs with reticulocyte counts. Investigations, such as osmotic fragility testing, cation studies, and red cell enzyme profiles, are reserved for the appropriate clinical scenarios. *Since transfusion may obscure the diagnosis of intrinsic red cell disorders, it may be useful to draw and save a few tubes of whole blood* (in citrate and heparin) just before transfusion.

      (2) **Therapy** varies with the condition (see Table 16-3). Secondary hemolysis usually resolves with treatment of the primary illness. (a) **Folate** supplementation (1 mg/day) should be provided in chronic hemolytic states to prevent megaloblastic crisis. (b) Although rare, **iron deficiency** due to chronic hemoglobinuria should be sought and treated appropriately. (c) **Transfusions** may be necessary in acute settings or in chronic hemolytic states marked by severe symptomatic anemia. (d) **Chronic** hemolysis is often associated with gallstone formation, and **cholecystectomy** may be required. (e) **Splenectomy** is frequently employed in disorders characterized by trapping (e.g., spherocytosis) to prolong red cell survival and decrease the level of anemia. This should be delayed as long as possible and appropriate measures taken to decrease the risk of infection (see sec.

Table 16-3. Causes of hemolytic anemia

Etiology	Diagnosis	Treatment
External	History, exam, smear, hemosideri-nuria	Supportive
Traumatic injury		
Thermal injury	Spherocytes	
Prosthetic valve		
Organ	Exam, cytopenias	
Sequestration	Hepatosplenomegaly	Splenectomy*
Erythrophagocytosis	Signs, symptoms, biopsy	Underlying condition
Vessel	History, exam, thrombocytopenia, smear	
Vascular malformation		
Microangiopathy	Signs, symptoms of associated condition	Underlying condition
Plasma		
Antibody	History, spherocytes, Coombs, mother-child blood type incompatibility	Steroids, cytotoxins, IVGG, splenectomy*
Toxin	History, signs, symptoms, spherocytes, toxic screen, renal tests, cultures	Underlying condition, supportive, detoxification
Electrolyte disturbance	Osmolarity, phosphate (spherocytes)	Electrolyte correction
Wilson's disease	History, exam, copper, ceruloplasmin	Penicillamine
Infection	Associated symptoms, cultures, titers	Antibiotics, supportive
Infantile pyknocytosis	Organomegaly, elevated SGOT, smear	Rarely necessary
Cellular	Family history, CBCs, smears	
Membrane defects	Characteristic morphology	
Spherocytosis	Osmotic fragility, cytoskeletal analysis	Splenectomy
Elliptocytosis	Osmotic fragility, cytoskeletal analysis	Splenectomy
Hydro(stomato)cytosis	Cation studies, osmotic fragility	Splenectomy*
Xerocytosis	Cation studies, decreased fragility	None necessary
PNH	Marrow dysfunction, Ham's, sugar water	Steroids
Abetali poproteinemia	Associated symptoms, acanthocytes	Rarely necessary
Liver disease	Associated symptoms, acanthocytes, targets	Underlying condition
Vitamin E deficiency	Prematurity, edema, thrombocytosis	Vitamin E supplements
Parasitic inclusions	History, thick smear	Antimicrobials
Enzymopathies	Family history, smears, enzyme analyses	Splenectomy*
G-6-PD deficiency	Spherocytes, Heinz prep, G-6-PD screen	Oxidant avoidance
Hemoglobinopathies	Family history, smears, electrophoreses	
Sickle cell disease	Sickle forms, sickle prep	Supportive
Thalassemia major	Basophilic stippling, targets	Splenectomy*
Hemoglobin C, E	Targets	Splenectomy*
Unstable hemoglobin	Basophilic stippling, Heinz prep	Splenectomy*
	Heat stability test, O_2 affinity	Oxidant avoidance

SGOT = serum glutamic oxaloacetic transaminase; PNH = paroxysmal nocturnal hemoglobinuria; IVGG = intravenous gamma globulin.* May be effective in certain cases.

I.B.3.c.(3)(b)(iii)). (f) **Medications** such as steroids or cytotoxic agents may be of value in antibody-mediated hemolysis.

(3) **Hereditary spherocytosis (HS)** is the most common form of hemolytic anemia in Northern Europeans. Although spherocytes are a characteristic feature of many hemolytic states, HS represents a group of inherited (usually autosomal dominant) disorders of RBC membrane protein structure.

   (a) **Evaluation** includes parental history. Splenomegaly is a prominent feature. Patients can present early in life (e.g., neonatal jaundice) or be asymptomatic, with the diagnosis suspected only on routine CBC evaluation. The mean corpuscular hemoglobin concentration (MCHC) is elevated and the smear reveals small, round RBCs that lack in central pallor (i.e., spherocytes).

   (b) **Diagnosis** is confirmed by demonstrating increased osmotic fragility. Membrane protein analysis is occasionally useful. **Treatment** is often unnecessary.

     (i) **Splenectomy** may be helpful for those with significant anemia.

     (ii) **Transfusions** are sometimes required, especially in young children for whom splenectomy is delayed and in the event of aplastic crisis.

     (iii) Folate supplementation should be given.

(4) **Sickle cell disease (SCD)**, which includes homozygous hgb S, doubly heterozygous hgb S/C, and hgb S/β-thalassemia, is especially common in populations of African descent. The incidence of heterozygosity (i.e., sickle trait) in African Americans is approximately 8 percent, with about 1 in 200–500 newborns affected with SCD. The greatest incidence of death is due to functional asplenia in infancy and early childhood in SCD. Mortality is markedly reduced by prophylactic antibiotics started early in the first year of life. Consequently, many states have recently adopted newborn screening programs to aid in early detection and institution of antibiotics.

   (a) **Etiology.** Hemoglobin S, consisting of two normal alpha and two abnormal β^s chains, has a propensity to polymerize, especially on deoxygenation. This leads to cellular abnormalities, which render the RBC misshapen, rigid, and adherent. With complete polymerization, the characteristic sickle form is produced.

   (b) **Evaluation.**

     (i) Newborns with SCD are asymptomatic due to the presence of hgb F. Symptoms of vasoocclusion can occur as early as 6 months of age, most commonly as *dactylitis* of the hands or feet.

     (ii) **Functional asplenia,** as demonstrated by the presence of Howell-Jolly bodies on peripheral smear, can develop early in life.

     (iii) Other manifestations of SCD include pallor, icterus, early hepatosplenomegaly (with eventual splenic atrophy), recurrent crises (see below), isosthenuria, and, with long-standing disease, osteonecrosis, chronic pulmonary disease, cardiomegaly, and renal insufficiency.

     (iv) **Laboratory findings** include severe anemia, bizarre RBC morphology (e.g., sickle forms), reticulocytosis, and direct hyperbilirubinemia. Exposure of blood to reducing agents induces sickling, the basis for many screening tests. Hemoglobin electrophoresis is used for confirmation.

   (c) **Therapy of specific syndromes**

     (i) **Painful or vasoocclusive crisis (VOC)** is the most common symptom in SCD. Musculoskeletal involvement is usual, although almost any tissue can be affected. Precipitating causes include infection, dehydration, exposure to cold, and hypoxia. **Treatment** consists of hydration, pain control, and reversal of the underlying trigger(s) if known. Mild episodes often respond to oral analgesics and fluids, whereas more severe bouts require hospitalization with intravenous (IV) support. Care must be taken to guard against fluid overload in older patients, who commonly have diminished cardiac function. Therapeutic options for pain control are reviewed elsewhere (see Chap. 1, p. 3). Particular efforts should be made to avoid deep sedation with resultant hypoventilation. **Note well: All SCD patients who require significant doses of narcotics should be maintained on oxygen saturation and cardiorespiratory monitors.** Red cell transfusion is not indicated for an uncomplicated pain crisis. VOC may mimic other complications of SCD that require a high index of suspicion for diagnosis (e.g., osteomyelitis, cholecystitis). Furthermore, patients with pain of the thorax or abdomen should be closely followed, since such symptoms are often the first signs of acute chest syndrome (see below).

   (ii) Aplastic crisis. Infection with parvovirus B19 results in transient suppression of RBC production. This is a common cause of aplastic crisis in SCD, characterized by a rapid drop in the hematocrit, the disappearance of reticulocytes, and a *decrease* in the serum bilirubin. Although these episodes are often self-limited, anemia can be severe enough to warrant transfusion. Patients with SCD and other chronic hemolytic conditions should be isolated from those potentially infected with parvovirus (e.g., fifth disease, aplastic crisis).

   (iii) Sequestration crisis due to the sudden pooling of blood in the spleen, or rarely the liver, is a life-threatening complication of SCD. Although most common in young children, this can occur later in life, especially in hgb S/C, in which early splenic infarction is unusual. The clinical presentation is one of rapidly developing shock and organomegaly. **Treatment** *requires immediate volume* resuscitation (see Chaps. 3 and 7) and reversal of anemia. In light of the high recurrence rate and associated mortality, *splenectomy* is usually performed after severe episodes. Patients with less critical events characterized by mild anemia and splenomegaly without cardiovascular insufficiency are sometimes managed expectantly. Chronic transfusions have been employed to delay the timing of splenectomy, although such therapy is of unproven overall benefit.

   (iv) Hyperhemolytic crisis is an infrequent symptom of SCD. Accelerated hemolysis may be seen in those with coexistent G-6-PD deficiency and infection or oxidant exposure. With severe anemia, transfusion may be necessary.

   (v) Megaloblastic crisis due to the increased folate requirements from rapid erythropoiesis can be prevented with prophylactic folic acid.

   (vi) Hypoxia is life-threatening in SCD since it promotes intravascular sickling with potential vital organ infarction (e.g., brain, lung, kidney, liver). **All patients seen for acute illness should be evaluated for possible hypoxemia. This is especially important when employing narcotics. Oxygen therapy and continuous oxymetric monitoring should be employed to maintain an O_2 saturation $\geq$ 98% at all times,** even if this requires intubation and artificial ventilation.

(vii) **Infection.** Due to splenic dysfunction, patients with SCD have increased susceptibility to bacterial infections, especially pneumococcus, meningococcus, *H. influenzae,* salmonella, and *Escherichia coli.* Severe infection, including septicemia, pneumonia, osteomyelitis, and urosepsis, is common in all ages. Consequently, episodes of fever require immediate medical attention. For a temperature ≥38.5°C, blood and urine cultures should be obtained and antibiotics administered parenterally (see Chap.14). **All** children with SCD should be treated with prophylactic antibiotics, most commonly penicillin, 125–250 mg bid. In addition, vaccination against pneumococcus at age two and *H. influenzae* during the first years of life is essential.

(viii) **Acute chest syndrome** is common and serves as a major risk factor for chronic lung disease and death in adolescents and adults with SCD. Mortality due to progressive respiratory failure and multiorgan infarction occurs. The syndrome is characterized by respiratory symptoms, chest or abdominal pain, fever, and an abnormal thorax examination. Although results of chest x-ray (CXR) are often normal at presentation, abnormal findings frequently develop. In severe episodes, multilobe involvement, hypoxemia, and anemia are common. Although the etiology is often unknown, respiratory infection, especially bacterial, viral, or *Mycoplasma* pneumonia, predisposes to the development of chest syndrome. Close monitoring and aggressive treatment are essential. Therapy should include hydration, analgesia, oxygen, and antibiotics. In addition to covering for common bacterial pathogens, erythromycin should be provided for the possibility of *Mycoplasma.* Although the role for transfusion is not completely defined, red cell exchange should be considered for those with severe involvement.

(ix) **Cerebrovascular disease** is a frequent complication of SCD. Infarction due to occlusion of large, often multiple cerebral vessels is the most common cause of stroke in children. Chronic transfusion to maintain hgb S below 30% dramatically reduces the otherwise high rate of recurrence. Such therapy may need to be lifelong. All patients with an acute cerebrovascular episode should undergo immediate RBC exchange.

(x) **Transfusion** (Table 16-4). Although blood transfusion can be lifesaving in SCD, **extreme caution is necessary to avoid hyperviscosity.** Unless the percent hgb S is lowered significantly, the Hct should probably not be raised above 25–30%. **Acute simple transfusion** is indicated when increased carrying capacity is desired, but no significant decrease in hgb S is necessary. **Chronic simple transfusion** is indicated when suppression of hgb S production is required. In practice, transfusion with 10–15 ml/kg packed RBCs every 3–4 weeks should be adequate to maintain hgb S ≤30%, which is the usual target. **Exchange transfusion** allows rapid and simultaneous adjustment of Hct and hgb S. Exchange should be employed when immediate restoration of circulation is vital to preserving life or organ function. Since major operations and general anesthesia may predispose to a variety of complications (e.g., acute chest syndrome), preoperative transfusion to lower hgb S has become standard practice. **Sensitization** to RBC antigens is a common problem in SCD. To prevent the development of potentially life-threatening anti-

Table 16-4. Indications for transfusion in SCD

Acute simple transfusion
Symptomatic anemia
Sequestration crisis
Aplastic crisis
Blood loss
Preoperative preparation*
Chronic transfusion
Cerebrovascular disease
Debilitating vaso-occlusive symptoms†
Complicated pregnancy†
Preoperative preparation*
Exchange transfusion
Severe acute chest syndrome
Cerebrovascular disease
Arterial hypoxemia syndrome
Refractory priapism
Eye surgery
Cerebral angiography
Preoperative preparation*

* under investigation
† selected patients

bodies, extended antigen-matched RBCs (especially C, D, E, c, e, and K antigens) should be employed if at all possible. These are mandatory in patients with prior sensitization.

(xi) **Hydroxyurea** has recently been shown to increase hgb F levels in patients with SCD. This agent may prove to be effective in decreasing certain complications.

(d) **Combined sickle hemoglobinopathies.** The presentation and complications of doubly heterozygous hgb S/C and hgb S/β-thalassemia are similar to those of homozygous sickle cell anemia. Diagnosis is made by hgb electrophoresis.

(5) **Hemoglobin C disease (homozygous condition)** is a mild disorder characterized by hemolysis and splenomegaly that is found most frequently in those of West African descent. Abdominal pain and cholelithiasis are common. **Laboratory features** include mild anemia, elevated MCHC, prominent targets and occasional intra-RBC crystals on smear, and a diagnostic hgb electrophoretic pattern. **Treatment** is symptomatic.

(6) **Enzymopathies.** Hemolytic disorders of RBC enzymes are most often autosomal recessive conditions. Although presentation may be at any age, neonatal jaundice is common. Diagnosis is confirmed by enzyme assay, although false-negative results are frequent in the setting of hemolytic crisis due to the preponderance of young, relatively enzyme-rich cells.

(a) **Glucose 6-phosphate dehydrogenase deficiency,** the most common of these disorders, is inherited in an X-linked recessive pattern and is frequent in those of Mediterranean and African descent. The A variety, observed largely in African Americans, requires oxidant stress (e.g., drugs, infection) for significant hemolysis to develop. Such exposure should be avoided (Table 16-5).

(b) **Pyruvate kinase (PK) deficiency** has an autosomal recessive pattern and is associated with spontaneous hemolysis, significant anemia, and characteristic burr cells on smear. Splenectomy may

Table 16-5. Agents associated with hemolysis in G-6-PD deficiency

Acetanilid
Doxorubicin
Fava beans
Furazolidone
Methylene blue
Nalidixic acid
Niridazole
Nitrofurantoin
Phenazopyridine
Primaquine
Sulfamethoxazole

be useful for severe cases. Folate supplementation is recommended and transfusions are sometimes necessary.

(7) **Autoimmune hemolytic anemia (AHA).** Possible causes include infection, collagen vascular disease (e.g., systemic lupus erythematosus [SLE]), malignancy (e.g., lymphoma), and medications (e.g., penicillin).

(a) **Evaluation.**

(i) History and physical examination are most often unrevealing, although icterus and splenomegaly may be present.

(ii) In addition to anemia and reticulocytosis, spherocytes are usually noted, and direct bilirubin and LDH are elevated.

(iii) **Diagnosis** of AHA is confirmed by the positive Coombs test. **"Warm" antibodies** (immunoglobulin G [IgG]) display a maximal reaction at around 37°C. **"Cold" antibodies** (IgM) react best at low temperature, fix complement, and agglutinate red cells. Patients with cold antibodies usually respond poorly to treatment and should avoid exposure to low temperatures.

(b) **Therapy**

(i) Secondary AHA often responds to treatment of the underlying condition or removal of the offending agent.

(ii) **Corticosteroids** are frequently useful in warm antibody–mediated hemolytic anemia. Prednisone (or methylprednisolone) is usually initiated at a dosage of 4–6 mg/kg/day until response is seen, and then, if possible, tapered fairly rapidly to 1–2 mg/kg/day. The dose should be reduced to the minimum required to maintain an acceptable hgb and reticulocyte count.

(iii) **High-dose IV gamma globulin (IVGG), splenectomy, and/or immunosuppressive agents** (e.g., cyclophosphamide) should be considered in patients who are resistant to or who require high doses of steroids. **Plasmapheresis** may be a useful adjunct when rapid reduction of the antibody titer is desired (e.g., severe, acute AHA).

(iv) **Blood transfusion may be hazardous** and should be used with extreme caution and only in the event of life-threatening anemia. High-dose IV steroids should be administered as far in advance of transfusion as possible. The unit of blood least reactive on crossmatch should be selected and infused extremely slowly and with close monitoring. In the setting of cold antibodies, blood should be given through a warmer to decrease the likelihood of immediate hemolysis.

(8) **Anemia of chronic illness.** Anemia, frequently mild, is a common

manifestation of numerous systemic conditions. Although usually normocytic, the MCV is occasionally low. The TIBC is frequently diminished. Treatment is aimed at the primary condition.

C. **Polycythemia,** or an increased RBC mass, is reflected in elevations in the hgb and Hct.

1. **Etiology.** In children, polycythemia is almost always secondary to chronic hypoxemia from congenital heart disease or pulmonary disorders (e.g., cystic fibrosis). Neonatal causes include maternal-fetal or excess placental transfusion, intrauterine hypoxia, maternal diabetes, and a variety of congenital disorders. Primary polycythemia (i.e., p. vera) is extremely rare in pediatric populations.

2. **Evaluation** should focus on the history and physical examination. Symptoms of hyperviscosity rarely develop until the Hct exceeds 55%. Headaches, dizziness, lethargy, exercise intolerance, visual disturbances, acrocyanosis, and vascular engorgement (plethora) are common. With extreme elevations (usually ≥70%), stroke may ensue. Extensive laboratory workup is rarely necessary. Venous rather than capillary sampling is required. Spun Hcts are more accurate than automated counters, which may underestimate the degree of elevation. Mild thrombocytopenia is commonly associated.

3. **Therapy**
   a. In the absence of adequate treatment for the underlying condition (e.g., cardiac repair), the only remedy for polycythemia is **phlebotomy.** Lowering the Hct is effective in alleviating symptoms of hyperviscosity and preventing recurrent stroke. Removal should be employed for symptoms or an Hct ≥65%.
   b. **Isovolumetric replacement is imperative** to prevent volume contraction and further impairment in microcirculatory perfusion. Normal saline or 5% albumin should be used.
   c. **Partial exchange transfusion** is the method of choice for newborns.
   d. For older children, **automated erythrocytapheresis** is preferred to manual removal, since the Hct can be adjusted rapidly and safely without altering the total blood volume.
   e. The Hct should rarely be decreased by more than 10 points at a time. The formula for determining the amount of removal is found in Table 16-8, found later in this chapter.
   f. **Chronic treatment** is usually necessary and is mandatory for those with a history of stroke.

II. **Bone marrow**
   A. **Primary marrow failure syndromes**
      1. **Aplastic anemia (AA) or pancytopenia** is characterized by diminished or absent production of all three blood cell lines.
         a. **Acquired AA,** although usually idiopathic, may be due to infection, drugs, radiation, or rare disorders.
            (1) **Evaluation** reveals mild to severe pancytopenia, reticulocytopenia, and varying degrees of hypoplasia or aplasia on marrow examination.
            (2) **Therapy.** The prognosis in severe AA is extremely poor, with mortality as high as 75 percent.
                (a) **Supportive care** including transfusion and antibiotics may be required. Potentially etiologic drugs should be eliminated.
                (b) **Bone marrow transplantation** offers the best chance for survival and is the treatment of choice for those with HLA-matched siblings. To decrease the risk of graft rejection, transfusions should be avoided if possible.
                (c) **Antithymocyte or antilymphocyte globulin or serum (i.e., ATG, ALG, ATS, ALS)** is often effective. ATG at a total dosage of 150 mg/kg should be given over 4–10 days. Serum sickness is a nearly universal side effect and relapse is common.
                (d) **Cyclosporine-A** has been effective in some patients with severe AA. Dosages starting at 6–9 mg/kg PO divided bid or tid are

adjusted according to serum levels or toxicity, or both. Common side effects include hepatic dysfunction, renal insufficiency, and immunosuppression.

    (e) Corticosteroids are often used in combination with ATG.

    (f) Other therapeutic modalities, such as **androgens, immunosuppressive agents,** and **hematopoietic growth factors,** may be helpful for individual patients.

  b. Fanconi's anemia is an autosomal recessive condition commonly associated with pigmentary, skeletal, renal, and developmental abnormalities that frequently culminates in malignancy, especially leukemia.

    (1) Evaluation. Diagnosis is usually suspected in the setting of cytopenia(s) and phenotypic features. The hematologic manifestations, characterized by progressive aplasia, usually do not appear until after infancy (median age of 7 years). Macrocytosis is universal even before the development of cytopenia. Surveillance for associated anomalies is necessary. **Diagnosis** is confirmed by demonstrating increased chromosomal breakage with exposure to diepoxybutane (DEB) or other agents that damage DNA. Prenatal diagnosis can be performed.

    (2) Therapy

      (a) Supportive care including transfusions and antibiotics is essential.

      (b) Androgens prolong survival, although many relapse off therapy and eventually become resistant. Oxymetholone at a dosage of 2–5 mg/kg/day is standard. Liver function should be monitored closely. **Corticosteroids** (e.g., prednisone) are often combined in an attempt to counterbalance androgen-induced growth acceleration. Both medications should be tapered slowly and maintained at the lowest possible dose.

      (c) Bone marrow transplantation can be curative, although severe morbidity and mortality associated with chemotherapy and radiation due to chromosomal sensitivity make modification of the preparative regimen essential. Recently, **umbilical cord blood transplantation** has been successfully performed.

      (d) Trials of **hematopoietic growth factors** offer promise in patients who are resistant to standard therapy and have no available marrow donors.

  c. Other rare forms of **constitutional AA** include aplasia in association with dyskeratosis congenita, Shwachman-Diamond syndrome, amegakaryocytic thrombocytopenia, and a variety of familial marrow failure syndromes.

2. Isolated cytopenias can involve any of the three cell lines. Only with rare exception do these evolve into pancytopenia.

  a. Pure red cell aplasia (PRCA) can be acquired or congenital.

    (1) Transient erythroblastopenia of childhood (TEC) is among the most common forms of PRCA.

      (a) Evaluation. This idiopathic disorder primarily affects otherwise healthy children from 1 month to 8 years (peak incidence, age 2). A preceding viral infection is commonly reported, although no specific organism has been shown to be associated with TEC. History and physical examination are unremarkable except for pallor of gradual onset. When a normal CBC from earlier in life is available, the diagnosis is fairly clear.

      (b) Therapy. The Hct has usually reached a nadir by the time of presentation and recovery most often occurs within a few months. Transfusion is sometimes needed.

    (2) Acquired PCA can also occur in association with viral infection, drugs, pregnancy, anti-RBC antibodies, thymoma, immunodeficiency, malignancy, and malnutrition. Most common is **aplastic crisis** in chronic hemolytic conditions due to parvovirus B19 (see sec. **I.B.5.b.1**).

(a) **Evaluation** should focus on a possible underlying cause. Evidence for parvovirus infection should be sought in patients with chronic hemolytic anemia or immunodeficiency.

(b) **Therapy.** Red cell recovery may follow drug removal, nutritional repletion, treatment of the underlying condition, or thymectomy as indicated. Splenectomy and a variety of immunosuppressive regimens have been employed in persistent PRCA with occasional success. With immunodeficiency, parvoviral infection may be chronic. IVGG is of benefit in this situation.

(3) **Congenital PRCA or Diamond-Blackfan anemia (DBA)**

(a) **Etiology.** This idiopathic disorder primarily affects white infants. *No* uniform pattern of inheritance has been established.

(b) **Evaluation.** The vast majority are noted to be pale at or soon after birth. Approximately 25 percent have associated congenital anomalies. Laboratory evaluation reveals macrocytic anemia (occasionally normocytic), reticulocytopenia, selective erythroid marrow hypoplasia or aplasia, normal or slightly diminished white blood cell (WBC) count, normal or slightly elevated platelet count, and normal chromosome studies.

(c) **Diagnosis.** The other major entity in the differential diagnosis of PRCA in early childhood is TEC. Although, DBA usually presents **before** and TEC **after** 1 year of age, there is significant overlap. Associated constitutional features may be indicative of DBA; however, these are absent in the majority of patients. Furthermore, although DBA is often associated with "fetal" erythropoiesis (e.g., macrocytosis, elevated Hgb F, and expression of the RBC antigen "i"), such features can also be seen in TEC during recovery. Thus, in the absence of a prior normal CBC to confirm TEC, the final diagnosis must await time. The absence of spontaneous improvement "confirms" DBA and warrants treatment.

(d) **Therapy. Corticosteroids** are effective in up to 75 percent of cases. Prednisone is begun at a dosage of 2 mg/kg/day, with a response usually seen within 1 month. Once the hgb and Hct have reached satisfactory levels, steroids should be tapered to the lowest possible qod dose. Nonresponders should be given a trial of prednisone at 4–6 mg/kg/day (or an alternative preparation at an equivalent dose). Steroid dependence is the rule. **Androgens, immunosuppressive agents, and hematopoietic growth factors** have met with anecdotal success. **Bone marrow transplantation** offers hope for those with suitable donors. When **chronic red cell transfusion** is required, close monitoring for iron overload is necessary.

b. **Neutropenia** (see sec. **IV.A.l**)

c. **Thrombocytopenia** is most commonly caused by peripheral destruction (see sec. **III.C.1**). Decreased platelet production may result from infection, drugs (e.g., trimethoprim, diuretics, chemotherapy), and a variety of inherited disorders.

(1) **Amegakaryocytic thrombocytopenia** is a rare congenital syndrome marked by absent megakaryocytes. Although present in infants, thrombocytopenia may go unnoticed until later in childhood. Macrocytosis and "fetal" erythropoiesis are common and progression to AA is the rule. Because of the extremely poor prognosis, marrow transplantation should be considered.

(2) **Thrombocytopenia with absent radii syndrome (TAR)** is another unusual familial condition. Thrombocytopenia develops in the first months of life. Transient leukocytosis is common and may raise the concern for leukemia. Physical and radiographic forearm features are pathognomonic. Although death from hemorrhage in the first year is frequent, those who survive usually demonstrate spontaneous improvement. Treatment is supportive.

B. Secondary marrow failure syndromes
   1. Leukemia. Primary hematopoietic malignancy (i.e., leukemia) almost always presents with signs and symptoms of cytopenias. **Leukemia** is the most common pediatric malignancy, occurring in approximately 1 in 20,000 children. All ages are affected, although the peak incidence is around age 4.
      a. Evaluation. The manifestations are protean. In addition to signs of cytopenia, anorexia, malaise, and fever are common. Leukemic infiltration can lead to adenopathy, gingival hyperplasia, hepatosplenomegaly, bone and joint pain, skin rash, increased intracranial pressure, focal neurologic deficits, testicular enlargement, and respiratory symptoms. Life-threatening presentations include hemorrhage, infection, and/or organ failure. The blood smear often reveals blasts. Bone marrow examination including histochemical stains, cytogenetics, and immunologic surface markers are required for accurate diagnosis.
      b. Therapy
         (1) Aggressive supportive care is essential. To prevent uric acid nephropathy, **allopurinol** (50–100 mg tid), IV **hydration**, and **alkalinization** (5% dextrose in water with $NaHCO_3$, 40–80 mEq/liter at 1.5–2.0 times maintenance, usually suffices) should be instituted immediately. Emergent broad-spectrum **antibiotics** and **transfusions** may be indicated.
         (2) Heparin is recommended during the initial therapy of certain forms of leukemia associated with disseminated intravascular coagulation (DIC).
         (3) Symptomatic hyperviscosity due to severe leukocytosis, especially CNS or pulmonary dysfunction, requires immediate **exchange transfusion** or **leukocytapheresis.**
         (4) Referral to centers familiar with specialized **chemotherapy and radiation therapy** protocols is necessary. Outcome varies with the type of leukemia and prognostic features.
         (5) Bone marrow transplantation is recommended for certain subtypes.
      c. Acute lymphoblastic leukemia (ALL) accounts for 75–80 percent of childhood leukemia. Survival rates vary significantly, but may be as high as 60–80 percent.
      d. Acute nonlymphoblastic leukemia (ANLL) includes seven subtypes **(M1–M7)** and accounts for about 20–25 percent of leukemia in childhood. Certain subtypes have characteristic features. M3 (acute promyelocytic) ANLL frequently presents with DIC, and M5 (acute monoblastic) with hyperleukocytosis or peripheral (e.g., skin) infiltration, or both. Historically, survival of ANLL has been significantly worse than in ALL. Recently, however, marrow transplantation has resulted in improved outcome for those with HLA-matched sibling donors.
   2. Metastatic malignancies, such as neuroblastoma, lymphoma, sarcomas, and malignant histiocytosis, may involve the marrow, resulting in cytopenia. Associated features are often telltale and include masses, pain, and radiographic findings. Biopsy of the bone marrow or primary tumor is required for pathologic diagnosis.
   3. Metabolic disorders characterized by marrow infiltration may cause cytopenia. Examples include **Gaucher's disease** and **osteopetrosis.**
   4. Infections involving the bone marrow can cause cytopenia. Examples include congenital TORCH infections, human immunodeficiency virus (HIV), Epstein-Barr virus (EBV), cytomegalovirus (CMV) fungus, and tuberculosis.
III. Coagulation
   A. Clotting factor deficiencies, single or multiple, are among the most common causes of bleeding.
      1. Hemophilia A is an X-linked recessive deficiency of factor VIII activity (F VIII:C) that affects approximately one in 5,000–10,000 males around the globe.
         a. Evaluation

(1) The severity of disease reflects the degree of deficiency. Family history is usually positive.

(2) Laboratory studies include a prolonged partial thromboplastin time (PTT) in the face of normal prothrombin time (PT), bleeding time, and platelet count.

(3) Diagnosis is confirmed by **F VIII:C assay.**

   (a) Mild deficiency: 5–30 percent of normal

   (b) Moderate deficiency: 1–5 percent of normal

   (c) Severe deficiency: <1 percent of normal

b. Therapy. Prompt initiation of F VIII replacement is essential. As the signs and symptoms of bleeding may be subtle, the maxim "when in doubt, treat" has appropriately evolved.

   (1) F VIII–containing products

   (a) Purified F VIII concentrates are the safest and most routine products for replacement. Monoclonal or recombinant preparations probably convey the lowest risk of transmission of hepatitis and HIV.

   (b) Fresh frozen plasma (FFP) is a nonspecific product, carries a variety of associated risks (see sec. **V.C**), and requires large volumes to correct factor deficiency. Consequently, FFP is rarely if ever used for hemophilia.

   (c) Cryoprecipitate, obtained by slow thawing of FFP, contains concentrated F VIII. As with FFP, it is rarely employed in this setting.

   (d) Deamino-D-arginine vasopressin (DDAVP) results in increased F VIII levels in some patients with hemophilia. Levels rarely increase to more than 2–3 times baseline and tachyphylaxis often develops after two to three doses. Consequently, DDAVP is **not** useful in major hemorrhage or when prolonged therapy is necessary. The major benefit is that DDAVP carries no risk of infection. A trial is required to demonstrate response **before** use in the management of bleeding. The dosage is 0.3 μg/kg (of the IV preparation at a concentration of 4μg/cc) IV over 30 minutes q12–24h for two to three doses. With repeated dosing, hyponatremia may develop.

   (2) Dose. In general, for **each unit per kilogram** of factor VIII concentrate administered, plasma levels will **rise by 2 percent.** The half-life of F VIII is 8–12 hours. Target levels depend on the severity of the hemorrhage, and the adequacy of replacement should be assessed by peak and trough F VIII levels and clinical response. The PTT should normalize when the F VIII level is raised above 40 percent.

   (a) Major bleeds require correction to **100 percent** and maintenance of **trough levels ≥50 percent.** A loading dose of 50 u/kg F VIII followed by 25 u/kg q12h usually suffices. Alternatively, in life-threatening situations, loading can be followed by continuous-infusion F VIII at 3–4 u/kg/hr titrated according to levels.

   (b) Minor bleeds should be treated with **30–50 percent** correction. F VIII, 25 u/kg followed by 10–15 u/kg q12/h, should be adequate.

   (c) Joint bleeds (hemarthroses). Consultation with hematologists, orthopedic surgeons, and physical therapists who specialize in hemophilia is essential. For **potential hemarthrosis** (e.g., mild trauma, normal examination) a single dose of 15–20 u/kg F VIII concentrate will often suffice. For **acute hemarthrosis** (swollen, painful joint) levels should be maintained above 30–50 percent for a few days until active bleeding stops. After the acute period, daily therapy with 25 u/kg may be necessary to prevent rebleeding during remobilization. **Elevation, ice, non–weight-bearing, and immobilization** (e.g., wraps, splints) are often helpful in minimizing the acute bleed. The joint should be slowly rehabilitated with early mobilization to prevent atrophy and contractures. **Joint aspiration** should be **avoided** if possible.

(d) **Forearm or calf bleeds**

(i) **F VIII** to maintain levels between **50 and 100 percent** should be administered for 7–10 days. Shorter courses may be adequate with early treatment and minimal bleeding.

(ii) **Close monitoring** for the development of **compartment syndrome** is mandatory. Fasciotomy, although associated with significant risks, may be necessary to preserve limb function.

(iii) **Ice and elevation** may be helpful.

(e) **Retroperitoneal or iliopsoas bleeds** require a high index of suspicion and confirmatory radiographs.

(i) **F VIII** to maintain levels between **50 and 100 percent** should be administered for 10–14 days.

(ii) **Close monitoring** for ongoing bleeding is critical since severe anemia may develop.

(iii) Early immobilization (i.e., traction) is often helpful.

(f) **Surgery** requires **100 percent correction** with close monitoring of levels for 10–14 days or as dictated by wound healing.

(g) **Dental extraction** requires **100 percent correction** for 5–7 days. **Epsilon–aminocaproic acid (Amicar)** in an initial dose of 200 mg/kg PO (5 gm maximum) followed by 100 mg/kg q6h (24 gm/day maximum) for 1 week should be added for procedures associated with significant oral bleeding. **Topical thrombin** may also be of benefit.

(h) **Head trauma or severe headache** requires levels of **100 percent** for a minimum of 48 hours. Cranial computed tomographic (CT) scan or magnetic resonance imaging (MRI) should be obtained in all cases. With documented central nervous system (CNS) hemorrhage, full dose replacement should be continued for at least 2 weeks. Long-term therapy is sometimes needed.

(i) **Hematuria,** if mild, usually resolves spontaneously with bed rest and hydration. Persistent hematuria due to kidney trauma may require a few doses of F VIII concentrate. **Prednisone** (2 mg/kg for 2–3 days) may be of benefit. **Amicar is contraindicated** because of the risk of clotting and genitourinary (GU) obstruction.

c. **Complications of therapy**

(1) **Inhibitors.** Anti–factor VIII antibodies develop in about 10–20 percent of patients who receive multiple concentrate infusions. **Expert advice should be sought in the management of bleeding in such patients.**

(a) The presence of inhibitors is suggested by inappropriately low F VIII levels despite replacement. **Diagnosis** is confirmed by inhibition assay. **One Bethesda unit of antibody inactivates one unit of F VIII.**

(b) **Patients with inhibitors should not receive factor VIII except in the event of life-threatening hemorrhage.**

(c) **Porcine F VIII** is useful for patients with **non–cross-reactive antibodies.**

(d) **Activated factor concentrates** that bypass F-VIII (e.g., FEIBA, Proplex) may allow coagulation to proceed.

(e) For life-threatening hemorrhage (e.g., CNS bleed, surgery), attempts can be made to overwhelm the inhibitor with large doses of F VIII. The **dose required** is roughly equal to the **(inhibitor level/ml)** × **(total plasma volume** × **2)**. This amount should be **added to the dose needed to achieve the desired correction** (i.e., 50–100% for major bleeds). This loading dose must then be followed by continuous-infusion maintenance F VIII. Massive doses may be required.

    (f) For mild bleeding, **local measures** (e.g., immobilization, ice, wraps) are the best treatment.

  (2) Infection. Patients with hemophilia have a high incidence of HIV and hepatitis C virus (HCV) due to past treatment with F VIII concentrates. (see sec. **A.1.d**).

  d. Prevention

    (1) antiplatelet medications (e.g., aspirin) are **prohibited.**

    (2) Trauma should be avoided, and, thus, hazardous and contact sports are contraindicated.

    (3) Prenatal diagnosis is available for known carriers.

2. Hemophilia B (Christmas disease) is an X-linked recessive deficiency of factor IX that is approximately one fourth as common as hemophilia A. **Therapy** is the same as for F VIII deficiency with a few exceptions.

  a. Many of the **F IX preparations** contain variable amounts of activated clotting factors. Consequently, to decrease the likelihood of thromboembolism, excessive doses should be avoided and Amicar should **not** be used in combination.

  b. Dose. In general, for **each unit per kilogram** of factor IX administered, plasma levels will **rise by 1 percent.** Thus, the usual dosage of factor required for minor bleeds is 30 units/kg, for major bleeds 50 units/kg, and for severe life-threatening hemorrhage 100 units/kg. The half-life of F IX is 24 hours.

3. Inherited deficiencies of other clotting factors, including **F I, II, V, VII, X, XI, XII, and XIII,** are much less common than hemophilia. Bleeding tendency and laboratory features vary markedly with the condition. **Replacement therapy,** when needed, is usually nonspecific (i.e., FFP), although purified factor concentrates (e.g., F VII) are being developed.

4. von Willebrand's disease (vWD) is the most common inherited bleeding disorder, affecting up to 1–3 percent of the population.

  a. Etiology. von Willebrand factor (vWF) is attached to F VIII and is essential in clot formation. Most subtypes of vWD are autosomal dominant conditions characterized by mild bleeding tendency.

  b. Evaluation

    (1) The family **history** is most often revealing. Epistaxis, mucosal bleeding, excessive bruising, and menorrhagia are *common symptoms.*

    (2) Laboratory evaluation usually includes a prolonged bleeding time and PTT, although these may vary over time. F VIII activity (VIII:C) (usually normal), antigen (vWF) (usually low), and ristocetin cofactor activity (RCoF) (decreased) are used for diagnosis. The platelet count is generally normal.

    (3) For accurate subtype **diagnosis,** ristocetin titration and vWF multimer analysis are often required.

  c. Therapy

    (1) Cryoprecipitate has historically been the standard form of replacement therapy on vWD. **FFP** is similarly effective, but requires 20 times more volume.

    (2) DDAVP causes the release of preformed vWF multimers and is sometimes effective in managing bleeding in vWD. The advantages, risks, and dosing are as outlined for hemophilia (see sec. **III.A.1.b.(1).(d)**) with the following exception: Ristocetin titration testing is essential before one administers DDAVP. Importantly, **DDAVP is contraindicated in type IIB vWD** since thrombocytopenia may be provoked.

    (3) F VIII concentrates that contain large vWF multimers have recently been used in the management of vWD. These carry less infectious risk than cryoprecipitate. A number of products are currently undergoing trials.

5. **Vitamin K deficiency** results in diminished production of factors II, VII, IX, and X and resultant prolongation of the PT, and less remarkably the PTT.
   a. **Etiology**
      (1) **Hemorrhagic disease of the newborn** (see Chap. 6)
      (2) **Malabsorption** of vitamin K can occur in any state characterized by fat malabsorption (e.g., cholestasis) and, rarely, with alterations in GI flora from antibiotics.
      (3) **Dietary inadequacy,** seen in patients on total parenteral nutrition with inadequate vitamin K supplementation, can result in symptomatic deficiency.
      (4) **Vitamin K antagonism** from drugs such as coumarin
   b. **Therapy**
      (1) **Prophylaxis** with **vitamin K₁** (0.5–1.0 mg IM) should be provided to all newborns at birth.
      (2) **Treatment** of older children with **vitamin K₁** (2.5–10.0 mg IM or slow IV) results in an increase in clotting factors and shortening of the PT within hours. Oral dosing can be provided except when malabsorption warrants otherwise.
      (3) **FFP** can be used in the event of acute hemorrhage. For initial hemostasis, 10 ml/kg is usually adequate.
6. **Liver disease** (see also Chap. 10)
   a. **Etiology.** The liver is the major site of synthesis of all coagulation factors except for F VIII.
   b. **Evaluation.** The vitamin K–dependent factors, especially F VII, are most sensitive. Thus, early or mild liver disease is characterized by a prolongation of the PT. More severe dysfunction results in elevations of the PT, PTT, and thrombin time (due to diminished fibrinogen).
   c. **Therapy**
      (1) **Vitamin K₁** should be administered. Doses of 1–5 mg (IM or slow IV) may be required on a daily basis.
      (2) If there is no response to vitamin K and in the event of bleeding, **FFP** should be given. In mild dysfunction, 10 ml/kg may be adequate; however, multiple infusions are often necessary. In such situations, **plasma or whole blood exchange** should be considered.
      (3) **Cryoprecipitate** should be employed for hypofibrinogenemia and bleeding.
      (4) **Platelets or DDAVP** may be helpful in treating quantitative or qualitative platelet defects.
7. **Disseminated intravascular coagulation (DIC)**
   a. **Etiology.** Severe infection is most often implicated with associated septicemia shock and acidosis. Extensive activation of coagulation results in severe microvascular thrombosis, tissue ischemia, microangiopathic hemolytic anemia, and depletion of both platelets and clotting factors. Fibrinolysis soon follows, exacerbating the hemorrhagic state.
   b. **Evaluation** often reveals bleeding from the GI tract, mucosa, and/or skin. Characteristic *laboratory features* include thrombocytopenia, microangiopathic hemolytic anemia, prolonged PT and PTT, diminished fibrinogen, and elevated fibrin split products. Factor levels, when measured, are low.
   c. **Therapy**
      (1) Aggressive **supportive care and reversal of the underlying condition(s)** are essential.
      (2) **Blood product support,** including packed red blood cells (PRBCs), FFP, platelets, and cryoprecipitate, is often required. **Plasma or whole blood exchange** may be helpful.
      (3) **Heparin** has *not* been clearly demonstrated to alter the course of DIC. It is sometimes employed, however, in patients with major thrombotic complications (e.g., purpura fulminans, arterial ischemia). Heparin is also used to prevent severe consumption during the initial therapy of M3 ANLL. The starting dose is 10–25 u/kg/hr by continuous IV

infusion. This should be used cautiously and titrated by the fibrinogen level (most sensitive), platelet count, and/or clinical response.

B. Hypercoagulable states that result in vascular thrombosis can be divided into primary and secondary conditions.

1. **Primary or inherited** prethrombotic disorders due to abnormalities of coagulation proteins are rare. Such conditions should be suspected when thrombosis occurs in young children (e.g., newborns), at unusual sites (e.g., CNS), in multiple family members, or recurrently in the absence of secondary conditions. Deficiency of natural anticoagulant proteins accounts for the majority of the known primary hypercoagulable states. The most common include deficiencies of protein C, protein S, and antithrombin III (AT-III), all of which are transmitted in an autosomal dominant fashion. **Evaluation** may reveal decreased levels of anti-thrombin III, protein S, or protein C. **Therapy** consists primarily of anticoagulation. Since coumarin therapy can cause a decrease in the levels of protein S and C, combined initial treatment with heparin is required to prevent skin necrosis in these two disorders. Adjunctive **FFP or AT-III replacement** may be required.

2. **Secondary or acquired** hypercoagulability is more common than primary deficiency. Associated conditions include sickle cell disease, thrombotic thrombocytopenic purpura (TTP), DIC, collagen vascular disease, malignancy, surgery, pregnancy, immobilization, myeloproliferative disorders (e.g., polycythemia vera), nephrotic syndrome, liver disease, paroxysmal nocturnal hemoglobinuria, metabolic disorders (e.g., homocystinuria, hyperlipidemia), use of vascular catheters or prosthetic devices (e.g., grafts, valves), hyperviscosity (e.g., polycythemia), and use of medications (e.g., asparaginase, oral contraceptives, coumarin, heparin). **Evaluation** should focus on the underlying disorder. **Treatment** of the primary condition is essential, whereas anticoagulation and/or thrombolysis may or may not be necessary.

C. Platelet Disorders

1. **Thrombocytopenia,** defined as a platelet count below 150,000/mm^3, is most commonly a result of **increased destruction** (see also sec. **II.A.2.c**).

   a. General **evaluation.** Many drugs are associated with isolated thrombocytopenia and a thorough history is essential. Petechiae, purpura, excessive bruising, and/or mucosal bleeding are common especially with counts below 20,000/mm^3 or trauma. *Laboratory features* include large platelets on smear and increased megakaryocytes on bone marrow.

   b. General **therapy.** Potentially causative agents should be withdrawn and antiplatelet agents should be avoided. To minimize bleeding, trauma and activities that cause increased intracranial pressure should be avoided. Platelet transfusion may be indicated (see sec. **V.B.5**).

   c. **Management of specific conditions**

      (1) **Hypersplenism** from any cause may result in platelet trapping, and is often accompanied by anemia and neutropenia. With irreversible hypersplenism and/or life-threatening cytopenia, splenectomy may be required.

      (2) **Drug-induced thrombocytopenia. Therapy** requires **drug withdrawal. Corticosteroids** may be helpful in the acute management of bleeding.

      (3) **Immune thrombocytopenic purpura (ITP)** due to the production of IgG platelet autoantibodies is a common childhood disorder.

         (a) **Etiology.** ITP is usually idiopathic, following viral infection. Rarely, ITP is secondary to a collagen vascular disorder.

         (b) **Evaluation.** The typical presentation is of a previously healthy child with bruising and petechiae, and a history of a preceding viral illness within the past month. Except for thrombocytopenia, the CBC is normal. Large platelets are commonly seen. Antiplatelet antibodies are often found, but not required since **diagnosis** is easily made on clinical grounds. Bone marrow aspiration to confirm the presence of increased megakaryocytes and rule out infiltrative processes is often performed. **This is strongly recommended before steroid therapy is instituted.**

(c) **Therapy.** No therapy has been shown to influence long-term outcome or mortality. Nonetheless, for those with bleeding or platelet counts <20,000mm^3, most recommend treatment.

   (i) **Corticosteroids** result in an increased rate of rise in the platelet count. In addition, vascular effects may decrease the risk of early bleeding. Standard practice is to initiate **prednisone** at a dose of 2 mg/kg/day for 5–10 days followed by a rapid taper over 3–4 days. The platelet count usually responds in 5–7 days. Many relapse off prednisone and can be successfully retreated. Recently, high-dose steroids (30 mg/kg/day) have been employed in the initial treatment of ITP.

   (ii) **Intravenous gamma globulin** at doses of 1 gm/kg/day for 2 days or 400 mg/kg/day for 5 days results in a slightly more rapid rise in the platelet count than standard-dose prednisone. Although this allows treatment without bone marrow, it is associated with increased cost, inconvenience, and the risk of allergic reactions. Consequently, many reserve IVGG for those with resistance, side effects, or contraindications to steroids.

   (iii) **Splenectomy** is curative for many with chronic ITP. This should be avoided in young children and precautions should be taken to minimize the risk of severe infection (see sec. **I.B.3.c.(3)(b)(iii)**).

   (iv) Additional therapeutic options usually reserved for patients with chronic ITP include vincristine, cyclophosphamide, and danazol. Recently, IV anti-Rh(D) globulin (RhoGAM) has been shown to be effective.

   (v) **Emergency management** of life-threatening hemorrhage should include high-dose IVGG and steroids, platelet transfusion, plasmapheresis, and/or splenectomy. Amicar may be useful for oral bleeding.

   (vi) **HIV** is commonly associated with ITP. Treatment with azidothymidine (AZT), steroids, IVGG, RhoGAM, and staphylococcal protein A column adsorption have all been shown to be effective. To decrease infectious complications, *chronic steroids and splenectomy should be avoided.*

d. **Outcome.** Of children with ITP, 75–80 percent fully recover by 6 months, and 90 percent have normal platelet counts by 1 year from diagnosis. The risk of chronicity increases with age. Mortality due to intracranial, pulmonary, or GI hemorrhage in acute ITP is less than 1 percent. Of those who die, 90 percent do so within the first few days of onset.

(4) **Neonatal immune thrombocytopenia** can result from **maternal auto- or isoantibodies.** Sensitization to platelet-specific antigens, most commonly PL^A

   (a) **Evaluation.** Infants usually present with severe petechiae and bruising related to birth trauma. CNS hemorrhage can be life threatening. Initial laboratory tests should include PT and PTT (to rule out DIC) and maternal platelet count. If these are normal, newborn antiplatelet antibody assay and maternal platelet typing should be performed to evaluate for possible isoimmune destruction. Notably, isosensitization may occur with first pregnancies.

   (b) **Therapy** is required for bleeding or a platelet count <20,000/mm^3. Spontaneous resolution occurs by 3–4 months. For **autoimmune thrombocytopenia,** treatment is as outlined for ITP and includes steroids and IVGG (see sec. **III.C.1.c.(3)(c)**). For **isoimmune thrombocytopenia,** transfusion with washed maternal or PL^{A1}-negative donor platelets is usually effective. **Family-donated** products should be irradiated to prevent transfusion-associated graft-versus-host disease (TAGVHO) (see sec. **V.C.2**). If suitable platelets are not available, steroids, IVGG, and/or random-donor platelet transfusion can be employed.

   (c) **Prevention.** For pregnant women with a prior history of iso- or autoimmune thrombocytopenia, many recommend fetal platelet count monitoring or elective cesarean section, or both, to prevent intracranial hemorrhage. Prenatal treatment with IVGG, steroids, and/or umbilical vein maternal platelet transfusion may be effective.

   2. **Qualitative platelet disorders** result in platelet-type bleeding, prolonged bleeding time, and abnormal aggregation studies in the absence of thrombocytopenia. **Secondary dysfunction** is most common (e.g., drugs, uremia, liver disease). **Congenital disorders of platelet function** are rare. **Therapy** varies with the condition, but may include platelet transfusion (see sec. **V.B.5.b.(3)**), Amicar, DDAVP, cryoprecipitate, FFP, and avoidance of trauma and anti-platelet medications.

IV. **White blood cells (WBCs)**
   A. **Neutrophils**, or polymorphonuclear (PMN) leukocytes, normally range between 1,500 and 8,000/mm³.
      1. **Neutropenia** is defined as an absolute neutrophil count (ANC) <1,000/mm³, where the ANC is equal to the (total WBC count) × (percent PMN + band forms). Severe neutropenia is defined as a count <500/mm³. In general, the risk of infection increases with the degree of neutropenia.
         a. **Etiology.** Neutropenia is due to either decreased marrow production or accelerated destruction (Table 16-6). Most common are transient, self-limited decreases related to viral infections or drugs.
         b. **Evaluation.** Children frequently present with recurrent fever and infection, especially stomatitis, adenitis, or sinopulmonary disease. *History* may be notable for periodicity, exposures, or affected family members. *Laboratory studies* should include twice-weekly CBCs for 4–6 weeks to evaluate for cyclic neutropenia. Past counts may suggest a congenital disorder. Bone marrow examination and antineutrophil antibodies may be required.
         c. **Therapy** varies with the condition (see Table 16-6) although certain general principles apply.
            (1) Medical evaluation and treatment are required for all febrile episodes (>38°C).
               (a) For those with an ANC <500/mm³, **empiric broad-spectrum parenteral antibiotics** should be provided (see Chap. 14).
               (b) Fungal, atypical, and opportunistic infections are common. Additional antimicrobial agents should be added as necessary.
               (c) **Granulocyte transfusion** is rarely indicated, but should be considered in cases of life-threatening or progressive infection.
            (2) **Prophylactic oral antibodies** should be considered. Trimethoprim/sulfamethoxazole (TMP/sulfa) combinations at a dose of 4–5 mg/kg/day of TMP are effective in cyclic or congenital neutropenia.
      2. **Disorders of neutrophil function** present similarly to neutropenic conditions.
         a. **Etiology.** Neutrophil dysfunction is most frequently secondary, although rare primary disorders exist (Table 16-7).
         b. **Evaluation.** Gamma globulin and complement levels should be analyzed. Specific assays of phagocyte function include prednisone stimulation (reserve and mobilization), opsonization and ingestion studies, Rebuck skin window (chemotaxis), nitroblue tetrazolium (NBT) reduction (superoxide generation), and flow cytometric analysis of neutrophil receptors.
         c. **Therapy.** The general principles of management of fever and infection are as outlined for neutropenia (see sec. **IV.A.1.c.**) Prophylactic antibiotics or IVGG, or both, are frequently beneficial. Specific treatment varies with the condition (see Table 16-7).

Table 16-6. Causes of neutropenia

Etiology	Diagnosis	Treatment
Decreased production		
Infection	Usually viral, transient acquired marrow injury; occasionally severe and protracted	Supportive
Kostmann's syndrome	Severe congenital neutropenia, AR inheritance, ANC <500/mm³, life-threatening infections	Prophylactic antibiotics, G-CSF, marrow transplant
Benign	Mild congenital neutropenia, ANC >500/mm³; infection is rare	Supportive
Cyclic	Oscillating neutropenia and symptoms usually q3 weeks; stomatitis is frequent	Prophylactic antibiotics; G-CSF increases nadir
Toxic	Drugs, radiation, chemotherapy, exposure history; may be severe	Agent removal, supportive
Nutrition	Severe B₁₂, folate, or copper deficiency	Nutritional repletion
Shwachman-Diamond	Neutropenia, exocrine pancreatic insufficiency, AR inheritance; may evolve to AA or leukemia	Supportive, pancreatic enzymes, ? growth factors, marrow transplant
Increased destruction		
Drug induced	Exposure history, especially antibiotics	Agent removal, supportive
Isoimmune neonatal	Severe congenital neutropenia, normal marrow, maternal anti-WBC antibodies, transient	Supportive
Autoimmune	Usually idiopathic and self-limited; may be severe; anti-WBC antibodies	Steroids, IVGG; treat underlying collagen vascular disorder

Key: AR = autosomal recessive; G-CSF = granulocyte colony stimulating factor

   3. **Neutrophilia** is usually reactive. Common etiologies include infection, inflammatory disorders, marrow invasion, exercise, and drugs (e.g., glucocorticoids, epinephrine). Rarely, asplenia, neutrophil receptor defects, or hereditary neutrophilia is responsible. Notably, newborns have markedly higher neutrophil counts than older children and adults.
V. Transfusion therapy
   A. All blood components have side effects and should not be administered without careful consideration of the indications, appropriate dose, and potential toxicities.
   B. Blood products
      1. Whole blood (WB)
         a. Contents. A unit of unmodified WB consists of 450 ml donor blood. The

Table 16-7. Causes of neutrophil dysfunction

Etiology	Diagnosis	Treatment
Depressed chemotaxis	Seen with chronic illness (e.g., renal failure) and infection (especially skin), antibody deficiency, excess IgE and/or IGA, complement disorders, and certain drugs; Rebuck is diagnostic	Treat underlying condition, IVGG, supportive; apheresis to lower IgE sometimes helpful
Opsonization disorders	Complement and antibody deficiencies	IVGG, supportive, plasma
Chédiak-Higashi disease	Recurrent, severe infection; giant granules; neutropenia; AR inheritance; albinism	Marrow transplant, supportive
Chronic granulomatous disease	Recurrent, severe infection (especially skin, lung) with catalase + organisms; usually X linked (sometimes AR); NBT test is diagnostic	Interferon gamma, supportive prophylactic antibiotics
Neutrophil adhesion disorders	Recurrent infection (especially omphalitis), elevated WBC, absent receptors by cytometry, AR inheritance, abnormal Rebuck	Marrow transplant, supportive
Nutritional	Severe phosphate or zinc deficiency	Repletion

Key: AR = autosomal recessive; NBT = nitroblue tetrazolium.

Hct is about 40%. WBCs, platelets, and plasma proteins lose function in storage. WB is an inefficient product with limited usefulness for replacement.

- b. **Indications**
    - (1) **Very fresh WB** that is unrefrigerated and <6 hours old is recommended for the treatment of *neonatal sepsis* with neutropenia. Double-volume exchange q12–24h is often required to maintain a measurable neutrophil count. **To prevent TAGVHD, blood must be irradiated.**
    - (2) **WB reconstituted** from PRBCs, FFP, and platelets is employed for most other indications including acute and/or large volume loss (e.g., trauma) and routine exchange transfusion (e.g., hyperbilirubinemia).
- 2. **Packed red blood cells (PRBCs)**
    - a. **Contents.** A unit of PRBCs consists of 200–250 ml with a Hct of 60–80% and variable amounts of WBCs and plasma.
    - b. **Indications**
        - (1) PRBCs are the standard product for treating most forms of acute and chronic anemia.
        - (2) **WBC removal** by filtration should be performed for those who require multiple transfusions to decrease the incidence and severity of sensitization to leukocyte antigens. This also decreases the risk of transmitting CMV.

(3) PRBCs washed in saline should be employed when plasma dilution is desired.

(4) Frozen/deglycerolized PRBCs are depleted of WBCs and plasma. They are primarily used for those who require lifelong transfusions and/or extended RBC antigen matching (e.g., SCD).

c. Dose (see Table 16-8)

(1) Most tolerate infusion rates of 10 ml/kg/hr.

(2) With volume intolerance, gradual correction can be achieved by infusing small aliquots (e.g., 5–10 ml/kg) over 4–6 hours. Diuretics may be helpful.

(3) When rapid correction is required, but is limited by fluid intolerance, partial exchange transfusion should be performed. Whole blood is removed in small aliquots and replaced with equal volumes of PRBCs. Automated exchange using a cell separator can be employed when large volumes are required.

3. Fresh frozen plasma

a. Contents. One unit consists of 250 ml with normal levels of clotting factors, albumin, and antibodies.

b. Indications. FFP should be used to replace clotting factors in the setting of bleeding and elevations of the PT or PTT. Because of potential side effects, **FFP should not be used solely for volume replacement.**

c. Dose

(1) 10 ml/kg raises the clotting activity by about 20 percent. Multiple doses may be required.

(2) Plasma exchange should be employed when large quantities are required and there is volume intolerance.

(3) The rate of transfusion is limited by citrate toxicity. Close monitoring

---

Table 16-8. Formulas for transfusion

1. Estimation of total blood volume (TBV)
   100 ml/kg neonates
   80 ml/kg infants and children
   65 ml/kg adults

2. Red blood cell volume (RCV)
   $RCV = TBV \times Hct$

3. RBC transfusion

   $$\text{Volume of PRBCs required (ml)} = \frac{(Hct_d - Hct_i)\,(TBV)}{Hct_{tx}}$$

   Example:
   To raise the Hct from 20 to 35% in a child with a TBV of 1,800 ml using PRBCs with an Hct of 75%:

   $$\frac{(.15)\,(1,800)}{.75} = 360 \text{ ml}$$

4. RBC removal for polycythemia

   $$\text{Volume of blood removed (ml)} = \frac{(Hct_i - Hct_d)\,(TBV)}{Hct_r}$$

5. RBC transfusion by manual partial exchange*

   $$\text{Volume of PRBCs required (ml)} = \frac{(Hct_d - Hct_i)\,(TBV)}{Hct_{tx} - \dfrac{(Hct_i + Hct_d)}{2}}$$

Key: Hct = Hematocrit (in fractional form, e.g., 40% = 0.40); Hct_i = initial Hct; Hct_d = desired Hct; Hct_{tx} = Hct of transfused cells (usually 0.7–0.8); Hct_r = Hct of blood removed from the patient (with manual phlebotomy, $Hct_r = Hct_i$).
* Adapted from P. I. Neiburg and J. A. Stockman, Rapid correction of anemia with partial exchange transfusion. *Am. J. Dis. Child.* 131:60, 1977.

of vital signs and ionized calcium levels is essential when large or rapid infusions are used.

4. **Cryoprecipitate**
   a. **Contents.** One unit contains approximately 300 mg fibrinogen and 80–100 units of F VIII in, and 75 units of F XIII 10–20 ml plasma.
   b. **Indications**
      (1) Bleeding in association with hypofibrinogenemia (<100 mg/dl)
      (2) Hemophilia A and vWD
      (3) Factor XIII deficiency
      (4) Bleeding due to uremia
   c. **Dose.** 0.3 u/kg should increase the fibrinogen by 200 mg/dl. Multiple doses may be required.

5. **Platelets**
   a. **Contents.** One unit contains 5.5×10^{10} platelets with variable quantities of WBCs and plasma. Single-donor apheresis products contain 6–8 units per bag.
   b. **Indications**
      (1) Thrombocytopenia with bleeding. The aim should be to raise the platelet count to a point where bleeding stops. Values between 50,000 and 100,000/mm^3 usually suffice. Counts >100,000/mm^3 should be maintained for high-risk situations, such as CNS, vascular, or surgical hemorrhage.
      (2) Prophylaxis for thrombocytopenia without bleeding. The risk of bleeding increases as the platelet count falls below 20,000/mm^3 Consequently, it has become routine to transfuse platelets prophylactically in the setting of severe thrombocytopenia. Exceptions include ITP or other antibody-mediated forms of platelet destruction. In addition, in those with chronic conditions such as aplastic anemia transfusion-related complications often develop, *making prophylactic transfusions difficult and potentially dangerous.*
      (3) Qualitative platelet disorders
         (a) In cases of acquired platelet dysfunction, platelet transfusion may be ineffective unless the underlying cause is reversed.
         (b) Bleeding in congenital platelet disorders usually responds to transfusion. Therapy should be gauged by hemostasis and shortening of the bleeding time.
      (4) Single-donor apheresis platelets and **WBC removal by filtration** should be employed for those who require multiple transfusions to decrease the incidence and severity of sensitization to leukocyte antigens.
      (5) Platelets washed in saline should be employed when plasma protein dilution is desired (e.g., maternal antibody removal).
   c. **Dose**
      (1) 0.1 u/kg normally increases the platelet count by 30,000–50,000/mm^3.
      (2) Repeat or larger doses are required in the event of ongoing destruction.
      (3) Refractoriness (persistent bleeding and/or thrombocytopenia) is common and posttransfusion platelet counts (10–60 minutes) should be obtained to assess the cause (Table 16-9).

6. **Albumin**
   a. **Contents.** Standard preparations consist of purified albumin 5% and 25%.
   b. **Indications**
      (1) Volume restoration
      (2) Hypoproteinemia
   c. **Dose**
      (1) The usual dose is 10 ml/kg of 5% or 2.5 ml/kg of 25% albumin.
      (2) Under normal circumstances, only about 40 percent remains in the intravascular space. Diuretics are sometimes used in combination with albumin 25% to manage extravascular fluid overload.

Table 16-9. Causes of platelet refractoriness

Continued bleeding despite appropriate increase in count
  Underlying disorder that impairs function of transfused platelets (e.g., uremia, drugs)
  Poor platelet quality (e.g., prolonged storage)
  Other causes of bleeding (e.g., DIC, vascular)
Inadequate increase in count
  Insufficient platelet dose
  Ongoing consumption (e.g., major hemorrhage)
  Sequestration (e.g., splenomegaly)
No increase in count
  Alloimmunization to HLA antibodies
  Antiplatelet antibody (e.g., ITP)

7. **Granulocytes**
    a. **Contents.** A unit contains approximately 5×10^{10} granulocytes with variable quantities of RBCs, platelets, and plasma.
    b. **Indications**
        (1) **Severe neutropenia** (ANC $< 500/\text{mm}^3$) without the expectation of rapid marrow recovery and life-threatening infection (especially gram negative or fungal)
        (2) **Sepsis neonatorum** with severe neutropenia. (see sec. **V.B.1.b.(1)**)
    c. **Dose**
        (1) Adolescents should receive 1 unit.
        (2) Children should receive 0.5–1.0 unit.
        (3) Neonates can be given small (e.g., 10 ml/kg) infusions or double volume WB exchange (see sec. **V.B.1.b.(1)**).
        (4) Transfusion should be repeated q 12–24 h until ANC recovery $> 500/\text{mm}^3$.
        (5) **To prevent TAGVHD, all WBC transfusions must be irradiated.**
  C. **Side effects** are associated with the transfusion of all blood products (see Table 16-10).
    1. **Transfusion reactions**
        a. **Acute hemolytic reactions**
            (1) **Etiology.** Major blood group (ABO) incompatibility results in isohemagglutinin and complement-mediated hemolysis. Such reactions are rare and due primarily to clerical errors. Occasionally, blood incompatible for "minor" RBC antigens results in immediate hemolysis when high-titer IgG antibodies are present from prior exposure.
            (2) **Evaluation.** Signs and symptoms include fever, rigors, shock, back pain, and hematuria. Direct Coombs test and repeat blood type and crossmatch are confirmatory.
            (3) **Therapy**
                (a) Immediate termination of transfusion
                (b) Intensive monitoring and supportive care including volume and cardiovascular resuscitation as necessary
                (c) Attempts to maintain renal blood flow with mannitol, furosemide, and/or dopamine (see Chap. 3)
                (d) Management of renal failure
                (e) Early plasmapheresis or exchange transfusion may be beneficial.
        b. **Delayed hemolytic reactions**
            (1) **Etiology.** These are due to sensitization to minor (non ABO) blood group antigens. IgG response usually occurs 7–10 days after transfusion. Such antibody development is particularly common in SCD.
            (2) **Evaluation.** Manifestations are usually more mild than with acute hemolytic reactions. Pallor, jaundice, myalgias, arthralgias, and low-grade fever are common. Laboratory features include hyperbili-

Table 16-10. Side effects of transfusion

Product	Blood group incompatibility	WBC sensitization	HCV	HIV	CMV	TAGVHD	Citrate
Whole blood	+	+	+	+	+	+	+
Packed red blood cells	+	+	+	+	+	+	±
Fresh frozen plasma	+	–	+	+	–	–	+
Cryoprecipitate	–	–	+	+	–	–	–
Platelets	±	+	+	+	+	+	–
Albumin	–	–	–	–	–	–	
White blood cells	+	+	+	+	+	+	±

HCV = Hepatitis C virus; HIV = Human immunodeficiency virus; CMV = cytomegalovirus; TAGVHD = Transfusion associated graft vs. host disease; WBC = white blood cell; † = side effect associated; – = side effect not associated; ± = side effect sometimes associated.

rubinemia, elevated LDH, anemia, positive Coombs test, and specific antibody analysis. Notably, with secondary anamnestic antibody production, severe intravascular hemolysis can occur.

 (3) Therapy varies with the severity of the reaction.
  (a) Antipyretics, analgesics, and observation usually suffice.
  (b) Severe reactions as outlined above **(V.C.1.a.(3))**
 (4) Prevention
  (a) Extended RBC antigen-matched blood should be provided for patients with known antibodies.
  (b) Many recommend the prophylactic use of PRBCs matched for minor antigens in chronic transfusion regimens (e.g., SCD, thalassemia major).
  (c) RhoGAM should be administered for PRBC or platelet transfusions that are mismatched for Rh(D).
c. Allergic reactions
 (1) Etiology. Usually due to sensitization to plasma proteins; however, prior transfusion is not required.
 (2) Evaluation. Urticaria, flushing, itching, angioedema, and rarely anaphylaxis can occur.
 (3) Therapy
  (a) Transfusion should be halted.
  (b) IV antihistamines (e.g., diphenhydramine, 1 mg/kg)
  (c) IV corticosteroids (e.g., methylprednisolone, 2 mg/kg) for severe reactions
  (d) Supportive care with fluids and epinephrine as needed
 (4) Prevention
  (a) Premedication with antihistamines or steroids or both, when the patient has a history of allergic reactions
  (b) Plasma-depleted platelets and PRBCs for patients with a history of severe reactions
d. Febrile reactions
 (1) Etiology. Primarily due to sensitization to leukocyte antigens. Prior exposure is required.
 (2) Evaluation. Symptoms consist primarily of fever and chills. Manifestations may be severe and mimic hemolytic or allergic reaction.

(3) Therapy
  (a) Termination of transfusion is only necessary for severe reactions.
  (b) Antipyretic agents are usually effective.
  (c) Severe chills or rigors should be treated with low doses of narcotics or steroids, or both.
(4) Prevention
  (a) Premedication with antipyretics should be provided for those with a history of reactions.
  (b) Leukodepleted platelets and PRBCs should also be employed.
e. Acute pulmonary reactions
  (1) Etiology. Respiratory symptoms developing during transfusion may be due to volume overload or any of the above described reactions. True pulmonary reactions may, however, result from leukoagglutination of WBCs, usually with granulocyte transfusion.
  (2) Evaluation. Patients may demonstrate mild tachypnea, dyspnea, and/or respiratory distress. CXR often reveals patchy infiltrates or pulmonary edema.
  (3) Therapy
    (a) Tranfusion should be halted.
    (b) Close monitoring of vital signs and oxygen saturation
    (c) Supplemental oxygen and respiratory support including artificial ventilation (see Chap. 3)
    (d) Glucocorticoids may be of benefit, although their role is unproven.
2. Transfusion-associated graft-versus-host disease
  a. Etiology. TAGVHD results when immunocompetent WBCs are transfused and proliferate in the recipient. The reaction against patient tissues is often *severe,* with reported mortality >80 percent. This occurs primarily in immunosuppressed patients, especially premature newborns, congenital immunodeficiency, marrow transplant, and those undergoing chemotherapy for oncologic disorders. In addition, transfusion of HLA-compatible products into immunocompetent hosts has been associated with this condition, presumably due to nonrecognition and nondestruction of transfused lymphocytes.
  b. Evaluation. Signs and symptoms are often nonspecific and include skin rash, fever, diarrhea, hepatitis, and cytopenias. A high index of suspicion is required and diagnosis is usually made by biopsy and/or HLA typing of lymphocytes.
  c. Therapy
    (1) Even with aggressive treatment, outcome is poor.
    (2) Immunosuppressive therapy, including steroids, ATG, monoclonal antibodies, and/or cytotoxic agents, should be considered.
  d. Prevention. Irradiation of cellular blood products with ≥2500 rads prevents TAGVHD. This should be employed in the following situations:
    (1) Potential suppressed immunity, including very low birth weight infants, immunodeficiency, malignancy, marrow or organ transplantation, bone marrow failure syndromes
    (2) All blood products from close family members or HLA-matched donors
    (3) All granulocyte transfusions including fresh WB exchange
3. Citrate toxicity
  a. Etiology. The major anticoagulants used to store blood contain large amounts of citrate, the action of which is to bind calcium and prevent clotting. With rapid or large volume infusion of citrate (i.e., plasma)-rich products, toxicity from systemic hypocalcemia is common. Neonates and those with renal insufficiency, hepatic dysfunction, acidosis, or shock are particularly at risk.
  b. Evaluation. Citrate toxicity should be suspected in the setting of substantial FFP use (e.g., exchange transfusion) or when rates exceed 0.25 ml/kg/min. Early symptoms include irritability, diaphoresis, chills, nau-

Table 16-11. Clinical uses of hematopoietic growth factors

Erythropoietin
Anemia
  Chronic renal failure
  HIV and AZT related
  Malignancy
  Prematurity
  Autologous blood donation
G-CSF
Neutropenia
  Chemotherapy related
  Kostmann's syndrome
  Cyclic
  Chronic
GM-CSF
Marrow failure
  Bone marrow transplant
  Myelodysplastic syndromes
  Peripheral stem cell collection
  Chemotherapy related

G-CSF = granulocyte colony stimulating factor; GM-CSF = granulocyte-macrophage colony stimulating factor.

sea, abdominal pain, vomiting, and paresthesias. Tachycardia, hypotension, and prolongation of the QT interval and QRS complex follow. With severe untreated toxicity, tetany, ventricular dysfunction, and cardiovascular collapse may ensue. *Diagnosis* can be rapidly confirmed by ionized calcium assay. With chronic FFP use and renal insufficiency, metabolic alkalosis may develop.

    c. Therapy
      (1) With the first suspicion of toxicity, transfusion should be interrupted and ionized calcium level checked.
      (2) Mild toxicity will usually resolve spontaneously. Infusion should be held until symptoms clear and should be resumed at a slower rate.
      (3) For significant toxicity, **IV calcium supplementation** is required (see Chap. 11).
    d. Prevention. Citrate toxicity can be avoided by close monitoring and prophylactic calcium replacement.
  D. Alternatives to transfusion. Much effort has been devoted to the development of therapies to decrease the risk of transfusion-related side effects. Blood substitutes, growth factors, and medications that modulate hgb production are currently undergoing human trials. A large number of **hematopoietic growth factors or cytokines** have recently been cloned, offering major promise for disorders marked by diminished blood cell production. Table 16-11 lists conditions that are potentially amenable to such therapy.

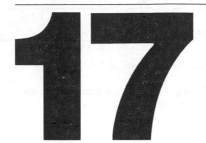

Allergic Disorders and Immunodeficiency

Linda Schneider

I. **Allergic disorders.** An allergic response is an "immediate" response involving antigen-specific, immunoglobulin E (IgE)-mediated degranulation of mast cells. Degranulation releases mediators such as histamine, eosinophil chemotactic factors of anaphylaxis, and platelet-activating factor. These mediators acutely cause increased vascular permeability and smooth muscle contraction. The result is manifest as anaphylaxis, asthma, and allergic rhinitis. In addition, mast cell degranulation triggers the synthesis and release of leukotrienes and interleukins. Leukotrienes are responsible for the late phase of the allergic response. Smooth muscle contraction and edema occur, as well as the recruitment of eosinophils, neutrophils, and lymphocytes, which may lead to chronic inflammation.

  A. **Anaphylaxis**

  1. **Etiology. Anaphylaxis** is the life-threatening clinical response caused by an immediate IgE-mediated reaction in a sensitized individual. **Anaphylactoid** reactions clinically resemble anaphylaxis, but are caused by direct mast cell activation or by non-IgE-mediated mechanisms. The most common causes of anaphylaxis/anaphylactoid reactions in children include antibiotics, foods, and stinging insects (Table 17-1).

  2. **Evaluation.** Anaphylactic reactions are systemic reactions that generally occur within minutes of exposure to precipitating agents.

  a. **Manifestations**

  (1) **General.** Prodromal symptoms include peripheral tingling or pruritus, warm sensation, malaise, and weakness.

  (2) **Cutaneous.** Diffuse flushing may occur as the initial symptom, followed by urticaria, angioedema, or both.

  (3) **Respiratory.** Symptoms may be as mild as sneezing and rhinorrhea, or as serious as laryngeal or upper airway edema with stridor, bronchospasm, or respiratory arrest.

  (4) **Cardiovascular.** Hypotension, tachycardia, or shock may occur.

  (5) **Gastrointestinal.** Nausea, vomiting, abdominal pain, and diarrhea may occur.

  3. **Diagnosis.** The diagnosis is primarily based on the clinical syndrome and a history consistent with exposure to a precipitating agent. Laboratory evaluation is not necessary for the acute diagnosis, but may be useful to rule out myocardial infarction, insulin reactions, or other syndromes that may mimic anaphylaxis. Evaluation for antigen-specific IgE may be useful to confirm or identify the precipitating agent and can be performed on a nonemergent basis.

  a. **Radioallergosorbent test (RAST)** is a semiquantitative assay for allergen-specific IgE. The advantage of this test is that it can be performed in vitro. However, the RAST is less sensitive than skin testing.

  b. **Skin tests.** The validity of the results must be individualized for each allergen. Skin tests are more reliable for pollens and inhalants than for foods or drugs.

  c. **Penicillin allergy.** If penicillin is implicated as a cause for anaphylaxis, skin testing can confirm sensitivity. RAST testing is not sufficient.

  4. **Therapy.** Once anaphylaxis is recognized, therapy should be instituted

Table 17-1. Major causes of anaphylaxis or anaphylactoid reactions

Antibiotics
    Penicillin, cephalosporins, tetracycline, streptomycin, and others
Biologicals
    Insect venoms, allergen extracts, gamma globulin, blood transfusions, antitoxins, antilymphocyte globulin, hormones, asparaginase, and others
Diagnostic agents
    Iodinated contrast media
Other drugs
    Aspirin, dextran plasma expanders
Foods
    Especially shellfish, peanuts, nuts, eggs, milk, fish, soy

immediately. If the responsible agent is being administered, it must be promptly discontinued (e.g., antibiotics, radiocontrast dye).

  a. General measures include administering oxygen, applying a tourniquet proximal to the site of an injection or insect sting, and administering isotonic fluids to treat hypotension.

  b. Pharmacologic measures

    (1) Epinephrine, 0.01 ml/kg of 1 : 1,000 solution, should be given SC, with a second dose administered at the site of a precipitating injection or insect sting.

    (2) Diphenhydramine, 1–2 mg/kg, should be given intravenously, intramuscularly, or PO q6h for at least 48 hours.

    (3) For the treatment of bronchospasm, laryngeal edema, and angioedema, see Chap. 3.

  c. Prophylaxis. To prevent recurrence, cautious avoidance of reexposure to the specific allergen implicated in the original episode is mandatory.

    (1) Anaphylaxis kits (e.g., EpiPen, Center Laboratories) should be given to all patients with a history of food or stinging insect anaphylaxis. In addition, these patients should wear a MedicAlert identification bracelet.

    (2) Insect venom immunotherapy should be considered for children with anaphylaxis precipitated by stinging insect venom. For children who experience only skin manifestations (generalized urticaria and/or angioedema), venom immunotherapy is not indicated.

    (3) Radiocontrast allergy. If future studies with contrast are absolutely required, pretreatment with diphenhydramine and corticosteroids is mandatory.

B. Asthma

  1. Etiology. Asthma is a reversible obstructive lung disease characterized by airway inflammation and hyperreactivity of the airways to various stimuli that results in recurrent episodes of wheezing and dyspnea. A number of factors can precipitate asthma (Table 17-2).

  2. Evaluation

    a. History. Asthma should be suspected in any child with a history of frequent or recurrent episodes of cough, dyspnea, wheezing, exercise intolerance, or "bronchitis." A careful history of inciting factors should be sought. A history of rhinitis, conjunctivitis, and atopic dermatitis suggests an atopic predisposition, as does a family history of allergic diseases. In the acutely wheezing child, the history should include duration of wheezing, probable precipitant, previous medications, and severity of previous attacks.

    b. Physical examination. The presence of physical findings depends to a great extent on the frequency of wheezing and on the state of the disease.

      (1) Asymptomatic patients may have normal examinations. In more

Table 17-2. Factors that precipitate asthma

Infections
  Viral (respiratory syncytial virus, adenovirus, influenza, parainfluenza,
    rhinovirus)
  Mycoplasma
  Bacteria (bronchitis, sinusitis, rarely pneumonia)
Allergens
  Seasonal pollens, animals, dust mites, molds
Irritants
  Smoke, solvents, air pollutants (ozone, sulfur dioxide, metabisulfite), cold air
Exercise
  In particular, running sports; seen less with swimming
Aspirin
  Prostaglandin-mediated, all nonsteroidal antiinflammatory agents may have
    similar effect. Nasal polyps may be present in aspirin triad (asthma, aspirin
    intolerance, and nasal polyps)

severe disease, wheezing and rhonchi may be heard even when the
patient feels well.

(2) Atopic predisposition may be suggested by edema of nasal mucosa,
allergic shiners, and eczema.

(3) The presence of clubbing, increased anteroposterior diameter of the
chest, recurrent sinusitis, or failure to thrive should prompt evaluation for disorders such as cystic fibrosis or immunodeficiency.

(4) Assessment of the acutely wheezing child should include vital signs;
peak flow; pulsus paradoxus; mental status (somnolence or agitation
suggests hypoxia); degree of dyspnea, i.e., retractions; and use of
accessory muscles, in addition to auscultation for breath sounds.

c. **Laboratory data**

(1) **Pulse oximetry** is a useful way to measure and monitor oxygen
saturation.

(2) **Arterial blood gases** may be useful in predicting impending respiratory failure. In the face of marked hyperventilation, a PCO_2 of 40 is
worrisome.

(3) **Complete blood count (CBC).** Eosinophilia suggests an extrinsic
precipitant. Neutrophilia may indicate a coincident bacterial infection or may reflect recent epinephrine therapy.

(4) **Radiologic evaluation**

(a) Chest x-ray may be helpful in differentiating bronchospasm from
other causes of acute wheezing (e.g., foreign body aspiration or
congestive heart failure). In severely ill patients, it may be useful
in diagnosing pneumomediastinum or pneumothorax.

(b) Other studies, such as a barium swallow, sinus films, and sinus
computed tomographic (CT) scan, should be considered on an
individual basis.

(5) **Allergy testing**

(a) Skin tests in children may be useful in identifying allergens. In
children with severe skin disease, RAST testing can be substituted, although it is less sensitive.

(b) Elevated total IgE levels suggest allergic disease, and determination may be useful in the evaluation of allergic bronchopulmonary aspergillosis.

(6) Tuberculin skin testing is useful in patients with a chronic cough and
in those considered for steroid therapy.

(7) Sweat testing is appropriate in patients with severe chronic wheezing,
particularly if they are failing to thrive.

(8) Pulmonary function testing (spirometry and peak flow measurement) can be performed in children 6 years of age or older and is useful in the following situations:

(a) Following asthmatic patients with acute exacerbation and determining those who require hospitalization or initiation of oral steroids

(b) Confirming the presence of reversible airway obstruction in patients during diagnostic evaluation

(c) Monitoring chronic asthmatic patients on maintenance bronchodilators and titrating their medications

3. **Therapy.** The goals of therapy are to reverse acute bronchospasm, and, in the patient with chronic disease, to minimize symptoms and hospitalizations, maximize school attendance, and allow normal activity. Treatment must be individualized: The patient should be aware of precipitants to avoid, and pharmacologic agents should be titrated according to symptoms. Prophylactic treatment should be used to minimize anticipated exacerbation.

a. **General measures**

(1) Avoid nonspecific respiratory irritants such as cigarette or wood/coal smoke, paint, aerosolized agents (e.g., hairspray, perfume), and air pollution.

(2) For the allergic patient, exposure to environmental allergens should be reduced.

(a) Dust/mite control measures

(i) Encase mattress, boxspring, and pillows in airtight plastic covers.

(ii) Wash bedding in hot (130°F) water weekly.

(iii) Remove dust collectors, e.g., furry toys, rugs, drapes, upholstered furniture, and carpeting, especially from the bedroom.

(iv) Use tannic acid solution or benzyl benzoate powder (Acarosan) to kill or alter the mite allergens in carpeting or upholstered furniture.

(v) Clean room at least weekly with damp dust cloth.

(b) Remove pets from the bedroom, preferably from the house.

(c) Use air conditioning to reduce pollen in patient's environment.

b. **Pharmacologic agents.** The pharmacologic treatment of asthma includes use of selective β_2-adrenergic agents, theophylline, cromolyn, and corticosteroids. These agents are discussed individually below, and their use in acute asthma, intermittent bronchospasm, and chronic asthma is then reviewed.

(1) **Beta-adrenergic agents.** These agents act rapidly, especially when administered by inhalation, and have limited side effects (primarily tremor, agitation, tachycardia). The selective β_2 agents are the mainstay of adrenergic therapy (Table 17-3). β_2-Adrenergic agents have a long duration of action and can be administered either orally or by inhalation. Inhaled beta agents are especially effective in exercise-induced asthma. The metered-dose inhalers are suitable for patients over 4–5 years of age, especially when used with a spacer device (e.g., InspirEase, Key Pharmaceuticals). In younger children, albuterol can be administered by nebulizer. When used on an outpatient basis, inhaled beta agents should be limited to fewer than six doses per day. Oral and inhaled beta agents can be used simultaneously for enhanced effect, although side effects are more frequent.

(2) **Theophylline** is a potent bronchodilator, but it has a small therapeutic window. Acute therapy usually involves IV aminophylline. In an outpatient setting, slow-release preparations (Table 17-4) are useful in eliminating the need for frequent dosing and in decreasing side effects associated with rising and falling serum levels. Suggested dosages are given in Table 17-5.

(a) Therapeutic levels are between 5 and 15 mg/ml, although sig-

Table 17-3. Some β_2 selective agents

Name	Forms available	Dose
Albuterol (Proventil, Ventolin)	Liquid, 2 mg/tsp Tablets, 2 or 4 mg Repetabs, 4 mg (long-acting, Proventil)	0.1 mg/kg/dose up to 4 mg tid
	Nebulizer solution, 0.5%	0.25–0.5 ml with saline or cromolyn tid–qid
	Nebulizer solution, 0.83%	3 ml (one-unit dose) tid–qid
	Metered-dose inhaler	2 puffs tid–qid
	Rotohaler (Ventolin)	1–2 capsules tid–qid
Pirbuterol (Maxair)	Metered-dose inhaler	2 puffs tid–qid
flunisolide	Aerobid	2–4 puffs bid
astemizole	Hismanal	10 mg PO qd
Triamcinolone	Nasacort	1–2 sprays in each nostril qd

nificant bronchodilatation occurs at lower levels. Because clearance varies greatly among children (Table 17-6), serum levels should be monitored. These levels should be obtained 1 hour after an IV dose and 2–6 hours after an oral dose of a long-acting theophylline.

(b) Side effects of theophylline are dose related and include poor sleep, poor concentration, agitation, abdominal pain, nausea, vomiting, headache, tremor, tachycardia, GI bleeding, arrhythmia, and seizures. In certain individuals, some side effects occur at levels below the therapeutic range especially with initial doses.

(3) **Cromolyn** works as a mast cell stabilizing agent in the prophylaxis of chronic asthma. It inhibits both the early and late asthmatic response. It is available as a solution for nebulization, as a metered-dose inhaler, or as a spin-haler. The nebulized form usually does not irritate the airway as the spin-haler powder form may, and therefore it can be given even in the face of acute wheezing. Cromolyn is a safe medication with almost no side effects. It is particularly effective in allergen-induced asthma, as well as in exercise-induced asthma.

(4) **Corticosteroids** act as antiinflammatory agents and decrease airway hyperreactivity.

(a) For an acute severe exacerbation, short-term use of oral or IV steroids is indicated. The equivalent of 1–2 mg/kg/day prednisone is given initially, divided into two to four doses. Three days of therapy are followed by tapering over 3–4 days.

(b) When prolonged therapy is anticipated, tapering to an alternate-day regimen substantially reduces side effects. Alternatively,

Table 17-4. Some long-acting theophylline preparations

Trade name	How supplied	Dose interval
Slo-bid Gyrocaps	50-, 75-, 100-, 125-, 200-, 300-mg capsules	q8–12h
Theo-Dur	100-, 200-, 300-mg tablets	q8–12h
Theo-Dur Sprinkle	50-, 75-, 125-, 200-mg capsules	q8–12h
Slo-Phyllin Gyrocaps	60-, 125-, 250-mg capsules	q8h

Table 17-5. Theophylline dosing according to age

Age (yr)	Total daily dose (mg/kg/24 hr)
1–9	24
9–12	20
12–16	18
Adults	13 (or 600–900 mg/day)

inhaled steroids (beclomethasone dipropionate [Beclovent, Vanceril], triamcinolone acetonide [Azmacort], and flunisolide [Aerobid]), administered as two to four puffs two to four times per day are effective as maintenance therapy. Their effectiveness is limited to long-term therapy because their onset of action is relatively slow. Side effects are minimal. The major complication is oral candidiasis. In order to prevent this, patients should be encouraged to use spacers and instructed to rinse the mouth after inhalation. Occasionally, beclomethasone may precipitate bronchospasm, and an alternate inhaled steroid should be prescribed.

c. Pharmacologic therapy
   (1) Acute therapy
      (a) Humidified oxygen
      (b) Adrenergic therapy
         (i) Nebulized therapy with albuterol, 0.1–0.15 mg/kg (maximum 5 mg) in 2 ml saline every 20 minutes for 1 hour
         (ii) If the patient is unable to generate peak flow or has decreased consciousness, SC epinephrine, 0.01 ml/kg (1 : 1,000), to a maximum of 0.3 ml every 20 minutes for a total of three doses
      (c) If symptoms improve substantially (peak expiratory flow rate > 60% predicted), the patient can be discharged on oral bronchodilators with good follow-up arranged. Patients already on bronchodilators should be placed on additional medications to prevent relapse. The increase in pharmacologic agents should be continued for 5–7 days after symptoms have abated.
   (2) Status asthmaticus. See discussion in Chap. 3.
   (3) Intermittent therapy. For the asthmatic patient who has infrequent short episodes of wheezing, use of beta-adrenergic agents prn may be sufficient.

Table 17-6. Factors that affect theophylline half-life

Decreased clearance
   Old age
   Very young age (<1 yr)
   Hepatic failure
   Viral illness
   Cimetidine and ranitidine
   Erythromycin, clindamycin
Increased clearance
   Young age (toddlers, school age)
   Cigarette smoking
   IV isoproterenol
   Phenobarbital, phenytoin, carbamazepine (Tegretol)
   High-protein diet

(a) Viral upper respiratory infections will prompt an exacerbation in most asthmatic patients. The anticipated wheezing can be prophylactically treated with oral or inhaled beta agents. This therapy should be continued for several days after symptoms resolve.

(b) Exercise-induced wheezing is minimized by inhaling albuterol or cromolyn 10–20 minutes before activity.

(4) Long-term. For patients with moderate to severe asthma, chronic antiinflammatory therapy is needed. For the patient with moderate asthma who has episodes of wheezing more than one to two times a week for extended periods, nebulized or inhaled cromolyn should be used for chronic therapy. Beta agonists can be used daily or prn. For the patient with severe asthma, beta agonists, theophylline, and cromolyn can be used simultaneously. If control of symptoms is not achieved, either inhaled corticosteroids or oral prednisone can be added. Alternative diagnoses and complicating factors (such as sinusitis) should be considered.

For further information on asthma management, the reader should see the NHLBI National Asthma Education Program's *Guidelines for the Diagnosis and Management of Asthma.*

C. Allergic rhinoconjunctivitis

1. Etiology. Allergic rhinitis is a symptom complex caused by IgE-mediated reactions to environmental allergens.

2. Evaluation

a. Onset may occur at any age with a seasonal or perennial pattern. The family history is often positive for allergic diseases.

b. Allergic rhinitis is distinguished from other forms of rhinitis by the presence of paroxysms of sneezing, clear rhinorrhea, nasal pruritus, and a positive response to antihistamines.

c. A careful **history** is important to correlate symptoms with allergen exposure. Note that late-phase reactions rather than immediate reactions may be prominent, rendering associations between exposure and onset of symptoms less clear.

d. **Physical examination** may reveal allergic shiners, transverse nasal crease, and Dennie's lines. Nasal polyps may be seen in patients with allergic rhinitis, although cystic fibrosis must be considered.

e. **Laboratory studies** often reveal peripheral blood and nasal eosinophilia, and elevated serum IgE. Skin tests and RAST testing are useful in confirming specific allergies.

3. Treatment

a. Avoidance of allergens and irritants [see **B.3.a(2)**]

b. **Pharmacologic measures**

(1) Antihistamines (H$_1$ antagonists) are most effective for rhinorrhea and sneezing. Prophylactic use before exposure is optimal. Side effects include mild anticholinergic effects and somnolence (except with terfenadine [Seldane], astemizole [Hismanal], and lovatidine [Claritin], which are nonsedating and approved for patients over 12 years). Multiple formulations exist, many in combination with decongestants (e.g., Dimetapp, Triaminic, Bromfed).

(2) Adrenergic drugs

(a) Local vasoconstrictors (e.g., Afrin) are effective in decreasing nasal congestion. These, however, should not be used for more than a few days, to avoid rebound edema (rhinitis medicamentosa).

(b) Oral adrenergic agents (e.g., Sudafed) are also effective in decreasing nasal congestion and can be used alone or in combination with antihistamines.

(c) Ophthalmic preparations (Naphcon-A, Vasocon-A) with antihistamines are available for treatment of **allergic conjunctivitis.**

(3) Cromolyn is available for use as a nasal spray (Nasalcrom). An ophthalmic preparation (Opticrom) was previously available. These agents have virtually no side effects.

(4) Topical steroids in the form of nasal sprays (e.g., beclomethasone [Beconase, Vancenase]; flunisolide [Nasalide]; triamcinolone [Nasacort]) are effective agents for treatment of allergic rhinitis. Side effects include transient nasal irritation and sneezing. Adrenal suppression has never been reported, even with continuous long-term use of these medications. The serious side effect of septal perforation is extremely rare.

(5) Immunotherapy should be considered for allergic rhinoconjunctivitis that is unresponsive to medical therapy.

D. Serum sickness

1. **Etiology.** Serum sickness is a vasculitic process that results from the deposition of circulating antigen-antibody complexes in the vasculature and secondary complement activation. The agents that most frequently cause serum sickness are drugs (penicillin, cefaclor), heterologous serum proteins (antilymphocyte globulin, antisnake venoms), and viral agents (hepatitis B, Epstein-Barr).

2. **Evaluation and diagnosis.** Laboratory tests are generally of little help, because serum sickness is a clinical diagnosis.

   a. The symptom complex occurs 7–14 days after exposure to the offending agent and may persist for weeks. It includes fever; urticaria; angioedema, usually about the face and neck; lymphadenopathy; splenomegaly; and arthralgia or arthritis. Less commonly, vasculitis occurs in other symptoms, causing GI, central nervous system (CNS), pulmonary, and renal symptoms.

   b. **Laboratory findings**

      (1) CBC may show leukocytosis, leukopenia, or eosinophilia. The erythrocyte sedimentation rate (ESR) is usually elevated.

      (2) Urinalysis rarely reveals proteinuria, microscopic hematuria, and hyaline casts.

      (3) Immune studies are notable for decreased serum complement (C3 and CH_{50}), elevated acute-phase reactants, elevated IgG levels, and occasionally the presence of immune complexes (e.g., Clq binding or Raji cell assays).

3. **Treatment.** Most cases of serum sickness are mild and resolve spontaneously within a few days to 2 weeks after the elimination of the offending agent. For prominent signs and symptoms, pharmacologic therapy is indicated.

   a. **Antihistamines.** Diphenhydramine (Benadryl) or hydroxyzine (Atarax) is useful in the symptomatic relief of urticaria and pruritus.

   b. **Nonsteroidal antiinflammatory agents** (such as ibuprofen) or **aspirin** reduce fever and usually alleviate joint symptoms.

   c. **Corticosteroid therapy** should be reserved for patients with major organ system involvement (e.g., renal or GI). Prednisone, 1–2 mg/kg/day in divided doses, should be initiated, with tapering after clinical improvement and discontinuation after a total course of 10–14 days.

   d. **Epinephrine,** SC, will decrease acute urticaria, wheezing, and laryngeal edema, but the effects are transient.

E. Urticaria. Approximately 15 percent of the population experiences at least one acute episode of urticaria or angioedema. Of these cases, only a small percentage progress to the chronic form, defined as recurrence of lesions over a period of 6 weeks. The incidence of **acute urticaria** is slightly higher in an atopic than in a nonatopic population, but the incidence of **chronic urticaria** is unaffected by hereditary background.

1. **Etiology**

   a. **Mechanism.** Although caused by a number of mechanisms, a final common pathway for urticaria or angioedema is release of the chemical mediators of immediate hypersensitivity.

b. Specific agents. It is difficult to estimate the frequency with which the cause of acute urticaria is identified because many persons with mild acute episodes may not seek medical assistance. Of those evaluated for chronic forms of the disease, however, it has been estimated that a cause is determined in fewer than 20 percent of cases. Causes and mechanisms of urticaria include: IgE mediated, complement mediated, direct mast cell–releasing agents, presumptive abnormalities of arachidonic acid metabolism, exercise-induced anaphylaxis, and physical causes (Table 17-7).

2. **Evaluation.** The clinical recognition of urticaria or angioedema rarely presents a problem. Urticaria consists of blanchable, transient, erythematous, edematous papules that are generally pruritic and range in size from 1–2 mm to several centimeters.

Urticaria and angioedema frequently coexist. Symptoms may last from hours to days. However, it is not unusual for patients with chronic urticaria or angioedema to have recurrent episodes for years. Both because of the long-term morbidity suffered by those whose symptoms recur over a prolonged period and the occasional association with a significant underlying disorder (see Table 17-7), evaluation of patients with chronic urticaria should be undertaken (Table 17-8).

3. **Therapy.** If the urticaria or angioedema is associated with a specific ingested or inhaled substance, avoidance is obviously the preferred approach. Simi-

Table 17-7. Etiology of urticaria and angioedema

Allergic
  Ingested allergens (foods, drugs)
  Injected allergenic drugs (e.g., penicillin, biologicals)
  Inhaled allergens (e.g., cat, pollens)
Complement mediated
  Serum sickness (drugs, infections)
  Vasculitis (systemic lupus erythematosus or other systemic rheumatic disease)
  Urticarial vasculitis (not associated with systemic disease)
Infections (hepatitis B, Epstein-Barr virus, parasites)
Direct mast cell–releasing agents
  Drugs (e.g., opiates, curare, hyperosmolar solutions)
  Radiocontrast media
Agents that affect arachidonic acid metabolism
  Nonsteroidal antiinflammatory agents (aspirin)
  Angiotensin-converting enzyme inhibitors
Exercise-induced anaphylaxis
Physical causes
  Dermatographism
  Cold
  Pressure
  Vibration
  Heat
  Solar
  Aquagenic
  Cholinergic
Neoplasms
Endocrine related (thyroid disorders with antithyroid antibodies)
Psychogenic
Idiopathic
Hereditary angioedema (urticaria does not occur)

Table 17-8. Urticaria and angioedema: laboratory evaluation

Suspected cause	Procedures
(General screening)	(CBC, urinalysis, chemical profile)
Vasculitis or complement related	Sedimentation rate, immunoglobulin analysis, antinuclear factor, quantitative complement (C3, C4, C1 inhibitor, CH_{50}), skin biopsy
Infections	Culture, stool for ova and parasites, hepatitis-associated antigen, x-rays (sinuses)
Allergic	Eosinophil count, IgE, skin testing and/or RAST for suspected allergen
Physical	
Cholinergic	Mecholyl test/stress induced
Dermatographism	Firm stroking of skin
Cold	Ice-cube application, cryoglobulins, cryofibrinogens, VDRL
Solar	Light exposure
Heat	Warm-water immersion
Hereditary angioedema and acquired angioedema with lymphoma and other neoplasms	C1 inhibitor, C1, CH_{50}, C4, C2

larly, with physical urticaria, avoidance of the precipitating factor, such as cold or sunlight, is advisable. Sunscreens have been beneficial in solar urticaria. Patients should avoid factors that enhance urticaria and angioedema in a nonspecific fashion; these include aspirin and other nonsteroidal antiinflammatory drugs (NSAIDs), alcohol, excessive heat, and tight, occlusive, or synthetic clothing.

    a. Antihistamines. Urticaria, whether acute or chronic, is best controlled by round-the-clock antihistamine therapy. In general, antihistamine dosages should be increased slowly, either to tolerance or until symptoms are controlled. There is no good evidence that any one antihistamine is more beneficial than another. Though hydroxyzine is often used for most forms of urticaria, cyproheptadine (Periactin) is suggested for the cold-induced type. A combination of H_1-type antihistamines from two groups may be additive in therapeutic effect and side effects. Addition of an H_2 antihistamine may be beneficial.

    b. Corticosteroids. There is no role for topical steroid therapy in this condition, and only rarely should systemic corticosteroid treatment be considered.

  F. Atopic Dermatitis (AD) is a chronic disease that follows a relapsing course. Over 85 percent of the patients with atopic dermatitis present during the first 5 years of life. In infancy chronicity is not yet apparent, and respiratory allergies are usually not found. The prevalence of AD appears to have increased from 3–4 percent in the 1960s to 10 percent in the 1990s.

    1. Etiology

      a. Multiple immunologic abnormalities are associated with atopic dermatitis. However, none is pathognomonic or universal. In general, the more severe the disease the more likely that immunologic abnormality is found. The immunologic abnormalities include type I and type IV hypersensitivity reactions, impaired immunoregulation of IgE, increased phosphodiesterase, impaired macrophage functions, and increased mast cell releasability. With appropriate allergen stimulation mast cells release mediators that lead to itching. Genetically determined cutaneous abnormalities or infections can also lead to itching. The physical trauma from scratching results in (IL-1 and IL-3), secretion of interleukins (IL-3, IL-4, IL-5, IL-6) and histamine-releasing factor, and other immunologic events, all of which perpetuate the reaction.

b. Triggers of atopic dermatitis include irritants, dry skin (xerosis), infections, allergens, sweating, changes in temperature, illness, fatigue, and emotional stress. Important irritants are wool and acrylic in clothing, perfumes and perfumed products, cosmetics, soaps, cleaning agents, alcohol-containing products, sand, tobacco smoke, paint, and citrus foods. Infections can worsen AD. Eczema herpeticum (disseminated herpes simplex virus) is a potentially serious and life-threatening complication.

c. **Defective cell-mediated immunity** may be noted in up to 80 percent of patients with AD, manifested by increased susceptibility to severe skin infections with viruses (e.g., herpes simplex), increased susceptibility to chronic dermatophyte infections, and decreased responsiveness to delayed-type hypersensitivity skin testing.

d. Diagnosis of food or inhalant allergies in patients with atopic dermatitis can be difficult since skin testing and RAST testing may yield false-positive results. In order to clarify whether a food is a trigger for atopic dermatitis, *double-blind placebo-controlled food challenges or elimination diets are required.*

2. **Diagnosis.** Table 17-9 lists the diagnostic criteria of Hanifin and Rajka. The major features include pruritus and a typical morphology and distribution. Acute lesions are characterized by erythema, edema, and vesiculation. Chronic lesions become eczematous, lichenified, and plaque-like. The skin distribution varies with age. In infancy the face and extensor surfaces of the arms and legs are involved. In the older child, the flexor surfaces of the extremities, neck, and upper trunk are commonly involved.

3. **Treatment**
   a. Moisturizers are the first line of topical therapy for AD, and are important to reduce and prevent the dry itchy skin that accompanies it. Petroleum products such as Vaseline or hydrated petrolatum are the best moisturizers. Nonperfumed skin creams can also be effective. Moisturizers should be applied to the skin immediately after a tepid bath (while the skin is still moist). A mild fragrance-free soap should be used and excessive scrubbing should be avoided.

   b. Tar preparations may act as antipruritics, disinfectants, antiinflammatory, and desquamating agents, when put in the bath or applied topically, are often beneficial in both the acute and chronic phases of AD.

   c. Avoidance of trigger factors is crucial to controlling AD. All-cotton clothing and bedding are less irritating than synthetic or wool fabrics. In some patients inhalant and food allergens can trigger a flare and should be avoided.

   d. Infections can worsen AD, and should be treated early with topical and/or oral antibiotics or antiviral agents.

   e. Emotional stress can exacerbate atopic dermatitis. In addition, the intense itching and skin appearance can lead to stress for the family and patient. Recognizing this stress and developing stress management techniques are often helpful. Lay organizations such as the Eczema Association for Science and Education and the Asthma and Allergy Foundation of America (AAFA) provide patients with information and support.

   f. **Topical steroids** should be used in conjunction with other forms of therapy especially emollients. For acute flares, a potent topical steroid, such as the difluorinated or the fluorochlorinated preparations, should be used for 7–10 days and then replaced with a midpotency topical steroid for 2–3 weeks until the lesions have resolved. Severely affected patients may require chronic use of a low-potency topical steroid in conjunction with lubricants. Fluorinated steroids should *not* be chronically applied to the

Table 17-9. Diagnostic criteria of atopic dermatitis

Children and adults
Must have 3 or more major features
Pruritus
Typical morphology and distribution
    Flexural lichenification or linearity in adults
    Facial and extensor involvement in infants and children
Chronic or chronically relapsing dermatitis
Personal or family history of atopy (asthma, allergic rhinitis, AD)
Plus 3 or more minor features
Xerosis
Ichthyosis/palmar hyperlinearity/keratosis pilaris
Immediate (type I) skin test reactivity
Elevated serum IgE
Early age of onset
Tendency toward cutaneous infection/impaired cell-mediated immunity
Tendency toward nonspecific hand or foot dermatitis
Nipple eczema
Cheilitis
Recurrent conjunctivitis
Dennie-Morgan infraorbital fold
Keratoconus
Anterior subcapsular cataracts
Orbital darkening
Facial pallor/facial erythema
Pityriasis alba
Anterior neck folds
Itch when sweating
Intolerance to wool and lipid solvents
Perifollicular accentuation
Food allergy
Course influenced by environmental/emotional factors
White dermatographism/delayed blanch

Source: From Hanifan and Rajka, Diagnostic features of atopic dermatitis. *Acta Dermatol. Venereol.* 92(Suppl):44, 1980.

face, genitals, axillae, inguinal region, or skin folds and they should not be used in infants. *Excessive or prolonged use of high-potency topical steroids can lead to local atrophy. Long-term application of steroids around the eyes or on the eyelids can lead to the development of glaucoma or cataracts.* Significant systemic absorption is a potential, albeit rarely clinically appreciated, hazard of topical steroids.

    g. Antihistamines may be helpful especially at night to control the itching associated with atopic dermatitis. Hydroxyzine and diphenhydramine are frequently prescribed. Nonsedating antihistamines such as astemizole and terfenadine occasionally provide relief for patients. Topical antihistamines should be avoided because of low efficacy and high likelihood of skin sensitization. In spite of the above therapies, some patients have recalcitrant or severe AD. For such individuals, short-term phototherapy using ultraviolet radiation (UVB or PUVA) is often beneficial. However, the usefulness of this therapy is limited by the long-term risks, inconveniences, and expense. A recent study has shown that cyclosporine (5 mg/kg/day) is an effective short-term therapy for refractory AD (J. M. Sowden et al., Double-blind, controlled, crossover study of cyclosporin in adults with severe refractory atopic dermatitis. *Lancet* 388:137–140, 1991). Two other immunomodulators, thymopentin and recombinant interferon gamma (IFN-g), have shown promising preliminary results for patients with severe AD and may be appropriate for chronic therapy. (D.Y.M. Leung et al., Thymopentin therapy reduces the clinical severity of atopic dermatitis. *J. Allerg. Clin. Immunol.* 85:927–933, 1990; and L. C. Schneider et al., Recombinant interferon-gamma therapy reduces the clinical severity of atopic dermatitis. *J. Allerg. Clin. Immunol.* 87:235, 1991). As the immunology of atopic dermatitis is better understood, specific cytokine or cytokine receptor antagonists may be important therapies for severe disease.

II. Immunodeficiency disorders

A. Etiology. The immune system can be divided into four components, and abnormalities may involve one or more components, resulting in a predisposition to recurrent infections. The immune system is composed of:

1. Humoral system (B lymphocytes)

2. T-lymphocyte system

3. Phagocytic system

4. Complement system

B. Evaluation

1. An immunodeficiency should be suspected if a child has an increased frequency of infection or infections of unusual severity, of prolonged duration, or with unusual complications. Unusual or opportunistic organisms may cause the infections.

  a. Although the normal child may have up to six respiratory infections in a year, the child with an immunodeficiency will have more prolonged infections and may not recover completely between infections.

  b. Chronic candidiasis or bronchiectasis, chronically draining ears, hearing loss, recurrent conjunctivitis, chronic cough, or diarrhea may be the presenting problem.

2. Abnormal humoral immunity will predispose to recurrent pyogenic infections, such as otitis, sinusitis, pneumonia, and meningitis caused by **pneumococcus, Haemophilus influenzae,** or **Streptococcus** species. Antibody is necessary for opsonization for phagocytosis of these organisms.

  a. Early complement components (C1, C4, C2, and C3) sequentially interact with antibody-coated bacteria. The opsonized bacteria are then phagocytized and destroyed by circulating or fixed phagocytic cells. The absence of specific antibody means that the rate of ingestion and destruction of pathogens is markedly reduced.

  b. IgG crosses the placenta and maternal IgG protects the infant for the first 3–4 months. There is a decline in transplacentally derived maternal IgG, followed by the onset of de novo IgG and IgM synthesis. Thus, the child with isolated antibody deficiency will often be asymptomatic for the first 4–6 months of life (Fig. 17-1). By approximately 5 years of age, adult levels of IgG, IgM, and IgA are present.

3. Immunity to many fungal and viral infections resides in cellular or T cell–mediated processes. Chronic candidiasis resistant to treatment in an infant, complications after viral infection or immunization, or an opportunistic infection may reflect such a deficiency.

4. In the majority of cases, historical information will permit a presumptive diagnosis of either a primary or a secondary immunodeficiency.

  a. Primary immunodeficiencies are:

   (1) Antibody-deficiency syndromes

    (a) X-linked agammaglobulinemia (XLA)

    (b) Common variable immunodeficiency

    (c) Selective IgA deficiency

    (d) Transient hypogammaglobulinemia of infancy

    (e) Selective IgG subclass deficiency

   (2) Primary T-cell deficiencies

    (a) DiGeorge's syndrome

    (b) Chronic mucocutaneous candidiasis

   (3) Combined T/B-cell deficiency

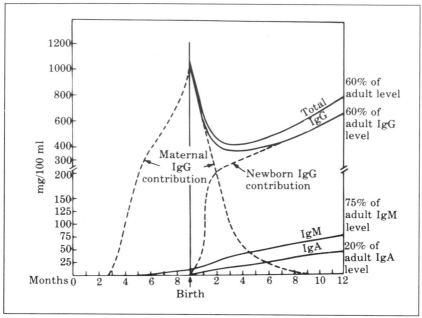

Fig. 17-1. Immunoglobulin (IgG, IgM, and IgA) levels in the fetus and infant in the first year of life. The IgG of the fetus and newborn infant is solely of maternal origin. The maternal IgG disappears by the age of 9 months, by which time the endogenous synthesis of IgG by the infant is well established. The IgM and IgA of the neonate are entirely endogenously synthesized because maternal IgM and IgA do *not* cross the placenta. (From E. R. Stiehm and V. A. Fulginiti, *Immunologic Disorders in Infants and Children.* Philadelphia: Saunders, 1973.)

    (a) Severe combined immunodeficiency disease (SCID)
    (b) Wiskott-Aldrich syndrome
    (c) Ataxia-telangiectasia
    (d) Hyper-IgE syndrome
    (e) Ommen's syndrome
  (4) Phagocytic disorders
  (5) Complement deficiencies
 b. **Secondary immunodeficiencies** may be associated with:
    (1) Viral infections such as human immunodeficiency virus (HIV), measles, rubeola, Epstein-Barr virus, and cytomegalovirus
    (2) Metabolic disorders such as malnutrition, uremia, and diabetes
    (3) Protein-losing states such as nephrotic syndrome and protein-losing enteropathy
    (4) Immunosuppressive agents, splenectomy, and malignancy
    (5) Prematurity
    (6) Miscellaneous disorders such as Down syndrome and histiocytosis
5. **Physical examination** should involve a search for the presence of lymphoid tissues (tonsils, lymph nodes, spleen), signs of infection, and incapacitation from chronic infection (hearing loss, failure to thrive, evidence of malabsorption). Skin involvement with eczema, candidiasis, telangiectasia, or petechiae should be noted.
6. The **laboratory evaluation** should be used to confirm a clinical suspicion based on the type of infection, the age of onset, family history, and physical examination.
   a. **Screening tests** such as a CBC with differential and an ESR are helpful as first steps. Nonimmunologic diseases should not be overlooked, and

tests such as a sweat test, or test for HIV in high-risk groups, should be performed.

b. B-cell function varies with age, and results must be interpreted accordingly.

(1) Total immunoglobulin levels, IgG, IgM, IgA, IgE. High levels of immunoglobulin suggest chronic granulomatous disease (CGD) or immotile cilia syndrome, and very high levels indicate acquired immunodeficiency syndrome (AIDS). Low IgG levels accompanied by low serum albumin suggest increased loss of all serum proteins, e.g., with protein-losing enteropathy.

(2) Specific antibody levels (to tetanus or diphtheria toxoids; isohemagglutinins; measles, rubella, or polio viruses; *H. influenzae* type B; and pneumococcus) Normal antibody levels to antigens rule out severe B-cell dysfunction.

(3) IgG subclass levels. In the face of normal or low normal total IgG levels and recurrent sinopulmonary infection, IgG subclass deficiency should be considered.

(4) Enumeration or peripheral blood B cells. Absence of B cells suggests XLA.

c. Tests for T-cell function

(1) CBC. Lymphopenia is suggestive of T-cell disorder. Thrombocytopenia and platelets with small size suggest Wiskott-Aldrich syndrome.

(2) Chest x-ray. Absence of a thymic shadow may indicate T-cell disease.

(3) Delayed skin tests to tetanus toxoid, diphtheria toxoid, *Candida*. Induration should occur at 48–72 hours. Negative tests are seen in 10–30 percent of normal individuals, and in patients receiving daily steroids. Such patients may be boosted with tetanus toxoid, and a tetanus skin test can be repeated 7 days later. A positive skin test rules out serious T-cell deficiency.

(4) T-cell subsets, and in vitro proliferation of T cells to mitogens and antigens. Absence of T cells is seen in SCID, and abnormal CD4/CD8 suppressor T-cell ratios are seen in AIDS and in disorders of immunoregulation.

d. Tests for complement include CH_{50} and determination of individual complement components. C4 levels are invariably reduced in hereditary angioneurotic edema (HANE), and this can be used as a screening test. C2 levels are reduced in acute attacks of HANE. The diagnosis of HANE is confirmed by determination of C1 inhibitor levels.

e. Tests for phagocytic function include nitroblue tetrazolium test, Rebuck skin window, spleen scan, bone marrow aspiration, phenotyping for CD11, and examination for presence of antineutrophil antibodies.

C. Diagnosis and therapy of specific disorders

1. General measures

a. Avoid administration of live virus vaccines, especially in children with suspected T-cell deficiencies or X-linked agammaglobulinemia.

b. In T-cell–deficient patients, **transfusion of blood products may induce the lethal complication of graft-versus-host disease.** Frozen washed red cells, platelets, or plasma should be irradiated with 5,000 rad to prevent this complication.

2. Antibody deficiency

a. Diagnosis

(1) X-linked agammaglobulinemia. Male children with this severe form of antibody deficiency present at approximately the sixth to twelfth month of life with recurrent infections with respiratory bacteria. Affected children have no significant IgG (<150 mg/dl), IgM, or IgA. B lymphocytes are absent from the peripheral blood. A tyrosine kinase that is important for B-cell maturation is missing or defective and consequently mature B cells are absent. This diagnosis can be made at birth by demonstrating the absence of B lymphocytes in the cord blood. Neutropenia, thrombocytopenia, and hemolytic anemia may occur. These patients are especially susceptible to enteroviral infections such as polio. **They should not receive live viral vaccines.**

(2) **Common variable agammaglobulinemia** is a term used to describe an inability to form specific antibody that is not due to X-linked agammaglobulinemia. Children with this condition are characterized by the presence of B lymphocytes that are incapable of the synthesis and/or secretion of normal immunoglobulin and antibody. Both boys and girls can be affected.

(3) In **IgA deficiency,** an IgA level less than 5 mg/dl is found, with normal levels of IgG and IgM and normal antibody responses. The lack of serum IgA is accompanied by absence of secretory IgA, and it is the latter that accounts for the sinopulmonary infections, diarrhea, or malabsorption seen. Secretory IgA is the primary protective antibody in secretions of the upper respiratory and GI tracts, and in breast milk. Nonetheless, most IgA-deficient individuals are asymptomatic. Symptomatic individuals should be screened for IgG_2 subclass deficiency, which may coexist.

(4) **Transient hypogammaglobulinemia of infancy.** In some infants there is a delay in immunoglobulin synthesis, so that the nadir of IgG seen at 3–4 months (approximately 300 gm/dl) is prolonged and continues to decrease (see Fig. 17-1). IgG levels remain low (often < 200 mg/dl), and IgM and IgA may be normal or low. During the time between the elimination of maternal IgG (6 months of age) and the onset of de novo synthesis (18–24 months), these children have little antibody protection and may suffer from recurrent infections caused by upper respiratory bacteria. The severity of these infections is not as great as that of infections in persons who have a lifelong inability to produce specific antibodies. Response to vaccination with tetanus and other protein antigens is usually normal. Wheezing, respiratory infections, and diarrhea may be the clinical symptoms.

(5) **IgG subclass deficiency.** IgG can be divided into four subclasses. Patients have been described who have normal total IgG levels but a marked reduction in IgG_2 or IgG_3, or both. These patients suffer from recurrent infections similar to those of individuals with absence of IgG. Many of these patients do not make specific antibodies on exposure to polysaccharide antigens (**pneumococcus, _H. influenzae_ type B** [Hib]). IgG_2 subclass–deficient patients do make normal responses to protein antigens and will respond to Hib conjugate vaccines. IgG_2 subclass levels are low in normal children less than 2 years old; therefore IgG subclasses should not be obtained until the patient is older than 2 years.

b. **Therapy**

(1) Prophylactic antibiotics can help reduce the frequency of recurrent bacterial infections. Antibiotics effective against probable pathogens can be administered for extended periods, or only during periods of increased risk for infection, as single daily doses or at full therapeutic doses. Side effects of frequent antibiotic usage include allergic reactions, bacterial resistance, diarrhea, and pseudomembranous colitis.

(2) Aggressive and immediate antibiotic treatment should be instituted for infection. Bronchiectasis should be managed with physical therapy, postural drainage, and antibiotics. Malabsorption and diarrhea should be treated with dietary restriction, and, if _Giardia_ infestation is demonstrated, the patient should be treated with metronidazole.

(3) In children with recurrent otitis media, audiologic evaluation is useful to identify possible impaired speech development.

(4) **Replacement gamma globulin** is highly effective in reducing the

frequency of infection in antibody-deficiency states. Patients with XLA or common variable agammaglobulinemia will require lifelong therapy with IV gamma globulin (IVGG). Rarely, IVGG is required for the other antibody-deficiency disorders.

(a) **IV gamma globulin** (Iveegam, Immuno AG; Gamimmune-N, Cutter; Sandoglobulin, Sandoz; Gammagard, Hyland-Baxter) can be used to administer large quantities (400–500 mg/kg every 3–4 weeks) of IgG. Trough IgG levels should be greater than 600 mg/dl. Some patients may require larger doses of IVGG even more frequently to prevent infections. Reactions to IVGG (fever, chills, nausea) can be treated by decreasing the infusion rate and pretreating with acetaminophen or aspirin and diphenhydramine on subsequent infusions.

(b) Patients with IgA deficiency may occasionally develop anaphylactic reactions to replacement gamma globulin. Gammagard, which has no IgA, can be safely administered to these patients.

(c) **Immune serum globulin (ISG)** is administered intramuscularly, given as a loading dose of 1.8 ml/kg and as a maintenance dose of 0.6 ml (100 mg)/kg every 3–4 weeks. ISG is rarely given, because IVGG provides higher IgG levels and is much less painful.

(5) Family members should be screened for immunodeficiencies.

3. **T-lymphocyte defects**
   a. **Pathophysiology.** T lymphocytes are derived from lymphoid stem cells that differentiate under the influence of the thymus into peripheral T lymphocytes, which are responsible for protection against viruses and fungi, and which regulate immunoglobulin synthesis.
   b. **Diagnosis**
      (1) **Congenital thymic asplasia (DiGeorge's syndrome).** This developmental abnormality of the third and fourth pharyngeal pouches results in absence of the thymus and parathyroid glands, cardiac defects, and a characteristic facies. Neonatal tetany (hypocalcemia), heart murmurs, and the absence of a thymic shadow should suggest the diagnosis. Decreased T cells and poor in vitro lymphocyte responses will be seen.
      (2) **Mucocutaneous candidiasis.** Patients with mucocutaneous candidiasis have recurrent *Candida albicans* infections of the fingernails and toenails, mouth, and vagina. They may have antibody deficiency disorders and/or associated autoimmune abnormalities that affect their adrenal and thyroid glands, leading to Addison's disease and hypothyroidism.
      (3) **Miscellaneous disorders.** Malnutrition, drug immunosuppression, and lymphocyte loss will cause T-cell dysfunction.
   c. **Therapy**
      (1) **DiGeorge's syndrome.** Most children have a partial defect and gradually acquire T-cell function without treatment. Transplantation of a fetal thymus corrects the immune defect, although this is rarely done. Irradiate all transfusions (see **1.b**) and avoid live viral vaccines until normal T-cell function is demonstrated.
      (2) **Mucocutaneous candidiasis.** Prophylaxis with oral ketoconazole is the therapy of choice.
      (3) **Associated endocrinopathies** must be treated.

4. **Combined (antibody and cellular) immunodeficiency**
   a. **Diagnosis**
      (1) **Severe combined immunodeficiency** may be inherited as an X-linked or autosomal recessive disorder, and the latter may be associated with absence of the enzymes adenosine deaminase (ADA) or nucleoside phosphorylase. Affected infants lack normal lymphoid stem cells and therefore do not have normal T-lymphocyte and B-lymphocyte immu-

nity. Frequently, they are clinically well for the first 2–3 months of life, and then the clinical triad of candidiasis, diarrhea, and pneumonitis develops. The male-female ratio is 3 : 1.

  (a) The **diagnosis** is confirmed by low immunoglobulin levels, absent antibody responses, and low numbers of circulating or cord blood T cells with abnormal in vitro responses. ADA should be assayed in red cells. With ADA deficiency the diagnosis can be made prenatally by the absence of enzyme activity in cultured amniotic fibroblasts.

  (b) Bony abnormalities may be seen on x-rays of the rib cage, pelvis, and spine in ADA deficiency.

  (c) If the child has inadvertently been given a nonirradiated transfusion or had a maternal-fetal transfusion, a graft-versus-host reaction may complicate the clinical picture with skin rash, diarrhea, hepatosplenomegaly, and failure to thrive.

  (2) **Wiskott-Aldrich syndrome** is an X-linked disorder characterized by eczema and T-lymphocyte abnormalities, including decreased T-lymphocyte function and an inability to make anticarbohydrate antibodies. Affected patients also have thrombocytopenia with platelets of reduced size and function. Patients are at risk of death due to bleeding and/or recurrent viral, fungal, and bacterial infection.

  (3) **Ataxia-telangiectasia** is diagnosed by the occurrence of ataxia, choreoathetosis, dysarthric speech, telangiectasis, sinopulmonary infection, and the frequently found IgA deficiency and abnormal T-cell function. Alpha fetoprotein is often elevated.

  (4) **Hyper-IgE syndrome.** These patients have elevated serum IgE levels and recurrent pyogenic infection, particularly skin abscesses due to *Staphylococcus aureus*. The IgE in some individuals contains specific antibody to *Staphylococcus*. The interaction of the specific IgE antibody with the *Staphylococcus* inhibits the opsonization of the bacteria by IgG antibody and blocks the phagocytosis and the destruction of *Staphylococcus* by circulating phagocytic cells. Laboratory evaluation often reveals poor specific antibody responses and poor T-cell proliferation to antigens.

  (5) **Ommen's syndrome.** Ommen's syndrome is a variant of SCID in which patients present with recurrent severe bacterial and fungal infections, hypereosinophilia, diffuse erythroderma, protracted diarrhea, failure to thrive, and hepatosplenomegaly. Lymphocyte counts are normal although clonal analysis reveals oligoclonality.

b. **Therapy**

  (1) Bone marrow transplantation is the treatment for severe immunodeficiency syndromes, such as SCID, Ommen's syndrome, and Wiskott-Aldrich syndrome. Bone marrow is harvested from a histocompatible donor and infused into the patient. Residual immune function in the recipient may be ablated just before transplant to allow engraftment. Complications of bone marrow transplantation include graft-versus-host disease and infection.

  (2) Patients with **bleeding and Wiskott-Aldrich syndrome problems** can be treated by splenectomy and placed on prophylactic (trimethoprim-sulfamethoxazole [Bactrim] or ampicillin) antibiotics to protect against bacterial sepsis. Excellent care of eczema is mandatory. The only definitive treatment is bone marrow transplantation.

  (3) Aggressive treatment with antibiotics is necessary. Multiple organisms may be responsible for clinical disease. Lung infiltrates may be secondary to *Pneumocystis,* which is treated with trimethoprim-sulfamethoxazole or, rarely, pentamidine if the former fails (see Chap. 15, p. 456).

  (4) Because of the antibody deficiency, all patients should receive intravenous gamma globulin therapy [see **2.b.4.(a)**].

(5) Siblings of affected SCID children should be isolated at birth and screened for SCID.
5. **Phagocytic and complement disorders**
   a. **Granulocyte disorders** (see Chap. 16, p. 485ff)
   b. **Complement abnormalities**
      (1) Deficiency of C1 associated with a lupus-like syndrome and susceptibility to bacterial infection
      (2) C2 deficiency associated with anaphylactoid purpura and systemic lupus erythematosus (SLE)
      (3) C3 deficiency and C3b inactivator deficiency associated with a history of recurrent pyogenic infections that mimic hypogammaglobulinemia. Can be inherited or acquired during nephritis or in disease in which C3 consumption occurs (SLE)
      (4) C4 deficiency with SLE
      (5) C5 deficiency associated with recurrent *Neisseria* infection and SLE
      (6) C7 deficiency with Raynaud's phenomenon, recurrent *Neisseria* infection
      (7) C6 and C8 deficiencies associated with recurrent *Neisseria* infections
      (8) Therapy for recurrent infections consists of appropriate antibiotics.
   c. **Splenic dysfunction.** The spleen is the site of a significant portion of the body's phagocytic capacity. Splenic hypofunction predisposes individuals to significant and overwhelming bacterial infection, particularly with respiratory bacteria.
      (1) Pathophysiology
         (a) The spleen can be congenitally absent, removed surgically, or hypofunctional as in sickle cell disease.
         (b) Patients who undergo splenectomy before the age of 2 have difficulty in processing carbohydrate antigens such as the capsular antigens of pneumococcus and *H. influenzae.*
      (2) Therapy
         (a) Antibiotics are indicated for infections. Because of the risk of overwhelming sepsis in patients with splenic absence or dysfunction, IV antibiotic administration should be instituted while awaiting cultures.
         (b) Prevention of infections
            (i) For patients at increased risk, prophylactic oral penicillin, 200,000 units bid, or ampicillin (or Augmentin), 250 mg bid, should be prescribed.
            (ii) It is important to educate parents about the risk of sepsis and the need to seek immediate medical attention at the first sign of infection. If prompt attention cannot be sought, the parents should be supplied with oral antibiotics that can be instituted at the first sign of infection.
            (iii) Patients who are hyposplenic should be immunized before splenectomy, if possible, with all available bacteria polysaccharide or conjugate vaccines.
6. **Hereditary angioneurotic edema.** This autosomal dominant disorder of dysfunction or deficiency of the inhibitor of the activated first component of complement results in unopposed C1 activation, consumption of C4 and C2, and release of a vasoactive peptide that causes subcutaneous and submucosal edema. Intermittent episodes of nonpruritic edema of the skin of the extremities and face occur after minor trauma or emotional stress, or without a precipitating cause. The swelling may involve the mucous membranes of the upper airway, causing **laryngeal obstruction and asphyxiation.** Abdominal pain with vomiting or diarrhea secondary to edema of the intestinal wall may occur without skin manifestations. Urticaria does not occur.
   a. **Diagnosis.** In the majority of patients, the level of C1 esterase inhibitor is decreased, but about 15 percent of persons with the disease have a

normal level of nonfunctional protein. In both groups, C4 levels are low and fall during attacks.

   b. Therapy

   (1) The major complication of acute attacks is laryngeal obstruction, and thus patients or parents should be instructed to seek medical attention without delay if hoarseness, voice changes, or difficulty in breathing or swallowing occurs. A tracheotomy will be necessary for laryngeal obstruction. Epinephrine and hydrocortisone are usually of little benefit in controlling the swelling, which contrasts with the relief they afford in anaphylaxis.

   (2) Administration of purified C1 esterase inhibitor is useful in acute attacks.

   (3) Androgens have been shown to increase the synthesis of C1 esterase. The routine use of danazol, 50–600 mg per day, or stanozolol, 2–24 mg per day, markedly decreases the frequency and severity of attacks.

Inflammatory Disorders

Robert Sundel

18

I. **Juvenile rheumatoid arthritis (JRA)** is a generalized systemic inflammatory disease.
   A. **Etiology** is unknown.
   B. **Evaluation.** There are five distinct modes of onset (Table 18-1). Laboratory findings in the systemic and polyarticular forms are reflective of generalized inflammation with elevated white blood count (WBC), erythrocyte sedimentation rate (ESR), platelet count, and anemia. Joint fluid reveals low viscosity and a WBC of $> 10,000/mm^3$ with a polymorphonuclear predominance.
   C. **Treatment**
      1. The **goal** is suppression of inflammation and prevention of deformity and disability.
      2. **Physical and occupational therapy** should maintain range of motion and functional joint positioning.
      3. **Antiinflammatory drugs**
         a. **Aspirin** (acetylsalicylic acid) is the traditional initial drug of choice in JRA. It provides symptomatic relief but does not arrest the progression of erosive arthritis.
            (1) The starting **dose** of 80 mg/kg/day in four doses to a maximum of 3,600 mg per day is adjusted to obtain salicylate levels of 20–30 mg/dl. Aspirin is given with food to avoid gastrointestinal irritation. Rectal and enteric-coated aspirin is erratically absorbed. Slow-release aspirin and the salicylate derivatives choline magnesium salicylate (Trilisate) and choline salicylate (Arthropan; both available in a liquid form) are sometimes useful in improving compliance and reducing GI toxicity.
            (2) Aspirin is **metabolized** by the liver and excreted by the kidney. At high dosages, small changes in dosage cause significant changes in level.
            (3) **Side effects**
               (a) **GI.** Nausea, abdominal pain, and diarrhea may occur, as may gastric ulcers and hemorrhage.
               (b) **Hepatic.** Liver enzyme elevations frequently occur. If mild and unaccompanied by associated symptoms, these elevations can be followed without change in therapy and will frequently resolve.
               (c) **Hematologic.** Bleeding time is elevated for up to 14 days after aspirin is stopped.
               (d) Aspirin is stopped when chickenpox or influenza develops, to reduce the risk of **Reye syndrome.** The Centers for Disease Control (CDC) recommends influenza vaccination for children receiving chronic aspirin therapy.
               (e) Patients with nasal polyps and asthma are likely to have **aspirin sensitivity** and should avoid aspirin.
            (4) **Signs of overdosage** include behavior change, tinnitus, lethargy, hyperventilation, dizziness, sweating, headaches, nausea, and vomiting.
         b. **Nonsteroidal antiinflammatory drugs (NSAIDs)** are indicated when no improvement on salicylates occurs within 1–2 months with adequate levels or if aspirin is contraindicated or poorly tolerated. Responses of

509

Table 18-1. Subgroups of juvenile rheumatoid arthritis

Subgroup	% of total	Sex ratio	Age at onset	Joints affected	Serologic and genetic tests	Extraarticular manifestations	Prognosis
Systemic onset	20	60% boys	Any age	Any joints	ANA negative, RF negative	High fever, rash, organomegaly, polyserositis, leukocytosis, growth retardation	25% severe arthritis
Rheumatoid factor Negative polyarticular	25	90% girls	Any age	Any joints	ANA 25%, RF negative	Low-grade fever, mild anemia, malaise, growth retardation	10–15% severe arthritis
Rheumatoid factor Positive polyarticular	5–10	80% girls	Late childhood	Any joints	ANA 75%, RF 100%	Low-grade fever, anemia, malaise, rheumatoid nodules	>50% severe arthritis
Pauciarticular with chronic iridocyclitis	35–40	80% girls	Early childhood	Few large joints (hips and sacroiliac joints spared)	ANA 50%, RF negative	Few constitutional complaints; chronic iridocyclitis in 50%	Severe arthritis uncommon; 10–20% ocular damage from iridocyclitis
Pauciarticular with sacroiliitis	10	90% boys	Late childhood	Few large joints (hips and sacroiliac involvement common)	ANA negative, RF negative, HLA-B27 75%	Few constitutional complaints; acute iridocyclitis in 5–10% during childhood	Some have ankylosing spondylitis at follow-up

ANA = antinuclear antibody; RF = rheumatoid factor; HLA-B27 = histocompatibility antigen-B27.

patients to the individual drugs of this class are somewhat variable; if one drug is ineffective in approximately 3–4 weeks, another should be tried. NSAIDs are well absorbed in the GI tract and excreted by the kidney.

(1) Specific agents

    (a) Tolmetin sodium is approved by the Food and Drug Administration (FDA) for use in children over 2 years of age. It is given at 20–40 mg/kg/day in three or four divided doses.

    (b) Naproxen has a low incidence of toxicity and is available in liquid form. It is approved by the FDA for use in children over 2 years of age. It is especially useful for adolescents with poor compliance because it requires dosing at 10–20 mg/kg/day in only two divided doses.

    (c) Indomethacin, 0.5–2.5 mg/kg/day, is given in three divided doses. Slow-release capsules of 75 mg are useful in alleviating severe morning stiffness. Indomethacin has a high incidence of CNS and gastric toxicity. It is approved for use in children over the age of 14 years.

    (d) Ibuprofen is generally well tolerated, but it requires dosing three or four times a day for a total of 30–40 mg/kg/day. A liquid form has recently been approved for use in children.

(2) Toxicity

    (a) Gastric. Dyspepsia, nausea, gastritis, diarrhea, and ulceration may occur. These are seen less frequently when NSAIDs are administered with food.

    (b) Hepatic. Elevation of liver enzymes is usually mild and reversible.

    (c) Hematologic. Reversible prolongation of bleeding time may occur. Anemia is a rare complication.

    (d) Renal. NSAIDs may cause fluid retention and can block the effect of some diuretics. They are contraindicated in patients with decreased glomerular filtration because they may precipitate acute renal failure; acute interstitial nephritis also has been reported.

    (e) Dermatologic. Rashes and oral ulceration may occur at high doses. Naproxen may cause a scarring photosensitive eruption, especially in fair-skinned children.

    (f) Patients with **aspirin sensitivity** should take NSAIDs with caution.

    (g) Central nervous system (CNS). Headaches, drowsiness, or dysphoria may limit the use of these agents.

c. Intraarticular steroids are indicated for severe inflammation of a few joints. Given no more often than every 3 months, the effects may persist from days to months. The primary risk is introducing infection into the joint space. A crystal synovitis may occur, lasting 1–2 days.

d. Oral steroids are indicated for severe systemic manifestations of JRA or for severe arthritis that prevents ambulation. They should be given in conjunction with a slow-acting remittive agent as a temporizing measure in as low a dose as possible.

4. Slow-acting remittive agents are drugs that slow or arrest bony erosion and cartilage loss. Time to onset of action may be months.

a. Hydroxychloroquine (Plaquenil) is an antimalarial agent with moderate antiinflammatory activity and possibly remittive effects. It is used at a dose of 4–7 mg/kg/day (400 mg/day maximum) in patients whose moderate synovitis is unresponsive to NSAIDs. It is contraindicated in patients with glucose 6-phosphate dehydrogenase (G-6-PD) deficiency. Regular ophthalmologic examinations are required to identify macular degeneration and corneal deposits, which require discontinuation of the drug. Gastric irritation and dermatitis may also occur, though they are reversible with cessation of the drug.

b. Gold salts at dosages up to 1 mg/kg/wk intramuscularly are used for severe or erosive arthritis and for synovitis that is unresponsive to NSAIDs and hydroxychloroquine. **Toxicities,** including dermatitis, mucositis, vasomotor reactions, eosinophilia, blood dyscrasias, and nephrotic syndrome, though reversible with discontinuation of the medication, may limit its use.

c. **Methotrexate** (5–10 mg/m^2/wk in one or two doses) is used for children who are unresponsive to or unable to tolerate gold therapy. It appears to function primarily as a steroid-like antiinflammatory agent. Acute toxicities may include bone marrow suppression, mucositis, chemical hepatitis, and gastritis. Data on potential disease-modifying effects as well as possible long-term toxicities are unavailable.

d. **Sulfasalazine** appears to have antiinflammatory effects, especially in the spondyloarthropathies. Toxicities at doses of 40–70 mg/kg/day in two or three divided doses include rash, gastritis, and bone marrow suppression.

II. **Seronegative spondyloarthropathy** is a chronic inflammatory arthritis of the peripheral joints and/or axial skeleton with enthesitis (inflammation of insertion of tendons into bone). This includes a group of disorders that have genetic and clinical similarities: juvenile ankylosing spondylitis, psoriatic arthritis, reactive arthritis, and inflammatory bowel disease (IBD)-associated arthritis.

A. **Etiology** is unknown.

B. **Evaluation**

1. **General clinical features** include asymmetric lower-extremity pauciarticular arthritis, usually presenting in older childhood (> 8 years); acute iridocyclitis; mucous membrane inflammation (pyuria, oral ulcerations); and skin lesions. Aortitis may occur. Boys are affected more commonly, more severely, and earlier than girls. Family history is frequently positive for one of the disorders listed above.

2. **General laboratory features** include a positive histocompatibility antigen HLA-B27 in many affected white patients and a positive HLA-B7 or B27 in a large percentage of black patients. Rheumatoid factor is negative, antinuclear antigen (ANA) is occasionally positive, and markers of acute inflammation may be normal or elevated.

C. **Diagnosis.** The specific illnesses included in this category present with the general features cited above and the following associated features:

1. **Juvenile ankylosing spondylitis (JAS)** is diagnosed by the finding of inflammatory involvement of the spine or sacroiliac joints.

2. **IBD-associated arthritis** may precede IBD by many months. The presence of weight loss, fever, anemia, abdominal pain, and hematochezia in a patient displaying the general features of this class of conditions should prompt consideration of IBD. This arthritis may occur as a nondeforming, nonerosive polyarthritis, which often correlates in activity with bowel inflammation and responds to symptomatic treatment with NSAIDs or sulfasalazine. Sacroiliitis, strongly associated with HLA-B27, has a poor prognosis even with aggressive chronic antiinflammatory therapy.

3. **Reactive arthritis** is generally a sterile pauciarticular inflammatory arthritis that follows bacterial infections of gastrointestinal or genitourinary sites. When associated with conjunctivitis and urethritis, the triad is termed *Reiter syndrome.* Reactive arthritis generally responds to NSAIDs in weeks to months, and chronic arthritis is rare.

4. **Psoriatic arthritis** is diagnosed by the characteristic skin or nail findings of psoriasis. Females are somewhat more likely than males to exhibit this condition, and presenting involvement is often pauciarticular, particularly of the distal interphalangeal joints. The illness may progress to polyarticular arthritis, or to a severe destructive disease.

D. **Treatment**

1. **Supportive care** with physical and occupational therapy is crucial in maintaining mobility. Special attention should be given to the axial skeleton. Custom-made shoe orthotics are helpful for Achilles tendon and plantar enthesitis.

2. **Drugs** (see sec. I.C.3)
   a. **Aspirin/NSAIDs.** Salicylates or NSAIDs are given initially. Indomethacin and tolmetin sodium seem to be more active in this form of arthritis than are other NSAIDs.
   b. **Intraarticular steroid injection** is used for severe inflammation of a few joints.
   c. **Remittive agents,** especially gold salts, are used for reactive arthritides that are unresponsive to NSAIDs.

III. **Lyme disease**
   A. **Etiology.** Lyme disease is a multisystem disease caused by the spirochete *Borrelia burgdorferi,* carried by the deer tick *Ixodes dammini.*
   B. **Evaluation.** Lyme disease may occur within weeks of the inciting tick bite, manifested initially by the characteristic rash of erythema chronicum migrans (ECM), a large expanding erythematous macule with central clearing. This may be accompanied by flu-like symptoms, including fever, lethargy, headache, neck pain, and myalgia. Late manifestations often occur without a history of antecedent tick bite or rash, sometimes years after exposure. Lyme arthritis usually involves the large joints (especially the knee) and is characterized by often recurrent attacks that last weeks to months.
   C. **Diagnosis** is made early in the disease by the appearance of ECM, or by positive antibody titers in the face of a consistent clinical history. Late disease is diagnosed by antiborrelial antibody titers plus characteristic clinical manifestations.
   D. **Treatment.** See Table 18-2.

IV. **Acute rheumatic fever (ARF)**
   A. **Etiology.** ARF occurs following streptococcal pharyngitis and is associated with the production of antistreptococcal antibodies, which cross-react with tissue antigens, causing injury.
   B. **Evaluation and diagnosis.** Diagnosis is made using the Jones criteria (Table 18-3).
   C. **Treatment**
      1. **Prevention.** ARF is avoided by treatment of group A streptococcal pharyngitis within 9 days of onset with benzathine penicillin, 1.2 million units IM, or penicillin V potassium, 50 mg/kg/day PO in four divided doses for 10 days. In penicillin-allergic patients, erythromycin, 30 mg/kg/day PO in four divided doses (maximum of 1,000 mg/day) for 10 days, is used.
      2. **Acute illness**
         a. **General.** Benzathine penicillin, 1.2 million units IM, or procaine penicillin G, 600,000 units intravenously daily for 10 days, is given. When the patient is allergic to penicillin, erythromycin is used.
         b. **Carditis**
            (1) **Without cardiomegaly.** Aspirin, 80 mg/kg/day in four divided doses, is given (see sec. I.C.3.a) until symptoms resolve and ESR normalizes.
            (2) **With cardiomegaly,** prednisone (see sec. V.C.2.c) is given at 1–2 mg/kg/day in three divided doses for 2–4 weeks; then aspirin therapy is begun.
         c. **Arthritis** is treated with aspirin as above.
         d. **Chorea** responds to rest and a quiet environment. Sedation with haloperidol may help in severe cases.
      3. **Prophylaxis.** Benzathine penicillin G, 1.2 million units IM, is given every 4 weeks. Penicillin-allergic patients are given either erythromycin, 500 mg per day in two doses, or sulfadiazine, 500 mg per day. Prophylaxis should be given for at least 5 years and should be continued throughout the patient's life in cases of chronic rheumatic heart disease or chorea.

V. **Systemic lupus erythematosus (SLE)** is an episodic multisystem disease characterized by circulating antibodies to nuclear and other tissue antigens (99% have a positive ANA). Autoantibodies and immune complexes seem important in mediating injury to tissues.
   A. **Etiology** is unknown.

Table 18-2. Complications and treatment of Lyme disease

Disease stage	Organ system	Treatment
Acute (stage 1)	General: malaise, flu-like symptoms Skin: Erythema migrans	Oral regimens: *children* < 9 yr: Amoxicillin 250 mg tid or penicillin V 250 mg qid for 10–30 days In case of penicillin allergy: erythromycin 250 mg tid for 10–30 days *adults:* tetracycline 250 mg qid, doxycycline 100 mg bid, or amoxicillin 500 mg qid, all for 10–30 days
Chronic (stage 2)	General: severe malaise and fatigue Skin: Annular rash Neurologic: meningitis, Bell's palsy, radiculoneuritis Cardiac: First-degree atrioventricular block (P-R interval < 0.3 sec) Musculoskeletal: migratory arthralgias and arthritis	Parenteral regimens: Penicillin G, 20 million U IV divided 6 times daily for 14–28 days, or ceftriaxone 2 gm daily for 14–28 days Oral regimens, as for early infection
Persistent (stage 3)	Skin: acrodermatitis chronica atrophicans Neurologic: chronic encephalomyelitis, spastic parapareses, ataxia Musculoskeletal: chronic arthritis, peripheral enthesopathy	Oral regimen for 1 month usually adequate Parenteral regimen, though duration of therapy not established Parenteral regimen as for stage 2 disease

Adapted from *Medical Letter on Drugs and Therapeutics* 30(769):65–66, 1988.

Table 18-3. Jones criteria (revised)*

Major manifestations	Minor manifestations	Supportive evidence
Carditis	Fever	Recent scarlet fever
Polyarthritis	Arthralgia	Throat culture positive for group A streptococci
Chorea	Previous rheumatic fever or rheumatic heart condition	
Erythema marginatum		
Subcutaneous nodules	Elevated ESR or positive CRP	Increased ASO or other streptococcal antibodies
	Prolonged P-R interval on ECG	

ESR = erythrocyte sedimentation rate; CRP = C-reactive protein; ASO = antistreptolysin O.
* Two major manifestations or one major and two minor manifestations with supportive evidence of recent streptococcal infection indicate a high probability of rheumatic fever.

Table 18-4. Criteria for systemic lupus erythematosus

Criterion	Definition
Malar rash	Fixed erythema, flat or raised, over the malar eminences, tending to spare the nasolabial folds
Discoid rash	Erythematous raised patches with adherent keratotic scaling and follicular plugging; atrophic scarring may occur in older lesions
Photosensitivity	Skin rash as a result of unusual reaction to sunlight by patient history or physician observation
Oral ulcers	Oral or nasopharyngeal ulceration, usually painless, observed by a physician
Arthritis	Nonerosive arthritis involving 2 or more peripheral joints, characterized by tenderness, swelling, or effusion
Serositis	(1) Pleuritis (convincing history of pleuritic pain or rub heard by a physician or evidence of pleural effusion) *or* (2) pericarditis (documented by ECG or rub or evidence of pericardial effusion)
Renal disorder	(1) Persistent proteinuria > 0.5 gm/day *or* (2) cellular casts — may be red cell, hemoglobin, granular, tubular, or mixed
Neurologic disorder	(1) Seizures (in the absence of offending drugs or known metabolic derangements, e.g., uremia, ketoacidosis, or electrolyte imbalance) *or* (2) psychosis (in the absence of offending drugs or known metabolic derangements, e.g., uremia, ketoacidosis, or electrolyte imbalance)
Hematologic disorder	(1) Hemolytic anemia with reticulocytosis, (2) leukopenia (< 4,000/mm^3 total on 2 or more occasions), (3) lymphopenia (<1,500/mm^3 on 2 or more occasions), *or* (4) thrombocytopenia (< 100,000/mm^3 in the absence of offending drugs)
Immunologic disorder	(1) Positive LE cell preparation, (2) anti-DNA (antibody to native DNA in abnormal titer), (3) anti-SM (presence of antibody to SM nuclear antigen), *or* (4) false-positive serologic test for syphilis known to be positive for at least 6 months and confirmed by *Treponema pallidum* immobilization or fluorescent treponemal antibody absorption test
Antinuclear antibody	An abnormal titer of antinuclear antibody by immunofluorescence or an equivalent assay at any point in time and in the absence of drugs known to be associated with "drug-induced lupus" syndrome

B. **Evaluation and diagnosis.** SLE is diagnosed when 4 of the 11 clinical criteria are present (Table 18-4).
C. **Therapy** is not curative, but often will prevent incapacitating symptoms and progressive tissue damage.
   1. **Supportive measures,** including rest and avoidance of triggering factors (drugs, sun, fluorescent light exposure, fatigue, and exposure to infection), help to avoid exacerbations. Hypertension and infectious complications must be vigorously treated. Raynaud's phenomenon is often responsive to avoidance of cold exposure, elimination of cigarettes and caffeine, and reduction of stress.
   2. **Drugs**
      a. **Aspirin/NSAIDs** (see sec. I.C.3) may control fever and arthritis. Hepato-

toxicity requiring discontinuation is relatively common in patients with SLE who are taking aspirin.

b. Plaquenil (see sec. I.C.4.a) may aid in controlling skin and joint manifestations, serositis, and malaise; however, it is not effective for renal, CNS, and hematologic disease.

c. Glucocorticoids

(1) Topical steroids are utilized for localized skin disease.

(2) Oral daily steroids are used for life-threatening or debilitating manifestations unresponsive to the above measures. Low-dose prednisone (0.5 mg/kg/day) is used for fever, dermatitis, or serositis. High-dose prednisone (0.5–2.0 mg/kg/day) is used for life-threatening end-organ involvement, such as cerebritis, hemolytic anemia, glomerulonephritis, severe serositis, myositis, or vasculitis. When inflammation is controlled, the steroid schedule is changed from every day to every other day. This dramatically reduces side effects.

(3) Pulse steroid therapy (methylprednisolone, 30 mg/kg IV on 3 consecutive days) is associated with faster clinical improvement and is used for rapidly progressive CNS or renal disease.

(4) Steroid toxicity

(a) Suppression of the hypothalamic axis may cause hypoadrenalism in times of stress.

(b) Immune suppression promotes susceptibility to infection and masks the signs and symptoms of infection.

(c) Changes in physical appearance, such as moon facies, buffalo hump, acne, striae, hirsutism, and bruising, are very disturbing to patients.

(d) Neurologic problems, such as euphoria, depression, psychosis, and pseudotumor cerebri, may be difficult to distinguish from neuropsychiatric manifestations of SLE, making management difficult.

(e) Metabolic effects, such as hyperglycemia, hypercholesterolemia, sodium retention, hypokalemia, and hypertension, are common.

(f) Musculoskeletal problems, including osteopenia, proximal myopathy, and aseptic necrosis, may lead to permanent disability.

(g) Ocular effects include glaucoma and cataracts.

d. Cytotoxic agents (cyclophosphamide, azathioprine, chlorambucil) are used for patients with severe prednisone toxicity or for individuals with life-threatening disease that is not controllable with corticosteroids. Intravenous cyclophosphamide boluses improve outcome in patients with diffuse proliferative glomerulonephritis. Controlled trials demonstrating efficacy of other agents are lacking.

3. Plasmapheresis is used for rapid removal of circulating immune complexes in conjunction with cytotoxic therapy. Its efficacy is unproven, though anecdotes report clinical improvement in acute life-threatening disease with its use.

VI. Juvenile dermatomyositis (JDMS) is a systemic disease with diffuse microangiitis involving skeletal muscle, skin, fat, the GI tract, and parts of the CNS.

A. Etiology is unknown. JDMS seems to develop after an acute viral infection in many children.

B. Evaluation. Clinical features include muscle weakness and tenderness, extensor surface skin rash, and constitutional symptoms. Arthritis may occur in some patients, and GI vasculitis is a potentially fatal complication of JDMS. Calcinosis and muscle atrophy may be severe long-term sequelae of prolonged muscle inflammation. JDMS is not associated with malignancy, unlike adult polymyositis.

C. Diagnosis is supported by elevated levels of muscle enzymes and typical findings on electromyogram (EMG) or magnetic resonance imaging (MRI). Muscle biopsy is indicated for confirmation of the diagnosis, and for prognostic evidence of extent of involvement.

D. Therapy

1. **Supportive measures** include **physical therapy,** positioning, and splinting to rebuild muscle strength and prevent contractures. Involvement of palatal-respiratory muscles requires vigorous suctioning, postural drainage, and attention to pulmonary function.

2. **Drugs**

   a. **Corticosteroids** (e.g., prednisone; see sec. **V.C.2.c**), 2 mg/kg/day in four divided doses, are prescribed until clinical improvement occurs, then tapered over 2–3 months to the lowest possible dose that maintains normal strength and muscle enzymes. A low dose of steroids is maintained for 1–3 years. If relapse occurs (rare after the first few years) high-dose corticosteroids are reinstituted. Bolus intravenous methylprednisolone may result in more rapid improvement.

   b. **Aspirin/NSAIDs** are used for arthritis associated with JDMS (see sec. **I.C.3**).

   c. **Cytotoxic agents** (methotrexate, cyclosporine-A) can be used in patients who are unresponsive to, or require continuous high-doses of, corticosteroids.

VII. Scleroderma is a systemic disease involving excessive fibrosis and vascular hyperreactivity. This condition often results in hidebound skin, Raynaud's phenomenon, and fibrosis of internal organs (including lungs, heart, GI tract, and kidneys).

A. Etiology is unknown.

B. Diagnosis is strongly suggested by one major or two minor criteria.

1. **The major criterion** is proximal scleroderma, i.e., hidebound and thickened skin with loss of appendages proximal to the wrists.

2. **Minor criteria** include sclerodactyly, digital pitting ulcers, or bibasilar pulmonary fibrosis.

C. Treatment. There is no cure for scleroderma; therapy is largely aimed at identifying and treating symptomatic organ involvement.

VIII. Mixed connective tissue disease (MCTD) is a condition with overlapping features of scleroderma, dermatomyositis, and/or SLE, and often associated with prominent arthritis.

A. Etiology is unknown.

B. Evaluation and diagnosis. Laboratory studies include acute-phase reactants. A high titer of ANA with elevated ribonucleoprotein (RNP) and extractable nuclear antigen (ENA) are characteristic of this disorder.

C. Treatment is based on the patient's predominant manifestations, which are treated like JRA, scleroderma, JDMS, or SLE.

IX. Necrotizing vasculitis is inflammation and necrosis of blood vessels, thought to be associated with the deposition of immune complexes in vessel walls (as in PAN), or with antiendothelial cell autoantibodies.

A. Mucocutaneous lymph node syndrome (MLNS) or **Kawasaki disease**

1. **Etiology.** MLNS appears to be caused by an as yet unidentified infectious agent.

2. **Evaluation and diagnosis.** The diagnosis of MLNS is made in an acutely ill child with 5 or 6 of the following criteria in the absence of alternative confirmed diagnoses (such as measles or scarlet fever):

   a. **Fever**

   b. **Rash** (polymorphic, not vesicular)

   c. Acute nonpurulent **cervical lymphadenopathy** (at least 1.5 cm)

   d. **Conjunctivitis** (bilateral, nonexudative)

   e. **Extremity changes** (including edema of hands and feet, erythema of palms and soles, or periungual desquamation)

   f. **Mucosal changes** (erythematous and fissured lips, red oropharynx, or strawberry tongue). **Laboratory** manifestations are not diagnostic and include evidence of acute inflammation with elevated ESR and C-reactive protein (CRP), leukocytosis, and thrombocytosis. Untreated, there is a 15–25 percent incidence of coronary aneurysm.

3. **Therapy**

a. Aspirin (see sec. I.C.3.a), 80–100 mg/kg/day until afebrile for 48 hours, then 3–5 mg/kg/day.

b. IV gamma globulin (IVGG), 2 gm/kg over 10–12 hours, dramatically reduces the incidence of coronary artery changes and the duration of acute inflammation. It is rarely associated with an anaphylactoid reaction or flushing, which respond to slowing the infusion rate, and with congestive heart failure secondary to the large infusion volume, which responds to diuretics (see Chap. 9, p. 245ff).

B. Polyarteritis nodosa (PAN)

1. **Etiology** is often idiopathic; PAN may follow an infectious illness (especially hepatitis B) or drug exposure.

2. **Evaluation.** PAN is characterized by systemic illness, including fever and malaise, with vasculitis involving one or more organs. Skin and renal involvement are common; liver, GI tract, cardiac, CNS, and musculoskeletal system involvement may occur.

3. **Diagnosis** is based on angiographic- or biopsy-proven vasculitis of medium-sized muscular arteries.

4. **Therapy** is similar to that in SLE, using steroids or cytotoxic agents to decrease progression to severe organ (especially kidney) injury.

C. Henoch-Schönlein purpura (HSP) is characterized by a maculopapular or purpuric rash of dependent portions of the body (typically legs and buttocks), arthritis or arthralgia, abdominal pain (possibly with GI hemorrhage or intussusception), and nephritis.

1. **Etiology** is unclear, but **HSP** often occurs after upper respiratory infection, streptococcal pharyngitis (approximately 30%), or gastroenteritis.

2. **Evaluation and diagnosis.** Laboratory findings are nondiagnostic and include elevated serum immunoglobulin (IgA), thrombocytosis, and normal complement levels. The diagnosis is usually made on clinical grounds; biopsy of newly affected skin often reveals perivascular deposition of IgA. Severe, prolonged renal involvement, including hematuria, hypertension, and occasionally uremia, may rarely (< 1%) progress to chronic renal failure.

3. **Treatment** is initially supportive.

   a. Salicylates or NSAIDs (see sec. I.C.3) are used to treat isolated arthritis.

   b. Corticosteroids (e.g., prednisone; see sec. V.C.2.c) at 1–2 mg/kg/day have been used for bowel involvement or severe arthritis that is unresponsive to aspirin. Nephritis is unresponsive to steroids.

X. Sarcoidosis is a chronic, multisystem granulomatous disease.

A. Etiology is unknown.

B. Evaluation

1. **In older children** (> 4 years) a multisystem disease develops, with noncaseating granulomas in the eye, lymph glands, muscle, liver, skin, and nervous system. Hilar adenopathy and pulmonary fibrosis are common.

2. **In younger children** (< 4 years) a maculopapular or nodular rash, arthritis (boggy, painless joint effusion with little limitation of motion), and uveitis, associated with fever and malaise, typically develop.

3. **Laboratory manifestations** include an elevated angiotensin II–converting enzyme (ACE) level and uptake in lacrimal and parotid glands on gallium scan. Systemic involvement is usually associated with elevated acute phase reactants.

C. Diagnosis depends on a biopsy of affected tissue revealing noncaseating granulomas without an infectious cause.

D. Treatment

1. Skin and joint manifestations are treated with NSAIDs or hydroxychloroquine.

2. Anterior uveitis is treated with topical steroid drops.

3. **Systemic symptoms and posterior iridocyclitis** are treated with prednisone (see sec. V.C.2.c), 1–2 mg/kg/day. For refractory eye disease, methotrexate may prevent progression to blindness.

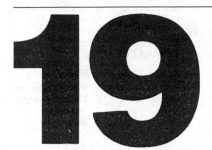

Neurology

Karl Kuban

I. **Disorders of mental status and intracranial hypertension**
   A. **Coma and acute increased intracranial pressure (ICP)** (see Chap. 3, p. 69ff).
   B. **Reye syndrome**
      1. **Etiology.** The cause is not understood, although it is probably a mitochondrial disease associated with influenza and varicella, and possibly aspirin use, that primarily involves the liver and brain.
      2. **Evaluation and diagnosis**
         a. Characteristically, an antecedent viral illness is followed by vomiting and progressive lethargy.
         b. **Examination.** Tachypnea, fever, lethargy, and stupor or coma are typical. Signs of elevated ICP and, more rarely, seizures may also be noted.
         c. **Laboratory findings**
            (1) Elevated serum **hepatocellular enzyme assays** (SGOT, SGPT, LDH) and elevated serum ammonia (arterial) are the laboratory hallmarks; one may also see metabolic acidosis and respiratory alkalosis as well as hypoglycemia and prolongation of the prothrombin time (PT) and partial thromboplastin time (PTT).
            (2) **A computed tomographic (CT) scan** or **magnetic resonance imaging (MRI) scan** may be necessary to rule out an intracranial mass.
            (3) **Liver biopsy** is generally performed when the diagnosis is in question. Features that may indicate the need for biopsy include an unusual age (16 years) and recurrent episodes, such as seen with disorders of carnitine metabolism.
      3. **Treatment**
         a. The primary intent is to maintain **cerebral perfusion pressure** (mean arterial pressure minus ICP) above 50 mm Hg and to avoid the complications of hepatic dysfunction. Both problems are directly related to the severity of the disease. Severity, in turn, is suggested by a number of prognostic variables. These include serum ammonia greater than 300 µg/dl, rapid clinical evolution through the stages of coma, posturing (decortication or decerebration), and an electroencephalographic (EEG) picture of deeper stages of coma.
         b. **Clinical staging and EEG grading of Reye syndrome.** See Table 19-1.
         c. **For the management of acute hepatic necrosis,** see Chap. 10, p. 288ff.
         d. **Cerebral support**
            (1) **Stage I or II clinically and grade 1, 2, or 3 by EEG**
               (a) An EEG is obtained q12h until EEG, or clinical stabilization, or improved grading is achieved. Progression to higher grades requires additional intervention [see **(2)**].
               (b) Initially, unless the patient is volume depleted, limit fluid to one-half maintenance; fluids should be chosen to prevent hypoglycemia and to avoid reducing serum osmolarity (in 5 or 10% dextrose in water [D/W] in normal saline), which may exacerbate cerebral edema. The goal is to elevate serum osmolarity to 290–310 mOsm.
               (c) Seizures should be treated with IV phenytoin (Dilantin) to avoid

Table 19-1. Clinical staging and EEG grading in Reye syndrome

Grade	Clinical description	EEG characteristics by age in years		
		<5	5–10	>10
1	Lethargic	Predominantly delta	Theta-delta	Predominantly theta
2	Agitated	Predominantly delta	Predominantly delta	Theta-delta
3	Decorticate	High-voltage delta	High-voltage delta	High-voltage delta
4	Decerebrate	Burst suppression and low voltage, (nearly) isoelectric		
5	Flaccid			

losing the ability to monitor the patient's level of consciousness (see Chap. 3, p. 67). Administer 15–20 mg/kg as a loading dose mixed in normal saline and given no more rapidly than 1 mg/kg/min.

(d) Electrolytes, osmolarity, blood sugar, and blood urea nitrogen (BUN) should be monitored q6–12h, and an arterial ammonia q12–24h. PT and PTT should also be repeated q12–24h.

(e) The head should be placed in the midline and elevated to 30 degrees to reduce the venous component of ICP.

(f) Lumbar puncture is relatively contraindicated in patients with Reye syndrome.

(2) **Stage III, IV, or V clinically and grade 4 or 5 by EEG.** In addition to the treatment outlines for stages I–II, the patient will require intracranial monitoring and possibly additional therapy, including intubation, hyperventilation, osmotic agents, and barbiturates (see Chap. 3, p. 71ff.)

C. **Chronic ICP**
 1. **Etiology.** The causes include hydrocephalus, brain tumors, brain abscess, arteriovenous malformations, and chronic subdural hematomas.
 2. **Evaluation**
    a. **Examination.** A lateralized examination suggests hemispheric brain tumor, subdural hematoma, abscess, or arteriovenous malformation. Asymmetric nystagmus, truncal or appendicular ataxia, and brainstem signs suggest a similar posterior fossa process. Nonlateralized and nonfocal signs suggest hydrocephalus and pseudotumor cerebri (see D and Chap. 3, p. 69).
    b. **Tests**
       (1) Cranial MRI scan or cranial CT scan
       (2) Lumbar puncture is contraindicated except in pseudotumor cerebri and simple communicating hydrocephalus.
       (3) Cranial sector scanning ultrasound can be used to evaluate the ventricular system and the cerebral hemispheres when the anterior fontanel is patent.
 3. **Treatment**
    a. Treat as in acute increased ICP (see Chap. 3).
    b. Posthemorrhagic hydrocephalus in premature newborns can be treated medically by daily lumbar puncture and removal of at least 10 ml cerebrospinal fluid (CSF). Serial lumbar punctures do **not** prevent the development of hydrocephalus.
    c. Most patients with progressive hydrocephalus will require a shunting procedure.

   d. When surgery is contraindicated, temporization may be achieved with furosemide (0.1–0.5 mg/kg q4–6h), glycerol or mannitol (0.25 gm/kg q6h), or acetazolamide (10 mg/kg q8–12h).
   e. Radiation in combination with chemotherapy or surgery is used as indicated for tumors or abscess.
D. Increased ICP without alteration of mental status: pseudotumor cerebri (benign intracranial hypertension)
   1. The **etiology** is unknown.
   2. Evaluation and diagnosis
      a. History. Headache is the rule. The patient may complain of visual loss or diplopia and, occasionally, nausea and vomiting.
      b. Examination. Papilledema, enlarged blind spot, visual scotoma, and sixth cranial nerve palsy may be seen. Other focal or lateralized neurologic signs, such as other cranial nerve palsies, hemiparesis, ataxia, and sensory deficits, diminish pseudotumor as a diagnostic consideration.
      c. Tests
         (1) A **cranial CT or MRI scan** must be performed to exclude hydrocephalus or a space-occupying lesion; the ventricles appear either normal in size or slit-like.
         (2) A **lumbar puncture** can be done after the absence of localizing signs and the presence of a normal CT or MRI scan have been established.
   3. Therapy. Untreated, persistent ICP may lead to permanent loss of vision.
      a. A single **lumbar puncture**, with removal of enough fluid to drop the pressure to approximately 150 mm H_2O or to 50 percent of the opening pressure, is often adequate. Symptoms (headache) are often dramatically alleviated following the lumbar puncture.
      b. Initially, some patients will require a series of lumbar punctures, daily at first, increasing the interval according to exacerbation of symptoms (headache) and rate of reaccumulation of CSF. Spinal puncture (low pressure) headache may complicate the clinical assessment. Spinal puncture headaches improve in the prone position and high-pressure headaches tend to improve in the upright position.
      c. When repeated lumbar punctures are not successful, **acetazolamide** (Diamox) can be initiated (10–25 mg/kg in 2–3 divided doses/day).
      d. Furosemide (Lasix), 0.1–0.5 mg/kg q4–6h, can be used if acetazolamide is not successful.
      e. If previous interventions are unsuccessful, a course of **dexamethasone** at 0.2–0.5 mg/kg/day is recommended. Corticosteroid dependency may result, however. A response to dexamethasone generally occurs within a few weeks. Improvement can be evaluated by the absence of headache and normalization of eye grounds (usually slower to resolve), as well as by lowering opening pressure on lumbar puncture. With normalization of opening pressure, dexamethasone can be given every other day and then tapered over 2–3 months.
      f. When all other modalities to control increased ICP fail, or when vision is acutely threatened, a **lumboperitoneal or ventriculoperitoneal** shunt may be necessary.
E. Attention deficit disorder (ADD) with (ADHD) or without hyperactivity (see also Chap. 20). The principal therapeutic concern is to properly identify the child who has an intrinsic inability to maintain attention, leading to a state of overactivity or inattention with consequent disruption of his or her educational program.
   1. The **etiology** is unknown.
   2. Evaluation and diagnosis
      a. History. In general, the early years are characterized by excessive activity, inability to sit quietly with a book or to watch a slow-moving television show, and unusual sleeping patterns. Girls are less likely than boys to have physical hyperactivity but still may have the other features of ADD.

b. Examination. There frequently are "soft neurologic signs," such as synkinesis, stress gait posturing, choreiform movements, and incoordination. However, these need not be present in order to make the diagnosis.

c. The **differential diagnoses** include hearing loss, petit mal seizures, chronic lead intoxication, and psychological responses to stress.

3. Therapy

a. Stimulant therapy will not be useful for the anxious or depressed child without ADD/ADHD. Its main purpose is to maximize attention. Some children will respond to only one of the available stimulant medications, and may do so either at very low or very high doses (Table 19-2). The following principles should be used in administering stimulant medications:

(1) Establish an educator and parental baseline with subjective and objective assessments. A Connor's hyperactivity scale is useful or one can use *Diagnostic and Statistical Manual of Mental Disorders* (3rd ed.) (DSM-III) criteria.

(2) Introduce small doses at first in the morning and at noon for methylphenidate (Ritalin) or dextroamphetamine (Dexedrine) and in the morning only for pemoline (Cylert), Ritalin-SR (slow release), or dextroamphetamine spansules.

(3) Increase the doses by ½ tablet/dose every 1–2 weeks after contact with parents and/or teachers until an optimal therapeutic effect is achieved, overdosage is recognized, or an exacerbation of symptoms is identified (see Table 19-2). Waiting a week before evaluation of effects tends to reduce the impact of placebo effects, the chance of good or bad days, etc.

(4) Overdosage of medication leads to withdrawal, weepiness, and somnolence. "Zombie-like" states usually imply overdosage symptoms. Appetite often is diminished while the child is on the medication (lunch most often). Most often children will make up for this at other meals.

(5) There is often a "coming down" or, more appropriately, "going up" effect as the medication wears off. At this time the child is excessively hyperactive and inattentive, and a very small dose of Ritalin in the late afternoon may ease the transition.

(6) Since the principal intent is to optimize education, in most circum-

Table 19-2. Drugs for attention deficit disorders[a]

Drug	Dosage (mg)	Dosage interval
Dextroamphetamine (Dexedrine)	2.5–15	8 AM, noon
Dextroamphetamine spansule (Dexedrine)	2.5–15	8 AM
Methylphenidate (Ritalin, Ritalin-SR)	2.5–20 20–40	8 AM, noon 8 AM
Pemoline[b] (Cylert)	18.75–112.5	8 AM
Desipramine[c] (Norpramin)	10–150	qhs

[a] Presence of a tic disorder or appearance of tics while on stimulant medication is a contraindication to its use or continued use.
[b] Liver functions must be monitored with Cylert.
[c] Must have baseline ECG and periodic reevaluations.

stances, medications can be given on school days or when optimal attention is necessary. It is useful to give the child medication on weekends during the initial weeks, so that parents can also assess drug efficacy. A follow-up educator's assessment is required to establish efficacy. Occasionally, the medication will help children with homework or in social activities and can be used at those times as well.

(7) Often, adjunctive behavior modification and counseling input are important. Many of these children have a poor self-image and have superimposed emotional difficulties. Some have an associated learning disability and will require a modified education plan. A hearing evaluation should be done, and an EEG evaluation is occasionally necessary.

(8) Summer drug holidays may be useful for reassessing the child's continued need for medication.

(9) Serial assessment of height, weight, and blood pressure is recommended.

(10) Rarely, children will respond to elimination of particular food additives as recommended in the Feingold diet.

b. **Antidepressant therapy.** A substantial experience with use of **desipramine** for ADD or ADHD has been accumulating over recent years. Desipramine has been used preferentially for children with concomitant Tourette's syndrome, when traditional stimulants are ineffective, or when substantial emotional problems coexist with ADD/ADHD. Baseline and periodic electrocardiograms (ECGs) are necessary and prolonged QT_c interval is a relative contraindication for its use (see sec. **VI.A**). **Side effects** include sedation and tachycardia. **Initial dosage** is 10 mg qhs with increments by 10 mg per day at weekly intervals until beneficial effect is attained or side effects interfere with its use. Doses in excess of 100 mg are rarely required. Response does not appear to be serum level dependent.

II. **Cranial nerve disorders**
   A. **Optic neuritis**
      1. **Etiology.** Optic neuritis may occur during or following an infection or may arise unrelated to infection, as with immune-mediated disorders or the first signs of a recurrent demyelinating disorder. It involves demyelination of the optic nerve head (papillitis) or the area behind the nerve head (retrobulbar neuritis).
      2. **Evaluation and diagnosis**
         a. **History.** The clinical history is that of lost vision; this may be unilateral or bilateral, and visual acuity may be reduced considerably. Associated ocular pain may be present.
         b. **Examination.** Visual acuity is reduced. With papillitis, papilledema is seen; with retrobulbar neuritis, the funduscopic findings are essentially normal. A careful neurologic examination may reveal other neurologic deficits to suggest a more disseminated disease.
         c. **Laboratory tests**
            (1) A **cranial CT or MRI scan** may be necessary to rule out raised ICP or chiasmatic region mass, which may lead to acute visual loss.
            (2) A **lumbar puncture** is necessary for similar reasons; CSF can be assessed for a more generalized involvement of the nervous system to include basic myelin protein and gamma globulins. (There may be a mild pleocytosis with optic neuritis.)
            (3) Somatosensory, brainstem, visual, and auditory evoked responses may identify more extensive white matter disease.
      3. **Therapy.** Optic neuritis is often self-limited. When the disease progresses, particularly to involve both eyes, **adrenocorticotropic hormone (ACTH)**, 60–80 units IV, given in two divided doses over 4–8 hours each, should be used; this is changed to IM ACTH gel after 3–7 days and then is slowly

tapered over 1–3 months. Patients must be carefully monitored for complications associated with the use of high-dose corticosteroids (see Chap. 11, p. 319ff). Concurrent antacid or H_2 blocker therapy is recommended.

B. Bell's palsy and facial palsy

1. **Etiology.** Facial nerve palsy may occur as a result of head injury, demyelination, tumor, hypertension, infection (including Lyme disease), or infarction. Idiopathic cases are termed **Bell's palsy.**

2. **Evaluation and diagnosis**

   a. **History.** Bell's palsy is preceded by an upper respiratory infection in approximately 75 percent of cases. Patients frequently complain of pain behind or in front of the ear for 1 or 2 days before or concurrent with the development of the facial weakness. The evolution of facial weakness occurs over a few hours. Rarely, Bell's palsy can recur one or several times. It occasionally recurs as part of Melkersson's syndrome.

   b. **Examination.** Mandatory findings in patients with Bell's palsy include weakness of both the lower and upper face, absence of other cranial nerve dysfunction, and normal blood pressure. Findings consistent with the diagnosis of Bell's palsy include hyperacusis of one ear, loss of taste on one side of the tongue, and unilateral overflow of tears or a dry eye.

   c. **Tests**

      (1) **Skull x-rays,** with attention to mastoid and petrous bones, are required to rule out infection or tumor.

      (2) A **complete blood count (CBC), heterophil antibodies,** and Lyme disease antibody titers may also be useful.

3. **Treatment**

   a. **Supportive.** Protection of the involved eye should include the use of a protective eye glass, and a methylcellulose eye lubricant is suggested if the eye is dry.

   b. **Specific.** If begun within 72 hours, a 10-day course of prednisone, starting with 0.75 mg/kg/day and reducing the dosage by 0.25 mg/kg/day every third day, may alleviate the pain associated with Bell's palsy, shorten recovery, and reduce instances of complete, permanent paralysis.

III. Spinal cord and cauda equina compression

A. Etiology. Spinal cord or cauda equina compression requires emergency intervention. It usually occurs because of trauma, tumor, infection, or hemorrhage. The process may be epidural, subdural, subarachnoid, subpial, or intramedullary.

B. Traumatic cord compression (see Chap. 3, p. 71).

C. Nontraumatic cord or cauda equina compression

1. **History.** Note should be made of the following:

   a. Previous history of tumor, bleeding diathesis, fever, or infections

   b. **Spinal pain** is often the most useful indication of the diagnosis and of localization of the compression. Most often, pain worsens with cough, a Valsalva maneuver, or percussion over the involved area.

   c. Alteration in bowel or bladder control

   d. Change in gait or lower-extremity weakness

   e. Perineal loss of sensation

   f. Differential points include paraspinal muscle spasm, vertebral bone pain, nerve root irritation (e.g., from ruptured disk), and other inflammatory spinal or paraspinal processes such as discitis.

2. **Physical examination**

   a. **General examination.** A stiff neck, particularly for both flexion and rotation, may suggest a lesion at the high cervical area. Pain provoked by straight leg raising may also help localize the problem. External evidence of trauma, bruits, or vascular malformations over the spine and vertebral tenderness to percussion may be sensitive localizing signs. Fever suggests epidural or subdural empyema.

   b. **Motor level**

      (1) **Tone and strength.** Generally, tone will be increased and strength

will be reduced at and below the level of a spinal lesion. Acutely, the tone may be decreased, increased, or normal.

(2) **Deep tendon reflexes.** The patient will be normoreflexive above the level of the lesion and hyperreflexive below it. Reflexes may be absent at the level of the lesion. In acute cord compression, one may note spinal shock presenting as total flaccidity and areflexia below the level of the lesion. An isolated asymmetric lost reflex at the knee or ankle suggests a trapped nerve and is most often seen with a herniated disk; however, other processes such as tumor and abscess can cause similar findings.

(3) **Plantars** are usually flagrantly extensor with spinal cord lesions.

c. **Sensory level.** One may discern a sensory level to touch, pain, or temperature. Absence of a sensory level, with loss of perianal sensation, suggests a cauda equina lesion.

d. **Lumbrosacral reflexes and signs.** A patulous anus and an absent anal, bulbocavernosus, or cremasteric reflex suggest a cauda equina lesion or spinal shock.

e. **Autonomic changes.** The presence of Horner syndrome suggests a lesion at the T1 level. Sweating is decreased or absent below the level of the lesion if it is above T10. Urinary retention is common.

3. **Laboratory tests**
   a. **Plain spine x-rays** of the suspected areas should be obtained. If a high cervical lesion is suspected, immobilization of the neck and open-mouth views of the odontoid may be necessary.
   b. **Bone scan** will occasionally be helpful to identify a bony problem such as osteomyelitis or a more benign disorder such as discitis.
   c. **Clotting studies** and **septic workup** should be obtained as indicated. A lumbar puncture is relatively contraindicated and should only be done as part of the myelogram, if necessary, after neurosurgical consultation.
   d. **MRI** of the spine is the diagnostic study of choice to evaluate anatomy and limits of the lesions. Occasionally, a myelogram will still be necessary and in the case of an arteriovenous malformation, arteriography may also be warranted.

4. **Treatment**
   a. **Dexamethasone (Decadron),** 0.5–1.0 mg/kg IV as a loading dose and 0.1–0.2 mg/kg q6h, should be administered as soon as a space-occupying lesion is suggested by a previous history of tumor or lytic lesions in bone or when there is evidence for active evolution. Antacid or cimetidine can be given concomitantly.
   b. For **epidural tumors,** radiation therapy has been shown to be as efficacious as decompressive laminectomy in most circumstances. However, hematoma, empyema, and bony impingement on the cord or the cauda equina most often require immediate surgical intervention.
   c. Appropriate antibiotics should be administered for empyema.
   d. Intermittent catheterization is used to treat urinary retention.

D. **Transverse myelopathy** usually presents as rapidly progressive segmental spinal cord dysfunction.
   1. The **etiology** includes postviral, vascular (involving ischemia in the distribution of the anterior spinal artery), or demyelinating disease.
   2. **Evaluation.** Proceed as for spinal cord compression; this is a diagnosis of exclusion.
   3. **Therapy is controversial and of equivocal efficacy.**
      a. Supportive therapy is the mainstay of treatment, depending on the level.
      b. A trial of **corticosteroids** may be helpful. Prednisone, 1 mg/kg/day, is often administered.
      c. **Plasmapheresis** may be useful.

IV. **Neuropathic diseases: Guillain-Barré syndrome (GBS; acute infectious polyneuritis)**

A. Etiology. This acute or subacute symmetric ascending disease of predominantly motor nerves is thought to be immune mediated.

B. Evaluation and diagnosis.

1. **History.** There is usually an antecedent viral illness or surgical procedure. Frequently, there are complaints of paresthesia and/or weakness of the lower extremities.

2. **Physical examination.** The cranial nerves are usually normal; bifacial weakness often appears later in the course. The Fisher variant (descending weakness with ataxia) may present with ophthalmoplegia or facial palsy early in the course of the disease. Distal hypotonia, symmetric weakness, and reduced deep tendon reflexes are most often noted. There should be absent extensor plantars, no sensory levels, and no perianal sensory loss.

3. **Laboratory tests.** CSF protein will usually be elevated **following** the first 48 hours of symptoms. Mild pleocytosis (up to 50–100 cells) does not exclude GBS.

C. Treatment. The therapy is largely symptomatic. There are, however, special considerations.

1. **Monitoring of respiratory status.** Compromise of the nerve roots innervating the phrenic nerve, C3, C4, and C5 may cause rapid respiratory embarrassment. Vital capacity must be monitored frequently, and a fall below 15 ml/kg warrants artificial ventilatory support. Compromise of C3, C4, and C5 is usually preceded by weakness of the upper extremities and occurs within the first 2 weeks of the onset of symptoms.

2. **Preparing patient and family.** It is critical that the patient and family be counseled that intubation may be necessary as routine support for the disease **before** urgent measures are required.

3. Substantial data in adults affirm the benefit of **plasmapheresis** in GBS as measured by rapidity of acute and long-term improvement, and it may reduce the risk for required ventilation support. There are more limited data from studies involving children, but similar benefits have been reported. Since plasmapheresis has inherent potential morbidity, we recommend its use in children when need for intubation, a procedure that also has potential inherent morbidity, appears likely by virtue of rapidity of evolution of symptoms or signs and/or involvement of lumbar and thoracic spinal segments. **Plasmapheresis** is generally also only used in the first 2 weeks of the disease. Treatments are given every other day for four to eight sessions. Each exchange involves the removal of 25–40 ml/kg plasma and replacement with Plasmanate or an equivalent solution.

4. **Corticosteroids.** The efficacy of corticosteroids in this disease is controversial and considered by some to lead to an increased incidence of relapse. On the other hand, corticosteroids are extremely effective for the relapsing form of polyneuritis.

5. Hypertension, thought to be mediated by the renin-angiotensin system, may occur. Propranolol and, if needed, an alpha-adrenergic blocker are recommended (see Chap. 8, p. 220).

6. **Physical therapy** to prevent contractures is important during the recovery phase.

V. Diseases of the neuromuscular junction and of muscle: myasthenia gravis

A. Etiology and evaluation. Myasthenia gravis is usually an immune-mediated disease involving the neuromuscular junction. It may occur as three clinical syndromes.

1. **Transient neonatal myasthenia gravis** is thought to occur because of passively transferred immunoglobulin G (IgG) antibodies. The signs and symptoms of weakness may be severe.

2. **Congenital myasthenia gravis** may present before birth with reduced fetal movements, postnatally, or up to several years following birth. The mother does not have myasthenia gravis. The symptoms are milder, though more persistent, than the transient disease.

3. **Juvenile myasthenia gravis** may occur any time during childhood and

usually presents with ptosis, diplopia or other bulbar symptoms and signs, and weakness.

B. Diagnosis. The response to anticholinesterase administration is the cornerstone of diagnosis. Repetitive nerve stimulation seeking a decremental response is confirmatory. The response to **edrophonium** (Tensilon), 0.2 mg/kg with a maximum of 10 mg, is transient, lasting less than 5 minutes, and may provoke profound cholinergic side effects. Therefore, neostigmine (Prostigmin) is used intramuscularly in neonates and occasionally in older children; 0.04 mg/kg neostigmine will elicit a response within 10 minutes and peak at 30 minutes. With either Tensilon or neostigmine, cardiac rhythm and blood pressure must be monitored, and atropine at 0.01 mg/kg/dose, with a maximum of 0.4 mg, must be available for intravenous injection.

C. Therapy

1. **Transient neonatal myasthenia gravis**
   a. **Supportive therapy** alone will be adequate only in a minority of patients.
   b. With feeding or respiratory difficulty, IM and oral neostigmine are helpful. The IM dosage range is 0.05–0.3 mg/kg; with oral doses it is 10 times higher. The frequency of administration can be ascertained clinically by respiratory function and force of the cry and may be necessary q1–12h. IM doses can be given 20 minutes before feedings.
   c. **Plasmapheresis** or **exchange transfusion** can be used for symptoms that are unresponsive to anticholinesterase therapy. Gamma globulin infusion has been reported to be effective as well.
2. **Congenital myasthenia gravis** can be managed as transient myasthenia in the neonatal period, although serious problems are not as evident. Plasmapheresis or exchange transfusion is not likely to be helpful. Chronic anticholinesterase treatment is often disappointing at any age.
3. **Juvenile myasthenia gravis**
   a. **Anticholinesterase drugs** are the cornerstone of management, both chronically, for cranial nerve dysfunction and weakness, and for acute respiratory embarrassment; neostigmine or pyridostigmine (Mestinon) is used, starting at 0.3–0.5 mg/kg and 1 mg/kg tid, respectively, with increasing dosage and adjustment of frequency of administration according to the response and its duration. Time span (sustained release) 180-mg tablets are available when dosing amounts permit their use.
   b. When anticholinesterase medications at higher doses are not effective, **prednisone** is warranted, starting at 0.5–1.0 mg/kg and increasing by 0.2 mg/kg up to 60 mg per day every other day until an optimal effect is achieved. The prednisone should subsequently be slowly tapered.
   c. **Thymectomy** may be effective therapy when other means of treatment have failed or when requirements for corticosteroids are prolonged, daily, and at high doses. Thymoma rarely occurs in childhood.
   d. **Plasmapheresis** has recently shown promise as a means of transiently improving severe symptoms and signs.
4. When using anticholinesterase medications, **overmedication may result in weakness, leading to the so-called cholinergic crisis.** Systemic cholinergic symptoms and signs suggest the proper diagnosis, and a Tensilon test distinguishes *cholinergic crisis* from *myasthenic crisis*. **Atropine,** 0.4 mg IV, is the treatment of choice for cholinergic crisis.

VI. Movement disorders

A. Gilles de la Tourette syndrome is characterized by multiple, complex tics occasionally associated with unusual vocalizations.

1. **Etiology.** This disease is thought to involve an alteration of dopaminergic neurotransmitter systems.
2. **Evaluation and diagnosis.** The diagnosis rests on the clinical identification of multiple, complex tics continuing for at least 6 months. Occasionally, this picture can be provoked by stimulant therapy. Children often have an associated ADD, learning disabilities, behavioral difficulties, or emotional problems as well.

3. Therapy

a. Discontinuation of stimulant drugs

b. **Pimozide** (Orap) or **haloperidol** (Haldol) is indicated when the frequency of movements has a negative impact on the child's physical, educational, social, or psychological well-being. Both medications are major tranquilizers and can produce side effects associated with phenothiazine at therapeutically effective doses.

   (1) Pimozide (Orap) produces sedation and lethargy, although less frequently than haloperidol. Generally, use of the smallest dosage that produces the desired effect is appropriate and the long half-life allows qhs administration. Dosing should be incremented slowly with changes instituted at weekly, every-other-weekly, or greater intervals depending on side effects. The starting dose is 1 mg.

   (a) **Major side effects** include dry mouth or sedation, or both, either of which may dissipate with time. Acute dystonic reactions occur 5–9 percent of the time and an initial dose of 0.5 mg benztropine at bedtime will prevent this side effect. After several weeks the benztropine can be discontinued. Doses should not exceed 20 mg per day or 0.3 mg/kg/day and most children require less than 8 mg per day.

   (b) A baseline ECG should be performed and QT_c greater than 0.44 seconds should prompt a cardiologic evaluation. ECG should also be performed during therapy and an increase of the QT_c 25 percent above baseline, development of T waves, a QT_c value of 0.47 seconds or greater, or a heart rate of less than 50 per minute should prompt a reduction in the pimozide dosage.

   (2) Haloperidol (Haldol) doses will range from 0.25 mg bid to as high as 4 mg tid. Initial doses should be small, 0.25 mg bid, and increased at weekly or greater intervals until satisfactory control is achieved or sedative side effects necessitate discontinuation or reduction of the drug.

c. Psychological counseling and modification of the educational program are often indicated.

B. Sydenham's chorea

1. The **etiology** is unknown.

2. **Evaluation** is that of acute rheumatic fever (see Chap. 14, p. 423).

3. The **diagnosis** rests on noting choreiform movements of the arms and fingers, unusual postures of the outstretched arm, facial grimacing, darting of the tongue, and an explosive speech pattern. The patients are frequently restless and emotionally labile. Hypotonia is present and deep tendon reflexes are pendular and may be "hung up" on repetitive tapping. Signs may be asymmetric or unilateral.

4. Therapy

a. **Prednisone therapy** (1–2 mg/kg/day) reportedly leads to improvement within a week.

b. **Haloperidol** (0.02–0.1 mg/kg/day in 2 divided doses) is reputed to be effective within 2 weeks.

c. **Phenobarbital** (3–5 mg/kg/day) or chlorpromazine (50–100 mg tid) can be used as a sedative for symptomatic relief from the movements.

d. A restful environment will help reduce external stimulation.

C. The **syndrome of opsoclonus-myoclonus (SOMy)** is also known as myoclonic encephalopathy of infancy.

1. Etiology. This syndrome is associated with neuroblastoma and encephalitis, or may be idiopathic. It is thought to occur because of inflammation of the brainstem or cerebellum, or both.

2. Evaluation and diagnosis

a. Evaluated in the same manner as occult neuroblastoma

b. **Physical examination.** The patients are most often irritable and photophobic. They usually have conjugate, chaotic, quick movements of the eyes in any direction of gaze, often aggravated when they are tired and noted during sleep. Jerking movements of the legs, particularly when attempts are made to place the child on his or her feet, are present. The child may appear markedly ataxic; similar movements may be noted at the upper extremities when reaching.

   c. **Laboratory evaluation.** In addition to tests necessary to evaluate neuroblastoma, these patients should first have a CT or MRI scan to rule out a posterior fossa mass and then a lumbar puncture to evaluate cells and protein, and to rule out enteroviral or arboviral infection.

3. **Therapy.** Treatment of the underlying neuroblastoma or waiting for a few weeks following a clear infectious cause may be all that is necessary. However, when SOMy persists, ACTH, given IM, is advocated (60–80 U/m², rapidly tapering to every other day and, subsequently, as clinically indicated, over 1–3 months). Some patients become ACTH dependent.

D. **Wilson's disease**
   1. **Etiology.** An autosomal recessively inherited inborn error of copper metabolism resulting in accumulation of copper in brain and liver
   2. **Evaluation**
      a. **History and examination.** May present with basal ganglia signs (tremor, rigidity, dystonia, chorea), psychiatric symptoms, a course of dementia, or liver disease (see Chap. 10, p. 290ff). A neurologic presentation is invariably associated with presence of Kayser-Fleischer rings of the cornea.
      b. **Ancillary evaluations**
         (1) Elevated urinary copper and diminished serum ceruloplasmin concentrations are usual but not invariable features. Liver biopsy is sometimes necessary and demonstrates elevated hepatic copper concentrations.
         (2) Slit-lamp examination is necessary to evaluate the presence of Kayser-Fleischer rings.
   3. Treatment with D-penicillamine as in Chap. 10, p. 290; see also Chap. 4, p. 117.

VII. **Paroxysmal disorders**
   A. **Seizures** represent a symptom complex and not a disease state. The tendency to have recurrent seizures in the absence of acute metabolic alterations or central nervous system (CNS) infection loosely defines epilepsy.
      1. **Etiology.** In the emergency room setting, the most important etiologic considerations include trauma, Trauma X, meningitis and encephalitis, space-occupying lesions, metabolic causes, cerebrovascular accidents, and toxic encephalopathies. Poor drug compliance or altered drug metabolism because of intercurrent illness is the most common cause of seizures in a patient with epilepsy.
      2. **Evaluation**
         a. The **history** should include questions about previous static or progressive neurologic or developmental dysfunction, symptoms of an infectious illness, or a history of headaches, early-morning vomiting, or visual alterations.
            (1) Precise details of the seizure, particularly observing the initial components of the seizures and deviations of the eyes and head, are important. The postictal assessment for eye position or weakness is also useful. The duration of the postictal state should be noted.
            (2) Absence of a return to baseline within 1 hour suggests either ongoing seizures or a response to administered medications, or is due to the underlying disease or a supervening problem.
            (3) A **family history** of febrile and nonfebrile seizures should be noted.
         b. **Physical examination.** A thorough neurologic examination should be performed, with particular attention to evaluation of mental status and

the fundi and a search for focal or lateralized signs. The general examination is relevant in particular to meningeal signs, trauma, and diseases of other body systems.

c. **Specific laboratory assessments** to include serum and CSF evaluation will depend on the clues to the cause provided by the history and physical findings.

   (1) An **awake and asleep EEG** should be done in all patients with seizures. An EEG is particularly useful for confirming the presence of paroxysmal discharges and in helping identify the possible focality of a discharge and space-occupying lesions, helping choose appropriate anticonvulsant medication, and helping determine when anticonvulsants should be discontinued. On occasion an EEG performed soon after a seizure will show only background slowing, which, if repeated after 7–10 days, will then demonstrate epileptiform activity.

   (2) A **cranial MRI scan** should be performed in patients with partial seizures, with otherwise unexplained loss of seizure control, with focal or lateralized abnormalities found on the neurologic examination, with focally abnormal EEGs, or with known or suspected specific white or gray matter neurologic diseases. A cranial CT scan is useful as a screen to identify cerebral calcifications associated with tuberous sclerosis, congenital infections, arteriovenous malformations, or cysticercosis. A CT scan is generally not indicated for patients with well-controlled primary generalized (grand mal) or pure absence (petit mal) seizures in whom the neurologic findings are normal.

d. The **differential diagnoses** include syncope, breath-holding spells (both may be followed by a brief, clonic seizure), decerebration, narcolepsy, complicated migraine, benign paroxysmal vertigo, and hysteria (pseudoseizures).

3. **Diagnosis**

a. **Grand mal (primary generalized, tonic-clonic)** seizures usually start without an aura or focal features. Characteristically, there is a tonic phase, usually lasting less than a minute, often associated with rolling up of the eyes. During this phase there may be little air exchange because of tonic contraction of the respiratory musculature, resulting in cyanosis. The tonic phase is followed by clonic jerking of the extremities, usually lasting 1–5 minutes, with associated improved air exchange. Hypersalivation, tachycardia, and metabolic and respiratory acidosis may be present. There is usually a postictal state lasting less than 1 hour.

b. **Focal motor seizures (partial seizures with elementary symptomatology).** Characteristically, focal motor seizures start in the hand or face and are associated with head and eye deviation toward the hemisphere opposite the seizure focus. They may start restricted to that area, without loss of consciousness, or they may generalize and quickly and phenotypically resemble grand mal seizures (secondary generalized, tonic-clonic seizures). Following the seizures, a Todd's paralysis or eye and head deviation **toward** the previously discharging hemisphere may be a clue to the focality.

c. **Temporal lobe or psychomotor seizures (partial seizures with complex symptomatology)** are preceded by an aura (e.g., emotional feelings, abdominal or head pain, feeling in the throat) about 50 percent of the time. These seizures may mimic other seizure types during various ictal episodes. Focal, motor, grand mal, or staring seizures may be present; at other times the seizures will appear more complex, with stereotyped, automatic behaviors, including, for example, running, lip smacking, laughing, and unusual movements of the face or hand. In general, there is a postictal state with full or partial amnesia for the seizure.

d. **Petit mal (primary generalized, absence seizures)** begin in childhood, usually occur after 3 years of age, and are characterized by staring with or without eyelid fluttering or head-nodding movements. The seizures are not preceded by an aura or followed by a postictal state and usually last for less than 30 seconds. They may occur many times a day and may be provoked by hyperventilation or stroboscopic lights. The associated EEG is specifically a 3-second spike-and-wave abnormality. It is important to differentiate these seizures from partial complex seizures because of implications of anticonvulsant treatment, causation, and prognosis. Occasional grand mal seizures occur in 10–20 percent of patients with typical petit mal seizures. By puberty the majority (75%) of patients no longer has seizures and has a normal EEG.

e. **Infantile spasms with hypsarrhythmic EEG.** Infantile spasms begin most often in the first year of life and are characterized by large myoclonic (salaam) spasms. This syndrome may occur as a consequence of various neurologic diseases or may arise without known antecedent problems. Development usually slows with the onset of spasms, and there is a high incidence of subsequent retardation, particularly among patients with antecedent neurologic disease.

f. **Mixed generalized seizures (atypical petit mal, petit mal variant, minor motor seizures).** This group of seizure disorders is typified by patients with Lennox-Gastaut syndrome, which is characterized by frequent, difficultly controlled seizures to include atonic, myoclonic (sudden muscle jerks), tonic and clonic seizures associated with an EEG pattern of atypical spike and waves (less than 3 per second spike and waves), multifocal spikes, and polyspikes. The age of onset is usually between 18 months and 5 years, and often follows infantile spasms. Patients often have developmental delay.

g. **Febrile seizures** occur between 6 months and 5 years of age in the context of fever, usually above 38.5°C (101.5°F), and most often as the temperature rises or at its peak. The seizures are usually phenotypically grand mal, although they may be tonic, atonic (limp), or clonic.

   (1) They are considered to be simple if they are single and last less than 15 minutes, and if no focal features are present during or following the fit. Implicit to the definition is an absence both of metabolic disarray and of nervous system infection. An EEG is unnecessary unless seizures are recurrent with atypical features (low-grade fever, complex seizure, abnormal examination).

   (2) Complex febrile seizures are multiple, prolonged, or focal.

   (3) All febrile patients with a first seizure *under 18 months* or *over 3 years* of age require **lumbar puncture** and a **metabolic screen,** as does any patient with complex febrile seizures, altered mental status, neurologic signs, meningeal signs, or uncertain follow-up.

   (4) **Risk factors** for subsequent development of epilepsy include:
      (a) Antecedent abnormal neurologic or developmental status
      (b) A family history of afebrile seizures
      (c) Complex febrile seizures

   (5) The presence of a single or no risk factor is associated with a less than 2 percent chance of the development of afebrile seizures. This contrasts with an approximately 6–10 percent occurrence with two or three risk factors. Further, each feature of seizure complexity (length > 15 minutes, multiple or focal) increases the risk of developing subsequent epilepsy. The presence of all three complex features is associated with near 50 percent risk of subsequent epilepsy.

4. **Therapy.** See also Table 19-3.
   a. **General principles**
      (1) **Acute seizure management. For management of status epilepticus,** see Chap. 3, p. 66ff.
      (2) **Acute seizure management: after the seizure**
         (a) **A history** and **physical examination** are required and will often help direct further course of therapy, depending on the cause.

Table 19-3. Drugs used for treatment of seizure disorders

Anticonvulsant	Half-life (hr)	Dosage (mg/kg/day)	Time/ day	Approx. thera- peutic range (μg/ml)	Common side effects
Phenytoin (Dilantin)	24–50	5 (5–12)[a]	bid	10–20 (5–10)[b]	Rash, hirsutism, gingival hyperplasia, hypertrichosis
Phenobarbital or mephobarbital (Mebaral)	60–92	3–5 (5–18)	qd	10–45	Lethargy, hyperactivity
Primidone (Mysoline)	6–14	5–25	tid	5–10	Lethargy, irritability
Carbamazepine (Tegretol)[c]	9–15	15–30	bid–tid	3–11	Lethargy, blurry vision, granulocytopenia
Ethosuximide (Zarontin)	20–60	20–30	bid	40–120	Nausea, hiccups
Valproic acid[c] (Depakene)	8–15	25–60	bid–tid	50–120	GI discomfort, tremor, alopecia
Clonazepam (Clonopin)	24–48	0.02–0.2	bid–tid	10–60	Lethargy, ataxia, hypersalivation

[a] Phenytoin is very poorly absorbed and/or has a very short half-life in the neonatal period; this problem gradually improves through the first years of life. [b] Depakene has interactions with phenytoin and phenobarbital. Total phenytoin will be reduced by approximately one-half and free phenytoin will be doubled. Thus, dosages of phenytoin should not be altered, and the therapeutic range should be considered to be between 5–10 μg/ml. Free Dilantin level (therapeutic: 1–2 μg/ml). Depakene also tends to increase phenobarbital levels. [c] Requires weekly CBC and liver functions for 2 weeks, then monthly for 3 months, then every 3–6 months.

    (i) In patients with probable febrile seizures, the treatment should be directed at the fever.

    (ii) The patient with serious head trauma or evidence of increased ICP and herniation may require mannitol, an immediate CT or MRI scan, and possible neurosurgical intervention.

    (iii) The febrile patient with meningeal signs will require lumbar puncture and antibiotic treatment.

    (iv) The patient with continued stupor or coma will require consideration of diseases such as Reye syndrome, metabolic disorders, or toxic ingestion.

  (b) A choice and mode of administration of anticonvulsant treatment should depend on:

    (i) The need for preservation of an optimal state of consciousness (meningitis, Reye syndrome, head injury, ingestion, stupor or coma of unknown cause). Phenytoin would be the drug of choice in such a circumstance.

    (ii) Seizure type (Table 19-4)

    (iii) Anticonvulsants that the patient is already taking (check MedicAlert tag)

    (iv) Urgency for need to control seizures (increased ICP and respiratory compromise would require IV administration of either lorazepam or diazepam; see Chap. 3, p. 67).

    (v) Recognize allergies (check the patient MedicAlert tag).

(3) Chronic management

    (a) The choice of anticonvulsant should be based on clinical and EEG assessment of the seizure type, with consideration of benefit-risk ratio of the drug.

    (b) A single drug at therapeutic level is more likely to be effective and cause fewer adverse reactions than multiple drugs at subtherapeutic levels.

Table 19-4. Anticonvulsant choice by seizure type

Seizure type	Principal drug of choice	Second-line or adjunctive drugs
Primary generalized (grand mal) seizures	Phenobarbital, mephobarbital (Mebaral) Phenytoin (Dilantin) Carbamazepine (Tegretol)	Valproic acid Acetazolamide (Diamox)
Partial elementary seizures (focal)	Phenobarbital Phenytoin Carbamazepine Primidone (Mysoline)	Valproic acid Methsuximide
Partial complex seizures (temporal lobe epilepsy)	Carbamazepine Phenytoin Primidone	Phenobarbital Valproic acid Acetazolamide Methsuximide
Primary generalized (petit mal, absence) seizures	Ethosuximide (Zarontin) Valproic acid (Depakene) Methsuximide (Celontin)	Acetazolamide Clonazepam (Clonopin) Phenobarbital
Infantile spasms	ACTH Valproic acid Clonazepam	Phenytoin Phenobarbital Acetazolamide
Febrile seizures	Phenobarbital	Valproic acid
Mixed generalized seizures	Phenobarbital Valproic acid Clonazepam	Acetazolamide Diazepam Ethosuximide Phenytoin ACTH Clorazepate (Tranxene) Lorazepam Methsuximide Carbamazepine Triple bromides Ketogenic diet
Neonatal seizures	Phenobarbital Phenytoin	Paraldehyde Valproic acid

ACTH = adrenocorticotropic hormone.

(c) The most effective level of the appropriate drug is established by increasing the dose until seizures are controlled, side effects are sustained, or the maximum therapeutic level is exceeded.

(d) It is often helpful to obtain peak (2–3 hr postdose) and trough (predose) blood levels in order to ascertain adequacy of levels throughout the day, establish frequency of dosing that may be required, and help in determining the utility of giving larger doses at certain times (such as hour of sleep to cover early-morning hours better).

(e) To alter anticonvulsant regimens, modify one drug at a time, allowing for reequilibration to the new level, which will depend on the drug's half-life. Reequilibration will usually require approximately five half-lives. Giving loading doses will substantially reduce the time to equilibration, but may cause greater number and degree of side effects.

(f) When substituting a new anticonvulsant for another, it is prudent to add the new anticonvulsant first and attain therapeutic levels before tapering away the previous medication.

(g) Discontinuation of an anticonvulsant, especially phenobarbital, carbamazepine (Tegretol), and the diazepines, should be done slowly, usually over a period of 1 to 6 months.

(h) When possible, tablets or capsules should be used in preference to liquid formulations. This is more likely to ensure uniformity of dosage. Most tablets can be crushed and mixed with food if necessary.

(i) In general, anticonvulsants can be discontinued when the patient has had no seizures for 2 years and has nonparoxysmal waking and sleeping EEGs. After 2 years of complete seizure control, a paroxysmal or epileptiform EEG predicts a recurrent incidence of approximately 50 percent; a nonparoxysmal/nonepileptiform EEG is associated with a 5–10 percent recurrence rate, usually within 6 months of discontinuation of medication.

(j) Patients with febrile seizures generally do not require prophylactic treatment unless seizures are frequent or are recurrently life threatening (status epilepticus). When phenobarbital is used, it should be continued for 1 year or until 3 years of age, after which the incidence of febrile seizures declines (see **3.g** for indications). Serum levels of at least 15 μg/ml are required for effective prophylaxis.

b. Specific anticonvulsant therapy (see Table 19-3)

(1) Phenobarbital

(a) The long half-life permits once-a-day dosing, usually best given at hour of sleep.

(b) It promotes hyperactivity/ADD in some children.

(c) Drug interactions

(i) Predictably reduces the *Tegretol* level when given concomitantly

(ii) Level will increase when *valproate* is added as a second drug

(d) Data related to reduced (3–6 pts) IQ scores in children treated with phenobarbital are controversial and inconclusive. (Any decisions to use pharmacologic interventions must always be based on an analysis of benefit-risk ratio.)

(2) Valproate (VPA)

(a) The relative short half-life requires tid/qid dosing.

(b) Valproate has been associated with liver necrosis in over 50 instances; the risk for this is enhanced under the age of 2, in the setting of multiple anticonvulsant medication use, and possibly by deficient baseline serum carnitine values. Bone marrow suppression may also occur.

    (c) Baseline ALT, ammonia, carnitine, and CBC values should be obtained and repeated frequently initially (weekly).

    (d) Serum ammonia is frequently mildly elevated in patients who are taking VPA; this should be a concern if ammonia values persistently climb or are associated with elevated liver function tests (ALT).

    (e) Concomitant administration of carnitine (Carnitor) increases serum carnitine values, limits ammonia elevations, and may reduce the likelihood of developing liver complications. Recommended Carnitor doses when baseline carnitine values are low when used in children under 2 years old, or when ammonia is elevated are 50–100 mg/kg/day (usually 75 mg/kg) as bid dosing.

    (f) Drug interactions

        (i) Serum *phenobarbital*, if given concomitantly, will increase 10–25 percent.

        (ii) *Valproate* will double the *free Dilantin* (usually 10% of total Dilantin), but drop the *total Dilantin* value by half; thus, generally Dilantin doses do not have to be altered, and therapeutic range is approximately 6–12 μg/ml. More accurate monitoring of Dilantin is achieved by obtaining free Dilantin levels (therapeutic: 1–2 μg/ml)

        (iii) Use with *clonazepam* will occasionally provoke an episode of status epilepticus.

  (3) Carbamazepine

    (a) The relative short half-life requires bid/tid/qid dosing.

    (b) The risk of irreversible hepatic necrosis or bone marrow suppression is minimal (on the order of 1/100,000); reversible dose-responsive or transient granulocytopenia is more common.

    (c) Drug interaction

        (i) *Tegretol* levels tend to drop in the face of most other anticonvulsants.

        (ii) Concomitant use of *erythromycin* will predictably markedly increase the serum Tegretol value, often prompting symptoms of toxicity.

    (d) Nongeneric formulary is preferred.

  (4) Diphenylhydantoin (Dilantin, phenytoin)

    (a) The half-life requires bid/tid dosing.

    (b) Use of Dilantin in the first few years of life leads to erratic and low serum levels at usual maintenance doses (see **B**).

    (c) Drug interactions

        (i) Valproate (see above)

        (ii) Tegretol (see above)

    (d) Nongeneric formulary is preferred.

B. Neonatal seizures

  1. Etiology. The causes can be categorized in the following manner:

    a. Metabolic. Hypoglycemia, hypocalcemia, hypomagnesemia, hyponatremia and hypoxemia

    b. Toxic. Maternal drug ingestion (withdrawal), inadvertent local anesthetic poisoning

    c. Hemorrhagic. Intraventricular, subdural, and subarachnoid hemorrhage

    d. Infectious. Bacterial, viral (TORCH)

    e. Effects resulting from inborn errors of metabolism. Organic acidemias, errors of amino acid metabolism, pyridoxine dependency, etc.

    f. Effects of asphyxia (hypoxia, ischemia). We specifically avoid the term *hypoxic-ischemic encephalopathy,* preferring to use the term **neonatal encephalopathy,** unless there is very clear and direct evidence of prenatal ischemia or postnatal hypoxia or ischemia, or both. Hypoxic-ischemic encephalopathy should never be a diagnosis of exclusion. Furthermore, even clear or direct evidence of compromised oxygen delivery to the fetu or the neonate does not preclude the presence of an underlying neurologic disorder that may have predisposed the fetus/neonate to the subsequent hypoxic or ischemic disturbance. Criteria traditionally used to identify past hypoxic-ischemic events, including abnormal fetal heart rate patterns, low Apgar scores, jitteriness, lethargy, and seizures, are not specific for hypoxic-ischemic events. Rather, hypoxic-ischemic events are an infrequent cause of any of these signs, and the vast majority of babies with these signs does **not** have long-term repercussions. **Continued presumptive use of the term *hypoxic-ischemic encephalopathy* impedes further search for other or underlying etiologies and tends to implicate the perinatal period as the time frame for the insult, with little or no firm substantiation.**

    g. Cerebral dysgenesis

    h. Benign familial seizures

2. **Evaluation**

    a. A full **perinatal history** and **neonatal examination** will help differentiate the causes.

    b. **Laboratory assessments** that are helpful include serum evaluation of blood sugar (Dextrostix), calcium, magnesium, sodium, CBC and cultures, and a toxic screen. A CSF examination, EEG with pyridoxine infusion, cranial ultrasound, and/or cranial CT scan are frequently important for diagnostic, therapeutic, or prognostic purposes.

3. **Diagnosis.** Seizures may be tonic, focal clonic, multifocal clonic, myoclonic, or, most commonly, subtle, which includes eye deviation, nystagmus, apnea, sucking movements, tongue thrusting, and bicycling and swimming movements. Spontaneous clonus and jitteriness should be differentiated from seizures.

4. **Therapy**

    a. As with older children with status epilepticus, attention must first be directed at **vital signs.**

    b. Therapy should subsequently be directed at the cause, in particular, when a metabolic factor such as hypoglycemia is recognized.

    c. Anticonvulsant therapy is required when glucose and pyridoxine administration (50–100 mg IV) is unsuccessful, or when the possibility of such a deficiency has been excluded.

    d. The cornerstone of therapy is **phenobarbital;** the patient can receive a loading dose of phenobarbital at 10–20 mg/kg administered over 5–10 minutes. **Phenytoin** can be used as a second drug at a loading dose of 20 mg/kg, and phenobarbital can be readministered at 10 mg/kg at hourly intervals for two further doses, if necessary, for ongoing seizures. After loading with phenobarbital and phenytoin, rectal **paraldehyde** is the next drug of choice. Rectal **valproate** is used on rare occasions.

    e. The **maintenance dose** of phenobarbital is 4–5 mg/kg/day in either once- or twice-a-day aliquots. Maintenance doses for **IV phenytoin** are 5–8 mg/kg/day, usually administered bid.

    f. Phenobarbital is well absorbed orally. Phenytoin, however, is very poorly absorbed orally and/or has an exceedingly short half-life in the first months of life and should, in general, be avoided if possible.

    g. Doses of phenytoin exceeding 10 mg/kg/day are occasionally necessary to maintain therapeutic serum levels when phenytoin must be maintained.

    h. Anticonvulsants can be discontinued at the time of discharge or at 3 months if the patient is no longer having clinical seizures, the EEG is not paroxysmal, and the neurologic findings are normal. Anticonvulsant levels should be monitored at the time of recurrent seizures, when side effects develop, and 3–4 weeks subsequent to an alteration of the maintenance dosage.

C. **Migraine headache.** The majority of childhood headaches not associated with acute illness is migrainous. Migraine occurs in 5 percent of children.

    1. **Etiology.** The neurologic symptoms associated with migraine are considered

to be a function of cerebrovascular constriction, leading to diminished cerebral blood flow to specific brain areas. The pain is thought to occur because of vasodilation, leading to stretching of intramural nerves.

2. **Evaluation and diagnosis.** Migraine headaches are typically periodic. They can be conveniently divided into classic (hemicranial, throbbing, and preceded by an aura), complicated (classic and a neurologic deficit), or common (no aura, generalized or bilateral head pain). Rarely, vomiting alone or abdominal pain alone is the only symptom of a migraine attack. Cyclic vomiting can be viewed as a form of migraine equivalent.

   a. **History and physical examination.** The diagnosis of migraine headache rests on identifying the intermittency of the headache. The majority of children has associated nausea and vomiting, photophobia, and sonophobia. Auras may include visual scotoma or scintillations, vertigo, malaise with associated pallor, perioral numbness, or alterations of perception. Neurologic findings may include confusional state, aphasia, brainstem signs, ataxia, hemiparesis, hemisensory loss, and loss of consciousness. In 90 percent of the children, a family member will have migraine, and many children will suffer from motion sickness.

   Headache is a symptom complex that may be provoked by many factors. Factors that may alert the clinician to a more serious illness include headaches that frequently occur during sleep, more often occur in the morning on waking, always occur on the same side of the head, often are associated with vomiting, and are associated with seizures. A focal or lateralized neurologic abnormality interictally, asymmetric cranial bruits, or evidence of elevated ICP at any time are also cause for concern and further evaluation. Such evaluation may include an EEG, cranial CT scan, and, occasionally, angiography. Headaches that persist day in and day out for long periods, particularly when also associated with substantial school absence, are often related to variable combinations of muscle tension, psychological-emotional issues, and conscious or subconscious secondary gain.

   b. **Laboratory evaluation.** The history and physical findings will determine which tests are necessary. The aim of the tests will be to rule out other causes of headache, which, of course, will depend on the clinical setting.

3. **Therapy.** The approach to treatment of migraine headache will depend on headache frequency, the degree of disability, and age. A diary may help identify provoking factors, such as certain foods, certain activities, or certain environmental variables.

   a. **Migraine-provoking agents,** such as chocolates, cheeses, nitrite-containing foods (processed meats), and MSG-containing foods, should be eliminated if they appear associated with headaches.

   b. **Other complicating factors,** such as emotional stress and withdrawal from chronic intake of caffeinated beverages, should also be evaluated.

   c. **Pharmacologic treatment** may be either symptomatic (Table 19-5) or prophylactic (Table 19-6). **Prophylaxis** is considered when the frequency is greater than once per week, leading to school absence; when such headaches are unresponsive to symptomatic treatment; or when side effects of the acutely administered medications lead to a similar or worse disability. Calcium-channel blockers have been used successfully as prophylaxis in adults and may be useful in children as well. Occasionally, prophylaxis with propranolol or ibuprofen can be used just before specific times when such activities are known to provoke migraine attacks (e.g., just before strenuous activity such as a soccer match).

   d. **Nonpharmacologic treatment.** Biofeedback and relaxation techniques have been useful in patients with common migraine or muscle tension–based headaches, and in those in whom emotional issues and anxiety provoke migraine attacks.

VIII. **Human immunodeficiency virus (HIV)-associated neurologic disease** (see Chaps. 14 and 16)

Table 19-5. Symptomatic treatment of migraine headache

Drug	Dosage and route of administration	Age 3–10 years	Age 11 years and older
Aspirin	Usual analgesic dosages PO or PR	Preferred	Preferred
Acetaminophen	Usual analgesic dosages PO or PR	Preferred	Preferred
Ibuprofen	Usual analgesic dosage PO	Preferred	Preferred
Fiorinal/Esgic (butalbital, 50 mg; caffeine, 40 mg; aspirin, 325 mg/acetaminophen, 300 mg)	Under 5 yr, ½ tablet; over 5, 1 tablet; age 11 yr and older, 1–2 tablets	Not preferred	
Ergotamine[a] tartrate (Ergomar)	2 mg, sublingual	Not preferred	Preferred
Cafergot[b] (ergotamine tartrate, 1.8 mg; caffeine, 100 mg)	PO: 1–2 tablets at onset of headache; 1 tablet q ½h to maximum of 4 PR: ½–1 suppository at onset; ½ tablet q½h to maximum of 2	Not preferred	Preferred
Midrin (isometheptene, 65 mg; acetaminophen, 325 mg/dichloralphenazone, 100 mg)	1–2 capsules immediately if needed, then repeat 1/hr to a maximum of 3/day (or 5/week)	Not preferred	Preferred

[a] Medication should not be used in renal or hepatic failure, hypertension, or with complicated migraine, and should be limited to 3 in 24 hr and 5 in 1 week. [b] Not to be taken with complicated migraine. Give no more than 6 PO tablets or 2 PR tablets in 24 hr. Limit to 8 PO tablets or 4 suppositories/week.

A. HIV has important direct effects on the nervous system. Acquired immunodeficiency syndrome (AIDS) should be viewed as the modern era's great imitator of other neurologic diseases.
B. **Clinical presentations**
   1. **Stroke/infarct.** This presentation may occur related to in utero cocaine exposure, thrombocytopenia due to an immune-mediated disorder, and arteriovenous inflammation related to an opportunistic infection such as *Aspergillus* or *Candida*.
   2. **Space-occupying mass.** This may occur related to hemorrhage from thrombocytopenia, infection from toxoplasmosis or other etiologies of cerebral abscess (e.g., fungal), and, much less likely, primary CNS tumor such as lymphoma, which occurs more commonly in the adult population.
   3. **Developmental delay.** This may occur as a result of congenital infection (e.g., cytomegalovirus [CMV]), prenatal influences of drugs to include cocaine and

Table 19-6. Prophylactic treatment of migraine headache

Drug	Dosage and route of administration	Age 3–10 years	Age 11 years and older
Phenobarbital	3–5 mg/kg/day qhs PO	Preferred	Not preferred
Phenytoin (Dilantin)	5 mg/kg/day bid PO	Preferred	Less commonly used or less effective than others
Propranolol[a] (Inderal)	(1) 0.5–3.0 mg/kg/day tid or qid (or bid for LA preparation)	Less commonly used or less effective than others	Preferred
Amitriptyline	0.2–0.5 mg/kg/day (in qhs dosages) PO	Not preferred	Preferred
Cyproheptadine	0.25 mg/kg/day bid/tid PO	Preferred	Preferred
Verapamil	40–80mg PO bid/tid	Not preferred	Preferred
Methysergide[b] (Sansert)	2 mg qd PO	Not preferred	Less commonly used or less effective than others
Biofeedback behavioral modification		Preferred	Preferred

[a] Not to be given to patients with asthma, sinus bradycardia with first-degree block, or congestive heart failure.
[b] May cause retroperitoneal fibrosis and vascular insufficiency. It is to be given only for brief periods (less than 5 months) in adolescence.

alcohol, malnourishment, neglect, and other socioeconomic factors. HIV may also directly affect the nervous system and continue to such a presentation.
4. **Degenerative disease.** This presentation most commonly occurs as a result of direct HIV infection, although opportunistic infections, cerebral tumors, and hydrocephalus may present similarly. Most often, the presentation is indolent with increasing apathy, failing academic work or loss of previously attained milestones, reduced language output, and social withdrawal. Gradually, the head circumference drops across percentiles, at times into the range of microcephaly, and motor tone first decreases and subsequently increases, usually starting in the lower extremities. The presentation can also occur subacutely evolving over weeks to months and more rarely acutely or catastrophically over hours to days or weeks.
5. **Epilepsy.** Seizures may occur as a result of opportunistic infections, tumors, infarcts, cerebral hemorrhage, and occasionally the HIV infection. HIV-caused seizures usually occur late in the course of the neurologic disease.
6. **Cerebral palsy.** Spasticity and dystonia may occur as a result of the same causes of the epilepsy syndrome noted above. When spasticity evolves in the first year or two of life, it may be difficult to know whether the findings are static and not related directly to HIV. Usually, diminished tone is followed by evolving spasticity starting in the lower extremities and subsequently the upper extremities. The neurologic findings are usually symmetric, and marked asymmetry should prompt a search for other treatable causes of increasing tone, such as an opportunistic infection.

7. **Acute cerebellar ataxia.** This may occur as a result of the HIV or can be a side effect of medication used to treat HIV, such as dideoxycytidine (DDC).
8. **Neuropathy/myopathy.** More often seen in adults with HIV but may also be caused by HIV treatment (e.g., DDC, dideoxyinosine)
9. **Myelopathy.** Vacuolar degeneration of the spinal cord has been reported in adults, but not in children to date.
C. **Diagnosis** (see Chaps. 6 and 14). Cerebrocortical and basal ganglia calcification and sulcal and ventricular widening suggestive of cerebral atrophy seen on **cranial CT** scan are consistent with the diagnosis of HIV. In addition to the CT scan, **cranial MRI** testing may be helpful in evaluating the cerebrum for evidence of infarct, hemorrhage, infection, and tumors when the CT scan is equivocal or abnormal.
D. **Therapy** (see Chap. 14)

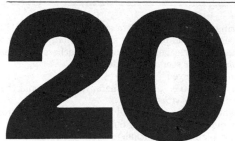

Behavior

David R. DeMaso and
Leonard A. Rappaport

I. Developmental problems
A. Poor school performance
1. The **etiology** includes the following:
   a. Physical disabilities and illness
   b. Developmental disability (overall developmental delay may not be recognized until school demands exceed abilities), neurodevelopmental dysfunction (dyslexia, attention deficit disorder, and learning disability)
   c. Emotional disorders, including individual or family problems and environmental deprivation
   d. Confounding factors, including poor school or class environment, unrealistic parental expectations, and excessive absences
2. **Evaluation and diagnosis**
   a. A full **history** by interview and supplemented by questionnaires (i.e., Connors, Anser system) should be obtained from the parents. It should include a description of the following:
      (1) Gestational and perinatal history
      (2) Developmental milestones
      (3) Description of early temperament
      (4) First hints of difficulties in functional areas
      (5) First school experience and subsequent experience
      (6) Functioning at home and in neighborhood
      (7) Medical problems
      (8) Rate of deterioration of performance
      (9) Lapses of attention
   b. The **school history** should be obtained from the parents and the school, and should include descriptions of current placement, current functioning, and the results of previous evaluations.
   c. A complete **physical examination,** including vision and hearing screens, should be performed.
   d. Some or all of the following **evaluations** can be performed by the pediatrician, school, or consultant, depending on their areas of expertise:
      (1) Neurodevelopmental examination
      (2) Educational evaluation, including achievement tests
      (3) Psychological testing, including:
         (a) Cognitive testing with standardized tests (e.g., WISC-R, WAIS, McCarthy)
         (b) Projective testing
      (4) Psychiatric interview
      (5) **Classroom observation** of the child
3. **Treatment**
   a. All physical disabilities or illnesses should be treated appropriately.
   b. In conjunction with parents and school, an individualized educational plan should be formulated to meet the child's needs. The plan should **always** include:
      (1) Description of present functioning and objectives for intervention
      (2) Classroom placement—ranges along a continuum from regular class-

room monitoring (least restrictive) to special private schools (most restrictive). Description of placement should include time per week, student-teacher ratio, specialized training of teachers or specialists, and description of other students in setting.

(3) Curriculum to be employed

(4) Other special services (i.e., physical therapy, occupational therapy, speech and language services, etc.)

(5) An objective and timely means of evaluating the success of proposed interventions (questionnaires every 6 months or yearly)

(6) All intervention plans should include:

    (a) A plan for remediation of areas of academic weakness

    (b) A parallel plan to circumvent areas of academic weakness (e.g., dictating a portion of a written assignment for a child with significant fine-motor planning problems, making Talking Books available to children with learning disabilities to convey content while basic skills are learned)

    (c) Every child needs some area of success in order to sustain his or her self-concept. Parents should strongly encourage an area of expertise (i.e., athletics, music, art, a collection).

  c. Children with significant emotional or family problems should receive psychological intervention.

  d. Medication may be appropriate for certain children with attention/activity problems (see sec. **II.A.4.c**).

B. School refusal (school phobia)

  1. The **etiology** includes separation anxiety or fear of school, which may reflect real school problems, such as a "class bully," a difficult teacher, or difficulty with new school material. School refusal may be a partial manifestation of a more pervasive social withdrawal in all spheres (see sec. **III.B.2**).

  2. Evaluation and diagnosis

    a. A child who has vague physical complaints with normal physical and laboratory findings should prompt the physician to ask about school absences.

    b. The **history** should emphasize the following:

      (1) Earlier separation problems

      (2) Previous undefined illnesses with prolonged school absence

      (3) The temporal pattern of symptoms. Children with school refusal often have more symptoms on Sunday night and Monday morning than at other times. They often are without symptoms on holidays and weekends.

      (4) Specific school problems that might be contributing to absences

    c. The longer the sustained absence and the older the child, the more serious and urgent the problem.

    d. The child who is not at school and also not staying at home (i.e., on street) usually has a conduct disorder.

  3. Treatment

    a. Reassure the child and parents **after** the physical examination and necessary laboratory tests that the symptoms do not represent serious disease.

    b. Tell the family that anxiety can cause physical discomfort and acknowledge that the child is experiencing the symptom.

    c. Suggest that school is the child's **job** and that there are few excuses acceptable for absences.

    d. Prepare the parents for possible escalation of symptoms when attendance is first enforced.

    e. If the child is to be permitted to stay home for illness, the child should be seen that morning for an examination by the physician.

    f. Help the family organize a specific plan for getting the child to school. The process may be slow, and desensitization techniques such as shortened school days can be helpful.

g. Try to ease the child's way back into school by speaking to the principal or teacher, or both, about decreasing any complicating stresses during the first few days.

h. Many children can be helped by their pediatrician. If, however, problems persist, or it is determined that school avoidance represents a more general social withdrawal, the child should be referred for further psychiatric evaluation and treatment. Adolescents almost always need referral.

C. Pervasive developmental disorder (infantile autism)
1. **Etiology.** Most likely, it is an organic brain disorder.
2. **Evaluation**
   a. These children manifest a pervasive development disorder. Their lack of attachment behavior is marked, although some improvement may be seen by age 5. Useful speech may eventually be gained in 50 percent of the children.
   b. **Associated behaviors** include stereotyped movements, tantrums, overactivity, and extreme fears.
   c. Mental retardation is present in 75 percent of cases.
   d. Seizures and electroencephalographic (EEG) abnormalities are common.
   e. Phenylketonuria, congenital rubella, hypsarrhythmia, and fragile X syndrome have been associated.
3. The **diagnosis** includes:
   a. Impaired social relationships manifested by lack of eye-to-eye gaze, discriminating people, cuddling, or smiling
   b. Impaired verbal and nonverbal communication, and imaginative activity, e.g., decreased comprehension, echolalia, and pronominal reversal
   c. Ritualistic phenomena with "an insistence on sameness"
   d. Onset usually before 30 months
4. **Treatment**
   a. A developmental-educational-psychological assessment of the child and the family is indicated. Skilled special education is needed in a structured and supportive environment. This frequently should occur in a full-day treatment setting, and occasionally in a residential setting. Unmanageability or danger to the child or others is an indication for a residential setting.
   b. **Behavioral treatment** has been a useful adjunct for social responses, communication, self-abusive behavior, and so on.
   c. **Neuroleptics** (e.g., chlorpromazine) have been useful in agitation and management, but do not correct global impairment. These drugs may decrease the seizure threshold, resulting in a possible exacerbation of seizures.
   d. About 60 percent remain handicapped and unable to lead an independent life. Good social adjustment is found in 15 percent, although relationship problems continue, with the other 25 percent somewhere in between these extremes. An improved prognosis is found in those with a higher IQ and speech by age 5 years. Long-term support is needed from the pediatrician.

II. Disruptive behavior problems
A. Attention deficit hyperactivity disorder (ADHD)
1. **Etiology.** The cause is thought to be related to abnormalities in neurotransmitters (norepinephrine, dopamine), but the exact nature of these abnormalities remains elusive. The most salient characteristic of these children is inattention to appropriate stimuli. Some, but not all, of these children are hyperactive.
2. **Evaluation**
   a. Requires a full history and physical examination, including information **directly** from the school. Visual, hearing, educational, or neurodevelopmental testing is often needed.
   b. While hyperactivity is often the most predominant symptom, other important symptoms include impulsivity, distractibility, inattentiveness, poor selection of salient information, insatiability, and inconsistency.

   c. The differential diagnosis includes:
   (1) Sensory deficit (vision and hearing)
   (2) Auditory processing or receptive language deficit
   (3) "Secondary attention deficit" from specific area of learning disability
        (see sec. **I.A**)
   (4) Emotional stresses or disorders (i.e., depression, anxiety, neglect)
   (5) Seizures (petit mal or atypical seizures)
   (6) Sleep disorders (see sec. **IV.D**)
   (7) Age-appropriate overactivity (i.e., active, but not haphazard or poorly
        organized behavior)
   (8) Illicit drug use
   (9) Mental retardation
   d. Parent and teacher questionnaires are helpful in diagnosis and in
      measuring treatment responses (Connors, Anser, etc.)
3. **Diagnosis.** Essential diagnostic features are: developmentally inappropriate
   degrees of inattention, impulsiveness, and hyperactivity. Diagnosis must
   first exclude other identifiable causes, although ADHD may coexist with
   other problems.
4. **Therapy**
   a. **Educational remediation** (academic underachievement is common)
   b. **Counseling.** Cognitive therapy aimed at teaching these children ap-
      proaches to increasing attention span and decreasing distractibility and
      impulsivity has appeared beneficial. Behavior modification programs
      within the home and classroom have had varying success.
   c. **Medication**
      (1) **Stimulant medications** have been shown to be beneficial in approxi-
           mately 75 percent of the children. A medication trial is necessary to
           tell which children will respond.
      (2) The positive effects of medication are most marked on behavior; the
           effect on academic or social functioning is less clear.
      (3) Teachers are the best source of information concerning medication
           response (i.e., questionnaires, telephone contact).
      (4) Stimulant medications
           (a) Methylphenidate (Ritalin), 5-, 10-, and 20-mg tablets; 20-mg
                sustained-release tablets
           (b) Dextroamphetamine (Dexedrine) 5-mg tablets; 5-, 10-, and 15-mg
                spansules (sustained release)
           (c) Pemoline (Cylert), 18.75- and 37.5-mg tablets
           (d) Recent studies have suggested that children respond differently
                to the three stimulants, and all should be tried before treatment
                failure has been accepted. Ritalin is most commonly used, but
                Dexedrine has the advantage of more dosage flexibility since it
                has several long-acting spansule dosages. Cylert is a long-acting
                preparation only.
           (e) There are two basic approaches to therapy (with no clear research
                that supports one over the other).
                (i) **Low-dosage approach.** Begin trial of chosen medication at
                     low dose. Increase slowly (on weekly or biweekly basis) until
                     there is a positive response (close teacher feedback is neces-
                     sary). Stop at first dose with positive response. Stop if there is
                     no response before toxicity.
                (ii) **Increase dosage** to a toxic level, then back up one dose.
           (f) Reports have indicated that maximal learning may occur at a
                lower dosage than that which provides the best behavior. This
                favors the low-dosage approach, but data are still unclear.
           (g) **Side effects**
                (i) Insomnia and decreased appetite (usually transient)
                (ii) Decreased growth: Monitor growth curves.
                (iii) Increased tics. It is unclear whether stimulants cause

Tourette's syndrome or exacerbate the underlying disease. One should not use a stimulant if the child has multiple or complex (movements plus verbal utterances) tics.

    (iv) Abdominal pain

    (v) Psychosis—rare and almost always reverts with withdrawal of medication

  (5) Other medications used—antidepressants (imipramine, desipramine)—may have a positive response in specific targeted populations.

  (6) Long-term follow-up studies have not supported the efficacy of stimulant medication alone in the treatment of ADHD. Positive follow-up studies support multimodal therapy, which includes stimulant medication, educational remediation, and counseling together.

  d. Diet. There has been decreasing support of diet as a significant cause of hyperactivity. The National Institutes of Health (NIH) Consensus Report (1982) suggests that diet may help a very small subgroup of children with ADHD.

  e. Megavitamins, antihistamines, sucrose avoidance, yeast, etc. There is no proven role for these much-publicized therapies.

B. Conduct disorders

  1. Etiology. Problematic parent-child relationships and child-rearing practices of varying severity are involved in these cases.

  2. Evaluation

    a. The parents or outside agency (e.g., school) usually present complaints of lying, fighting, truancy, bullying, and/or legally defined delinquent acts such as stealing and fire setting. The behaviors, occurring more frequently in boys than in girls, are persistent, troublesome, and socially disapproved.

    b. Isolated delinquent acts **without** obvious social or school impairments are common and of little significance. Fire setting between the ages of 4 and 7 years may occur out of curiosity rather than pathology. An adolescent's oppositional behavior may reflect a move toward independence and may not violate major societal rules.

    c. Emotional disorders such as depression may be present, but can be overshadowed by the troublesome behavior.

    d. Learning disabilities are frequently associated, along with a history of temperament extremes.

    e. Comorbid ADHD is common.

  3. Diagnosis. These are conditions in which **repetitive, persistent** behaviors violate either the basic rights of others or major age-appropriate societal norms or rules (lasting at least 6 months).

  4. Treatment

    a. Prevention is important. Early prenatal education about the temperamentally difficult infant may be helpful. Counseling and advice should be offered around firm and consistent discipline techniques. Infant intervention programs or parent-effectiveness training groups may be available.

    b. Supervised recreational experiences, such as organized social clubs (e.g., Big Brothers or Sisters) and job placements, can be beneficial. A supportive relationship (i.e., caring and empathetic with firm age-appropriate limits) can be established with, for example, a physician, school counselor, or member of the clergy.

    c. Referral to a child psychiatrist is recommended for the child who is persistently out of control. Treatment is most helpful when the problems are responses to emotional difficulties.

    d. For the resistant child it may be necessary for the parents to go to the **juvenile court** to obtain court supervision via probation. Frequently, a psychiatric evaluation can be ordered.

    e. A **residential placement** may be needed, either when parents are unable to provide needed firm structure or when the child's behaviors are extreme.

    f. Assessment of a child's **social attachment** (e.g., has friendships in peer group for more than 6 months, extends to others with no immediate advantage, does not blame or inform on friends, and/or is concerned for the welfare of others) can be helpful in determining responses to intervention. Children with better attachments have a better prognosis.

C. Drug and alcohol abuse

  1. Etiology. Frequently, the substance abuser grows up in a family environment of inconsistency and rejection. The needs of the child are met erratically. Low self-worth, feelings of inferiority, and hostility are often present. Drugs are utilized to provide relief from this situation. There also may be unclear hereditary components along with contributing sociocultural factors (e.g., peer pressure).

  2. Evaluation

    a. A complete **drug and alcohol history** should be obtained, including types, amounts, and frequency. Include any evidence of physical tolerance or dependence.

    b. School performance is frequently poor, and conduct problems are common.

    c. A **family history** of substance use should be sought.

    d. Evidence of parental inconsistency and rejection may be obtained.

    e. In the drug-abusing child, the substance may be taken for pleasure rather than for curiosity. **Frequently, multiple drugs are used.**

  3. Diagnosis. A pattern of pathologic substance use that causes impairment in social or school functioning (for at least 1 month)

  4. Treatment. Once abuse is established, treatment is difficult and frustrating, with only modest success.

    a. Prevention by **early recognition** is important. Significant family or school problems are indications to pursue a family substance-abuse history. Early family counseling referral can be helpful to the young child.

    b. Efforts should be made to keep school a **positive learning experience,** which includes an evaluation for a learning disability.

    c. The goal is to establish a **supportive relationship** with a significant adult, such as a physician, school counselor, social worker, or member of the clergy. The substance abuser will be difficult to engage and may have frequent relapses. The relationship needs to be firm, consistent, and nonrejecting.

    d. Additionally, a **group treatment program,** such as Alcoholics Anonymous, may help to improve peer relationships. Referrals can be made to community outpatient and inpatient detoxification treatment programs.

III. Emotional disorders

  A. Eating disorders

    1. Anorexia nervosa

      a. Etiology. Anorexia nervosa is a symptom complex with different psychiatric diagnoses. It is an increasingly common disorder found in women of the higher and middle socioeconomic class (rarely men) between 10 and 30 years of age. The clinical course varies greatly and is often frustrating. Mortality ranging from 5–20 percent has been reported.

      b. Evaluation

        (1) Early symptoms

          (a) A self-imposed diet that gradually leads to drastic caloric reduction and marked weight loss

          (b) A preoccupation with food without loss of appetite

          (c) An intense fear of gaining weight and a distorted body image

        (2) Later findings

          (a) Feelings of incompetence and being out of control

          (b) Eating binges, self-induced vomiting, laxative or diuretic abuse, and/or excessive exercising

        (3) Before making the diagnosis, any physical illness that would account for the weight loss, such as inflammatory bowel disease or endocrine disorders, must be excluded. Psychiatric illnesses, such as schizophrenic disorders and depressive disorders, must be ruled out.

(4) **Physical manifestations** include hypothermia, hypotension, lanugo, and dependent edema. Both primary and secondary amenorrhea occur. Late findings include osteoporosis and growth retardation.

(5) **Laboratory findings** are normal until the later stages of malnutrition. Leukopenia, lymphocytosis, low erythrocyte sedimentation rate, and low fibrinogen levels then occur. Low serum lactic dehydrogenase estrogens and triiodothyronine (T_3) have been found, along with incomplete suppression of adrenocorticotropic hormone (ACTH) and cortisol levels by dexamethasone.

c. **Diagnosis** (adapted from *Diagnostic and Statistical Manual of Mental Disorders* [3rd ed.] [*DSM III-R*]. Washington, DC: American Psychiatric Association, 1987)

(1) Intense fear of becoming fat, which does not decrease as weight loss progresses

(2) Distortion of body image

(3) Refusal to maintain weight over a minimal normal weight for age and height

(4) Body weight is less than 85 percent of the mean weight for age on pediatric growth charts.

d. **Treatment**

(1) Before drastic weight loss, patients may respond to **encouragement, kindly firmness, and nutritional education.**

(2) If there is no response, **psychiatric consultation** is indicated. Management requires a collaboration between pediatrics and psychiatry.

(3) Outpatients should be seen medically at least once a week for **weight monitoring.** Encouragement and support, along with firm and unchanging weight expectations, are indicated.

(4) Although an outpatient program can be attempted and may succeed, **hospitalization** is often necessary. Indications include severe malnutrition, vital-sign instability, acute dehydration, electrolyte imbalance (e.g., hypokalemic alkalosis), and/or outpatient treatment failure.

(5) **Care during hospitalization** (adapted from The Children's Hospital Anorexia Nervosa and Assorted Eating Disorders Clinic)

(a) The standard protocol treats nutritional aspects and not associated family or personality problems.

(b) Psychiatric consultation is recommended in establishing both emotional and nutritional treatment programs.

(c) On admission, a weight range is calculated using the Frisch tables, giving minimum ideal body weight at which 10 percent of patients would be expected to regain menses. Add 10 lb to establish the range. (See R. E. Frisch et al., *Hum. Biol.* 45:469–483, 1973.)

(d) The patient is expected to gain 0.2 kg per day or 1.4 kg per week. Baseline actual weight will be taken on the morning following admission. Dehydrated patients' baseline weight will not be tabulated until 24 hours after admission.

(e) Patients may exceed, but may not drop below, daily expected weight gain (i.e., if patient gains 0.4 kg on one day, she does not have to gain another 0.2 kg over her previous high weight, but does need to achieve 1.4 kg for the week).

(f) Weight should be measured by staff each morning after voiding. Vital signs are taken each morning. Normal signs include temperature above 97°F, pulse above 60 mm Hg, and a systolic blood pressure of 80 or above.

(g) A regular house diet is ordered for the first 24 hours.

(h) A nutritional consult should be ordered immediately to determine preadmission caloric intake and intake necessary to gain 1.4 kg per week. Using calculated caloric intake for weight gain, a selected diet is then ordered.

(i) If vital signs are low, the patient is placed on bed rest; if all signs are normal after 4 hours, then room rest; if normal after another 4 hours, then ad lib activity on the floor is allowed. When signs are stable for 48 hours, outside or vigorous activity can be permitted as long as expected weight gain is met.

(j) Liquid food supplements are started if weight is below the expected weight for that day. Begin with 500 calories of Ensure or Sustacal taken under supervision between meals (midmorning, midafternoon, midevening). They are given by nasogastric tube if not taken orally within 15 minutes. These must be regarded as medicines, the taking of which is nonnegotiable and not a replacement for meals or minimum daily fluid intake. They should be increased by one can each day if weight goal is not met, up to a maximum of eight cans per day. Bed rest is enforced for 1 hour after the supplement is received.

(k) If a patient requires an intravenous line, it should not be removed until the patient is taking 32 oz fluids plus supplement orally.

(l) Vomiting or laxative abuse should be monitored by periodic electrolyte determinations. If necessary, making the bathroom inaccessible for 2 hours after meals may help to control vomiting.

(m) Constipation is relieved by eating, although stool softeners may be needed.

(n) Neuroleptics and tricyclic antidepressants have been used with limited success.

(o) Before discharge, assess the patient's readiness to assume free-choice eating versus a need for a prescribed diet.

(p) Individual psychotherapy or family therapy, or both, are indicated both during and after discharge. Group therapy is being used increasingly.

2. **Bulimia nervosa**
   a. **The etiology** is not known. Both psychological and organic theories have been proposed.
   b. **Evaluation**
      (1) This disorder occurs predominantly in late adolescence, with a chronic and intermittent course over years. It is seldom incapacitating. Binges are usually planned and done secretly. Most of the patients weigh within a normal range.
      (2) **Anorexia nervosa**, epileptic equivalent seizures, central nervous system (CNS) tumors, Klüver-Bucy–like syndromes, and Kleine-Levin syndrome must be excluded.
   c. **Diagnosis** (adapted from *DSM III-R*)
      (1) Recurrent episodes of rapid consumption of a large amount of food, usually over a 2-hour period
      (2) Awareness that the eating pattern is abnormal and fear of not being able to stop voluntarily
      (3) Regularly engages in either self-induced vomiting, use of laxatives/diuretics, strict dieting, or exercise to prevent weight gain
      (4) Minimum average of two episodes a week for at least 3 months
      (5) Persistent overconcern with body shape and weight
   d. **Treatment**
      (1) **Psychotherapy** and **behavioral treatment** may be used with some success. Psychiatric consultation is recommended.
      (2) **Dehydration** and **electrolyte imbalance** (hypokalemia) secondary to the vomiting, cathartics, or diuretics may need correction.
      (3) **Tricyclic antidepressants** are being given clinical trials.

3. Obesity
   a. Etiology. Social, emotional, learning, genetic, and physical activity factors and/or fat cell size and number have been implicated.
   b. Evaluation
      (1) Childhood-onset obesity tends to be severe, with onset more likely at 0–4 and 7–11 years.
      (2) Obesity **need not** denote a psychiatric disturbance. However, it is often associated with emotional disorders (often, a body image disturbance). There is no specific personality type.
      (3) Weight gain secondary to craniopharyngioma, pituitary tumor, Prader-Willi syndrome, Laurence-Moon-Biedl syndrome, ovarian dysfunction, and Cushing syndrome must be excluded.
   c. Diagnosis. *Obesity* is a marked increase in body fat, resulting in a weight more than 20 percent above mean weight for age on pediatric growth charts.
   d. Treatment
      (1) The **prognosis** for sustained weight loss is poor. Prevention via early recognition and nutritional advice is important. Inappropriate use of food to calm a child's discomfort should be discouraged.
      (2) Successful treatment requires high motivation and **family involvement.** Important components include a balanced low-calorie diet and increased physical activity. Though not ideal, behavioral treatment programs involving positive reinforcement for stepwise weight reduction have been the most effective.
      (3) **Group support,** such as Weight Watchers, may be helpful.
      (4) Individual **psychiatric treatment** may be needed.
4. Pica
   a. Etiology. A specific nutritional deficit and/or unmet needs from the parental relationship are postulated
   b. Evaluation
      (1) Pica occurs most frequently between the ages of 18 months and 5 years. The normal infant hand-to-mouth reactions are not included. Ingestion ranges from paint to hair to dirt, with no aversion to food.
      (2) Developmental disability, mineral deficiencies such as iron deficiency, child neglect, poor parent-child relationships, infantile autism, and schizophrenic disorders may be associated.
      (3) Complications depend on the material ingested and include lead poisoning, alopecia, intestinal parasites, and intestinal obstruction (e.g., trichobezoar).
   c. Diagnosis requires evidence of regular eating of a nonnutritive substance.
   d. Treatment
      (1) **Improved observation and supervision** of the child are usually indicated. Improved parental care may occur with direct advice to increase attention to the child. Social service or psychiatric consultation might then be considered if there is no response.
      (2) When factors besides inadequate supervision are present, specific therapy should be attempted.
      (3) Offending agents, such as paint containing lead, should be removed from the child's environment.
      (4) Behavioral treatment using positive reinforcement has had some success.
B. Phobic disorders
   1. Etiology. Psychoanalytic theory assumes displacement of anxiety from an unconscious conflict onto a feared object. **Learning theory** describes learning an irrational response to a benign situation.
   2. Evaluation
      a. Fear of animals, insects, the dark, noise, and death are commonly encountered. Rarely is a phobia the only symptom if an emotional

disorder is present. Self-limited phobic fears in the preschool child are
well known.
  b. School phobia is common on school entrance and again during early
  adolescence.
  c. Social phobias (fear of certain social situations) usually begin after
  puberty.
  d. Agoraphobia can be seen in late adolescence and can be associated with
  a history of school phobia.
  e. Parental anxiety may play a significant contributing role in the child's
  anxiety.
3. **Diagnosis (adapted from *DSM III-R*).** A phobia is a persistent and irrational
  fear of a specific object, activity, or situation. The fear and subsequent
  aversive behavior are significant sources of distress or interfere with social
  and school functioning.
4. **Treatment**
  a. Reassurance given to the parents can help alleviate parental anxiety and
  indirectly reduce the child's anxiety.
  b. Psychiatric consultation is indicated when the phobia becomes disabling.
  c. Behavioral treatment is the treatment of choice for simple phobias. More
  complex phobias often require environmental changes, behavioral treatment, and psychotherapy (individual or group) in various combinations.
  d. Agoraphobia associated with discrete anxiety attacks may respond to
  antidepressant medications.
C. Depressive disorders
1. **Etiology.** Both biologic and psychosocial factors are involved.
2. **Evaluation**
  a. Children should be asked about their affective state (e.g., "Do you ever
  feel really sad or unhappy?" "Do you cry often?"). Severity, frequency, and
  setting should be assessed. Asking about suicide (e.g., "Do you ever think
  about hurting yourself?") will not precipitate the event, but will relieve
  a child in addition to allowing intervention.
  b. Particular indications for an **affect history** include parental rejection,
  physical illness, sudden loss, conduct disorders, school refusal and school
  problems, and sleep disturbances.
  c. Depression in a child is often associated with parental depression.
  d. A history from **different sources** (e.g., child, parent, or school) is helpful.
  A disparity is not unusual (e.g., the parents may be unaware of their
  child's depression).
  e. Transitory depressive moods without disabling effects at home or school
  are common in children.
  f. Infectious diseases (e.g., influenza), hypothyroidism, or medications may
  cause depressed moods.
3. **Diagnosis** (adapted from *DSM III-R*)
  a. A prominent and persistent depressed mood (e.g., "sad," "blue," "down in
  the dumps," or "low," or a persistently sad facial expression) or marked
  lack of interest or pleasure in almost all usual activities
  b. At least three of the following are required for a depressive period:
    (1) Insomnia or hypersomnia
    (2) Appetite changes and significant weight loss or gain
    (3) Low energy level or chronic tiredness
    (4) Feelings of inadequacy or worthlessness
    (5) Decreased effectiveness at school or home
    (6) Decreased attention, concentration, or ability to think clearly
    (7) Social withdrawal; less active or talkative than usual
    (8) Irritability or excessive anger toward parents or caretakers
    (9) Inability to respond with pleasure to praise or rewards
    (10) Pessimistic attitude toward the future or brooding about past events
    (11) Tearfulness or crying

(12) Negative affect on awakening (e.g., tired, drowsy, sick, or irritable) that improves over the next few minutes or hours

(13) Recurrent thoughts of death or suicide

    c. Symptoms must be present almost daily for at least 2 weeks.

  4. Treatment

    a. A **supportive relationship** should be established, ranging from environmental manipulations (e.g., school changes or parent education) to individual meetings.

    b. **Psychiatric consultation** is recommended for evaluation and treatment of persistent depression.

    c. **Antidepressants** have been used successfully, but require close monitoring along with ongoing psychological treatment. Sleep disturbances and diurnal affect variations may be clues to a drug-responsive depression.

D. Overanxious disorders

  1. Etiology. Excessive states of anxiety may relate to temperamental variation, or chronic environmental stress, or both.

  2. Evaluation

    a. The history is elicited by asking what kind of things the patient worries about.

    b. Precipitating stresses include high performance pressure, damage to self-esteem, or feelings of lack of competence.

    c. Accident proneness, hypermaturity, excessive conformity, and difficulty getting to sleep are common symptoms.

    d. Parental anxiety often contributes to the child's worries.

    e. Worries may focus on separation from those to whom the child is attached.

  3. Diagnosis (adapted from *DSM III-R*). The predominant disturbance is generalized and persistent anxiety or worry lasting at least 1 month, as manifested by at least four of the following:

    a. Unrealistic worry about future events

    b. Preoccupation with appropriateness of past behavior

    c. Overconcern about competence (e.g., school, social, athletic)

    d. Somatic complaints, such as headaches or stomachaches, with no established physical basis

    e. Excessive need for reassurance about worries

    f. Marked self-consciousness

    g. Marked feelings of tension or inability to relax; shakiness, trembling, restlessness, or fidgeting

    h. Autonomic hyperactivity (e.g., sweating, heart pounding, dry mouth, diarrhea, high resting pulse and respiration rate)

  4. Treatment

    a. Anxiety may be responsive to support, reassurance, and/or advice to the child and the parents. If the child is unresponsive to this supportive relationship and there is interference with school, home, and/or play, psychiatric consultation can be helpful.

    b. **Acute anxiety** may be helped by benzodiazepines, hydroxyzine, or diphenhydramine.

    c. If motivated, the child (usually 7 years or older) can be instructed in the use of **meditative or relaxation techniques.** The patient is told to practice twice a day and to use the techniques during acute upsets. The following outlines sample instructions given and demonstrated to the child:

      (1) Arrange a quiet and comfortable place.

      (2) Close your eyes and think about "doing nothing."

      (3) Relax your head, neck, and shoulders slowly.

      (4) Exhale slowly after a medium-deep breath and let "relaxation or calmness" flow through your body down to your hands and feet.

      (5) Repeat a single word (e.g., *calm, relax, one*) after each exhalation and feel "relaxation."

(6) Continue to focus on the repetition of a single word, and observe the relaxation for about 5–10 minutes.

E. Conversion disorders

1. **Etiology.** Psychological theory assumes "conversion" of anxiety into a physical dysfunction to lessen conscious anxiety.

2. **Evaluation**

   a. Motor or sensory disturbances along with symptoms complicating a physical illness are common presentations.

   b. A **previous history** of undiagnosable physical symptoms, conversion reactions, or both, is helpful.

   c. A **coexisting organic illness** does not rule out the diagnosis.

   d. **Emotional stress** before the symptom and/or exposure to a person with similar physical symptoms is frequent.

   e. The **differential diagnosis** includes systemic lupus erythematosus and multiple sclerosis, both of which may present with conversion-like symptoms.

3. **Diagnosis** (adapted from *DSM III-R*)

   a. The predominant disturbance is a loss or alteration in physical functioning, suggesting a physical disorder.

   b. The symptom cannot be explained by a known pathophysiologic mechanism and is not under voluntary control.

   c. **Psychological factors** are judged to be involved, as shown by one of the following:

      (1) The temporal relationship between an environmental stimulus that is related to a psychological conflict or need and the initiation of a symptom

      (2) The symptom enables the patient either to avoid a noxious activity or to gain support from the environment that otherwise might not be forthcoming.

4. **Treatment**

   a. **Psychiatric consultation** is indicated. Successful treatment has been obtained with psychotherapy, suggestion, environmental manipulation, and direct symptom approach (e.g., hypnosis).

   b. **Support of the family** is helpful, frequently by reassurance about symptoms that are not medically serious.

   c. In 10–30 percent of patients with a diagnosis of conversion disorder, **organic illness** will be misdiagnosed. Ongoing pediatric follow-up in conjunction with a psychiatric investigation is indicated.

IV. Behavior with physical manifestations

A. Nonorganic failure to thrive

1. **Etiology.** Indicators of risk include a "temperamentally difficult" child, parental isolation or unavailability, disordered parent-child interactions, and/or psychosocial stressors.

2. **Evaluation**

   a. **Organic causes** are investigated simultaneously by history and physical examination, because there is an increase in secondary physiologic disorders. There is frequently a mixed organic and nonorganic cause. Organic risk factors include minor congenital anomalies, prenatal malnutrition, prematurity, and ongoing medical illness.

   b. Determine **growth patterns** by obtaining previous weights, heights, and head circumferences. Typically, weight falls off growth curve before height and head circumference. Premature infants who had appropriate weight for gestational age have normal growth. Growth charts should be corrected for prematurity to 24 months. About 35 percent of small-for-gestational-age infants are below the 5th percentile at age 4 years.

   c. Take a **social history** to determine interference with adequate caretaking. Risk factors include economic stress, disorganized families, social isolation, parental depression, and history of parental loss.

d. Observe feeding and nonfeeding situations between parent(s) and child, looking for decreased, inconsistent, or nonmutual interactions.

e. Assess the child's **development,** including a social responsivity, because delays are common. A child's temperament may frustrate the caretaker. Rapid weight gain early during hospitalization is supportive of a nonorganic cause, but failure to gain does not rule out the diagnosis.

3. Diagnosis is confirmed by evidence that disturbances of interaction interfere with feeding behavior. These disturbances can range from an obvious lack of care to much caring, but maladaptive parent-child feeding interactions.

4. Treatment

a. The initial goal is nutritional rehabilitation and treatment of any associated medical problems. Screen children for anemia and lead levels.

b. Nonorganic risk factors need to be addressed simultaneously with medical issues. Parents should be actively involved in the investigation and treatment. Remember that the inability to feed one's child is frustrating and guilt provoking.

c. Restoring adequate caretaking may reverse the situations. In other instances, a child's maladaptively learned feeding responses may respond to behavioral or family treatment. The interactional difficulties must be directly addressed with parents. Psychiatric or social service consultation is indicated.

d. Developmental stimulation of the child through community infant-stimulation programs can be helpful.

e. Close pediatric follow-up is indicated, given the risk for subsequent behavior problems, cognitive delays, school difficulties, and slow growth.

f. Remember that frequently the cause is neither nonorganic nor organic, but rather a dynamic interaction between social, psychological, and physiologic factors.

B. Encopresis

1. Etiology includes:

a. Chronic constipation with concomitant leakage secondary to the loss of internal sphincter competence

b. Psychosocial stresses

c. Hirschsprung's disease, or aganglionic megacolon (very rare cause)

d. Neurologic abnormalities, including spinal cord lesions, autonomic dysfunction, or seizures

e. Muscle disorders, including amyotonia congenita and cerebral palsy

f. Organic causes of severe constipation (i.e., hypothyroidism)

2. Evaluation

a. In most cases a detailed **history and physical examination** will be sufficient to rule out pathologic causes. Nighttime accidents are rare and suggest emotional or neurologic abnormalities. Abdominal and rectal examinations are helpful in estimating the amount of stool retention. Detailed neurologic or motor examinations may be indicated if underlying neuropathy or myopathy is suspected.

b. Rarely, **laboratory evaluation** may be indicated to rule out underlying abnormalities as suggested by history or physical examination (e.g., hypothyroidism, hypercalcemia, disaccharidase deficiency, malabsorption).

c. A **plain film of the abdomen** can be helpful in assessing the degree of stool retention, and can be used in patient education.

d. **Anal manometry or rectal biopsy** may be indicated in the rare case of suspected Hirschsprung's disease.

e. A **urinalysis** and **urine culture** should be done in the initial evaluation of girls with encopresis because of the increased incidence of associated urinary tract infections.

3. The **diagnosis** is confirmed by the occurrence on a regular basis of deposition of stools in a child's underwear after the age of 4. Primary encopresis applies to cases in which bowel continence has never been achieved, and secondary encopresis applies to cases in which incontinence occurs in those who were once fully trained for at least 6 months.

4. **Treatment**

a. **Education.** It should be explained that the lack of control is not the child's fault. A physiologic explanation of a distended colon that has lost sensation and muscle tone is helpful. Some families may have difficulty dealing with stresses, and referral for psychiatric or psychological therapy may be necessary, preferably after a period of initial medical intervention.

b. **Conditions to facilitate** the development of regular bowel habits should be established, including easy access to bathrooms, privacy, and toilet seating with foot support for younger children.

c. **Initial catharsis** is aimed at completely disimpacting the bowel. The following is recommended for the average 7-year-old child (appropriate adjustments should be made for larger and for smaller children).

   (1) **Home treatment** is practical in almost all cases after education. **For moderate to severe retention** (majority of patients), go through three to four cycles (9–12 days total) as follows:

   (a) **Day 1.** Hypophosphate enemas (Fleet, adult size)

   (b) **Day 2.** Bisacodyl (Dulcolax) suppositories

   (c) **Day 3.** Bisacodyl tablet once

   More recently **polyethylene glycol** electrolyte solution (**Golitely**), given orally at a starting dose of 40 ml/kg over 6 hours, has been used. Encopretic patients may require increased dose and duration of treatment.

   (2) **Inpatient treatment** for severe retention, when home compliance is poor, or when parental administration of enemas is psychologically stressful

   (a) High normal saline enemas (750 ml for a 7-year-old) bid for 3–7 days

   (b) Bisacodyl suppositories bid for 3–7 days

   (c) Use of the bathroom for 15 minutes after each meal

d. The **maintenance phase** is aimed at establishing a consistent bowel pattern after initial catharsis is complete. Exacerbations should be expected during this phase, and the child should be monitored closely to minimize discouragement. The most common reason for failure of therapy is either too much or too little medication. Doses for individual children should be titrated to a particular end point (e.g., two soft bowel movements/day).

   (1) **Mineral oil** (at least 2 tbsp) or other stool softener (docusate sodium) should be used bid, usually for 4–6 months. Light mineral oil is generally better tolerated than regular mineral oil. In most cases, **mineral oil should not be used in children less than 5 years old because of the risk of aspiration.** If used in younger children, mineral oil should be mixed with a food such as yogurt, but **never** be put in a bottle.

   (2) In severe cases or during relapses, an **oral laxative** (senna or danthron) can be added. In severe cases, laxatives can be used daily for 2–3 weeks, then on alternate days for 1 month (given between mineral oil doses). Relapses may require a shorter course.

   (3) The child should sit on the toilet for 5 minutes twice a day at the same time each day (usually postprandially). Timing should be consistent. This is essential and needs constant reinforcement.

   (4) Multiple vitamins bid between mineral oil doses are suggested, although they are probably not necessary.

   (5) **High-roughage diet,** usually bran cereal

e. **Close long-term follow-up** for support, compliance, and associated symptoms is needed. Visits should take place every 4–8 weeks initially, and a physician should be available by phone to make dosage adjustments when necessary.

   f. Parents and patients should be warned of the **possibility of relapses.** Signs of relapse include large-caliber stools, increased mineral oil leakage, abdominal pain, decreased frequency of defecation, and soiling. It is important for parents to react to relapses without being punitive or blaming the child.

   g. For refractory cases, **biofeedback techniques may be useful.**

C. **Enuresis.** There is a male predominance in enuresis at all ages and an increased familial incidence. By age 5, approximately 92 percent of children have achieved daytime dryness, 80 percent nighttime dryness. It is not until age 12 that 95 percent of children achieve nighttime dryness.

   1. **Etiology**
      a. **Organic factors** include structural abnormalities of the genitourinary tract (i.e., ectopic ureter), urinary tract infections, diabetes mellitus, neurologic abnormalities, and diabetes insipidus, in both diurnal and nocturnal cases.

      b. **Diurnal**
         (1) Bladder spasm-urge syndrome. In this syndrome the patient has unpredictable attacks of a sudden urge to void (most common cause).
         (2) Giggle micturition. Sudden involuntary, uncontrollable, and complete emptying of the bladder on giggling in a person (usually female) who is otherwise continent.
         (3) Vaginal reflux. Reflux of urine, usually in overweight girls, into vagina with subsequent leakage, leading to constant wetness of underwear.

      c. **Nocturnal.** No clear cause but seems to have multifactoral etiology related to the following:
         (1) Genetic factors. If one parent had enuresis, there is a 40 percent chance of the child having enuresis; if both parents had enuresis, there is a 70 percent chance for each child.
         (2) Arousal from sleep. Parents report that children with enuresis seem more difficult to arouse, although sleep cycles are normal.
         (3) Small functional bladder capacity. Children with enuresis seem to be able to hold less urine volume in their bladder before voiding (normal bladder capacity, 10 ml/kg; adult, 350–500 ml).
         (4) Maturational delay
         (5) A more recently proposed theory involves decreased nocturnal secretion of vasopressin, the antidiuretic hormone.
         (6) Constipation can worsen enuresis by decreasing functional bladder capacity.
         (7) Psychological factors. Stress appears to exacerbate enuresis. The mechanism is unclear.

   2. **Evaluation and diagnosis**
      a. **History.** A detailed history should be taken to elucidate the following points: the pattern of wetting; the time of day wetting occurs; the number of times per night; the number of nights per week; the number of daytime voidings; periods of dryness; sleeping abnormalities, including snoring; dysuria; polyuria; description of urinary stream; family history; worsening during periods of personal or family stress; toilet training efforts; parental response to wetting; how the child views the problem; how wetting has affected the child's social relationships and social activities; why the parents have sought help at this time; medications the child is taking.

      b. **The physical findings** are normal in the majority of cases. Special attention should be given to the following points: height and weight; blood pressure; genitalia, including locating the urethral meatus; palpation of the abdomen for an enlarged bladder; fecal impaction; abdominal or costovertebral angle tenderness; observation of the urinary stream, including the ability to start and stop it (anatomic and neurologic abnormalities); spine abnormalities; and neurologic findings in the lower extremities, including strength, tone, deep tendon reflexes, and sensation (may be associated with bladder innervation abnormalities). Bladder capacity should be measured.

   c. **Laboratory evaluation** should include:

     (1) A urinalysis in **all cases.** Urine cultures are indicated in girls and sometimes in boys.

     (2) Radiologic studies only if anatomic abnormalities, recurrent urinary tract infections, or an abdominal mass is suspected.

     (3) Blood urea nitrogen (BUN), creatinine, and creatinine clearance if renal disease is suspected

     (4) Cystoscopy and cystometrogram in rare cases

     (5) An EEG if a seizure disorder is suspected

     (6) Rarely, sleep studies

3. Treatment

   a. **Organic causes** for enuresis should be treated appropriately.

   b. **Therapy for idiopathic enuresis is highly controversial.** In all cases it is important to decrease the blame and guilt feelings of the child as well as the struggle between parents and child. Explain that many other children have the same problem. It is helpful to involve the child actively in any therapeutic modality, and he or she should become involved in caring for him- or herself.

     (1) Reassurance is sufficient treatment in many cases, especially with younger children, since a large proportion will have spontaneous resolution.

     (2) Conditions should facilitate dryness. These include easy access to bathrooms during the school day, privacy, and a light in the bathroom at night.

     (3) Conditioning devices are commercially available.* These new alarms attach to the underwear and are easy to use. They have 60–70 percent efficacy with a low relapse rate. They appear to be the therapy of choice in enuresis.

     (4) Behavior modification (see sec. **VII**) is helpful for a number of children. A system of rewards for dry nights or dry days can be instituted. Regular times for voiding can be helpful (often done in combination with alarm).

     (5) Bladder training exercises to stretch the bladder and increase its capacity may be helpful. Once a day children are asked to hold onto their urine for as long as possible.

     (6) Self-awakening techniques that the child does him- or herself, and **dry bed training,** which is a more intensive program involving parents to teach the child to wake at night, have both been reported to be successful in some cases. These are effective in younger children when intervention is being requested.

     (7) Medication

       (a) Imipramine has been shown in controlled studies to decrease the frequency of enuresis in approximately 60 percent of children. It can be particularly helpful on a short-term basis for control of nocturnal enuresis when symptoms may prevent visiting friends overnight, going to camp, and so on. In some cases a pattern of dryness can be established that may persist after the medication is tapered.

         (i) The **dose** is approximately 1 mg/kg 1 hour before bedtime (15–25 mg for children under 12 years of age, 50 mg for

---

* One such device is the Palco Wet-Stop, available from Palco Laboratories, 5026 Scotts Valley Drive, Scotts Valley, CA 95066 (money-back guarantee).

children over 12). If there are no effects after 10–14 days, the dosage can be increased to a maximum of 50 mg for younger children and 75 mg for older children.

(ii) Medication should be given for a maximum of 4 months. The drug should be tapered over 4–6 weeks for best results. Relapses off medication are common (up to 60%).

(iii) **Side effects** of imipramine include mood, sleep, and gastrointestinal disturbances. **Life-threatening cardiac arrhythmias may occur with overdosage,** and care must be taken to prevent unsupervised administration.

(b) **Desmopressin** is a synthetic analogue of the antidiuretic hormone vasopressin, and reduces urine production by increasing water reabsorption in the distal tubules, resulting in more concentrated urine. Improvement is seen in 60 percent of children, but most studies show a relapse in 80 percent when treatment is discontinued. As with imipramine there is a role for short-term treatment.

(i) **Desmopressin** is administered **intranasally,** the starting dose being 20 μg (one spray into each nostril). The maximum dose is 40 μg, with doses being increased by 10 μg each week. Duration of action is 12 hours.

(ii) The treatment period has generally been 12 weeks, although in more recent studies desmopressin has been used for longer periods. Tapering is achieved by reducing the dosage by one spray (10 μg) every 2 weeks.

(iii) Side effects include **headaches, abdominal pain, nausea,** and **nasal irritation.** There is a theoretical complication of **hyponatremia** secondary to water retention, but this has not been reported in studies using desmopressin for nocturnal enuresis. It is contraindicated in patients with **hypertension or cardiac disease.**

(8) **Relapses** are common, and parents should be counseled so that they can react to relapses without being punitive or blaming the child.

D. **Sleep disorders**

1. **Non–rapid-eye-movement (NREM) parasomnias: disorders of arousal.** These include confusional arousals, sleep walking, and sleep terrors.

a. The **etiology** is unclear but there is frequently a positive family history. Episodes occur in the first third of the night during a transition from deep (stage 3/4) NREM sleep to another sleep stage. All have in common that the child is often confused and unresponsive to his or her environment, exhibits autonomic features (tachycardia, sweating, pupillary dilatation), and has retrograde amnesia of the episode.

b. **Evaluation and diagnosis**

(1) **Confusional arousals** are most common in the first 3 years of life, and may present as unexplained crying or moving in the crib. The child looks confused or agitated, and may have verbal (talking, crying, or screaming) motor (thrashing around in bed or walking around the room), or autonomic features.

(2) **Sleep walking** occurs at least once in 15–30 percent of healthy children, with 2–3 percent having more frequent episodes. It is most common between 6 and 12 years, with most children having outgrown it by 15 years. Episodes usually involve the child calmly walking around the house, although sometimes the child may display unusual behavior such as urinating on the floor.

(3) **Sleep terrors** are most common between 5 and 7 years and have a prevalence of around 3 percent. They usually begin with a terrified scream accompanied by an intense autonomic response. The child generally looks fearful and may run around as if running away from

something. Efforts to console the child often make the episode worse. Episodes may be brief or may last up to 45 minutes. Sleep terrors differ from nightmares in the following characteristics:

	Sleep terrors	Nightmares
Sleep stage	NREM	REM
Time of night	First ⅓	Mid to last ⅓
Wakefulness	Unrousable	Easily roused
Amnesia	Yes	No
Family history	Yes	No
Return to sleep	Easy	Difficult

c. Treatment
  (1) As these episodes are self-limiting, often no specific intervention is necessary other than giving an explanation and recommending a decrease in physical contact during the episode. The event should be allowed to run its course with the parent protecting the child if necessary.
  (2) Episodes may be precipitated by stress, fatigue, and illness in susceptible individuals.
  (3) Regularizing the sleep schedule to avoid sleep deprivation may also help.
  (4) Basic safety precautions should be taken to ensure that the sleep-walking child does not harm him- or herself (secure windows, alarms on outside doors).
  (5) When arousals are disruptive or dangerous, pharmacologic therapy (benzodiazepines or tricyclic antidepressants) or relaxation mental imagery can be used.
  (6) Scheduled awakening before the time that the event typically occurs has been found to be successful in some cases.
  (7) If events are unusual (early morning, or history of tonic-clonic movements, etc.), nocturnal seizures should be ruled out.
2. Delayed sleep initiation and maintenance are problems frequently seen in young children.
  a. The **etiology** is multifactorial and one or more of the following may be present.
    (1) Inappropriate sleep associations occur when a child learns to fall asleep in a particular way, such that those conditions need to be present all the time for the child to fall asleep. Examples include rocking, feeding, or pacifiers, all of which must be reestablished if the child is to fall back asleep after waking. Another example is that of the child who falls asleep in the parents' bed but then is moved, so that he or she wakes in a completely different environment.
    (2) Feedings during the night can also contribute to frequent nighttime wakings, either by continued wet diapers or the patterned response of learning to be hungry at certain times. Most healthy full-term babies can sleep through the night without a feeding by 5–6 months.
    (3) Erratic scheduling can also contribute to difficulties in falling asleep or nighttime wakings. This includes daytime naps, as well as times of going to bed and waking.
    (4) Poor and inconsistent **limit setting**, both at bedtime and nighttime wakings, can also contribute to the problem.
  b. Diagnosis and evaluation
    (1) A very detailed history should be taken, including sleep schedules during the day and weekends, the current sleep environment (where does the child sleep, is anyone else present) and bedtime routines.

(2) A detailed family and social history is important to examine the presence of other contributing problems (for example, marital problems, maternal depression).

(3) Careful sleep charting is often very useful, particularly in chaotic families where it is difficult to know exactly what is happening.

(4) Physical examination

c. Treatment

(1) A detailed explanation should be given to parents about the etiology of the problem in a noncritical manner.

(2) Strategies to deal with inappropriate sleep associations should be discussed. For example, putting a child into the crib while still awake or partially awake instead of rocking him or her to sleep; introduction of a regular nighttime routine; elimination of a nighttime bottle

(3) If frequent feeding is a problem, then either cutting down the amount of fluid given over 7–10 nights or, if nursing, decreasing the amount of time that one feeds the child over successive nights, can be discussed.

(4) The importance of a regular routine both during the night and day needs to be explained to parents.

(5) Education about consistent limit setting should be provided, but it is important that methods employed must be acceptable to the parents (e.g., using a gate to help the child learn to stay in his or her room). Behavior modification charts using stickers can be employed to help motivate youngsters as young as 3–4 years of age.

(6) Close follow-up by appointment or telephone is necessary to support and guide families while changes are taking place.

3. Narcolepsy is a syndrome of **excessive daytime sleepiness (EDS)** and abnormalities of rapid-eye-movement (REM) sleep. Usual onset is between 15 and 35 years, with occurrence before puberty being unusual. Men and women are affected equally, with prevalence in the United States estimated between 1 in 1,000 and 1 in 10,000.

a. The precise **etiology** is unclear but narcolepsy is strongly linked to class II HLA antigens located on chromosome 6. Among adults with narcolepsy the DR2 antigen was found in 85 percent of patients, as compared with a prevalence of 25 percent among healthy control subjects.

b. Evaluation and diagnosis

(1) One or more of the following is present.

(a) EDS, which is more pronounced in sedentary situations. This symptom is usually the most common presentation in children.

(b) Cataplexy is an abrupt loss of muscle tone that is brought on by excitement or emotion.

(c) Hypnagogic hallucinations are visual or auditory hallucinations that accompany either the onset of sleep or awakening.

(d) Sleep paralysis is motor paralysis (with the exception of respiratory muscles) that occurs either at the onset of sleep or at awakening.

(e) All four symptoms are present in approximately 10 percent of cases. Generally, **EDS** and **cataplexy** are the most common symptoms.

(2) Narcolepsy is associated with the occurrence of REM sleep within the first 10 minutes of sleep onset.

(3) The diagnosis is confirmed by a **Multiple Sleep Latency Test,** which looks at multiple nap recordings to assess sleep latency and the presence of sleep-onset REM. Ideally, this is preceded by an all-night sleep study to rule out the possibility of REM sleep deprivation the night before. This is also important to exclude conditions such as obstructive sleep apnea or nocturnal seizures, which may also present with EDS.

    c. Treatment
      (1) Referral to a sleep clinic or specialist is helpful, as this condition is lifelong and often requires medication.
        (a) Stimulant medication to help EDS
        (b) Tricyclic antidepressants at nighttime to help control hypnagogic hallucinations, sleep paralysis, and cataplexy
      (2) Scheduled naps lasting 20–30 minutes to help daytime alertness are a useful strategy irrespective of medication usage.
      (3) Educating parents and teachers about narcolepsy is essential to the well-being of the child, both socially and physically.
      (4) Driving and swimming pose a risk for these patients, and should be monitored closely until the symptoms are under control.
  4. Obstructive sleep apnea syndrome is a potentially lethal condition characterized by multiple obstructive or mixed apneas during sleep, associated with repetitive episodes of inordinately loud snoring or excessive daytime somnolence.
    a. The **etiology** is unclear, but it is thought to be secondary to anatomic predisposition (e.g., large tonsils or adenoids, Pierre Robin syndrome) with possibly a CNS component.
    b. Evaluation and diagnosis
      (1) The **history** should evaluate the following:
        (a) EDS
        (b) Loud **intermittent** snoring during sleep, with frequent episodes of apnea
        (c) Enuresis
        (d) Poor school performance
        (e) Naps that do not decrease sleepiness
        (f) Often, tape recording sleep can be helpful.
      (2) Physical examination should include an upper airway examination. An ear, nose, and throat examination and x-rays to detect upper airway obstruction are indicated when the diagnosis is suspected from the history.
      (3) An **ECG** should be done to detect right ventricular hypertrophy, cor pulmonale, and arrhythmias.
      (4) A **sleep study** with full monitoring of the ECG, respiratory pattern, EEG, and PO_2 should be performed.
    c. Treatment
      (1) Avoid all forms of sedation; they may exacerbate the apnea.
      (2) Surgery to remove obstruction (e.g., adenoids, tonsils) has been attempted with varying success. After operation, these patients should be monitored closely in an intensive care unit until the airway is clearly stabilized.
      (3) Tracheostomy cures the problem, but the cost-benefit ratio must be considered.
      (4) Weight loss is often beneficial in obese patients.
      (5) The use of medication is controversial and its merits unproved.
V. Chronic illness
  A. Chronic illness in a child constitutes a major and prolonged stress for the entire family. The psychological reactions of the family, including the child, occur in phases with indistinct transitions. These are as follows:
    1. Shock and disbelief. Regressive behaviors, unrealistic fears, and, most commonly, denial are prominent (lasting weeks to even months).
    2. Protest and anguish. Guilt, depression, anger, and sorrow can occur. There is mourning for lost normality and dashed hopes. The young child may experience illness as a punishment for being "bad" or may become bitter at illness-related treatments or restrictions. The adolescent may fear "loss of control" or "being different." Blaming parents or physicians is common.
    3. Restitution. This phase ideally represents awareness of new limitations, development of adequate social patterns, constructive use of strengths, and

a denial that is consistent with hope. Families usually adapt well. However, increased emotional problems are found in chronically ill children when compared with control groups.
B. Evaluation
1. History should emphasize the child's previous **adaptive** capacities (e.g., school performance problems, poor peer relations, or difficult reactions to loss) or family relationship problems.
2. **Maladaptive** responses by the child include overdependence, noncompliance, overanxiousness, aggressiveness, and/or withdrawal. Overprotection, indulgence, rejection, and/or blaming may be parental responses.
C. Treatment
1. A long-term **supportive relationship with the family** may allow anxieties and frustrations to be expressed.
2. **Clear and honest explanations** regarding the diagnosis, prognosis, and management should be given to both parent and child. Repeated explanations, especially at the time of the initial diagnosis, are commonly needed.
3. **Siblings** often feel guilt, or resentment, or both, about the sick child. Parents should be encouraged to keep the siblings informed, with the physician's assistance if necessary.
4. **Parents** should be encouraged to minimize as much as possible the "sick child" role. Chronically ill children still need discipline.
5. If available, **group meetings** for parents and children who have experienced similar problems can be helpful.
6. **Compliance** is a frequent problem, especially for the adolescent. The following approach is recommended:
   a. Early education regarding the illness and clear explanations about the management are preventive. Reassurance and positive verbal feedback regarding compliance are helpful.
   b. If compliance becomes a problem, verify the situation (e.g., blood levels). The results then should be discussed directly with the patient. A behavioral treatment program with a positive reinforcement system (e.g., awards, stickers, praise) may then be attempted.
   c. If the preceding measures are unsuccessful or time constraints make step 2 difficult, then psychiatric consultation may be necessary.
VI. Separation experiences
A. Death of a parent, sibling, or significant other. As in chronic illness (see sec. **V**), a child's grief is phasic, with indistinct transitions. The stages are: shock and disbelief, protest and anguish, and detachment and reorientation toward a new relationship. The child's reaction is intimately connected to that of the parents or surviving parent: The more distraught child usually has a parent who also has not resolved the loss. The finality of death is not fully understood until approximately age 10 years. Prior to this, reversibility is possible in the child's view. The child frequently attributes the incident to something he or she "has done." Crying, sleep difficulties, anxiety, irritability, regression, depression, preoccupation with the deceased, feeling the presence of the deceased, or somatic concerns can be observed. The duration can be from weeks to a year. Reactions going beyond 1 year denote an unresolved grief reaction. **Treatment** is as follows (see Chap. 1, p. 10):
1. The parents can be encouraged to be as open as possible with their explanations and their own individual reactions. It is beneficial and reassuring to the child to be told exactly what has happened and what will take place. Evasive information will only ultimately further confuse the child. Parents should be encouraged to state their genuine beliefs about the type of survival after death when asked by the child.
2. When death is impending, it is helpful to inform the child about the upcoming loss and allow visitation if possible.
3. Reassurances are important for the child at the time of the death. The child should be informed that he or she will be taken care of, that the child will not die, that he or she does not have the same illness that caused the death, and

that no one else is going away. It is important that the child be reassured that no one, in particular the child, is to blame for the loss.

4. It is helpful to the child to attend the funeral. Attendance can provide meaningful information to the child, and he or she can observe the appropriate expression of emotions. A supportive adult relationship should be provided to the child during the ceremonies. For the younger child, attendance at a portion of the funeral may be arranged.

5. The parents should be told that the child will often ask very painful questions. Direct questions about death are frequent and repeated.

6. The child and the family may benefit by referral for counseling. This can be offered routinely to each family when such a loss has occurred. Referral is also indicated when there appears to be a "block" in the mourning process, evidenced by a continued yearning for the lost person over years.

B. **Hospitalization.** Emotional distress during a hospitalization is most marked between the ages of 6 months and 4 years and is related to separation from familiar figures and the strange environment. There is concern about desertion or punishment. Beginning at age 4 years, there is increasing concern over the illness and treatment and about injury to one's body. Fear of death coincides with understanding of finality by age 10 years.

Immediately following hospital discharge, a child may manifest hostility, clinging, anxiety, and so on, for weeks. This is more frequent when prior parent-child relationships are problematic. There is an increased risk of emotional problems if there are multiple separations or if the hospitalization lasts longer than 1 week. **Treatment** is as follows (see also Chap. 1):

1. Physician support with careful explanation of treatment plans to both parents and child is crucial.

2. Encourage familiar home routines. For the infant or toddler, overnight visits by the parents are beneficial, whereas for the older child, frequent visiting may be sufficient.

3. Encourage normalization of activity as much as possible. This can range from "playroom" usage to game playing to school work.

4. Consultation with a child psychiatrist can be useful for the particularly problematic or withdrawn child.

5. When hospitalization is elective, prehospitalization preparation, including visiting the hospital, can be helpful both to the child and the parents.

6. Following discharge, the parents should return to setting the same limits and discipline as they did prior to the hospitalization.

C. **Divorce.** The effect of this increasingly common event depends on the age of the child. Preschool children may be grief stricken and wonder if they themselves can be divorced. The older child will also be hurt though may be more easily reassured. The adolescent tends to separate himself or herself from the situation. At all ages, however, there is questioning about whether the child caused the divorce. Psychological difficulties will depend more on marital discord or disturbed parent-child relationships than on the separation itself. **Treatment** is as follows:

1. Encourage the parents to relate specific and honest facts about the divorce to their children. Their children often need to know that both parents still love them, that the divorce is not the children's fault, and that they will be cared for. Repeated explanations are frequently needed and requested by the child.

2. Recommend that the child be kept out of ongoing disputes between the parents. If possible, the child should not be involved in the adversary system of the court.

3. Allow ventilation of feelings about the divorce by parent or child.

4. Visitation should not be used by one parent against the other.

5. The noncustodial parent can be advised to "go where the child goes" (e.g., to a school activity) when visiting the older child who wants to be with friends.

6. A counseling referral is indicated for the child and family who are having disabling distress.

D. **Working parents.** There is a lack of evidence for a relationship between employment and maternal deprivation. Most parents work out of economic necessity. The crucial factor for the child is the quality of care. Substitute care that is caring, predictable, and meets a child's need does not appear harmful to the child. Work may be an important stress reducer for some parents, thus improving the quality of time spent with the children. It can be helpful for one parent to remain at home until an infant's behavior becomes stable.

VII. **Behavioral treatment program.** The brief program outlined in five steps (see **A–E**) is based on the principle of **operant conditioning** (behavior is determined in part by its consequences). If a behavior is followed by a rewarding event (**positive reinforcement**), it tends to be strengthened and occurs more frequently. If the behavior is followed by no event (**extinction**) or by an aversive event (**punishment**), it tends to be weakened and occurs less frequently. These principles have been applied to a wide range of behaviors (e.g., enuresis, atopic dermatitis scratching, medicine compliance, eating disorders). A good relationship with a motivated or interested family is important for success.

   A. **Specify the target behavior.** A detailed history is needed regarding the behavior to be modified, including environmental antecedents and consequences of this behavior (e.g., scratching might be the target, with an important consequence being parent attention).

   B. **Measure the target behavior (baseline).** Have the family record the frequency, time, and duration of the behavior. This is an **important step** to allow later determination of the effectiveness of the intervention (e.g., scratching occurs so many times per hour).

   C. **Choose the reinforcer(s).** Together with the family, search for a reward or reinforcer that will maintain a new behavior. This is done by looking for what the child likes (e.g., toys, money, stickers) or what the child does a lot (e.g., play computer games).

   D. **Arrange the contingency**

      1. An arrangement is made in which access to the reinforcer is contingent on producing the new behavior (e.g., reinforcement is given in response to a specified reduction in scratches per hour).

      2. The reinforcer is maximally effective when it immediately follows the behavior to be strengthened (e.g., stickers might be given for a specified time with no scratching or a reduction in scratching).

      3. In beginning the program the reinforcers must be easily obtainable. Later, the requirements to gain the reinforcer can be increased. A major problem in the failure of programs is making the reinforcement too difficult to obtain at first (e.g., no scratching for 10 min might be required at first; later, 20 min might be required).

      4. The use of stickers, stars, or points that can be posted on a chart or pasted in a book is useful. These can later be turned in for reinforcers (e.g., 10 points may gain a new toy).

      5. Reinforcers definitely include social approval and praise for desired behaviors. Ignoring the nondesired behavior can also be used.

   E. **Monitor the progress**

      1. The programs usually need repetition to become effective. Recording the child's progress, as in step 4, will allow evaluation of effectiveness.

      2. As the new behavior is established, other reinforcers (e.g., social approval) become important, so that the formal program can be gradually phased out.

      3. In the long run, the use of punishment is not an effective intervention.

      4. These programs can be highly effective with specified behaviors. However, for difficulties in establishing an effective program, the lack of time required to arrange a program, or complex behavior problems, a psychological consultation is indicated.

Formulary

The following formulary is adapted from that used at The Children's Hospital. Generic names are used almost exclusively except in the few cases (e.g., Mucomyst) in which the trade name is so widely known that confusion might result if the trade name were omitted. Some widely used drugs or formulations such as decongestants are included for the convenience of the reader. Their inclusion does not imply our endorsement but rather our recognition of their use. Doses are included, again for convenience. In all cases, doses should be checked against the text for indications, age, duration, and other specific considerations.

Our thanks go to The Children's Hospital Department of Pharmacy for its permission to adapt the formulary.

Name (generic)	Available Preparations	Dosage	Special Considerations
Acetaminophen	Drops: 100 mg/mL — 15 mL btl Solution: 160 mg/5 mL — 4 oz btl Suppository: 125 mg, 650 mg Tablet: 80 mg (chewable), 325 mg	65 mg/kg/24 hr in 4–6 divided doses	
Acetazolamide	Capsule: 500 mg Injection: 500 mg — vial Tablet: 125 mg, 250 mg	**Diuretic:** Parenteral or oral: 5 mg/kg/24 hr daily or every other day **Epilepsy, glaucoma:** Oral: 8–30 mg/kg/24 hr in 3–4 divided doses	
Acetylcysteine sodium (Mucomyst)	Solution: 20% — 10 mL vial 10% — 10 mL vial	**Pulmonary mucolytic:** 3–5 mL by nebulization 3–4 times/day **Acetaminophen ingestion:** Oral: 140 mg/kg once; then 70 mg/kg/dose q4h for 17 doses; repeat dose if emesis occurs within 1 hr of dose	
Actifed*	Solution: 2.5 mL and 5 mL u/d,† and 120 mL btl Tablet: Combination product	Children, 4 mo–2 yr: 1.25 mL tid–qid 2–4 yr: 2.5 mL tid–qid 4–6 yr: 3.75 mL tid–qid 6–12 yr: 5 mL or ½ tablet tid–qid 12 yr: 1 tablet tid–qid	Contains: Per 5 mL Per Tablet Triprolidine HCl 1.25 mg 2.5 mg Pseudoephedrine HCl 30 mg 60 mg Do not exceed 4 doses in 24 hr
Acyclovir	Capsule: 200 mg Injection: 500 mg, 1 gm — vial Ointment: 5% — 15 gm tube	**Mucosal and cutaneous herpes simplex or varicella zoster in immunocompromised patients:** Infants: See p. 176	

*Trade name
†Unit dose

Name (generic)	Available Preparations	Dosage	Special Considerations
		Herpes simplex encephalitis and varicella zoster: 30 mg/kg/24 hr (1,500 mg/m²/24 hr) in 3 divided doses given over 30–60 min for 7–14 days	
Adenosine	Solution, 6 mg/vial	0.1 mg/kg, may repeat after 5 minutes at twice the dose (must be rapid IV push) **HSV:** 30 mg/kg/24 hr in 3 divided doses for 7 days in patients with normal renal function	Dosage and frequency should be adjusted in patients with acute or chronic renal impairment
Albuterol	Oral inhal: 90 μg/dose — 17 gm aerosol container Syrup: 0.4 mg/mL Tablet: 2 mg, 4 mg Solution for inhalation 0.5%: 5 mg/mL — 20 mL	*Oral:* Children: 2–6 years: 0.1–0.2 mg/kg/dose 3 times/day; maximum dose not to exceed 4 mg 3 times/day 6–12 years: 2 mg 3–4 times/day; maximum dose not to exceed 24 mg/day (divided doses) Children > 12 years and Adults: 2–4 mg 3–4 times/day; maximum dose not to exceed 8 mg 4 times/day Inhalation MDI: Albuterol 90 μg/spray 17 gm (Proventil, Ventolin): Children < 12 years: Administer 1–2 inhalators 4 times/day using a tube spacer Children > 12 years and Adults: Administer 1–2 inhalations every 4–6 hours	

Name (generic)	Available Preparations	Dosage	Special Considerations
		Inhalation: NICU patients: 5–20 breaths of ½ or full strength 0.083% albuterol every 4–6 hours (can be given more frequently according to need) Neonates, Infants, and Children ≤ 12 years: 5–20 breaths of full strength 0.5% albuterol or 0.02–0.03 mL/kg to a maximum of 1 mL 0.5% albuterol diluted in 2–3 mL normal saline until nebulized every 4–6 hours (can be given more frequently according to need) Children > 12 years and Adults: 5–20 breaths of full strength 0.5% albuterol or 0.5–1 mL 0.5% albuterol diluted in 2–3 mL normal saline until nebulized every 4–6 hours (can be given more frequently according to need)	
Alcohol, dehydrated (ethanol 100%)	Injection: 2 mL — ampul	**As a metabolic blocking agent in an ethylene glycol or methanol ingestion:** Parenteral, IV: *Loading dose:* 0.6 mg/kg either as a 10% IV or a 20–50% oral solution *Maintenance dose:* 110–130 mg/kg/hr adjusted as needed to provide a serum concentration ≥ 100 mg/dL	

Name (generic)	Available Preparations	Dosage	Special Considerations
Allopurinol	Injection: 500 mg — vial (investigational) Tablet: 100 mg, 300 mg	**Hyperuricemia:** Oral: 10 mg/kg/24 hr in 3–4 divided doses; after 48 hr of treatment, titrate dose according to serum uric acid levels	Do not exceed 600 mg/24 hr Inhibits inactivation of 6-mercaptopurine and azathioprine (requires that doses of these agents be reduced by 60–75%) Avoid use with iron supplements
Aluminum carbonate	Capsule: 600 mg Suspension: 400 mg/5 mL — 360 mL btl Tablet: 500 mg		2.8 mg sodium per capsule 2.1 mg sodium per tablet 2.4 mg sodium per 5 mL
Aluminum hydroxide	Capsule: 500 mg Suspension: 600 mg/5 mL — 30 mL u/d, 150 mL Tablet: 300 mg, 600 mg		
Aluminum phosphate	Suspension: 4% — 120 mL btl		12.5 mg sodium per 5 mL
Amantadine HCl	Capsule: 100 mg Solution: 50 mg/5 mL — 16 oz btl	Children, 1–9 yr: 4–8 mg/kg/24 hr in 2–3 divided doses to a maximum of 150 mg/24 hr 9–12 yr: 100 mg–200 mg/day in 2 divided doses	Useful for prophylaxis of influenza in an epidemic setting when it is too late to immunize; continue for at least 10 days following a known exposure Useful therapeutically to reduce duration of symptoms and to decrease small airway disease
Aminophylline	Injection: 25 mg/mL — 10 mL vial Solution: 105 mg/5 mL — 8 oz btl Tablet: 100 mg	Neonates: Apnea (aminophylline concentration 2 mg/mL, pharmacy prepared): Loading dose: 5 mg/kg; dilute dose in 1-hour IV fluid via syringe pump over 1 hour	Approximately 85% of the aminophylline dose is anhydrous theophylline Therapeutic level: Asthma: 10–20 µg/mL Neonatal apnea: 6–13 µg/mL

Name (generic)	Available Preparations	Dosage	Special Considerations
		Maintenance: 2 mg/kg every 8–12 hours or 1–3 mg/kg/dose every 8–12 hours; administer IV push 1 mL/minute (2 mg/minute) Wheezing: 4–6 mg/kg every 6 hours Theophylline levels should be drawn every 4–6 hours initially (longer intervals are OK when infant is stable) Treatment of acute bronchospasm in patients > 6 months of age: Loading dose (in patients not currently receiving theophylline): Based on aminophylline: 6 mg/kg over 20–30 minutes; administration rate should not exceed 25 mg/minute Based on theophylline: 4.7 mg/kg over 20–30 minutes; administration rate should not exceed 20 mg/minute Maintenance dosage, approximate (first 12 hours): Children 6 months to 9 years: Aminophylline: 1.2 mg/kg/hr; theophylline: 0.95 mg/kg/hour Children 9–16 years and young adult smokers: Aminophylline: 1 mg/kg/hour; theophylline: 0.79 mg/kg/hour	

Name (generic)	Available Preparations	Dosage	Special Considerations
		Older patients and patients with cor pulmonale: Aminophylline: 0.6 mg/kg/hour; theophylline: 0.47 mg/kg/hour Patients with CHF or liver failure: Aminophylline: 0.5 mg/kg/hour; theophylline: 0.39 mg/kg/hour Second 12-hour period: Dosage should be adjusted according to serum level	
Amikacin	Injection: 250 mg/mL — 4 mL vial	Newborn: 15 mg/kg/24 hr in 2 divided doses Children: 22.5 mg/kg/24 hr or 750 mg/m^2/24 hr in 3 divided doses to a maximum of 1.5 gm/24 hr	Allowable predose level < 10 μg/mL; allowable 1 hr postdose range: 15–35 μg/mL Dilute to 2.5 mg/mL in D$_5$W or NS and infuse over 30 min
Aminocaproic acid	Injection: 250 mg/mL — 20 mL vial Solution: 1.25 gm/5 mL — 16 oz btl Tablet: 500 mg		See text
Amitriptyline	Tablet: 10 mg, 25 mg, 50 mg	**Depression,** daily dose range: 0.5–5.0 mg/kg/24 hr (older adolescents 3.5 mg/kg/24 hr); increase by 0.5 mg/kg/24 hr every 3 days **Attention deficit disorder,** daily dose range: 0.2–0.5 mg/kg/24 hr in 1 or 2 divided doses	Not recommended in children < 12 yr old In many patients the long half-life permits single daily dosing at bedtime, thereby utilizing the sedative effect

Name (generic)	Available Preparations	Dosage	Special Considerations
Ammonium chloride	Tablet: 500 mg	**Urinary acidification:** 75 mg/kg/dose qid to a total of 2–6 gm/24 hr **Refractory hypochloremic metabolic alkalosis:** Calculate the dose from following formula: Ammonium chloride (mEq) = chloride deficit (mEq/liter) × (0.3 × wt in kg)	Use with caution in infants Do not use in patients with liver disease Administer ½ to ⅔ of the calculated dose, then reevaluate
Amobarbital sodium	Injection: 250 mg — ampul	**Seizures:** Parenteral, IV: 3–5 mg/kg/dose **Sedation:** 2 mg/kg/24 hr in 4 divided doses	For IV use dilute to a 10% solution and infuse not faster than 1 mL/min Amobarbital should be injected within 30 minutes after opening vial to minimize hydrolysis **Drug interactions** Probenecid, allopurinol
Amoxicillin	Capsule: 250 mg, 500 mg Suspension, oral: 25 mg/mL (150 mL); 50 mg/mL (150 mL)	Oral: Children: 20–40 mg/kg/day in 3 divided doses Adults: 250–500 mg 3 times/day; maximum dose: 2–3 gm/day	
Amoxicillin and clavulanate	Suspension, oral: Amoxicillin trihydrate 50 mg and clavulanic acid 12.5 mg/mL (75 mL) Tablet: 250 = Amoxicillin trihydrate 250 mg and clavulanic acid 125 mg	Oral: Dosage should be calculated and prescribed based on the amoxicillin component Children < 40 kg: 20–40 mg/kg/day in 3 divided doses Adults: 250–500 mg every 8 hours	**Contraindications:** Known hypersensitivity to amoxicillin or clavulanic acid (penicillins), infectious mononucleosis, concomitant use of disulfiram **Adverse reactions:** Diarrhea, nausea, vomiting, rash **Drug interactions:** Allopurinol, disulfiram

Name (generic)	Available Preparations	Dosage	Special Considerations
Amphotericin B	Injection: 50 mg/vial	The dilution for amphotericin B infusions is 0.1 mg/mL in D₅W Test dose: 0.1 mg/kg/dose to maximum of 1 mg, infuse over 30–60 minutes; if test dose tolerated, give therapeutic dose Initial therapeutic dose: 0.25 mg/kg; daily dose can then be increased to 0.5–0.6 mg/kg the next day Severely ill patients: The full dose can be given after the test dose Maintenance dose: 0.5 to 1 mg/kg/day given once daily; infuse over 2–6 hours; once therapy established, amphotericin B can be administered on an every-other-day basis at 1–1.2 mg/kg/dose; maximum dose: 1.5 mg/kg in children Adults: IV: 1 mg/kg/day **or** 1.5 mg/kg every other day	**Additional information** Do not administer through filters smaller than 1 μ
Ampicillin	Injection: 1 gm — vial	**Infection:** Neonates: Premature, < 1 week: 50–100 mg/kg/24 hr in 2 divided doses Premature, > 1 week: 100 mg/kg/24 hr in 3 divided doses Term infants < 1 week: 150–250 mg/kg/24 hr in 3–4 divided doses Infants and Children: 100–400 mg/kg/24 hr in 4–6 divided doses	3 mEq sodium per gm

573

Name (generic)	Available Preparations	Dosage	Special Considerations
		Meningitis: Neonates: < 1 week: 100–200 mg/kg/24 hr in 2 divided doses >1 week: 200–400 mg/kg/24 hr in 3–4 divided doses Infants and Children: 300–400 mg/kg/24 hr in 4–6 divided doses	
Ampicillin and sulbactam	Powder for injection: 1.5 gm = ampicillin sodium 1 gm and sulbactam sodium 0.5 gm; 3 gm = ampicillin sodium 2 gm and sulbactam sodium 1 gm	Dosage should be calculated and prescribed as the ampicillin dosage Uncomplicated urinary tract infection: 100 mg/kg/ day (ampicillin) in 4 divided doses Cellulitis, skeletal and abdominal infection, and to rule out sepsis: 200 mg/kg/day (ampicillin) in 4 divided doses; maximum dose: 2 gm (ampicillin) every 6 hours	Should not be used to treat meningitis; once culture results are available, other antibiotics may be more appropriate
Amrinone	Solution: 20 mg/amp	Load 1–3 mg/kg over 15 minutes; infusion of 5–20 µg/kg/min	
Amyl nitrite vaporol	Ampul: 12/box	**Cyanide poisoning:** Inhale contents of vaporol 30 sec out of every min; use a new vaporol every 3 min	Consult with the Poison Control Center for management of cyanide poisoning
Ascorbic acid	Injection: 500 mg/mL — 1 mL ampul Drops: 35 mg/0.6 mL Tablet: 100 mg, 250 mg	**Urine acidification:** 2–8 gm/m² in 6 divided doses **Dietary supplement:** 50–60 mg/day	

Name (generic)	Available Preparations	Dosage	Special Considerations
Aspirin	Chew-tab: 75 mg Suppository: 125 mg, 600 mg Tablet: 300 mg	Children: Analgesic and antipyretic: Oral, rectal: 10–15 mg/kg/dose every 4–6 hours Antiinflammatory: Oral: 80–100 mg/kg/day in 3–4 divided doses Kawasaki disease: Oral: 100 mg/kg/day in 4 divided doses; after fever resolves: 3–5 mg/kg/day once daily	**Reference range:** Salicylate blood levels for antiinflammatory effect: 150–300 µg/mL; analgesic and antipyretic effect: 30–50 µg/mL Avoid overdosage, particularly in infants Strong association with Reye syndrome
Azathioprine	Capsule: 10 mg (special prep) Injection: 5 mg/mL (20 mL) Tablet: 50 mg	*Initial,* renal transplant, parenteral or oral: 3–5 mg/kg/24 hr *Maintenance,* oral: 1–3 mg/kg/24 hr Rheumatoid arthritis: Oral: 1 mg/kg/day for 6–8 weeks; increase by 0.5 mg/day every 4 weeks until response, or up to 2.5 mg/kg/day	Reduce dose to ¼–⅓ of usual dose if allopurinol is given concurrently
Aztreonam	Injection: 2 gm	Neonates: IV: Postnatal 0–7 days: < 2 kg: 60 mg/kg/day in 2 divided doses > 2 kg: 90 mg/kg/day in 3 divided doses Postnatal 7–30 days: <2 kg: 90 mg/kg/day in 3 divided doses >2 kg: 120 mg/kg/day in 4 divided doses Infants > 1 month and children: IV: 90–120 mg/kg/day in 3–4 divided doses Cystic fibrosis: 150–200 mg/kg/day; maximum 6–9 gm/day	

Name (generic)	Available Preparations	Dosage	Special Considerations
Beclomethasone dipropionate	Nasal inhal: 42 µg/inhalation — 16.8 gm aerosol Oral inhal: 42 µg/inhalation — 17 gm aerosol container	Children, 6–12 yr: 1–2 inhalations 3–4 times/day Children > 12 yr: 2 inhalations 3–4 times/day	Do not exceed 10 inhalations/24 hr
Bisacodyl	Tablet: 5 mg Suppository: 10 mg	*Oral:* Children 3–12: 5 mg/dose Children ≥ 12 years and Adults: 5–15 mg/day as a single dose *Rectal suppository:* Children 2–11 years: 5–10 mg/day as a single dose Children ≥ 12 years and Adults: 10 mg/day as a single dose	Swallow tablet whole; do not crush or chew Do not administer milk or antacids within 1 hr of receiving tablet **Do not use in children < 2 yr old**
Bretylium tosylate	Injection: 50 mg/mL — 10 mL ampul	**Usual dosage: 5 mg/kg bolus IV** followed by additional doses of 5 mg/kg every 6 hours for up to 48 hours	
Brompheniramine maleate	Ex-tab: 8 mg, 12 mg Solution: 2 mg/5 mL — 480 ml btl Tablet: 4 mg	Solution or tablet: Children < 2 yr: not recommended 2–6 yr: 0.5 mg/kg/24 hr in 3–4 divided doses; do not exceed 6 mg/24 hr >6 yr: 2–4 mg/dose 3–4 times/day Ex-tab: Children < 6 yr: not recommended >6 yr: 8 mg 2–3 times/day	
Calcifediol	Capsule: 20 µg, 50 µg	**Chronic renal failure — dialysis patients:** *Initial:* 300–350 µg weekly (given daily or on alternate days)	Titrate by adjusting dose at 4-week intervals

Name (generic)	Available Preparations	Dosage	Special Considerations
Calcitonin	Injection: 400 units — vial	**Patients with normal calcium:** 20–100 µg daily or 50–200 µg on alternate days **Paget's disease:** IM or SC: Initial: 100 units daily Maintenance: 50 units/day or 50–100 units every 1–3 days **Hypercalcemia:** 4 units/kg every 12 hours; after 1–2 days may increase to 8 units/kg every 12 hours until more specific treatment is established	
Calcitriol	Capsule: 0.25 µg	Oral: individualize dosage to maintain Ca^{++} levels of 9–10 mg/dL; adjust dose at 4- to 8-week intervals **Renal failure:** Children: Initial: 15 ng/kg/day Maintenance: 5–40 ng/kg/day: 0.25–2 µg/day has been used (with hemodialysis); 0.014–0.041 µg/kg/day (not receiving hemodialysis) Adults: 0.25 µg daily or every other day; may require 0.5–1 µg daily **Hypoparathyroidism/pseudohypoparathyroidism:** Children < 1 year: 0.04–0.08 µg/kg/day Children > 1 year and Adults: 0.25 µg/day	Dose should be titrated to maintain Ca^{++} levels of 9–10 mg/dL; adjust dose at 4–8 week intervals

Name (generic)	Available Preparations	Dosage	Special Considerations
		Most children 1–5 years require 0.25–0.75 µg/day Most children > 6 years and adults require 0.5–2 µg/day **Hypocalcemia in premature infants:** 1 µg/day for 5 days **Vitamin D dependent rickets:** 1 µg/day **Vitamin D resistant rickets** (familial hypophosphatemia): 2 µg/day; initial: 15–20 ng/kg/day; maintenance: 30–60 ng/kg/day	
Calcium chloride	Injection: 100 mg/mL — 10 mL vial (27 mg/mL elemental calcium)	**Cardiac arrest:** Infants and children: 20 mg/kg/dose or 0.2 mL/kg/dose IV; may repeat in 10 minutes if necessary	**Do not administer IM or SC**
Calcium glubionate	Solution: 1.8 gm/5 mL — 16 oz btl	**Neonatal hypocalcemia:** 1,200 mg/kg/24 hr in 4–6 divided doses Children, *maintenance:* 600–2,000 mg/kg/24 hr in 4 divided doses to maximum of 9 gm/24 hr	115 mg elemental calcium per 5 mL
Calcium gluconate	Injection: 100 mg/mL — 10 mL vial (9 mg/mL elemental calcium)	**Cardiac arrest:** Infants and children: 100–200 mg/kg/dose **Hypocalcemic tetany:** Infants and children: 100–200 mg/kg/dose IV for 1 dose, then an infusion of 500 mg/kg/24 hr	
Calcium lactate	Tablet: 300 mg	**Maintenance (or mild hypocalcemia):** Infants: 400–500 mg/kg/24 hr in 3 to 4 divided doses	42 mg elemental calcium (18%) per tablet

Name (generic)	Available Preparations	Dosage	Special Considerations
Captopril	Tablet: 12.5 mg, 25 mg, 50 mg, 100 mg	See text	
Carbamazepine	Chew-tab: 100 mg Tablet: 200 mg	See text	**Discontinue if evidence of significant bone marrow depression**
Cefaclor	Capsule: 250 mg Suspension: 125 mg/5 mL — 75 and 150 mL btl 250 mg/5 mL — 75 and 150 mL btl	20–40 mg/kg/24 hr in 2–3 divided doses to a maximum of 2 gm/24 hr	
Cefazolin	Injection: 1 gm — vial	Infants > 1 month and children: 50–100 mg/kg/24 hr in 3 divided doses **Prophylaxis:** 40 mg/kg/24 hr in 3 divided doses for 1 day	2.4 mEq sodium per gm
Cefoxitin	Injection: 1 gm — vial	Neonates, < 1 week: 40 mg/kg/24 hr in 2 divided doses Children: 80–160 mg/kg/24 hr in 4 divided doses	2.3 mEq sodium per gm
Ceftazidime	Injection: 1 gm — vial	Neonates: 60 mg/kg/24 hr in 2 divided doses Infants and children: 100–150 mg kg/24 hr in 3 divided doses **Cystic fibrosis:** 300 mg/kg/24 hr	2.3 mEq sodium per gm
Ceftriaxone	Injection: 1 gm — vial	50–100 mg/kg/24 hr in 1 or 2 doses to a maximum of 4 gm/24 hr	3.6 mEq sodium per gm May be given IM or IV, qd or q12 hr No dosage adjustment is necessary for patients with impaired renal or hepatic function

Name (generic)	Available Preparations	Dosage	Special Considerations
Cephalexin	Capsule: 250 mg Suspension: 125 mg/5 mL — 100 mL and 200 mL btl 250 mg/5 mL — 100 mL and 200 mL btl	25–50 mg/kg/24 hr in 4 divided doses	
Chloral hydrate	Capsule: 250 mg, 500 mg Solution: 500 mg/5 mL — 16 oz btl	Oral or rectal, **sedative:** 15–25 mg/kg/dose to a maximum of 2 gm/dose **Hypnotic:** 50 mg/kg/dose	When given orally, the solution should be well diluted with water or milk
Chloramphenicol	Capsule: 250 mg Injection: 1 gm — vial Ophthal oint: 1% — 3.5 gm tube Ophthal sol: 0.5% — 7.5 mL drop btl Suspension: 150 mg/5 mL — 60 ml btl	Premature infants, < 4 weeks: 25 mg/kg/24 hr in 2 divided doses Term infants, < 1 week: 25 mg/kg/24 hr in 2 divided doses Infants, 1–4 weeks: 50 mg/kg/24 hr in 2 divided doses Infants, > 4 weeks and children: 75 mg/kg/24 hr in 4 divided doses	Draw drug level at 1 hr postdose and adjust dosage as necessary Therapeutic range: 15–25 μg/mL
Chloroquine phosphate	Tablet: 250 mg (= 150 mg base), 500 mg (= 300 mg base)	Dosage calculated using base **Amebiasis:** 10 mg/kg/24 hr qd to a maximum of 300 mg/24 hr for 21 days **Malaria, treatment:** 10 mg/kg once, to a maximum of 600 mg/dose, then 5 mg/kg qd for 2 days **Malaria, prophylaxis:** 5 mg/kg once a week to a maximum of 300 mg/dose; begin 1 week before and for the duration of exposure and continue for the following 6 weeks.	Parenteral form not recommended Administer with food

Name (generic)	Available Preparations	Dosage	Special Considerations
Chlorothiazide	Injection: 500 mg — 20 mL vial Suspension: 250 mg/5 mL — 8 oz btl	Children < 6 mo, oral: 30 mg/kg/24 hr in 2 divided doses > 6 mo: 20 mg/kg/24 hr in 2 divided doses	
Chlorpheniramine	Capsule: 8 mg, 12 mg Solution: 2 mg/5 mL — 230 mL btl Tablet: 4 mg	Solution or tablet: 0.35 mg/kg/24 hr in 4–6 divided doses Capsule: 0.2 mg/kg/24 hr bid-tid	
Chlorpromazine	Conc sol: 30 mg/mL — 120 mL btl Injection: 25 mg/mL — 1 mL ampul Solution: 10 mg/5 mL — 120 mL btl Suppository: 25 mg Tablet: 10 mg, 25 mg, 50 mg	Parenteral, IM: 1.5–2.0 mg/kg/24 hr in 4–6 divided doses Oral: 2 mg/kg/24 hr in 4–6 divided doses Rectal: 2–4 mg/kg/24 hr in 3–4 divided doses	SC injection is not advised The IV route is only for severe hiccups and surgery
Cholestyramine	Powder: 9 gm u/d pkt (440 mg/gm powder)	Children, < 6 yr: Initiate therapy with small doses and adjust as needed; no dose has been established > 6 yr: 240 mg/kg/24 hr in 3–4 divided doses	Do not take in dry form. Mix with water or other fluids May bind with other drugs given concurrently
Cimetidine	Injection: 150 mg/mL — 2 mL vial Solution: 300 mg/5 mL — 237 mL btl Tablet: 200 mg, 300 mg	20–40 mg/kg/24 hr in 4 divided doses	
Ciprofloxacin hydrochloride	Tablet: 250 mg Injection: 2 mg/mL (20 mL)	Children: 20–30 mg/kg/day in 2 divided doses	Dilute to 1–2 mg/mL; infuse over 60 minutes

Name (generic)	Available Preparations	Dosage	Special Considerations
Clindamycin	Capsule: 150 mg Injection: 150 mg/mL — 6 mL vial Top sol: 1% — 60 mL btl	Parenteral, IM or IV: Neonates, < 1 mo: 15–20 mg/kg/24 hr in 3 divided doses Children, > 1 mo: 15–40 mg/kg/24 hr in 3–4 divided doses Oral: Children, > 1 mo: 10–25 mg/kg/24 hr in 3–4 divided doses	Not recommended in children < 18 years of age; modify dosage in patients with renal impairment
Clonazepam	Tablet: 500 µg, 1 mg, 2 mg	Children: 10–30 µg/kg/24 hr in 2–3 divided doses to a maximum of 50 µg/kg/24 hr	
Clotrimazole	Top cream: 1% — 30 gm tube Vag cream: 1% — 45 gm tube Top sol: 1% — 30 mL squz btl Vag supp: 100 mg, 500 mg	Vaginal cream: 1 applicatorful at bedtime for 7–14 days Vaginal supp: 1 suppository intravaginally at bedtime for 7 days or 2 at bedtime for 3 days (only if not pregnant)	
Codeine	Injection: 30 mg/mL — 1 mL vial Solution: 15 mg/5 mL — 500 mL btl Tablet: 15 mg, 30 mg	**Analgesic:** 0.05–1 mg/kg PO or IM q3–4h **Antitussive:** 1–1.5 mg/kg/day in 4–6 divided doses	
Cosyntropin	Injection: 250 µg — vial	Children, < 2 yr: 125 µg Children, > 2 yr: 250 µg	Administered as single dose over 2 minutes; may need retest
Cromolyn sodium	Capsule: 20 mg Inhal sol: 20 mg/2 mL — 60/box	Children, > 2 yr: capsule: 20 mg via spin-haler inhaled qid	

Name (generic)	Available Preparations	Dosage	Special Considerations
	Inhal oral: 800 μg/spray (8.1 gm)	Children, > 2 yr: solution: 20 mg by nebulizer qid	
Cyanocobalamin	Injection: 100 μg/mL — 1 mL syringe and 10 mL vial; 1 mg — 1 mL syringe and 10 mL vial	**Vitamin B$_{12}$ deficiency:** 100 μg qd for 10 days followed by 100 μg monthly maintenance	
Cyclosporine	Capsules: 25 mg, 100 mg Injection: 50 mg/mL Solution, oral: 100 mg/mL (50 mL)	Children and Adults: Cyclosporine doses should be adjusted to maintain whole blood HPLC trough concentrations between 100–200 ng/mL *Oral:* Initial: 14–18 mg/kg/dose daily beginning 4–12 hours before organ transplantation Maintenance: 5–10 mg/kg/day *IV:* Initial: 1–6 mg/kg/day in divided doses every 12 hours	Protect IV solution from light; use contents of oral solution within 2 months after opening Do not administer liquid from plastic or styrofoam cups; mixing with milk, chocolate milk, or orange juice, preferably at room temperature, improves palatability; stir well and drink at once, do not allow to stand before drinking; rinse with more diluent to ensure that the total dose is taken; after use, dry outside of pipette; do not rinse with water or other cleaning agents
Cyproheptadine	Solution: 2 mg/5 mL — 16 oz btl Tablet: 4 mg	Children, 2–14 yr: 0.25 mg/kg/24 hr in 2–3 divided doses; do not exceed 12 mg/24 hr	
Dantrolene	Capsule: 25 mg, 50 mg Injection: 20 mg — vial Suspension: 25 mg/5 mL — 120 mL btl	**Chronic spasticity:** Oral: Initiate 0.5 mg/kg bid, increase by 0.5 mg/kg up to as high as 3 mg/kg 3–4 times a day	Monitor liver function including frequent AST or ALT Safety of dantrolene has not been established in children < 5 yr **Concurrent use of MAO inhibitors contraindicated**

583

Name (generic)	Available Preparations	Dosage	Special Considerations
		Malignant hyperthermia: IV: Rapid IV push of 1 mg/kg and continuing until symptoms subside or the maximum cumulative dose of 10 mg/kg has been reached **Preoperatively (in susceptible individuals):** Oral: 4–8 mg/kg/24 hr in 3–4 divided doses for 1–2 days before surgery **Postcrisis:** Oral: 4–8 mg/kg/24 hr in 4 divided doses for 1–3 days to prevent recurrence of the manifestations of malignant hyperthermia	
Deferoxamine	Injection: 500 mg — vial	Children: Acute iron intoxication: IV: 15 mg/kg/hour continuous infusion; maximum: 6 gm/24 hours Chronic iron overload: IM: 20–25 mg/kg/day IV: 500 mg to 2 gm with each unit of blood transfused SC: 20–40 mg/kg/day over 8–12 hours	
Demerol compound*	Injection: 1 mL and 2 mL — syringe (special prep) combination product	0.1 mL/kg to a maximum of 2 mL	Each mL contains: Meperidine, 25 mg Chlorpromazine, 6.25 mg Promethazine, 6.25 mg

Name (generic)	Available Preparations	Dosage	Special Considerations
Desmopressin (DDAVP)	Solution: 100 μg/mL — 2.5 mL drop btl Injection: 4 μg/mL — 10 mL vial	Diabetes insipidus: 3 months to 12 years: Intranasal: 2.5–30 μg/day in 1 or 2 divided doses; allow diuretic phase between doses to avoid water intoxication Hemophilia: > 3 months: IV: 0.3 μg/kg by slow infusion 30 minutes preop Nocturnal enuresis: ≥ 6 years: Intranasal: Initial: 20 μg at bedtime; range: 10–40 μg	Titrate dose to achieve control of excessive thirst and urination
Dexamethasone	Injection: 4 mg/mL — 1 mL syringe and 5 mL vial Ophthal oint: 0.05% — 3.5 gm tube Ophthal sol: 0.1% — 5 mL drop btl Solution: 500 μg/5 mL — 10 mL u/d and 120 mL btl Tablet: 500 μg, 1.5 mg, 4 mg Turbinaire: 0.142% — 12.6 gm aerosol	**Antiinflammatory or immunosuppressive:** 0.03–0.2 mg/kg/24 hr in 2–4 divided doses **Cerebral edema:** *Initial:* 1.5 mg/kg/dose *Maintenance:* 1.5 mg/kg/24 hr in 4 divided doses for 5 days; taper slowly over the next 5 days and discontinue **Airway edema:** 0.25–0.5 mg/kg/dose qid as needed for croup or beginning 24 hr before planned extubation, then continue for 4–6 doses **Shock:** 3–6 mg/kg/dose q4–6h for a maximum of 48–72 hr	

585

Name (generic)	Available Preparations	Dosage	Special Considerations
Dextroamphetamine sulfate	Capsule: 10 mg, 15 mg Tablet: 5 mg	**Hyperkinesis, attention deficit:** Children, > 6 yr: 5 mg in morning for 2 days; then 5 mg in morning and at noon for 2 days; increase by 5 mg/day at 2–4 days interval to gain optimal response Dose range: 5–80 mg/24 hr Children, 3–6 yr: use ½ of the above dose	Not recommended for treatment of hyperkinesis, attention deficit in children < 3 yr
Diazepam	Injection: 5 mg/mL — 2 mL syringe Tablet: 2 mg, 5 mg	Children: Sedation or muscle relaxation: Oral: 0.12–0.8 mg/kg/day in divided doses every 6–8 hours IM, IV: 0.04–0.3 mg/kg/dose every 2–4 hours; maximum: 0.6 mg/kg within an 8-hour period if needed Status epilepticus: IV Infants ≥ 1 month and Children ≤ 5 years: 0.05–0.5 mg/kg/dose every 15–30 minutes to a maximum total dose of 5 mg, repeat in 2–4 hours as needed Children > 5 years: 0.05–0.3 mg/kg/dose every 15–30 minutes to a maximum total dose of 10 mg, repeat in 2–4 hours as needed **or** 1 mg every 2–5 minutes to a maximum of 10 mg	**Rapid IV injection may cause apnea** IV rate should not exceed 5 mg/min Do not mix diazepam with other drugs or IV solutions Diazepam injection is not approved for use in infants < 30 days of age

Name (generic)	Available Preparations	Dosage	Special Considerations
Diazoxide	Injection: 15 mg/mL — 20 mL ampul Suspension: 50 mg/mL — 30 mL btl	**Hypertensive crisis:** Parenteral: Children: 3–5 mg/kg dose IV push within 30 sec; repeat in 20 min if no effect observed; then, q3–10h as needed **Hyperinsulinemic hypoglycemia:** Oral: Infants and Newborns: 8–15 mg/kg/24 hr in 2–3 divided doses Children: 3–8 mg/kg/24 hr in 2–3 divided doses	
Dicloxacillin	Capsule: 125 mg, 250 mg, 500 mg Suspension: 62.5 mg/5 mL, 100 mL, and 200 mL btl	25–50 mg/kg/24 hr in 4 divided doses **Osteomyelitis:** Up to 100 mg/kg/24 hr in 4 divided doses	Disagreeable taste limits use of suspension
Digoxin	Injection: 100 µg/mL — 1 mL ampul; 250 µg/mL — 2 mL ampul Solution: 50 µg/mL — 2 oz drop btl Tablet: 125 µg, 250 µg	*Digitalization* is accomplished by giving 50%, 25% and 25% of total digitalizing dose at 8–12 hr intervals *Maintenance* doses are divided in 2 doses approximately 12 hr apart	Maximum dose in children: 0.25 mg/24 hr Digoxin should be ordered in "mg" doses carried to not more than 2 decimal places The oral solution should be ordered in "mL" followed by "mg" in parentheses

Oral Digoxin Doses

Age	Total digitalizing dose/kg/24 hr	Maintenance dose/kg/24 hr
Premature	0.03–0.04 mg/kg	0.0075–0.01 mg/kg
Term newborn	0.04–0.05 mg/kg	0.01–0.013 mg/kg
Infants, < 2 yr	0.06–0.08 mg/kg	0.015–0.02 mg/kg
Children, > 2 yr	0.04–0.06 mg/kg	0.01–0.015 mg/kg

Name (generic)	Available Preparations	Dosage	Special Considerations
Dimenhydrinate (Dramamine)	Injection: 50 mg/mL — 1 mL cart Tablet: 50 mg	Parenteral, IM: 5 mg/kg/24 hr in 4 divided doses Oral: 5 mg/kg/24 hr in 4 divided doses	Injection must be further diluted for IV use with 10 mL 0.9% sodium chloride and injected over a period of 2 min
Dimercaprol	Injection: 100 mg/mL — 3 mL ampul	**Lead toxicity, IM:** **Moderate poisoning:** 2 mg/kg/dose 6 times a day or up to 12 mg/24 hr for 2–3 days **Severe poisoning:** 4 mg/kg/dose 6 times a day for 5–7 days **Arsenic, mercury, or gold toxicity, IM:** **Mild:** Days 1 and 2: 3 mg/kg/dose qid Day 3: 3 mg/kg/dose bid Days 4–14: 3 mg/kg/dose qd **Severe:** Days 1 and 2: 3 mg/kg/dose 6 times a day Day 3: 3 mg/kg/dose qid Days 4–14: 3 mg/kg/dose bid	

Dimetapp*	Tablet: combination product
	Solution: 4 oz btl
		Solution: Children, 1–6 mo: 1.25 mL tid–qid
		2–4 yr: 3.75 mL tid–qid
		4–12 yr: 5 mL tid–qid
		>12 yr: 5–10 mL tid–qid
		Tablet: Children > 12 yr: 1 tablet bid
			Contains:
			
			       Per Per
			       Ex-tab 5 mL
			Brompheniramine 12 mg 2 mg
			Phenylpropa-
			  nolamine 75 mg 12.5

Diphenhydramine	Capsule: 25 mg, 50 mg Injection: 50 mg/mL — 1 mL syringe	5 mg/kg/24 hr in 4 divided doses; do not exceed 300 mg/24 hr	**Concurrent use of MAO inhibitors is contraindicated**

Name (generic)	Available Preparations	Dosage	Special Considerations
Dobutamine	Solution: 12.5 mg/5 mL — 4 oz btl Injection: 250 mg — vial	2.5–15.0 µg/kg/min based on patient's response	Dilute in D_5W or NS to 250–1,000 µg/mL Inactivated by alkaline (e.g., sodium bicarbonate) solutions **Concurrent administration with mineral oil is contraindicated**
Docusate sodium (Colace)	Capsule: 50 mg, 100 mg Conc sol: 10 mg/mL — 30 mL drop btl Syrup: 4 mg/mL	Infants and children < 3 yr: 10–40 mg/24 hr in 1–4 divided doses 3–6 yr: 20–60 mg/24 hr in 1–4 divided doses 6–12 yr: 40–120 mg/24 hr in 1–4 divided doses Adolescents: 50–200 mg/24 hr in 1–4 divided doses	
Docusate and casanthranol (Peri-Colace)	Capsule: Combination product Solution: 16 oz btl	Syrup: 5–10 mL at bedtime	Contains: Per Cap / Per 5 mL Docusate 100 mg / 20 mg Casanthranol 30 mg / 10 mg
Dopamine	Parenteral sol: 40 mg/mL	3–20 µg/kg/min IV; titrate to desired response	Inactivated by alkaline (e.g., sodium bicarbonate) solutions
Doxycycline	Capsule: 50 mg, 100 mg, 300 mg Tablets: 100 mg Oral sol: 50 mg/5 mL Parenteral: 100, 200 mg/mL	Children ≥ 8 yrs: 2–4 mg/kg/day in 1–2 divided doses	Do not exceed 200 mg/day

Name (generic)	Available Preparations	Dosage	Special Considerations
Droperidol	Injection: 2.5 mg/mL	**Premedication or induction of anesthesia:** Children, 2–12 yr: IM or IV: 0.09–0.165 mg/kg	Dosage should be individualized according to patient's age, weight, physical status, underlying pathogenic condition, and other drugs, and the type of anesthesia used
Edetate calcium disodium (EDTA)	Injection: 200 mg/mL	**Mild to moderate lead poisoning:** 25–50 mg/kg **Severe lead poisoning:** up to 75 mg/kg/24 hr not to exceed 1.5 gm daily **Usual dosage:** Children: Asymptomatic lead toxicity: Initial: Up to 50 mg/kg/24 hours in a continuous IV drip if possible or in 2–4 divided doses for 5 days Subsequent courses: Up to 50 mg/kg/24 hours in a continuous IV drip if possible or in 2–4 divided doses for 3–5 days Symptomatic lead toxicity or lead encephalopathy: Initial: Up to 75 mg/kg/24 hours in a continuous IV drip if possible or in 6 divided doses for 5–7 days; give with dimercaprol (BAL) Subsequent courses: As for asymptomatic toxicity above	

Name (generic)	Available Preparations	Dosage	Special Considerations
Edrophonium (Tensilon)	Injection: 10 mg/mL	**Myasthenia gravis test:** 0.2 mg/kg as a single dose IV: Infants: Initial: 0.1 mg; if no response follow with an additional 0.4 mg for a maximum total dose of 0.5 mg Children: Diagnosis: Initial: 0.04 mg/kg followed by 0.16 mg/kg; if no response; maximum total dose: 10 mg Titration of therapy: 0.04 mg/kg one time; if strength improves, an increase in neostigmine or pyridostigmine dose is indicated Reversal of nondepolarizing neuromuscular blocking agents: 1 mg/kg/dose	**May precipitate cholinergic crisis**
Epinephrine	1:1,000 (aqueous): 1 mg/mL 1:200 (Susphrine*): 5 mg/mL 2.25% (racemic) 1:10,000 (aqueous): 100 µg/mL	1:1,000 (aqueous): 0.01 mL/kg/dose SC (max. single dose 0.3 mL) 1:200 (Susphrine*): 0.005 mL/kg/dose SC (max. single dose 0.15 mL) 2.25% (racemic): 0.05 mL/kg; 1 dose diluted to 3 mL with 0.9% NaCl via nebulizer 1:10,000: 0.1 mL/kg; 1 dose; may be given via endotracheal tube	

Name (generic)	Available Preparations	Dosage	Special Considerations
Erythromycin	Erythromycin ethylsuccinate: Susp: 200, 400 mg/5 mL Drops: 100 mg/2.5 mL Tabs: 200 mg, 400 mg Erythromycin lactobionate: Vials: 500 mg, 1,000 mg Erythromycin estolate: Tabs: 500 mg Chewable tabs: 125 mg, 250 mg Drops: 100 mg/mL Capsules: 125 mg, 250 mg Susp: 125, 250 mg/5 mL Erythromycin stearate: Tabs: 125 mg, 250 mg, 500 mg	Parenteral, IV: 20–40 mg/kg/24 hr in 4 divided doses Oral: 30–50 mg/kg/24 hr in 4 divided doses	GI side effects common May cause elevated digoxin, theophylline, and carbamazepine levels Estolate causes hepatotoxicity in adults but rarely in children
Esmolol	Solution: 100 mg/vial	0.5 mg/kg bolus; infusion of 50–200 µg/kg/min	
Ethacrynic acid	Injection: 50 mg — vial Tablet: 25 mg	Parenteral, IV: 0.5–1.0 mg/kg/dose Oral: 25 mg/24 hr; increase in 25 mg increments every 2–3 days as needed to a maximum of 2–3 mg/kg/24 hr	
Ethambutol	Tablet: 100 mg, 400 mg	Children, > 12 yr: 15–25 mg/kg/24 hr as a single daily dose	Not recommended for children < 12 yr
Ethosuximide	Capsule: 250 mg Solution: 250 mg/5 mL	Children > 6 yr, initial: 250 mg/24 hr in 2 divided doses Maintenance: Increase dose by 250 mg every 4–7 days to maximum of 1.5 gm/24 hr	Collect blood sample at steady state (6–24 hr after dose) The ideal serum concentration is 40–100 µg/mL

Name (generic)	Available Preparations	Dosage	Special Considerations
Fentanyl		Children: Sedation for minor procedures/analgesic: 1–3 years: IM. 2–3 µg/kg/dose, may repeat after 30 minutes to 1 hour; IV: 0.2–0.5 µg/kg/dose 3–12 years: IM: 1–2 µg/kg/dose, repeat after 30 minutes to 1 hour; IV: 0.5–1 µg/kg/dose Continuous analgesic: 1–3 µg/kg/hour	
Ferrous gluconate (11.6% Fe)	Solution: 300 mg (35 mg Fe/5 mL) Tablet: 320 mg (37 mg Fe) Capsule: 325 mg (38 mg Fe) Capsule (SR): 435 mg (50 mg Fe)	See Ferrous sulfate	
Ferrous sulfate (20% Fe)	Drops: 75 mg (15 mg Fe/0.6 mL) Syrup: 90 mg (18 mg Fe/5 mL) Elixir 220 mg (44 mg Fe/5 mL) Tablet: 300 mg (60 mg elemental Fe)	**Therapeutic:** 6 mg/kg/24 hr (elemental iron) in divided doses tid **Prophylaxis:** Preterm infant: 2 mg/kg/24 hr (elemental iron) in divided doses q8–12h Term infant: 1 mg/kg/24 hr (elemental iron) in divided doses q8–12h	
Folic acid	Injection: 5 mg/mL Oral sol: 250 µg/5 mL Tablet: 1 mg	1 mg daily regardless of age	

Name (generic)	Available Preparations	Dosage	Special Considerations
Furosemide	Injection: 10 mg/mL Oral sol: 10 mg/mL Tablet: 20 mg, 40 mg, 80 mg	Premature newborns: Parenteral, IM or IV: 1–2 mg/kg/dose q12–24h Oral: Not recommended Infants and children: Parenteral, IM or IV: 1 mg/kg/dose q2h; may increase by 1–2 mg/kg/dose after 2 hr to a maximum of 6 mg/kg/dose qd–bid Oral: 2 mg/kg/dose of q6–8 hr; increase by 1–2 mg/kg/dose after 6–8 hr to a maximum of 6 mg/kg/dose qd–bid	May cause hypokalemic metabolic alkalosis and volume depletion Prolonged use in premature infants may result in nephrocalcinosis
Gamma benzene hexachloride	Shampoo: 1% Lotion: 1% Cream: 1%	Shampoo: use ≤ 30 mL/application Lotion: apply to skin, leave on for 12–24 hr, then wash off	
Gentamicin	Injection: 10 mg/mL, 40 mg/mL Intrathecal: 2 mg/mL Ophthal oint: 0.3% Ophthal sol: 0.3%	Neonates, < 1 week: 5 mg/kg/24 hr in 2 divided doses >1 week: 7.5 mg/kg/24 hr in 3 divided doses Children, < 5 yr: 7.5 mg/kg/24 hr in 3 divided doses 5–10 yr: 6 mg/kg/24 hr in 3 divided doses >10 yr: 4.5 mg/kg/24 hr in 3 divided doses Ophthal oint: Apply bid–tid Ophthal sol, **severe infection:** up to 2 drops every hr **Mild infection:** 1–2 drops 6 times a day	Allowable predose level: < 2 μg/mL Allowable 1-hr postdose range: 4–8 μg/mL

Name (generic)	Available Preparations	Dosage	Special Considerations
Gentian violet	Solution: 1%	**Oral moniliasis:** Apply tid for 3 days	
Glucagon	Injection: 1 mg/mL	Neonates: 0.03 mg/kg/dose q4h as needed Children: 0.03–0.1 mg/kg/dose, repeated in 20 min as needed	Do not exceed 1 mg/dose
Griseofulvin, microsize	Suspension: 125 mg/5 mL Tablet: 125 mg, 250 mg, 500 mg	Children: 10 mg/kg/24 hr in 2–4 divided doses with meals	
Guaifenesin (Robitussin)	Solution: 100 mg/5 mL — 8 oz btl	Children, 2–5 yr: 2.5–5.0 mL 6 times a day Children > 5 yr: 5–10 mL 6 times a day	
Guanethidine	Tablet: 10 mg, 25 mg	Infants and newborns: Not recommended Children, *Initial:* 0.2 mg/kg/24 hr; increase by 0.2 mg/kg/24 hr every 7–10 days; *maximum:* 3 mg/kg/24 hr	Orthostatic hypotension can occur frequently
Haloperidol	Conc sol: 2 mg/mL Injection: 5 mg/mL Tablet: 1 mg, 2 mg, 5 mg, 10 mg	Children: Oral: 3–12 years: Agitation or hyperkinesia: 0.01–0.03 mg/kg/day once daily Tourette's disorder: 0.05–0.75 mg/kg/day in 2–3 divided doses Psychotic disorders: 0.05–0.15 mg/kg/day in 2–3 divided doses IM: 1–3 mg/dose every 4–8 hours; maximum, 0.1 mg/kg/day	Dose should be individually adjusted to patient Not recommended for children < 3 yr of age Oral dosage range is 2–100 mg/24 hr

Name (generic)	Available Preparations	Dosage	Special Considerations
Heparin sodium	Injection: 10 units/mL, 1,000 units/mL Vial: 20,000 units/mL	Infants and children: *Initial:* 50 units/kg IV bolus *Maintenance:* 15–25 units/kg/hr as continuous infusion	
Hepatitis B immune globulin	Injections: 5 mL — vial	IM: 0.06 mL/kg to a maximum of 3–5 mL, given within 7 days of exposure	Indicated for postexposure prophylaxis only Administer by deep IM injection only
Hydralazine	Injection: 20 mg/mL Tablet: 10 mg, 25 mg, 50 mg, 100 mg	**Hypertensive crisis:** Parenteral, IM, or IV: 0.1–0.2 mg/kg/dose 4–6 times a day **Chronic hypertension:** Oral: 0.75–1 mg/kg/24 hr in 2–4 divided doses	
Hydrochlorothiazide	Tablet: 25 mg, 50 mg, 100 mg	Infants, < 6 months: 2–3 mg/kg/24 hr in 2 divided doses Children: 2 mg/kg/24 hr in 2 divided doses	
Hydrocortisone	Cream: 0.5%, 1% Injection: 50 mg/mL Ointment: 1% Oral Susp: 10 mg/5 mL Tablet: 5 mg, 10 mg, 20 mg	**Physiologic replacement:** IM or IV: 0.25–0.35 mg/kg/day once daily Oral: 0.5–0.75 mg/kg/day in 3–4 divided doses	See text
Hydrocortisone acetate	Injection: 50 mg/mL — 10 mL vial Tablet: 25 mg	**Antiinflammatory or immunosuppressive:** Parenteral, IM: 1–5 mg/kg/24 hr in 1–2 divided doses Oral: 2.5–10 mg/kg/24 hr in 3–4 divided doses **Physiologic replacement:** Parenteral, IM: 0.25–0.35 mg/kg/24 hr	

Name (generic)	Available Preparations	Dosage	Special Considerations
Hydroxychloroquine	Tablet: 200 mg	Oral: 0.5–0.75 mg/kg/24 hr in 3 divided doses	
Hydroxyzine	Tablet: 10 mg, 25 mg, 50 mg, 100 mg Capsule: 25 mg, 50 mg, 100 mg Syrup: 10 mg/5 mL Suspension: 25 mg/5 mL Vials: 25, 50 mg/mL	Oral: 2–4 mg/kg/24 hr in divided doses q6h Parenteral: 0.5–1.0 mg/kg/dose q4–6h IM as needed	For IM administration in children, injections should be made in the midlateral muscles of the thigh
Ibuprofen	Tablet: 200, 400, 600, 800 mg	Oral: Fever: 20 mg/kg/day in 3 divided doses Oral: JRA: 35 mg/kg/24 hr in 4 divided doses	
Imipenem/cliastatin (Primaxin)	Injection: 500 mg	IV infusion: Dosage recommendation based on imipenem component: Children < 12 years: 60–100 mg/kg/day in 4 divided doses Dosing adjustment with renal impairment: See table	Final concentration should not exceed 5 mg/mL; infused over 30–60 minutes Contains 3.2 mEq of sodium per gram

Creatinine Clearance mL/min/1.73 m^3	Frequency	% Decrease in Daily Maximum Dose
30–70	q6h	50
20–30	q8h	63
5–20	q12h	75

Name (generic)	Available Preparations	Dosage	Special Considerations
Imipramine	Tablet: 10 mg, 25 mg, 50 mg	**Depression:** *Initial:* 0.5 mg/kg/24 hr for 2–3 days; increase by 0.5 mg/kg/24 hr every 1–2 weeks **Enuresis:** 0.5–2.0 mg/kg/24 hr	Not recommended for children < 6 yr; except for enuresis
Immune globulin IM (gamma globulin)	Injection: 2 mL — vial	**Hepatitis A case contacts:** 0.02 mL/kg/dose **Travelers:** 0.02–0.05 mL/kg/dose (dependent on length of stay) **Immunoglobulin deficiency:** 0.6 mL/kg/dose given every 3–4 weeks; double dose at onset of therapy; some patients may require more frequent injections	Administer by deep IM injection only
Immune globulin IV	Injection: 3 gm — vial; 6 gm — vial	**Immunodeficiency syndrome:** 0.2 mg/kg/dose by IV infusion once a month **Idiopathic thrombocytopenic purpura (ITP)** **Kawasaki disease:** 400 mg/kg/dose by IV infusion on 5 consecutive days	
Indomethacin	Capsule: 25 mg, 50 mg Injection: 1 mg vial	**Closure of ductus arteriosus:** IV only; a course of therapy is 3 IV doses given at 12–24 hr intervals; dosage according to age is as follows: < 48 hr: 1st dose: 0.2 mg/kg 2nd dose: 0.1 mg/kg 3rd dose: 0.1 mg/kg	Administer oral doses with food or milk Insufficient data to recommend an oral dose for patients < 14 yr of age Monitor renal and hepatic function before and during use

Name (generic)	Available Preparations	Dosage	Special Considerations
		2–7 day: 1st dose: 0.2 mg/kg 2nd dose: 0.2 mg/kg 3rd dose: 0.2 mg/kg > 7 day: 1st dose: 0.2 mg/kg 2nd dose: 0.25 mg/kg 3rd dose: 0.25 mg/kg **Arthritis:** 0.5–2.0 mg/kg/24 hr PO in 3 divided doses	
Ipecac syrup	Solution: 1.4 mg/mL	Children, < 1 yr: 5–10 mL followed by 200 mL water > 1 yr: 15 mL followed by 200 mL water; repeat once in 20 min *only* if no emesis occurs	If emesis does not occur within 30 min of initial dose, ipecac must be removed via gastric lavage
Iron dextran	Injection: 50 mg/mL	Individualized doses according to weight are recommended *Maximum daily dose:* Infants, < 5 kg: 0.5 mL Children, < 10 kg: 1 mL >10 kg: 2 mL	Inject IM by "Z" technique and never inject into the arm or other exposed areas
Isoetharine	Solution: 1%	0.25–0.5 mL diluted to 2 mL in NS nebulized up to 6 times a day as needed	
Isoniazid	Injection: 100 mg/mL — 10 mL vial Tablet: 50 mg, 100 mg, 300 mg Syrup: 50 mg/mL	**Active tuberculosis:** 10–20 mg/kg/24 hr in 1–2 divided doses **Prophylaxis:** 10 mg/kg/24 hr given daily	Follow LFTs; supplemental pyridoxine (1–2 mg/kg/day) is recommended
Isoproterenol HCl	Injection: 200 μg/mL — 5 mL ampul	Parenteral: 0.05–2 μg/kg/min; increase slowly if necessary	

Name (generic)	Available Preparations	Dosage	Special Considerations
	Solution: 0.5%–10 mL btl Oral inhal: 0.25%–22.5 mL aerosol (Mistometer)	Oral inhal: 1–2 puffs q6h Aerosol: 0.01 mL/kg/dose diluted in 2 mL NS q4h as needed	
Kanamycin sulfate	Capsule: 500 mg Injection: 250 mg/mL — 2 mL vial	Parenteral: IM or IV: Newborn < 1 week and < 2 kg: 15 mg/kg/24 hr in 2 divided doses < 1 week and > 2 kg: 20 mg/kg/24 hr in 2 divided doses > 1 week and < 2 kg: 20 mg/kg/24 hr in 2 divided doses > 1 week and > 2 kg: 30 mg/kg/24 hr in 3 divided doses Children: 30 mg/kg/24 hr in 3 divided doses to a maximum of 1.5 gm/24 hr	Administer IV over 30–60 min Follow serum levels
Ketoconazole	Tablet: 200 mg	Children, < 20 kg: 50 mg daily 20–40 kg: 100 mg daily > 40 kg: 200 mg daily	Closely monitor patients for liver toxicity
Lactase	Solution: 16,000 units/mL — drop btl	Add 4–10 drops per quart of milk depending on level of lactose conversion desired	Each 5 drop dosage contains not less than 1,000 nlu (neutral lactase units) of beta D-galactosidase derived from *Kluyveromyces lactis* yeast 4–5 drops hydrolyzes approximately 70% of the lactose in 1 quart of milk at refrigerator temperature, at 42°F (6°C) in 24 hr, or will do the same in 2 hr at 85°F (30°C); additional time and/or enzyme required for 100% lactose conversion

Name (generic)	Available Preparations	Dosage	Special Considerations
Lactulose	Solution: 3.3 gm/5 mL — 30 mL u/d and 64 oz btl	Infants: 2.5–10 mL/24 hr in 3–4 divided doses Children and adolescents: 40–90 mL/24 hr in 3–4 divided doses Chronic therapy: 30–45 mL 3–4 times a day	1 quart of milk contains approximately 50 gm lactose Titrate dose to produce 2–3 soft stools per day
Levothyroxine sodium	Injection: 200 µg — vial Tablet: 25 µg, 50 µg, 100 µg, 150 µg, and 200 µg	Children: Oral: 0–6 months: 8–10 µg/kg/day 6–12 months: 6–8 µg/kg/day 1–5 years: 5–6 µg/kg/day 6–12 years: 4–5 µg/kg/day >12 years: 2–3 µg/kg/day IV, IM: 75% of the oral dose	
Lidocaine	Injection: 0.5% — 50 mL vial; 1% — 2 mL, 5 mL, and 30 mL ampul; 2% — 2 mL ampul; 20 mg/mL — 5 mL syringe; 40 mg/mL and 50 mL vial Jelly: 2% — 30 mL tube Ointment: 5% — 35 gm tube Top sol: 4% — 50 mL btl Oral viscous sol: 2% — 100 mL squz btl	Parenteral, **antiarrhythmic:** *Loading dose:* 1 mg/kg/dose IV push; may repeat in 10 min to desired effect or for total 3 doses *Maintenance:* 20–50 µg/kg/min infusion Oral solution: Children, < 3 yr: 2.5 mg 6–8 times a day > 3 yr: 5 mL 6–8 times a day	
Lindane	Cream: 1% — 60 gm tube Lotion: 1% — 60 mL btl Shampoo: 1% — 60 mL btl	Cream and lotion: apply and leave on 8–12 hr, then wash off thoroughly; may repeat in 1 week, if necessary	

Name (generic)	Available Preparations	Dosage	Special Considerations
		Shampoo: use 15–30 mL and lather for 4–5 min, then rinse thoroughly; may repeat in 1 week, if necessary	
Lithium carbonate	Capsule: 300 mg	Dosage should be individualized to the patient's response and serum levels. *Initial:* 300 mg bid; increase by 300 mg at 5–7 day interval with serum levels 4–5 days after dose change *Maintenance:* 300 mg tid or qid; adjust dose to achieve therapeutic levels; most clinicians recommend a steady state level between 0.5–1.5 mEq/L	Doses in children < 12 yr of age have not been established; however, The Children's Hospital recommendations are ½ the adult dosage (shown)
Lomotil*	Solution: 60 mL drop btl Tablet: 2.5 mg	Children, 2–5 yr: 2.5 mg 3 times a day 5–8 yr: 2.5 mg 4 times a day 8–12 yr: 2.5 mg 5 times a day	Contraindicated in children < 2 yr of age due to decreased margin safety Reduce dose as soon as initial control of symptoms is achieved Do not exceed recommended dose; if no response in 48 hr, Lomotil will not be effective Combination product: contains: diphenoxylate, 2.5 mg; atropine sulfate, 0.025 mg
Loperamide	Capsule: 2 mg	Acute diarrhea: 0.04–0.8 mg/kg/day in 2–4 divided doses Chronic diarrhea: 0.08–0.24 mg/kg/24 hr in 2–3 divided doses	Discontinue if no improvement seen in 48 hr Maximum dose = 2 mg No data on long-term use in children

Name (generic)	Available Preparations	Dosage	Special Considerations
			If more than 2–3 sprays/dose are required, give doses more frequently rather than in larger amounts Titrate dose to control excessive thirst and urination
Lorazepam	Injection: 2 mg/mL (1 mL, 10 mL); 4 mg/mL (1 mL, 10 mL) Tablet: 0.5 mg, 1 mg, 2 mg	Anxiety and sedation: Infants and Children: Oral, IV: Usual: 0.05 mg/kg/dose (range: 0.02–0.09 mg/kg) every 4–8 hours Adults: Oral: 1–10 mg/day in 2–3 divided doses: usual dose: 2–5 mg/day in divided doses Preoperative: Adults: IM: 0.05 mg/kg administered 2 hours before surgery: maximum: 4 mg/dose IV: 0.044 mg/kg 15–20 minutes before surgery: usual maximum: 2 mg/dose Status epilepticus: Slow IV Neonates: 0.05 mg/kg over 2–5 minutes; may repeat in 10–15 minutes (see Warnings regarding benzyl alcohol) Infants and Children: 0.1 mg/kg IV over 2–5 minutes, do not exceed 4 mg/single dose; may repeat second dose of 0.05 mg/kg IV in 10–15 minutes if needed	

Name (generic)	Available Preparations	Dosage	Special Considerations
Lypressin	Solution: 185 μg/mL — 8 mL squz btl	Adolescents: 0.07 mg/kg IV over 2–5 minutes; maximum: 4 mg/dose; may repeat in 10–15 minutes 1–2 nasal sprays qid and at bedtime	
Maalox	Suspension: 5 oz btl Tablet	See text	0.06 mEq (1.35 mg) sodium per 5 mL suspension 0.03 mEq (0.84 mg) sodium per tablet Acid neutralizing capacity of 2.7 mEq/mL or 8.5 mEq/tablet
Magnesium citrate	Solution: 10 oz btl	0.5 mL/kg (to a maximum of 200 mL)/dose; may repeat q4–6h until liquid stool results	Contraindicated in renal failure
Magnesium gluconate	Tablet: 500 mg	3–6 mg/kg/day; maximum: 400 mg/24 hr divided into 3–4 doses	27 mg elemental magnesium per tablet
Magnesium hydroxide	Suspension: 15 mL and 30 mL u/d, and 480 mL btl	0.5 mL/kg/dose	May change rate of absorption of orally administered drugs; thus, use caution when scheduling doses of other oral medication
Magnesium sulfate	Injection: 500 mg/mL — 2 mL vial (= 4 mEq/mL) Powder: 16 oz btl	**Hypomagnesemia:** Parenteral, IV, or IM: 25–50 mg/kg/dose 4–6 times a day for 3–4 doses; may repeat if hypomagnesemia persists **Anticonvulsant:** Parenteral, IV or IM: 20–40 mg/kg/dose **Cathartic:** Oral: 250 mg/kg/dose 4–6 times a day	Injection must be further diluted for IV use Contraindicated in renal failure

Name (generic)	Available Preparations	Dosage	Special Considerations
Malt soup extract (Maltsupex)	Powder: 16 oz btl Solution: 5.3 gm/5 mL — 16 oz jar	Infants, bottle fed: ½–2 heaping tbsp/day mixed in formula Breastfed: 1–2 tsp in 2–4 oz water or juice 1–2 times/day Children: 1–2 tbsp in 8 oz liquid 1–2 times/day	
Mannitol	Injection: 25%–50 mL vial	**Anuria or oliguria (test dose):** Children: 500–1,000 mg/kg/dose over 3–5 min **Neurosurgery preop:** 1.5–2.0 gm/kg infused over 30–60 min **Acute intracranial hypertension (cerebral edema):** 250 mg/kg IV push over 3–5 min as needed; response is better if furosemide is given concurrently with or 5 min before the first dose; dose may be increased to 1 gm/kg/dose	
Mebendazole	Chew-tab: 100 mg	**Pinworms:** 100 mg once; repeat in 2 weeks if not cured **Roundworms, whipworms, hookworms:** 100 mg bid for 3 days; repeat in 3 weeks if infestation persists	Dosing guidelines are for patients ≥ 2 yr of age
Meclizine HCl	Chew-tab: 25 mg	**Motion sickness** Children > 12 yr: 25–50 mg qd	May repeat dose q24h for duration of journey
Menadiol sodium diphosphate	Tablet: 5 mg	5 mg qd	Water-soluble vitamin K analogue

Name (generic)	Available Preparations	Dosage	Special Considerations
Meperidine	Injection: 50 mg/mL — 1 mL ampul; 100 mg/mL — 1 mL ampul Solution: 50 mg/5 mL — 16 oz btl Tablet: 50 mg	1–1.5 mg/kg/dose every 3–4 hours as needed; maximum: 100 mg/dose See also Table 1-1	Approximately 50% of an oral dose is absorbed When given IV may precipitate seizures in patients with seizure disorders
Mephenytoin	Tablet: 100 mg	3–15 mg/kg/24 hr in 3 divided doses	
Mephobarbital	Tablet: 30 mg, 50 mg, 100 mg	6–8 mg/kg given at bedtime	
Metaproterenol	Inhal sol: 5% — 10 mL drop btl Inhal powder: 1.5% — 15 mL aerosol inhaler Solution: 10 mg/5 mL — 16 oz btl Tablet: 10 mg, 20 mg	Children, < 6 yr: 1.3–2.6 mg/kg/24 hr in 3–4 divided doses 6–9 yr and < 27 kg: 10 mg tid–qid > 27 kg: 20 mg tid–qid	
Metaraminol bitartrate	Injection: 10 mg/mL — 1 mL ampul	IM: 0.1 mg/kg/dose as needed IV bolus: 0.01 mg/kg as needed IV drip: begin with 5 µg/kg/min	
Methadone	Injection: 10 mg/mL — 1 mL ampul Solution: 1 mg/mL — 500 mL btl	**Analgesia:** SC or oral: 0.1–0.15 mg/kg/dose given every 4 hours	Antitussive dose is ¼ the analgesic dose
Methenamine mandelate	Tablet: 5 mg Ex-tab: 500 mg Suspension: 250 mg/5 mL — 16 oz btl	Children, < 5 yr: 50 mg/kg/24 hr in 4 divided doses to a max. of 250 mg/dose 6–12 yr: 500 mg qid	Acid urine (pH ≤ 5.5 or less) is essential for antibacterial action Ascorbic acid can be used to achieve urine acidification

Name (generic)	Available Preparations	Dosage	Special Considerations
Methimazole	Tablet: 5 mg	*Initial:* 0.4 mg/kg/24 hr in 3 divided doses *Maintenance:* 0.2 mg/kg/24 hr in 3 divided doses, beginning when patient is euthyroid	
Methyldopa	Injection: 50 mg/mL — 5 mL vial Suspension: 250 mg/5 mL — 16 oz btl Tablet: 125 mg, 250 mg	Parenteral, IV: 5–10 mg/kg/dose q6–8h to a total dose of 20–40 mg/kg/24 hr Oral: *Initial:* 10 mg/kg/24 hr in 2–4 divided doses *Increment:* 5–10 mg/kg/24 hr at intervals of 2–7 days *Maximum:* 40 mg/kg/24 hr in 2–4 divided doses	Positive Coombs test in 10–20% of patients receiving methyldopa Monitor hepatic function, white cell and differential blood count
Methylene blue	Injection: 1% — 10 mL ampul	**Methemoglobinemia:** 1–2 mg/kg/dose IV, slowly over 5–10 min; may repeat in 1 hr if needed **NADH-methemoglobin reductase deficiency:** 1.5–5 mg/kg/24 hr; do not exceed 300 mg/24 hr; give with 5–8 mg/kg/24 hr ascorbic acid in 3–4 divided doses	Contraindicated in G-6-PD deficiency May discolor urine and feces
Methylphenidate	SR-Tablet: 20 mg Tablet: 5 mg, 10 mg	Children > 6 years: Attention deficit disorder: Oral: Initial: 0.3 mg/kg/dose or 2.5–5 mg/dose given before breakfast and lunch; increase by 0.1 mg/kg/dose or by 5–10 mg/day at weekly intervals; usual dose: 0.5–1 mg/kg/day; maximum dose: 2 mg/kg/day or 60 mg/day	Schedule II controlled substance; however, a 60-day supply may be prescribed for hyperkinetic children

Name (generic)	Available Preparations	Dosage	Special Considerations
Methylprednisolone	Injection: 40 mg, 125 mg, 500 mg vial	**Antiinflammatory or immunosuppressive:** 0.16–0.8 mg/kg/24 hr in 2–4 divided doses **Shock:** 30 mg/kg/dose q6h until clinical signs of shock abate for maximum of 48–72 hr **Status asthmaticus:** *Initial:* 1–2 mg/kg/dose *Maintenance:* 0.5–1 mg/kg/dose qid up to 5 days before changing to oral prednisone	
Metoclopramide	Injection: 5 mg/mL — 2 mL and 10 mL ampul Solution: 5 mg/5 mL — 16 oz btl Tablet: 10 mg	Parenteral, **antiemetic:** 0.5–2.0 mg/kg/dose 30 min prior to chemotherapy and repeated 2 hr for 2 doses, then q3h for 3 doses	If extrapyramidal symptoms should occur, inject diphenhydramine IM
Metronidazole	Injection: 5 mg/mL — 100 mL vial Tablet: 250 mg	**Anaerobic bacterial infection:** *Loading dose:* 15 mg/kg; then 30 mg/kg/24 hr in 4 divided doses **Amebiasis:** 35–50 mg/kg/24 hr in 3 divided doses for 10 days	Injectable dosage form contains 24 mEq sodium per gm No alcohol should be ingested for 24 hr after the dose
Metyrapone	Tablet: 250 mg	15 mg/kg/dose q4h for total of 6 doses; minimum dose of 250 mg recommended	Used to test hypothalamic-pituitary ACTH function

Name (generic)	Available Preparations	Dosage	Special Considerations
Mezlocillin	Injection: 4 gm—vial	Newborn, < 1 week: 150 mg/kg/24 hr in 2 divided doses Infants and children: 300 mg/kg/24 hr in 4 divided doses	1.85 mEq sodium per gm
Miconazole	Injection: 10 mg/mL (20 mL)	Children: IV: 20–40 mg/kg/day divided every 8 hours	
Midazolam hydrochloride	Injection: 1 mg/mL, 5 mg/mL	Children: Preoperative sedation: IM: 0.07–0.08 mg/kg 30 minutes to 1 hour before surgery IV: 0.035 mg/kg/dose, repeat over several minutes as required to achieve the desired sedative effect, up to a total dose of 0.1–0.2 mg/kg Conscious sedation: IV: 0.1–0.2 mg/kg, follow loading dose with a 2 μg/kg/minute continuous infusion, titrate to desired effect using 0.4–6 μg/kg/minute	
Morphine sulfate	Injection: 2 mg/mL — 1 mL cart; 5 mg/mL — 1 mL vial; 10 mg/mL — 1 mL vial Oral sol: 10 mg/5 mL — 500 mL btl	IM or SC: 0.1–0.2 mg/kg/dose repeated q4h as needed to a max. single dose of 15 mL IV: Use ½ the IM dose (⅔ of an oral dose is absorbed)	
Mylanta*	Chew-tab: combination product Suspension: 30 mL u/d and 5 oz btl		Each chew-tab or 5 mL suspension contains: Aluminum hydroxide, 200 mg Magnesium hydroxide, 200 mg Simethicone, 20 mg

Name (generic)	Available Preparations	Dosage	Special Considerations
Mylanta-II*	Chew-tab: combination product Suspension: 5 oz btl		Mylanta contains an insignificant amount of sodium per daily dose and is considered dietetically sodium free Each chew-tab or 5 mL suspension contains: Aluminum hydroxide, 400 mg Magnesium hydroxide, 400 mg Simethicone, 40 mg Mylanta-II contains an insignificant amount of sodium per daily dose and is considered dietetically sodium free
Nadolol	Tablet: 40 mg, 80 mg	1–2 mg/kg/24 hours in 1–2 divided doses	Dose once daily Adjust dose in renally impaired patients
Nafcillin	Injection: 1 gm — vial	Neonates, < 1 mo: 60 mg/kg/24 hr in 4–6 divided doses Children: 100–200 mg/kg/24 hr in 4–6 divided doses	2.9 mEq sodium per gm Oxacillin is preferred in neonates
Naloxone HCl	Injection: 20 μg/mL — 1 mL ampul; 400 μg/mL — 1 mL ampul	Neonates and children, IM, IV, SC: 0.01 mg/kg	Repeat dose in 2–3 min as needed If no improvement after 3 doses, a nonopioid drug should be suspected
Naproxen	Tablet: 250 mg	5–7 mg/kg/dose every 8–12 hours	
Neomycin	Oral sol: 125 mg/5 mL — 16 oz btl Tablet: 500 mg	50–100 mg/kg/24 hr in 4–6 divided doses	A daily dose > 1 gm should be avoided

Name (generic)	Available Preparations	Dosage	Special Considerations
Neostigmine	Injection: 250 µg/mL ampul; 1 mg/mL — 10 mL vial	**Myasthenia gravis test dose:** IM: 0.04 mg/kg/dose once	
Neutra-Phos*	Capsule: combination product Powder: 64 gm btl	Children, < 4 yr: Begin at 60 mL qid Children, > 4 yr: Begin at 75 mL (or 1 capsule) qid; do not exceed 600 mL/24 hr	Do not swallow whole capsule Empty contents of 1 capsule in 75 mL water. The resulting solution contains: Phosphorus, 8 mmol Sodium, 7.125 mEq Potassium, 7.125 mEq
Nitrofurantoin	Capsule: 50 mg Suspension: 25 mg/5 mL — 16 oz btl Tablet: 50 mg	5–7 mg/kg/24 hr in 4 divided doses; reduce to 2.5–5.0 mg/kg/24 hr after 10–14 days	Administer with meals Avoid usage in neonates < 1 week old Avoid in renal failure
Nitroprusside	Injection: 50 mg — vial	0.5–5 µg/kg/min as a constant infusion	Dissolve contents of 50 mg vial in 2–3 mL of D_5W; then further dilute it in 500 mL of D_5W to produce 100 µg/mL solution for infusion Wrap solution bottle in aluminum foil; discard after 24 hr Monitor serum cyanide levels and acid-base balance
Norepinephrine bitartrate	Injection: 1 mg/mL — 4 mL ampul	Begin at 2.0 µg/kg/min; titrate to desired blood pressure; max. dose 6 µg/kg/min	Each mL of solution contains 1 mg of base Avoid extravasation; administer into large catheterized vein
Nystatin	Cream: 100,000 units/gm — 15 gm tube Ointment: 100,000 units/gm — 15 gm tube	Infants, premature: 50,000 units (0.5 mL) by mouth 4 times/day Infants: 100,000 units (1 mL) by mouth 4 times/day	

Name (generic)	Available Preparations	Dosage	Special Considerations
	Powder: 100,000 units/gm — 15 gm squz btl Suppository: 100,000 units Suspension: 100,000 units/mL — 60 mL drop btl and 16 oz btl Tablet: 500,000 units	Children: 200,000–300,000 (2–3 mL) by mouth 4 times/day	
Opium, tincture (opium, deodorized)	Tincture: 16 oz btl	**Analgesia:** 0.01–0.02 mL/kg/dose q3–4h **Diarrhea:** Children: 0.005–0.01 mL/kg/dose q2–4h; do not exceed 6 doses/24 hr	Contains 10 mg/mL anhydrous morphine
Ortho-Novum 1/35 28* (or Norinyl 1/35 28)	Tablet: combination product	1 tablet qd	Each peach tablet contains: Norethindrone, 1 mg Ethinyl estradiol, 35 μg Each green tablet contains inert ingredients
Ortho-Novum 1/50 28* (or Norinyl 1/50 28)	Tablet: combination product	1 tablet qd	Each yellow tablet contains: Norethindrone, 1 mg Mestranol, 50 μg Each green tablet contains inert ingredients
Ovral-28*	Tablet: combination product	1 tablet qd	Each tablet contains: Norgestrel, 0.5 mg Ethinyl estradiol, 50 μg
Oxacillin	Injection: 1 gm — vial	Neonates, < 1 week: 100 mg/kg/24 hr in 2 divided doses >1 week: 200 mg/kg/24 hr in 4 divided doses	

612

Name (generic)	Available Preparations	Dosage	Special Considerations
		Infants and children: 150–200 mg/kg/24 hr in 6 divided doses	
Oxybutynin	Solution: 5 mg/mL — 16 oz btl Tablet: 5 mg	Children, > 5 yr: 5 mg bid up to a max. of 5 mg tid	
Oxycodone		See Table 1-1	
Oxymetazoline	Solution: 0.05% — 20 mL drop btl Spray: 0.05%–15 mL squz btl	Children, > 6 yr: 2–3 drops or 1–2 sprays each nostril bid	Rebound rhinitis is common Do not use longer than 3–5 days
Pancrelipase	Ex-cap: combination product Pancrease Pancrease MT-4 Pancrease MT-10 Pancrease MT-16	Children, < 1 year: 2,000 units of lipase with meals Children, 1–6 years: 4,000–8,000 units of lipase with meals and 4,000 units with snacks Children, 7–12 years: 4,000–12,000 units of lipase with meals and snacks	To protect enteric coating, microspheres should **not** be crushed or chewed

	Lipase (units)	Pro-tease (units)	Amy-tase (units)
Entenc-coated micro-spheres			
Pancrease	4,000	25,000	20,000
Entenc-coated micro-tablets			
MT-4	4,000	12,000	12,000
MT-10	10,000	30,000	30,000
MT-16	16,000	48,000	48,000

Name (generic)	Available Preparations	Dosage	Special Considerations
Paraldehyde	Injection: 5 mL — ampul	IM, oral, rectal: **Sedative:** 0.15 mL/kg/dose **Hypnotic or anticonvulsant:** 0.3 mL/kg/dose	Avoid IV administration To ensure a fresh solution, use ampuls of paraldehyde for IM, oral, or rectal use Dilute oral solution well
Paramethadione	Capsule: 300 mg	Children, < 2 yr: 300 mg/24 hr 2–6 yr: 600 mg/24 hr > 6 yr: 900 mg/24 hr	Adjust subsequent doses by response Divide into 3–4 doses/day
Paregoric	Tincture: 16 oz btl	**Analgesic:** 0.25–0.5 mL/kg/dose qd–qid **Antidiarrheal:** 0.1 mL/kg after each loose stool up to 4 times a day	Contains 0.4 mg/mL morphine
Pemoline	Tablet: 18.75 mg, 37.5 mg	Children, > 6 yr: *Initial:* 37.5 mg as a single dose in the morning; dose may be increased by 18.75 mg/24 hr at weekly intervals until a desired clinical response is achieved; dosage in children should not exceed 112.5 mg/24 hr	Beneficial effects may not become evident until the third or fourth week of therapy This drug should be discontinued periodically to reassess the patient's condition
Penicillamine	Tablet: 250 mg	≤ 30 mg/kg/24 hr *Rheumatoid arthritis:* Children: Initial: 3 mg/kg/day (≤ 250 mg/day) for 3 months, then 6 mg/kg/day (≤ 500 mg/day) in divided doses twice daily for 3 months; maximum: 10 mg/kg/day in 3–4 divided doses *Wilson's disease:* Children: 20 mg/kg/day in 4 divided doses	

Name (generic)	Available Preparations	Dosage	Special Considerations
Penicillin G, benzathine	Injection: 600,000 units/mL — 1 mL and 2 mL cart	*Cystinuria:* Children: 30 mg/kg/day in 4 divided doses *Lead poisoning:* Children: 10–30 mg/kg/day in 2–3 divided doses Newborn, IM: 50,000 units/kg/24 hr once Infants and children, < 30 kg, IM: 600,000 units once Children, > 30 kg, IM: 1.2 million units once	
Penicillin G potassium	Injection: 1,000,000 units and 5,000,000 units — vial Tablet: 200,000 units	**Infection:** Newborn, < 1 week: 50,000 units/kg/24 hr in 2–3 divided doses Infants: 75,000 units/kg/24 hr in 3 divided doses Children: 25,000–100,000 units/kg/24 hr in 4–6 divided doses **Meningitis:** Newborn, < 1 week: 200,000–300,000 units/kg/24 hr in 2–3 divided doses Infants: 200,000–300,000 units/kg/24 hr in 4 divided doses Children: 200,000–400,000 units/kg/24 hr in 6 divided doses	
Penicillin G procaine	Injection: 600,000 units/mL — 1 mL and 2 mL cart, and 4 mL syringe	Newborn, IM: 50,000 units/kg/24 hr daily Children, IM: 100,000–600,000 units/24 hr in 1–2 divided doses	When used to treat gonorrhea, simultaneously dose with probenecid (25 mg/kg)

Name (generic)	Available Preparations	Dosage	Special Considerations
Penicillin G sodium	Injection: 5,000,000 units — vial	**Infection:** Newborn, < 1 week: 50,000 units/kg/24 hr in 2–3 divided doses Infants: 75,000 units/kg/24 hr in 3 divided doses Children: 25,000–100,000 units/kg/24 hr in 4–6 divided doses **Meningitis:** Newborn, < 1 week: 200,000–300,000 units/kg/24 hr in 2–3 divided doses Infants: 200,000–300,000 units/kg/24 hr in 4 divided doses Children: 200,000–400,000 units/kg/24 hr in 6 divided doses	250 mg = 400,000 units Administer on empty stomach 1 hr before or 2 hr after meals
Penicillin V	Solution: 125 mg/5 mL — 200 mL btl; 250 mg/5 mL — 200 mL btl Tablet: 250 mg	25–50 mg/kg/24 hr in 4 divided doses	
Penicilloyl-polylysine	Injection: 0.2 mL — ampul	0.01–0.02 mL intradermally (sufficient to raise the smallest perceptible bleb)	Skin test material should always be applied first by the scratch technique
Phenazopyridine	Tablet: 100 mg, 200 mg	Children, 6–9 yr: 12 mg/kg/24 hr in 2–3 divided doses 9–12 yr: 100 mg tid	Phenazopyridine is an azo dye and produces an orange to red color in urine
Phenobarbital	Injection: 60 mg — vial Solution: 20 mg/5 mL — 2.5 mL, 3.75 mL, 5 mL, and 7.5 mL u/d, and 16 oz btl Tablet: 15 mg, 30 mg, 100 mg	IV, oral: **Sedative:** 2 mg/kg 3 times/day **Anticonvulsant:** 3–5 mg/kg/dose	

Name (generic)	Available Preparations	Dosage	Special Considerations
Phensuximide	Capsule: 250 mg, 500 mg Suspension: 300 mg/5 mL — 16 oz btl	1–3 gm/24 hr in 2–3 divided doses	
Phentolamine mesylate	Injection: 5 mg — ampul	*Test dose* (pheochromocytoma): 1 mg	
Phenytoin	Chew-tab: 50 mg Capsule: 30 mg, 100 mg Injection: 50 mg/1 mL — 2 mL and 5 mL vial Suspension: 30 mg/5 mL — 8 oz btl; 125 mg/5 mL — 8 oz btl	IM, IV, oral: 5–7 mg/kg/24 hr in 1 or 2 divided doses *Status epilepticus: IV:* Loading dose: Neonates: 15–20 mg/kg in a single or divided dose Infants, Children, Adults: 15–18 mg/kg in a single or divided dose Maintenance anticonvulsant: Neonates and Infants: 5–8 mg/kg/day in 2 divided doses Children and Adults: 4–7 mg/kg/day in a single dose or in 2 divided doses *Anticonvulsant: Oral:* Loading dose: 20 mg/kg; based on phenytoin serum concentrations and if no doses had been administered in the previous 24 hours; on the average, for every 1 mg/kg administered, serum level will increase by 1 µg/mL Maintenance dose: Neonates: 5 mg/kg/day in divided doses every 12 hours	Ideal serum concentration is 10–20 µg/mL Select a blood sample at steady state (6–12 hr after dose) Clinically significant interactions may occur when other drugs are administered with phenytoin Suspension must be shaken before each dose

Name (generic)	Available Preparations	Dosage	Special Considerations
		Infants > 10 days to Children ≤ 3 years: 8–10 mg/kg/day in divided doses every 8–12 hours Children ≥ 4 years and Adults: 5–8 mg/kg/day in divided doses every 12–24 hours *Arrhythmias:* Loading dose: IV push: 1.25 mg/kg every 5 minutes for 12 doses; total loading dose: 15 mg/kg Maintenance dose: Children: Oral: IV: 2–5 mg/kg/day in 2 divided doses Adults: Oral: 250 mg 4 times/day for 1 day, 250 mg twice a day for 2 days, then 300–400 mg/day in divided doses 1–4 times/day	
Physostigmine salicylate	Injection: 1 mg/mL — 2 mL ampul	**Anticholinergic poisoning:** 0.5 mg slowly over 2–3 min; repeat in 2–5 min if no effect; once effect is accomplished, lowest total effective dose every 30–60 min slowly for recurrence of symptoms	Consult Poison Control Center IV rate not to exceed 0.5 mg/minute
Phytonadione	Injection: 2 mg/mL — 0.5 mL ampul; 10 mg/mL — 1 mL ampul Tablet: 5 mg	**Hemorrhagic disease of newborn:** **Prophylaxis,** IM or SC: 0.5–1 mg within 1 hour of birth **Treatment,** IM or SC: 1 mg **Oral anticoagulant–induced hypoprothrombinemia:** 2.5–10 mg; repeat in 12–48 hr if needed	Avoid IV route whenever possible

Name (generic)	Available Preparations	Dosage	Special Considerations
Potassium chloride	Tablet: 750 mg Injection: 2 mEq/mL — 10 mL vial Oral powder: 20 mEq pkt Solution: 5 mEq, 10 mEq, 15 mEq, 20 mEq, and 30 mEq u/d; 5 mEq/5 mL — 120 mL btl	*Maintenance:* 1–2 mEq/kg/24 hr *Replacement:* Up to max. of 4 mEq/kg/24 hr; replace over 3–7 days to avoid hyperkalemia	Max. concentration of 40 mEq/L when infused into peripheral vein May give higher concentrations via central line **with caution**
Potassium iodide	Solution: 1 gm/mL — 30 mL drop btl	1 drop per year of age tid	Give with food or milk after meals Dilute 1:10 (100 mg/mL) before administering
Potassium phosphate	Injection: 5 mL — vial	*Maintenance* or **hypophosphatemia:** 1–3 mmol/kg/24 hr	Each ml contains: Potassium, 4.4 mEq Phosphorus, 3 mmol
Pralidoxime	Injection: 1 gm — vial	20–50 mg/kg/dose after initial treatment with atropine; may be repeated q8–12h as needed	Consult Poison Control Center
Prednisone	Tablet: 1 mg, 5 mg, 20 mg, 50 mg	See text for specific dose up to 2 mg/kg/24 hr	
Primidone	Suspension: 250 mg/5 ml — 8 oz btl Tablet: 250 mg	Children, < 8 yr: 125 mg at bedtime for 1 week; increase to 125 mg bid the next week, and by 125 mg increments at weekly intervals to a maximum of 1.25 gm/m²/24 hr in 2–4 divided doses Children, > 8 yr: 250 mg at bedtime for 1 week; increase to 250 mg bid	**History of varicella susceptibility should be obtained** Select a blood sample at steady state between doses after 24 hr

Name (generic)	Available Preparations	Dosage	Special Considerations
		for the next week; continue increasing by 250 mg increments at weekly intervals to a maximum dose of 2 gm/24 hr in 2–4 divided doses	
Probenecid	Tablet: 500 mg	**Uricosuric:** Children, < 2 yr: Not recommended 2–14 yr: *Initial:* 25 mg/kg for 1 dose *Maintenance:* 40 mg/kg/24 hr in 4 divided doses	
Procainamide	Capsule: 250 mg, 375 mg, 500 mg Injection: 100 mg/mL vial	Parenteral, IM: 20–30 mg/kg/24 hr in 4–6 divided doses; do not exceed 4 gm/24 hr < 1 yr: IV, *Loading dose:* 3–7 mg/kg slowly over 30 min > 1 yr: IV, *Loading dose:* 5–15 mg/kg slowly over 30 min; continue at 20–80 μg/kg/min by continuous infusion Oral: 15–50 mg/kg/24 hr in 6 divided doses	Monitor Q-T interval and blood pressure closely
Prochlorperazine	Injection: 5 mg/mL — 2 mL ampul Solution: 5 mg/5 mL — 120 mL btl Suppository: 2.5 mg, 5 mg, 25 mg Tablet: 5 mg	Parenteral, IM: Children, > 10 kg: 0.2 mg/kg/24 hr in 3–4 divided doses Oral or rectal: Children, > 10 kg: 0.4 mg/kg/24 hr in 3–4 divided doses	Not recommended for use in children < 2 yr of age or weight < 10 kg Children seem prone to develop extrapyramidal reactions, even on moderate doses; therefore, use lowest effective dose **Do not use IV**

Name (generic)	Available Preparations	Dosage	Special Considerations
Promethazine	Injection: 25 mg/mL — 16 oz btl Suppository: 25 mg Tablet: 12.5 mg, 25 mg	**Antihistamine:** 0.1 mg/kg/dose q6h during the day and 0.5 mg/kg/dose at bedtime **Motion sickness:** 0.5 mg/kg/dose, 30–60 minutes before departure, q12h **Nausea and vomiting:** 0.25–0.5 mg/kg/dose q4–6h as needed **Sedative or preop:** 0.5–1.0 mg/kg/dose q6h as needed	
Propranolol	Injection: 1 mg/mL — 1 mL ampul Tablet: 10 mg, 40 mg	See text for specific dosage	
Propylthiouracil	Tablet: 50 mg	*Initial:* 5–7 mg/kg/24 hr in 3 divided doses *Maintenance:* ⅓ to ⅔ of initial dose, beginning when patient is euthyroid	
Pseudoephedrine	Solution: 30 mg/5 mL — 120 mL and 473 mL btl Tablet: 30, 60 mg	5 mg/kg/24 hr in 4 divided doses	Effect noted in 15–30 min; peaks in 30–60 min
Psyllium hydrophilic	Powder: 500 mg/gm — 210 gm btl	4–10 gm qd–tid	0.43 mEq sodium per 6.4 gm (6.4 gm = 1 tsp)
Pyridostigmine bromide	Ex-tab: 180 mg Injection: 5 mg/mL — 16 oz btl Tablet: 60 mg	**Myasthenia gravis,** Oral: 7 mg/kg/24 hr in 4–6 divided doses	
Pyridoxine	Injection: 100 mg/mL — 10 mL vial Tablet: 25 mg, 50 mg	**Neuritis,** treatment: 10–50 mg qd **Prophylaxis:** 1–2 mg/kg daily **Isoniazid-induced deficiency:** 100 mg qd for 2 weeks	

Name (generic)	Available Preparations	Dosage	Special Considerations
Pyrimethamine	Tablet: 25 mg	**Malaria (chloroquine-resistant):** < 10 kg: 6.25 mg qd for 3 days 10–20 kg: 12.5 mg qd for 3 days 20–40 kg: 25 mg qd for 3 days > 40 kg: 25 mg twice daily for 3 days **Toxoplasmosis:** *Loading dose:* 2 mg/kg/dose qd for 3 days *Maintenance:* Consult infectious disease specialist	
Quinidine gluconate	Ex-tab: 300 mg Injection: 80 mg/mL — 20 mL vial	See Quinidine sulfate dosing information	Equivalent to 62% anhydrous quinidine If used with digoxin, reduce digoxin dose by ½ IV use not recommended; use only if drug cannot be given orally
Quinidine sulfate	Tablet: 200 mg	Parenteral, IV: 2–10 mg/kg/dose q3–6h as needed Oral: 15–60 mg/kg/24 hr in 4 divided doses	Equivalent to 83% anhydrous quinidine If used with digoxin, reduce digoxin dose by ½ IV use not recommended; use only if drug cannot be given orally
Quinine sulfate	Capsule: 300 mg	**Malaria, uncomplicated attack (chloroquine-resistant):** 25 mg/kg/24 hr in 3 divided doses for 3 days	For severe malaria attack IV therapy is recommended; however, IV dosage form is unavailable commercially in the United States except from CDC

Name (generic)	Available Preparations	Dosage	Special Considerations
Rabies immune globulin	150 units/mL — 2 mL vial	Parenteral, IM: 20 units/kg	Indicated for all persons suspected of exposure to rabies except those previously immunized with vaccine Should be given as promptly as possible after exposure, but may be administered up to 8 days after first dose of vaccine Should be administered in conjunction with vaccine Give ½ dose IM; other ½ should be infiltrated around site of bite
Rabies vaccine (human)	Injection: 1 pack	*Postexposure dose*, IM: 5 doses of 1 mL each; the first dose should be administered as soon as possible after exposure in conjunction with rabies immune globulin: an additional dose should be given on each of days 3, 7, 14, and 28 after the first dose	WHO currently recommends a sixth dose 90 days after the first dose
Ranitidine hydrochloride	Injection: 25 mg/mL Solution: 75 mg/5mL Tablet: 150 mg	Children: Oral: 2–3 mg/kg/dose every 12 hours IV: 1 mg/kg/dose every 8 hours	
Reserpine	Tablet: 0.1 mg, 0.25 mg	0.01–0.02 mg/kg/24 hr in 2 divided doses	See text for use in hypertensive crisis
Riboflavin (vitamin B$_2$)	Tablet: 10 mg	5–10 mg daily	

Name (generic)	Available Preparations	Dosage	Special Considerations
Rifampin	Capsule: 150 mg, 300 mg	**Meningococcal disease prophylaxis:** 10–20 mg/kg/24 hr in 2 divided doses to a max. of 600 mg/24 hr for 2 days (4 doses) **Haemophilus influenzae type B prophylaxis:** 20 mg/kg/24 hr as a single dose to a max. of 600 mg/24 hr for 4 days **Tuberculosis:** 10–20 mg/kg/24 hr qd	Administer 1 hr before or 2 hr after meals Stains urine orange Stains soft contact lenses Interferes with oral contraceptives Not used during pregnancy
Selenium sulfide lotion	Suspension: 2.5%–120 mL btl	As shampoo: Massage 5–10 mL into wet scalp, leave on scalp 2–3 minutes, rinse thoroughly and repeat; shampoo twice weekly for 2 weeks, then every week or 2 weeks As lotion (for tinea versicolor): leave on for 10 min, then rinse; use daily for 7 days	
Senna fruit	Granules: 110 mg/gm — 170 gm can Solution: 218 mg/5 mL — 8 oz btl Suppository: 652 mg Tablet: 187 mg	Solution: children, 1 mo–1 yr: 1.25–2.5 mL bid 1–5 yrs: 2.5–5 mL bid 5–15 yrs: 5–10 mL bid Tablet: children, > 35 kg: 1 tablet bid	
Sodium bicarbonate	Injection: 1 mEq/mL — 10 mL and 50 mL syringe, and 50 mL vial Oral sol: 1 mEq/mL — 128 oz btl (special prep) Tablet: 300 mg	**Cardiac arrest:** Infants and children: 1–2 mEq/kg initially, then as indicated by blood gases	See text for specific usage

Name (generic)	Available Preparations	Dosage	Special Considerations
Sodium fluoride	Chew-tab: 2.2 mg Gel: 1.1% 60 gm tube Solution: 5.5 mg/mL — 30 mL drop btl	Based on fluoride concentration in drinking water, < 0.3 ppm f: Children, 0–2 yrs: 0.25 mg qd 2–3 yr: 0.5 mg qd 3–12 yr: 1 mg qd 0.3–0.7 ppm f: ½ the above dose > 0.7 ppm f: fluoride supplements contraindicated	Each 2.2 mg sodium fluoride is equivalent to 1 mg of elemental fluoride (on which the doses are based)
Sodium polystyrene sulfonate (Kayexalate)	Powder: 454 gm btl Suspension: 15 gm/60 mL — 16 oz btl	Oral: 1 gm/kg/dose qid Rectal: 1 gm/kg/dose q2–6h	Effective exchange rate = approximately 1 mEq potassium/gm resin Rectal route is less effective than oral
Spectinomycin HCl	Injection: 4 gm — vial	IM: 40 mg/kg/dose once	
Spironolactone	Tablet: 25 mg	Infant guidelines: Dose at 1.5–3.0 wt(kg) mg/kg/24 hr < 5 6.25 mg daily or every other day 5–10 12.5 mg daily or every other day 10–20 12.5 mg bid > 20 25 mg qd	Tablets are scored
Streptomycin	Injection: 1 gm — vial	Newborn, IM: 20–30 mg/kg/24 hr in 2 divided doses for 10 days Children, IM: 20–40 mg/kg/24 hr in 2 divided doses for 10 days Maximum dose 2 gm/24 hr	Used principally as therapy for tuberculosis

Name (generic)	Available Preparations	Dosage	Special Considerations
Succimer	Capsule: 100 mg	Oral: 30 mg/kg/day for 5 days followed by 20 mg/kg/ day for 14 days	Treatment of lead poisoning in children with blood levels > 45 μg/dL. It is not indicated for prophylaxis of lead poisoning in a lead-containing environment.
Sulfadiazine	Tablet: 500 mg	**Bacterial infection:** Newborn: **Not recommended** Children: *Loading dose:* 75 mg/kg/ dose once; then 150 mg/kg/24 hr in 4 divided doses to a max. of 4 gm/24 hr **Malaria (chloroquine-resistant):** 100–200 mg/kg/24 hr in 4 divided doses to a max. of 2 gm/24 hr for 5 days **Toxoplasmosis:** 25 mg/kg 4 times/ day for 3–4 weeks given with pyrimethamine 2 mg/kg/day for 3 days, then 1 mg/kg/day for 3–4 weeks	Used together with pyrimethamine and quinine for chloroquine-resistant strains of *P. falciparum*
Sulfasalazine	Tablet: 500 mg	*Initial:* 40–60 mg/kg/24 hr in 3–6 divided doses *Maintenance:* 20–30 mg/kg/24 hr in 4 divided doses	
Sulfisoxazole	Suspension: 500 mg/5 mL — 16 oz btl Tablet: 500 mg	Newborn: **Not recommended** Oral: children, > 2 months: 120–150 mg/kg/24 hr in 4 divided doses to a max. of 6 gm/24 hr	May cause orange-yellow discoloration of urine and skin
Sulfobromophthalein	Injection: 50 mg/mL — 3 mL ampul	IV: 2–5 mg/kg dose	For testing the functional capacity of the liver

Name (generic)	Available Preparations	Dosage	Special Considerations
Terbutaline	Injection: 1 mg/mL — 1 mL ampul Tablet: 2.5 mg, 5 mg Aerosol, oral: 0.2 mg/activation (10.5 gm)	Oral: Children, < 12 yr: *Initial:* 0.05 mg/kg/dose tid, increased gradually as required; max. of 0.1 mg/kg/dose tid or total of 5 mg/24 hr Children, > 12 yr: *Initial:* 2.5 mg tid *Maintenance:* Usually 5 mg or 0.075 mg/kg/dose tid Parenteral, SC: Children, < 12 yr: 0.01 mg/kg/dose to a max. of 0.3 mg/dose q15–20 min for 3 doses Children, > 12 yr: 0.25 mg/dose, repeated in 15–30 min if needed once only; a total dose of 0.5 mg should not be exceeded within a 4-hr period Inhalation: 2 every 4–6 hours	
Terfenadine	Tablet: 60 mg	Oral: Children ≤ 12 years: 15–30 mg/dose twice daily Children > 12 years and Adults: 60 mg twice daily	
Tetanus immune globulin	Injection: 5 mL — vial	IM: 250 units	Indicated in tetanus-prone injuries in a nonimmunized person or in a person immunized > 10 yr ago
Tetracycline	Capsule: 250 mg	Oral: Children, > 8 yr: 25–50 mg/kg/24 hr in 4 divided doses not to exceed 3 gm/day	Use of tetracyclines in childhood (to 8 yr of age) **may cause permanent discoloration and enamel hypoplasia of the teeth**

Name (generic)	Available Preparations	Dosage	Special Considerations
Theophylline (6–8 hr)	Capsule: 60 mg, 126 mg, 250 mg	**Asthma:** Children, < 9 yrs: 12–24 mg/kg/24 hr in 3–4 divided doses 9–12 yr: 12–20 mg/kg/24 hr in 3–4 divided doses 12–16 yr: 10–18 mg/kg/24 hr in 3–4 divided doses >16 yr: 10–13 mg/kg/24 hr in 3–4 divided doses	Give 1 hr before or 2 hr after meals Do not give with dairy products or antacid Therapeutic levels: **bronchial asthma,** 10–20 µg/mL; **status asthmaticus,** maintain at 16–20 µg/mL; **neonatal apnea,** 7–23 µg/mL Slo-phyllin Gyrocaps frequently require q6h dosing in children Drug interactions: when given with cimetidine, erythromycin, propranolol, or phenytoin, increased theophylline blood levels have been demonstrated
Theophylline (8–12 hr)	Ex-cap: 50 mg, 100 mg, 300 mg Ex-cap: 75 mg (sprinkle) Ex-tab: 100 mg, 200 mg, 300 mg	**Asthma:** Children, < 9 yr: 12–24 mg/kg/24 hr in 2–3 divided doses 9–12 yr: 12–20 mg/kg/24 hr in 2–3 divided doses 12–16 yr: 10–18 mg/kg/24 hr in 2–3 divided doses >16 yr: 10–13 mg/kg/24 hr in 2–3 divided doses	Therapeutic levels: **bronchial asthma,** 10–20 µg/mL; **status asthmaticus,** maintain at 16–20 µg/mL Patients should be started on extended release capsules whenever possible Slo-bid
Thiamine	Injection: 100 mg/mL — 10 mL vial Tablet: 10 mg, 100 mg	Dietary supplement, Thiamine deficiency: IM, IV (if critically ill): 10–25 mg/dose daily Maintenance: Oral: 5–10 mg/day for 1 month	Minimum daily requirements of this water-soluble vitamin range from 0.3 mg in an infant to 1.5 mg in an adult male; the arbitrary dose of 10 mg is both safe and effective

Name (generic)	Available Preparations	Dosage	Special Considerations
Thioridazine	Conc sol: 100 mg/mL — 120 mL drop btl Tablet: 10 mg, 15 mg, 25 mg, 50 mg	Children, > 2 yr: Oral initially: 0.5–1 mg/kg/24 hr in 3–4 divided doses individualized to patient (at minimum of 3 mg/kg/24 hr)	
Thyroid	Tablet: 15 mg, 30 mg, 60 mg, 120 mg	*Initial:* 4 mg/kg/24 hr in a single daily dose	
Ticarcillin	Injection: vial	Newborns, < 1 week, < 2 kg: 150 mg/kg/24 hr in 2 divided doses > 2 kg: 200 mg/kg/24 hr in 3 divided doses Newborns, > 1 week, < 2 kg: 200 mg/kg/24 hr in 3 divided doses > 2 kg: 300 mg/kg/24 hr in 3 divided doses Neonates, children: 200–300 mg/kg/24 hr in 6 divided doses	5.2 to 6.5 mEq sodium per gm
Tobramycin	Injection: 40 mg/mL — 2 mL vial, 60 mg, and 80 mg syringe Ophthal oint: 0.3%–3.5 gm tube	Neonates, < 1 week: 5 mg/kg/24 hr in 2 divided doses > 1 week: 7.5 mg/kg/24 hr in 3 divided doses Children, < 5 yr: 7.5 mg/kg/24 hr in 3 divided doses 5–10 yr: 6 mg/kg/24 hr in 3 divided doses > 10 yr: 4.5 mg/kg/24 hr in 3 divided doses Children with cystic fibrosis: Usual dose: 7.5 mg/kg/ day in 3 divided doses; range: 6–10 mg/kg/day in 3 divided doses Ophthal oint: Apply bid–tid	Allowable predose level (trough): 0.5–2 μg/mL; allowable 1-hr postdose range (peak): 4–8 μg/mL Obtain drug levels after third dose; peak levels are drawn 30 minutes after the end of a 30-minute infusion; the trough is drawn just before the next dose

Name (generic)	Available Preparations	Dosage	Special Considerations
Tolazoline	Injection: 25 mg/mL vial	**Neonatal pulmonary hypertension:** Parenteral, IV: *Loading dose:* 1–2 mg/kg over 10 min *Maintenance:* 1–2 mg/kg/hr	Administer with meals or milk to minimize GI side effects
Tolmetin	Tablet: 200 mg	Children, > 2 yr: *Initial:* 15 mg/kg/24 hr in 3 divided doses; increase in increments of 5 mg/kg/24 hr at intervals of 1 week until therapeutic effect or adverse reaction is noted *Maximum:* If wt > 60 kg: 30 mg/kg/24 hr	
Triamterene	Capsule: 50 mg, 100 mg	2–4 mg/kg/24 hr in 1–2 divided doses	
Trifluoperazine (Stelazine)	Tablet: 1 mg, 2 mg, 5 mg	Children 6–12 years: Psychoses: Hospitalized or well-supervised: 0.2–0.5 mg/kg/24 hr in 2 divided doses	100 mg chlorpromazine = 10 mg trifluoperazine
Trihexyphenidyl	Solution: 2 mg/mL — 16 oz btl Tablet: 2 mg	**Drug-induced extrapyramidal disorders:** 1–15 mg/24 hr in 1–4 divided doses	
Trimethadione	Capsule: 300 mg Chew-tab: 150 mg	40 mg/kg/24 hr in 3–4 divided doses	Maintenance dosage should be the least amount of drug required to maintain control
Trimethaphan camsylate	Injection: 50 mg/mL — 10 mL ampul	Individualize doses	Dilute to 1 mg/mL in D_5W and administer by IV infusion
Trimethobenzamide (Tigan)	Capsule: 100 mg, 250 mg Injection: 100 mg/mL — 2 mL ampul Suppository: 100 mg, 200 mg	Oral: 20–45 kg: 100 mg tid-qid Rectal: Children < 20 kg: 100 mg tid-qid	Do not use injection IV Trimethobenzamide is *hepatotoxic*

Name (generic)	Available Preparations	Dosage	Special Considerations
Trimethoprim (TMP)-sulfamethoxazole	Injection: 5 mL vial Suspension: 2.5 mL and 5 mL u/d, 100 mL and 473 mL btl Tablet: combination product	Newborn: **Not recommended** Children: > 2 months: 8 mg TMP/kg/24 hr in 2 divided doses **Serious gram-negative infection or** *P. carinii*: 20 mg TMP/kg/24 hr in 3–4 divided doses *P. carinii* **prophylaxis:** 10 mg TMP/kg/24 hr in 2 divided doses 3 times/week	Concentrations: trimethoprim, 80 mg/5 mL of injection, 40 mg/5 mL of suspension, 80 mg/tablet; sulfamethoxazole, 400 mg/5 mL of injection, 200 mg/5 mL of suspension, 400 mg/tablet Also known as Co-trimoxazole
Tromethamine (Tham)	Injection: 500 mL — vial	Depends on buffer base deficit; when deficit is known: tromethamine mL of 0.3 M solution = body weight (kg) x base deficit (mEq/L); when base deficit is not known: 2–4 mL/kg/dose IV Metabolic acidosis with cardiac arrest: IV: 3.5–6 mL/kg into large peripheral vein	Administer through central vein whenever possible Must not be given for period greater than 24 hr **Contraindicated** in anuria, uremia, chronic respiratory acidosis, and salicylate intoxication
Valproic acid	Tablet: 125 mg, 250 mg, 500 mg Solution: 250 mg/5 mL — 16 oz btl	15 mg/kg/24 hr in 1–3 divided doses; increased in weekly intervals by 5–10 mg/kg/24 hr; max. dose 60 mg/kg/24 hr	Dose divided bid is preferable Monitor for hepatotoxicity
Vancomycin	Injection: 500 mg — vial Oral sol: 250 mg/5 mL (special prep)	Parenteral, IV: neonates, < 1 week: 30 mg/kg/24 hr in 2 divided doses Infants and children: 40–60 mg/kg/24 hr in 4 divided doses Oral: 10–50 mg/kg/day in 3–4 divided doses not to exceed 2 gm/day	Check serum levels

Name (generic)	Available Preparations	Dosage			Special Considerations
Varicella-zoster immune globulin	Injection: 125 units — vial	Wt(kg)	Dose	No. of vials	Administer by deep IM injection only
		0–10	125 units	1	Use within 72 hours of exposure
		10–20	250 units	2	
		20–30	375 units	3	
		30–40	500 units	4	
		40–50	625 units	5	
Vasopressin, aqueous	Injection (aqueous): 20 units/mL ampul	*Diabetes insipidus:* IM, SC: (Highly variable dosage) Children: 2.5–5 units 2–4 times/day *GI hemorrhage:* IV continuous infusion: Children: Initial: 0.1–0.3 units/ minute, then titrate dose as needed			Do not confuse with injection in oil Titrate dose based on serum and urine osmolality in addition to fluids balance
Vasopressin tannate, in oil	Injection in oil: 5 units/mL ampul	Children: 1.25–2.5 units every 1 to 3 days			Do not confuse with aqueous injection Titrate dose to achieve desired control of excessive thirst and urination
Verapamil	Injection: 5 mg/2 mL — 2 mL ampul Tablet: 80 mg, 120 mg	Parenteral, IV: 0.1 mg/kg/dose IV push over 2 minutes; may be repeated once Oral: 4–10 mg/kg/24 hr in 3 divided doses			Contraindicated in children < 1 yr of age IV use contraindicated in patients taking beta blockers
Vidarabine	Ophthal oint: 3%–3.5 gm tube	Apply 1 cm of ointment 5 times a day at 3-hr intervals; continue application for 5–7 days after healing seems to be complete			

Name (generic)	Available Preparations	Dosage	Special Considerations
Vitamin A	Capsule: 25,000 units, 50,000 units Injection: 50,000 units/mL — 2 mL vial Solution: 50,000 units/mL — 30 mL drop btl	Deficiency: Infants < 1 year: 10,000 units/kg/day for 5 days, then 7,500–15,000 units/day for 10 days Children 1–8 years: 5,000–10,000 units/kg/day for 5 days, then 17,000–35,000 units/day for 10 days Children > 8 years and Adults: 100,000 units/day for 3 days, then 50,000 units/day for 14 days Malabsorption syndrome (prophylaxis): Children > 8 years and Adults: 10,000–50,000 units/day of water-miscible product Dietary supplement: Infants up to 6 months: 1,500 units Children: 6 months to 3 years: 1,500–2,000 units/day 4–6 years: 2,500 units/day 7–10 years: 3,300–3,500 units/day Children > 10 years and Adults: 4,000–5,000 units/day	3 drops = 0.1 mL
Vitamin ADC drops	Solution: 50 mL drop btl	Infants and children, < 2 yr: 1 mL daily	
Vitamin ADC with fluoride drops	Solution: 50 mL drop btl	Infants and children, < 2 yr: 1 mL daily	0.25 mg fluoride per mL

Name (generic)	Available Preparations	Dosage	Special Considerations
Vitamin B complex	Capsule Injection: 2 mL — ampul Solution: 12 oz btl	1 capsule daily	1 capsule = 10 mL of solution
Vitamin E	Capsule: 100 units, 400 units Solution: 50 units/mL — 30 mL drop btl	Vitamin E deficiency: Treatment: Neonates, premature and low birth weight: 25 units/day results in normal levels within 1 week Children with malabsorption syndrome: 1 unit/kg/day of water miscible vitamin E to raise plasma tocopherol concentrations to the normal range within 2 months Adults: 60–70 units/day Prevention: Neonates, low birth weight: 5 units/day Neonates, if full term: 5 units/liter formula Adults: 30 units/day Cystic fibrosis, β-thalassemia, sickle cell anemia may require higher daily maintenance doses: Cystic fibrosis: 100–400 units/day Sickle cell: 450 units/day β-Thalassemia: 750 units/day	

Name (generic)	Available Preparations	Dosage	Special Considerations
Warfarin	Injection: 50 mg — vial Tablet: 2 mg, 5 mg	Infants and Children: 0.1 mg/kg/day; range: 0.05–0.34 mg/kg/day; adjust dose to achieve the desired prothrombin time Infants < 12 months may require doses near high end of range	
Xylose, D	Powder: 100 gm btl	500 mg/kg/dose in a 10% aqueous solution	
Zinc sulfate	Capsule: 220 mg	Zinc deficiency: 0.5–1 mg/kg/24 hr of elemental zinc divided 1–3 times/day	55 mg elemental zinc per 220 mg capsule Administer with food or milk

Index

Abdomen
abscess in, antibiotics in, 372
assessment in newborn, 125
blunt trauma of, 85
pain in, 43–44
Abortion, 351
Abscess
abdominal, antibiotics in, 372
brain, 409–410
intracranial pressure increase
in, 520
epidural, 72
peritonsillar, 57–58, 402
retropharyngeal, 58, 402
Absence seizures, 530–531
Abuse and neglect of children,
76–78
assessment of child and family in,
77–78
diagnosis of, 76–77
management of, 77
problems in, 76
rape and sexual abuse in, 78–81,
351. See also Sexual abuse
Accident prevention, 29
Acel-imune, 28
Acetaminophen
analgesic properties of, 4
antipyretic properties of, 34
dosage of, 5
in migraine headache, 538
toxic effects of, 4, 109–111
N-acetylcysteine in, 105, 111
Acetazolamide, 247
in pseudotumor cerebri, 521
Acetest, 353
Acetoacetate, urinary, tests for, 353
N-Acetylcysteine, in acetaminophen
poisoning, 105, 111
Acetylsalicylic acid. See Aspirin
Acid-base balance, 198–199
abnormalities in, 199–201
Acid ingestion, caustic burns from,
105–106
Acid maltase deficiency, symptoms
of, 157

Acid-phosphatase test in sexual
abuse or rape, 70
Acidemias, organic, 170
Acidosis
in acute renal failure, 230–231
in biochemical disturbances, 352
in cardiorespiratory arrest, management of, 49
diabetic ketoacidosis, 332–334
in hyaline membrane disease, 149
lactic acid, 201
in meconium aspiration, 150
metabolic, 200–201
renal tubular, 226–229
distal, 228
hypokalemia in, 233
proximal, 226–228
rickets in, 322
type IV, 228–229
respiratory, 199
in salicylate poisoning, 109
in total parenteral nutrition, 271
treatment of, 360
Aciduria, paradoxical, 197, 201
Acquired immunodeficiency syndrome, 435–437. See also HIV
infection
ACTH
deficiency of, 307
treatment of, 308
ectopic production by tumors, 318
serum levels in adrenal insufficiency, 315
therapy with
in opsoclonus-myoclonus syndrome, 529
in optic neuritis, 523–524
Actinomyces israelii in pelvic inflammatory disease, 414
Acute care, 48–98
in apparent life-threatening
events, 75–76
arterial lines in, 96–97
in cardiac failure, 64–66
cardiopulmonary resuscitation in,
48–51

Plumbism. *See* Lead poisoning
Pneumatosis intestinalis in necrotizing enterocolitis, 189
Pneumococcal vaccine, 26
Pneumococci
antibiotics affecting, 369
in bacteremia, 74
in epiglottitis, 55
in meningitis, 407
in osteomyelitis, 420
in otitis media, 399
in pneumonia, 406
and vaginitis, 341
Pneumocystis pneumonia, 456–457
in HIV infection, 437
prevention of, 456–457
treatment of, 456
Pneumocytosis, 442
Pneumograms in apnea, 154
Pneumomediastinum, neonatal, 151, 152
Pneumonia, 62, 405–407
antibiotics in, 369, 370, 372
cryptococcal, 428
in foreign body aspiration, 62
in HIV infection, 436, 437
neonatal, 183–184
Pneumocystis, 456–457
treatment of, 406–407
Pneumopericardium, neonatal, 151, 152
Pneumothorax, 62–63
from cardiopulmonary resuscitation, 51
in central venous pressure line placement, 96
in cystic fibrosis, 64
neonatal, 151–152
in positive pressure ventilation, 95
tension, 63
Poisoning, 99–121
acetaminophen, 109–111
and agents with low toxicity, 106
antidotes in, 104–105
caustics, 105–106
elimination enhancement in, 102–104
emergency management in, 99
gastrointestinal decontamination in, 101–102
hydrocarbon, 106–108
iron, 108
lead, 113–121
prevention of, 29
salicylate, 108–109
signs and symptoms in, 100–101
substance abuse, 112–113

supportive therapy in, 99–101
theophylline, 111
tricyclic antidepressants, 111–112
Poliovirus vaccine
killed virus in
for immunodeficient patients, 25
side effects of, 26
oral attenuated
contraindications to, 25
recommended schedule for, 23–24
side effects of, 26
Polyarteritis nodosa, 518
Polycose
for infant feeding, 129
in nutritional deficiencies, 267
Polycystic ovary syndrome, amenorrhea in, 344–345
Polycythemia, 470
neonatal, 169
Polydipsia
in diabetes insipidus, 309
in diabetes mellitus, 325
Polyglandular deficiency syndrome, autoimmune type 1, 319
Polymyxin B, metabolism and excretion of, 378
Polyneuritis, acute infectious, 525–526
Pompe's disease, symptoms of, 157
Pork tapeworm, 440, 449–450
Portagen
for infant feeding, 131
in nutritional deficiencies, 267
Positive pressure breathing in pneumothorax, 63
Postmortem examination in metabolic diseases, 358
Potassium, 196–197
in body fluids, 206
in foods and beverages, 232–233
in formulas for infant feeding, 130–131
hyperkalemia, 197
in acute renal failure, 230
in chronic renal failure, 232–233
in neonates, 186
hypokalemia, 197
in chronic renal failure, 233
in neonates, 186
in theophylline poisoning, 111
losses in dehydration, 205
maintenance requirements, 204
replacement therapy
in diabetic ketoacidosis, 333–334
in salicylate poisoning, 109

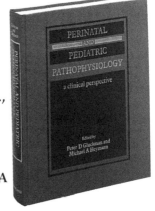
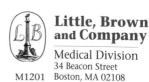

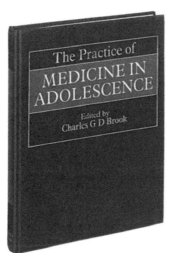

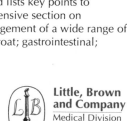

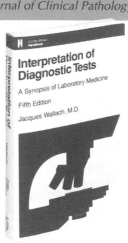
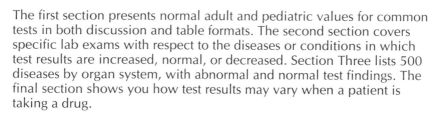

The Little, Brown Spiral® Manual Series
The Little, Brown Handbook Series
AVAILABLE AT YOUR BOOKSTORE

THE LITTLE, BROWN HANDBOOK SERIES

Visit your local bookstore or call 1 (800) 343-9204 for these and other Little, Brown Medical Publications. In Canada, check with your local bookstore or contact Copp Clark Pitman, Ltd., 2775 Matheson Blvd., East, Mississauga, Ontario, Canada L4W 4P7

For further information write to Little, Brown and Company, Medical Division, 200 West Street, Waltham, MA 02254